AF371260

Biological and Pharmacological Activity of Plant Natural Compounds

Biological and Pharmacological Activity of Plant Natural Compounds

Editors

Raffaele Pezzani
Sara Vitalini

MDPI • Basel • Beijing • Wuhan • Barcelona • Belgrade • Manchester • Tokyo • Cluj • Tianjin

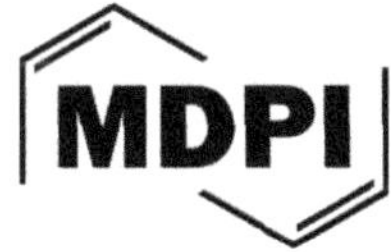

Editors
Raffaele Pezzani
University of Padova
Italy

Sara Vitalini
Milan State University
Italy

Editorial Office
MDPI
St. Alban-Anlage 66
4052 Basel, Switzerland

This is a reprint of articles from the Special Issue published online in the open access journal *Molecules* (ISSN 1420-3049) (available at: https://www.mdpi.com/journal/molecules/special_issues/Nat).

For citation purposes, cite each article independently as indicated on the article page online and as indicated below:

LastName, A.A.; LastName, B.B.; LastName, C.C. Article Title. *Journal Name* **Year**, *Volume Number*, Page Range.

ISBN 978-3-0365-0304-2 (Hbk)
ISBN 978-3-0365-0305-9 (PDF)

Contents

About the Editors . . . . **vii**

Raffaele Pezzani and Sara Vitalini
Editorial to the Special Issue "Biological and Pharmacological Activity of Plant Natural
Compounds"
Reprinted from: *Molecules* **2021**, *26*, 63, doi:10.3390/molecules26010063 . . . . **1**

Jianmei Zhang, Stephanie Triseptya Hunto, Yoonyong Yang, Jongsung Lee and Jae Youl Cho
Tabebuia impetiginosa: A Comprehensive Review on Traditional Uses, Phytochemistry, and
Immunopharmacological Properties
Reprinted from: *Molecules* **2020**, *25*, 4294, doi:10.3390/molecules25184294 . . . . **5**

**Aline T. de Carvalho, Marina M. Paes, Mila S. Cunha, Gustavo C. Brandão, Ana M. Mapeli,
Vanessa C. Rescia, Silvia A. Oesterreich and Gustavo R. Villas-Boas**
Ethnopharmacology of Fruit Plants: A Literature Review on the Toxicological, Phytochemical,
Cultural Aspects, and a Mechanistic Approach to the Pharmacological Effects of Four Widely
Used Species
Reprinted from: *Molecules* **2020**, *25*, 3879, doi:10.3390/molecules25173879 . . . . **21**

**Mehdi Sharifi-Rad, Raffaele Pezzani, Marco Redaelli, Maira Zorzan, Muhammad Imran,
Anees Ahmed Khalil, Bahare Salehi, Farukh Sharopov, William C. Cho and Javad Sharifi-Rad**
Preclinical Activities of Epigallocatechin Gallate in Signaling Pathways in Cancer
Reprinted from: *Molecules* **2020**, *25*, 467, doi:10.3390/molecules25030467 . . . . **87**

**Lúcio Ricardo Leite Diniz, Marilia Trindade de Santana Souza, Joice Nascimento Barboza,
Reinaldo Nóbrega de Almeida and Damião Pergentino de Sousa**
Antidepressant Potential of Cinnamic Acids: Mechanisms of Action and Perspectives in
Drug Development
Reprinted from: *Molecules* **2019**, *24*, 4469, doi:10.3390/molecules24244469 . . . . **117**

**Ana Damjanović, Branka Kolundžija, Ivana Z. Matić, Ana Krivokuća, Gordana Zdunić,
Katarina Šavikin, Radmila Janković, Jelena Antić Stanković and Tatjana P. Stanojković**
Mahonia aquifolium Extracts Promote Doxorubicin Effects against Lung Adenocarcinoma Cells
In Vitro
Reprinted from: *Molecules* **2020**, *25*, 5233, doi:10.3390/molecules25225233 . . . . **129**

Jisu Song, Heejung Seo, Mi-Ryung Kim, Sang-Jae Lee, Sooncheol Ahn and Minjung Song
Active Compound of *Pharbitis* Semen (*Pharbitis nil* Seeds) Suppressed KRAS-Driven Colorectal
Cancer and Restored Muscle Cell Function during Cancer Progression
Reprinted from: *Molecules* **2020**, *25*, 2864, doi:10.3390/molecules25122864 . . . . **143**

**Xin Zhang, Yamei Li, Zhengping Feng, Yaling Zhang, Ye Gong, Huanhuan Song, Xiaoli Ding
and Yaping Yan**
Multifloroside Suppressing Proliferation and Colony Formation, Inducing S Cell Cycle Arrest,
ROS Production, and Increasing MMP in Human Epidermoid Carcinoma Cell Lines A431
Reprinted from: *Molecules* **2020**, *25*, 7, doi:10.3390/molecules25010007 . . . . **157**

**Jae Il Lyu, Jaihyunk Ryu, Chang Hyun Jin, Dong-Gun Kim, Jung Min Kim, Kyoung-Sun Seo,
Jin-Baek Kim, Sang Hoon Kim, Joon-Woo Ahn, Si-Yong Kang and Soon-Jae Kwon**
Phenolic Compounds in Extracts of *Hibiscus acetosella* (Cranberry Hibiscus) and Their Antioxidant
and Antibacterial Properties
Reprinted from: *Molecules* **2020**, *25*, 4190, doi:10.3390/molecules25184190 . . . . **171**

Sabina Lachowicz, Anna Michalska-Ciechanowska and Jan Oszmiański
The Impact of Maltodextrin and Inulin on the Protection of Natural Antioxidants in Powders
Made of Saskatoon Berry Fruit, Juice, and Pomace as Functional Food Ingredients
Reprinted from: *Molecules* **2020**, *25*, 1805, doi:10.3390/molecules25081805 . . . . **183**

Trina H. García, Claudia Quintino da Rocha, Livan Delgado-Roche, Idania Rodeiro,
Yaiser Ávila, Ivones Hernández, Cindel Cuellar, Miriam Teresa Paz Lopes, Wagner Vilegas,
Giulia Auriemma, Iraida Spengler and Luca Rastrelli
Influence of the Phenological State of in the Antioxidant Potential and Chemical Composition
of *Ageratina havanensis*. Effects on the P-Glycoprotein Function
Reprinted from: *Molecules* **2020**, *25*, 2134, doi:10.3390/molecules25092134 . . . . **203**

Adil Farooq Wali, Muneeb U Rehman, Mohammad Raish, Mohsin Kazi, Padma G. M. Rao,
Osamah Alnemer, Parvaiz Ahmad and Ajaz Ahmad
Zingerone [4-(3-Methoxy-4-hydroxyphenyl)-butan-2] Attenuates Lipopolysaccharide-Induced
Inflammation and Protects Rats from Sepsis Associated Multi Organ Damage
Reprinted from: *Molecules* **2020**, *25*, 5127, doi:10.3390/molecules25215127 . . . . **217**

Nam-Hun Kim, Hong-Ki Kim, Ji-Hak Lee, Seung-Il Jo, Hye-Min Won, Gyeong-Seok Lee,
Hyoun-Su Lee, Kung-Woo Nam, Wan-Jong Kim and Man-Deuk Han
Juglone Suppresses LPS-induced Inflammatory Responses and NLRP3 Activation in
Macrophages
Reprinted from: *Molecules* **2020**, *25*, 3104, doi:10.3390/molecules25133104 . . . . **233**

Lindaiane Bezerra Rodrigues Dantas, Ana Letícia Moreira Silva, Cícero Pedro da Silva Júnior,
Isabel Sousa Alcântara, Maria Rayane Correia de Oliveira, Anita Oliveira Brito Pereira Bezerra
Martins, Jaime Ribeiro-Filho, Henrique Douglas Melo Coutinho, Fabíolla Rocha Santos
Passos, Lucindo José Quintans-Junior, Irwin Rose Alencar de Menezes, Raffaele Pezzani and
Sara Vitalini
Nootkatone Inhibits Acute and Chronic Inflammatory Responses in Mice
Reprinted from: *Molecules* **2020**, *25*, 2181, doi:10.3390/molecules25092181 . . . . **245**

Nomadlozi Blessings Hlophe, Andrew Rowland Opoku, Foluso Oluwagbemiga Osunsanmi,
Trayana Georgieva Djarova-Daniels, Oladipupo Adejumobi Lawal and
Rebamang Anthony Mosa
A Lanosteryl Triterpene (RA-3) Exhibits Antihyperuricemic and Nephroprotective Effects
in Rats
Reprinted from: *Molecules* **2020**, *25*, 4010, doi:10.3390/molecules25174010 . . . . **259**

Danijela Stanisic, Leticia H. B. Liu, Roney V. dos Santos, Amanda F. Costa, Nelson Durán
and Ljubica Tasic
New Sustainable Process for Hesperidin Isolation and Anti-Ageing Effects of Hesperidin
Nanocrystals
Reprinted from: *Molecules* **2020**, *25*, 4534, doi:10.3390/molecules25194534 . . . . **269**

About the Editors

Raffaele Pezzani is both a biologist and a physician with a Ph.D. in Neuroscience from the University of Padova, Italy. He has authored or co-authored more than 60 scientific publications and has been cited more than 800 times. He has also served as an editorial board member and as an editor of reputable and impactful journals. He is the principal investigator of his research group in Padova and has long lasting and effective experience (more than 20 years) in biology and medicine. Fields of expertise: endocrinology; oncology; phytotherapy; nutraceutics.

Sara Vitalini is a biologist with a Ph.D. in Plant Biology and Crop Production from the University of Milano, Italy. She has authored or co-authored more than 60 peer-reviewed papers and serves as a regular referee, editorial board member and guest editor of some international journals. Her research group is mainly concerned with ethnopharmacology, pharmaceutical biology and phytochemistry. Fields of expertise: bioactivity; medicinal plants; natural products; phytochemicals.

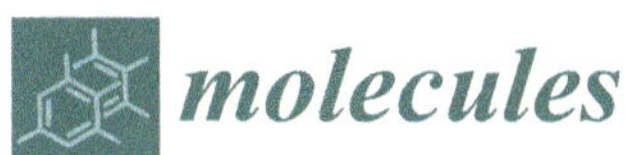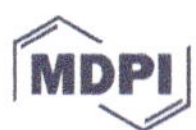

Editorial

Editorial to the Special Issue "Biological and Pharmacological Activity of Plant Natural Compounds"

Raffaele Pezzani [1,2,*] and Sara Vitalini [3,*]

1 Endocrinology Unit, Department of Medicine (DIMED), University of Padova, 35128 Padova, Italy
2 Associazione Italiana per la Ricerca Oncologica di Base, 35128 Padova, Italy
3 Department of Agricultural and Environmental Sciences, Milan State University, via G. Celoria 2, 20133 Milan, Italy
* Correspondence: raffaele.pezzani@unipd.it (R.P.); sara.vitalini@unimi.it (S.V.)

Received: 22 December 2020; Accepted: 23 December 2020; Published: 25 December 2020

Plant natural products are a valuable source of compounds with a healthy potential effect on living organisms, including animals and humans. These natural compounds are commonly called phytochemicals, specifically indicating their origin from the plant kingdom. It is frequently reported that phytochemicals merge with phytotherapeutics, which are molecules with a keen effect on health. This Special Issue entitled *"Biological and Pharmacological Activity of Plant Natural Compounds"* focused its attention on such plant-derived products and aimed to expand our knowledge on bioactive effects in preclinical models.

This Special Issue consisted of 4 reviews and 11 research articles that substantially contributed to the mission of *Molecules*, i.e., to increase scientists' and readers' perspectives and knowledge on plant natural products.

The first review evaluated *Tabebuia impetiginosa* (Mart. ex DC.) Mattos, an Amazonian plant traditionally used against fever, malaria, bacterial and fungal infections, and skin diseases [1]. The work emphasized that the main effect of this plant could derive from its anti-inflammatory activity together with the presence of immunomodulatory compounds. In addition, the authors suggested that even if the biological effects of *T. impetiginosa* are clearly detectable, future research needs to better characterize its mechanisms of action, which until now remain elusive.

The comprehensive work of De Carvalho and collaborators explored the phytochemical composition, biological and toxicological properties of four fruit species, i.e., *Talisia esculenta, Brosimum gaudichaudii, Genipa americana,* and *Bromelia antiacantha* [2]. They reported that these plants demonstrated anti-inflammatory, antitumor, and photosensitizing properties, in addition to providing key molecules with pharmacological and healthy activity.

Another review investigated the wide spectrum of biological activities of epigallocatechin gallate (EGCG), the main bioactive component of tea [3]. The mechanism of action along with signaling pathways and its pharmacological properties (antioxidative, anti-inflammatory, and antitumor) were reported, suggesting that EGCG could play a key role in the future treatment or prevention of cancer.

Interestingly, the work of Diniz and co-authors evaluated the antidepressant effects of cinnamic acids [4]. Such molecules, as reported in different animal model experiments of behavioral disorders, indicated their potential applicability as antidepressant drugs, given their low costs in certain cases. Cinnamic acids could have a future in the treatment of depression and other psychiatric conditions.

In addition to reviews, 11 preclinical studies were performed, ranging from the pharmacological effects to the biological impact on cell processes and/or signaling pathways.

Mahonia aquifolium (Pursh) Nutt. is a plant with potential anticancer effects. It has been studied in association with doxorubicin in lung cell models demonstrating stimulating antiproliferative results [5].

M. aquifolium extract showed apoptosis activation, cell cycle modulation, and a decrease in the invasion process. Furthermore, the synergistic effects of this plant extract and doxorubicin (with the subsequent decrease in toxic effects) suggested its potential application in higher models.

Seeds of *Pharbitis nil* (L.) Choisy, a traditional plant used in East Asia to treat inflammation and cancer, were used in cell models of colorectal cancer to evaluate the antiproliferative effects of the purified extract [6]. Cell cycle modulation and apoptosis induction were observed, with changes in the RAS/ERK and AKT/mTOR pathways. In addition, the extract preserved muscle cell function, suggesting the seeds of *P. nil* as a promising novel nature-derived drug against colorectal cancer.

Four different secoiridoids were studied for their potential anticancer effects on human epidermoid carcinoma (A431) and non-small cell lung cancer (A549) cell lines [7]. One of these compounds, multifloroside showed the highest inhibitory activity against A431 cells, with the ability to suppress colony formation, induce S cell cycle arrest, and increase reactive oxygen species (ROS) production and mitochondrial membrane potential.

A work on the phenolic compounds from 18 different *Hibiscus acetosella* accessions were assessed for their antibacterial activity and antioxidant activity (associated with the level of anthocyanins) [8]. For the first time, the antibacterial activity of *H. acetosella* was shown on the Gram-negative *Pseudomonas aeruginosa* and on the Gram-positive *Staphylococcus aureus*, reserving an antimicrobial perspective in higher organisms for these compounds.

Another work evaluated the influence of maltodextrin and inulin (used as a carrier) on the quantitative and qualitative composition of the polyphenolic profile of *Amelanchier alnifolia* Nutt. fruit, juice, and pomace powders, in order to study the polyphenol profile and antioxidant properties [9]. The results showed the strong effect of the processing and matrix composition on the preservation of the antioxidant properties of *A. alnifolia*. The authors claimed that properly designed high-quality powders are necessary to obtain valuable nutraceutical additives for future use in humans.

Ageratina havanensis (Kunth) R. M. King and H. Robinson was used as a basis to compare the quantitative chemical composition of extracts in its flowering and vegetative stages [10]. This plant, typical to the Caribbean and Texas, was also studied for its antioxidant activity and to evaluate its effects on P-glycoprotein (P-gp) function. The results showed the content of major flavonoids of *A. havanensis*, its antioxidant effects, and the ability to inhibit P-gp. Thus, this plant species is a source of new potential inhibitors for drug efflux.

In an animal study, Wali and colleagues showed the protective effect of zingerone (ZIN) against lipopolysaccharide-induced oxidative stress, DNA damage, and cytokine storm [11]. They reported the strong antioxidative effect of ZIN, with the restoration of plasma enzymes and attenuated plasma proinflammatory cytokines and sepsis biomarkers. Thus, ZIN appears to be a convincing candidate for validation in future clinical trials for its anti-inflammatory and antioxidant properties.

Similar to ZIN, juglone (5-hydroxyl-1,4-naphthoquinone), a well known black walnut (*Juglans nigra*) derivative, was evaluated as an anti-inflammatory compound in a mouse macrophage cell model (J774.1 cells) [12]. The results showed that juglone could reduce inflammatory cytokine production and NLRP3 inflammasome activation in macrophages, indicating this molecule to be a possible therapeutic tool to control inflammation.

Another potential anti-inflammatory compound was nootkatone (NTK), a sesquiterpenoid found in the essential oils of many species of the *Citrus* genus, tested in mice models of acute and chronic inflammation [13]. The authors reported that NTK was effective in reducing IL1-β and TNF-α production, COX-2 activity, and that it could antagonize the H1 receptor in acute assays. However, further studies are necessary to understand its mechanism of action in chronic inflammation.

Furthermore, renal diseases were investigated in in vivo models. Hlophe et al. analyzed the effects of a plant-derived lanosteryl triterpene, known as RA-3 [14]. The compound was able to reduce blood urea nitrogen, creatinine, uric acid, and xanthine oxidase biomarkers in rats, suggesting antihyperuricemic and nephroprotective properties. Moreover, antioxidant status with a decrease in malondialdehyde content was observed, again indicating the potential role of RA-3 in renal diseases.

Hesperidin (HSP), one of the principal bioflavonoids of *Citrus* fruits, was extracted from orange bagasse and tested to eliminate dark eye circles in in vitro artificial 3D skin [15]. The most effective methods for HSP nanonization were explored, and this nanonized compound was found to be the most skin-friendly and could be potentially used in cosmetics.

Overall, this Special Issue significantly contributes to stressing the importance of the biological and pharmacological activities of plant natural compounds. The aforementioned preclinical results revealed novel molecules with exciting properties that could potentially be useful for further human studies, for nutritional purpose, and for therapeutic aid.

Funding: This research received no external funding.

Conflicts of Interest: The authors declare no conflict of interest.

References

1.   Zhang, J.; Hunto, S.T.; Yang, Y.; Lee, J.; Cho, J.Y. Tabebuia impetiginosa: A Comprehensive Review on Traditional Uses, Phytochemistry, and Immunopharmacological Properties. *Molecules* **2020**, *25*, 4294. [CrossRef] [PubMed]

2.   De Carvalho, A.T.; Paes, M.M.; Cunha, M.S.; Brandão, G.C.; Mapeli, A.M.; Rescia, V.C.; Oesterreich, S.A.; Villas-Boas, G.R. Ethnopharmacology of Fruit Plants: A Literature Review on the Toxicological, Phytochemical, Cultural Aspects, and a Mechanistic Approach to the Pharmacological Effects of Four Widely Used Species. *Molecules* **2020**, *25*, 3879. [CrossRef] [PubMed]

3.   Sharifi-Rad, M.; Pezzani, R.; Redaelli, M.; Zorzan, M.; Imran, M.; Ahmed Khalil, A.; Salehi, B.; Sharopov, F.; Cho, W.C.; Sharifi-Rad, J. Preclinical Activities of Epigallocatechin Gallate in Signaling Pathways in Cancer. *Molecules* **2020**, *25*, 467. [CrossRef] [PubMed]

4.   Diniz, L.R.; Souza, M.T.; Barboza, J.N.; Almeida, R.N.; Sousa, D.P. Antidepressant Potential of Cinnamic Acids: Mechanisms of Action and Perspectives in Drug Development. *Molecules* **2019**, *24*, 4469. [CrossRef]

5.   Damjanović, A.; Kolundžija, B.; Matić, I.Z.; Krivokuća, A.; Zdunić, G.; Šavikin, K.; Janković, R.; Stanković, J.A.; Stanojković, T.P. Mahonia aquifolium Extracts Promote Doxorubicin Effects against Lung Adenocarcinoma Cells In Vitro. *Molecules* **2020**, *25*, 5233. [CrossRef] [PubMed]

6.   Song, J.; Seo, H.; Kim, M.-R.; Lee, S.-J.; Ahn, S.; Song, M. Active Compound of Pharbitis Semen (Pharbitis nil Seeds) Suppressed KRAS-Driven Colorectal Cancer and Restored Muscle Cell Function during Cancer Progression. *Molecules* **2020**, *25*, 2864. [CrossRef] [PubMed]

7.   Zhang, X.; Li, Y.; Feng, Z.; Zhang, Y.; Gong, Y.; Song, H.; Ding, X.; Yan, Y. Multifloroside Suppressing Proliferation and Colony Formation, Inducing S Cell Cycle Arrest, ROS Production, and Increasing MMP in Human Epidermoid Carcinoma Cell Lines A431. *Molecules* **2020**, *25*, 7. [CrossRef] [PubMed]

8.   Lyu, J.I.; Ryu, J.; Jin, C.H.; Kim, D.-G.; Kim, J.M.; Seo, K.-S.; Kim, J.-B.; Kim, S.H.; Ahn, J.-W.; Kang, S.-Y.; et al. Phenolic Compounds in Extracts of Hibiscus acetosella (*Cranberry hibiscus*) and Their Antioxidant and Antibacterial Properties. *Molecules* **2020**, *25*, 4190. [CrossRef] [PubMed]

9.   Lachowicz, S.; Michalska-Ciechanowska, A.; Oszmiański, J. The Impact of Maltodextrin and Inulin on the Protection of Natural Antioxidants in Powders Made of Saskatoon Berry Fruit, Juice, and Pomace as Functional Food Ingredients. *Molecules* **2020**, *25*, 1805. [CrossRef] [PubMed]

10.   García, T.H.; Rocha, C.Q.; Delgado-Roche, L.; Rodeiro, I.; Ávila, Y.; Hernández, I.; Cuellar, C.; Lopes, M.T.; Vilegas, W.; Auriemma, G.; et al. Influence of the Phenological State of in the Antioxidant Potential and Chemical Composition of Ageratina havanensis. Effects on the P-Glycoprotein Function. *Molecules* **2020**, *25*, 2134. [CrossRef] [PubMed]

11.   Wali, A.F.; Rehman, M.U.; Raish, M.; Kazi, M.; Rao, P.G.M.; Alnemer, O.; Ahmad, P.; Ahmad, A. Zingerone [4-(3-Methoxy-4-hydroxyphenyl)-butan-2] Attenuates Lipopolysaccharide-Induced Inflammation and Protects Rats from Sepsis Associated Multi Organ Damage. *Molecules* **2020**, *25*, 5127. [CrossRef] [PubMed]

12.   Kim, N.-H.; Kim, H.-K.; Lee, J.-H.; Jo, S.-I.; Won, H.-M.; Lee, G.-S.; Lee, H.-S.; Nam, K.-W.; Kim, W.-J.; Han, M.-D. Juglone Suppresses LPS-induced Inflammatory Responses and NLRP3 Activation in Macrophages. *Molecules* **2020**, *25*, 3104. [CrossRef] [PubMed]

13. Bezerra Rodrigues Dantas, L.; Silva, A.L.; da Silva Júnior, C.P.; Alcântara, I.S.; Correia de Oliveira, M.R.; Oliveira Brito Pereira Bezerra Martins, A.; Ribeiro-Filho, J.; Coutinho, H.D.; Rocha Santos Passos, F.; Quintans-Junior, L.J.; et al. Nootkatone Inhibits Acute and Chronic Inflammatory Responses in Mice. *Molecules* **2020**, *25*, 2181. [CrossRef] [PubMed]

14. Hlophe, N.B.; Opoku, A.R.; Osunsanmi, F.O.; Djarova-Daniels, T.G.; Lawal, O.A.; Mosa, R.A. A Lanosteryl Triterpene (RA-3) Exhibits Antihyperuricemic and Nephroprotective Effects in Rats. *Molecules* **2020**, *25*, 4010. [CrossRef] [PubMed]

15. Stanisic, D.; Liu, L.H.B.; dos Santos, R.V.; Costa, A.F.; Durán, N.; Tasic, L. New Sustainable Process for Hesperidin Isolation and Anti-Ageing Effects of Hesperidin Nanocrystals. *Molecules* **2020**, *25*, 4534. [CrossRef] [PubMed]

Publisher's Note: MDPI stays neutral with regard to jurisdictional claims in published maps and institutional affiliations.

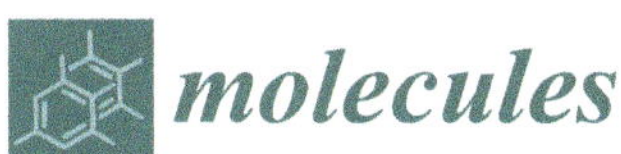 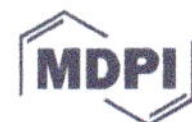

Review

Tabebuia impetiginosa: A Comprehensive Review on Traditional Uses, Phytochemistry, and Immunopharmacological Properties

Jianmei Zhang [1,†], Stephanie Triseptya Hunto [1,†], Yoonyong Yang [2], Jongsung Lee [1,*] and Jae Youl Cho [1,*]

1   Department of Integrative Biotechnology, and Biomedical Institute for Convergence at SKKU (BICS), Sungkyunkwan University, Suwon 16419, Korea; zhangjianmei1028@163.com (J.Z.); stephunto@gmail.com (S.T.H.)
2   Biological and Genetic Resources Assessment Division, National Institute of Biological Resources, Incheon 22689, Korea; tazemenia@korea.kr
*   Correspondence: bioneer@skku.edu (J.L.); jaecho@skku.edu (J.Y.C.); Tel.: +82-31-290-7861 (J.L.); +82-31-290-7868 (J.Y.C.)
†   These authors contributed equally to this work.

Academic Editors: Raffaele Pezzani and Sara Vitalini
Received: 29 August 2020; Accepted: 16 September 2020; Published: 18 September 2020

Abstract: *Tabebuia impetiginosa*, a plant native to the Amazon rainforest and other parts of Latin America, is traditionally used for treating fever, malaria, bacterial and fungal infections, and skin diseases. Additionally, several categories of phytochemicals and extracts isolated from *T. impetiginosa* have been studied via various models and displayed pharmacological activities. This review aims to uncover and summarize the research concerning *T. impetiginosa*, particularly its traditional uses, phytochemistry, and immunopharmacological activity, as well as to provide guidance for future research. A comprehensive search of the published literature was conducted to locate original publications pertaining to *T. impetiginosa* up to June 2020. The main inquiry used the following keywords in various combinations in titles and abstracts: *T. impetiginosa*, Taheebo, traditional uses, phytochemistry, immunopharmacological, anti-inflammatory activity. Immunopharmacological activity described in this paper includes its anti-inflammatory, anti-allergic, anti-autoimmune, and anti-cancer properties. Particularly, *T. impetiginosa* has a strong effect on anti-inflammatory activity. This paper also describes the target pathway underlying how *T. impetiginosa* inhibits the inflammatory response. The need for further investigation to identify other pharmacological activities as well as the exact target proteins of *T. impetiginosa* was also highlighted. *T. impetiginosa* may provide a new strategy for prevention and treatment of many immunological disorders that foster extensive research to identify potential anti-inflammatory and immunomodulatory compounds and fractions as well as to explore the underlying mechanisms of this herb. Further scientific evidence is required for clinical trials on its immunopharmacological effects and safety.

Keywords: *Tabebuia impetiginosa*; Taheebo; traditional uses; immunopharmacology; immunological disorders

---

1. Introduction

Historically, people have used natural products such as plants, animals, microorganisms, and other biological resources to assuage and cure diseases [1]. Many of the commercial drugs (such as atropine, teniposide, aescin, digoxin, silymarin, and so on) available today were initially developed from plants and other biological resources used in traditional medicines [2,3]. Therefore, knowledge of the traditional use of natural products plays a large role in drug discovery and development.

Tabebuia impetiginosa (Mart. Ex DC. Mattos) is a plant belonging to the family Bignoniaceae, which is mainly distributed in the Amazon rainforest and other tropical regions of Central and Latin America [4]. It is not only a decorative plant but also has high pharmaceutical value. *T. impetiginosa* has been used as a traditional medicine to treat various diseases and has antinociceptive, anti-edematogenic, antibiotic, and antidepressant effects [5–7]. Moreover, the inner bark of this tree can be made into poultice or concentrated tea to treat various skin inflammatory diseases [8]. Several categories of compounds have been isolated and identified from *T. impetiginosa*, principally quinones, flavonoids, naphthoquinones, and benzoic acids [9–12]. In recent years, many investigations have demonstrated that extracts or compounds isolated from *T. impetiginosa* reveal an extensive range of pharmacological activities such as anti-obesity, antifungal, anti-psoriatic, antioxidant, anti-inflammatory, and anti-cancer activities [4,7,13–18]. It is particularly prominent in immunopharmacology. Typically, the mechanism of anti-inflammatory activity of extract from the inner bark of *Tabebuia* was studied through a molecular biological approach. Nevertheless, the clinical applications of *T. impetiginosa* have been poorly researched, and there is a void of information on its mechanisms of action.

As far as we know, no review in the literature provides a comprehensive summary of *T. impetiginosa*. Thus, in an attempt to provide a basis for the in-depth exploration and clinical application of this plant, we reviewed the traditional medicinal uses, botany, immunopharmacology, phytochemistry, and ethnopharmacology of *T. impetiginosa*, in addition to perspectives and possible directions of future research. Furthermore, this review will be conducive to identifying the information gaps important for future research into *T. impetiginosa*.

2. Methodology

A scientific literature review regarding the traditional uses, phytochemistry, anti-inflammatory, anti-cancer, antioxidant, and anti-autoimmune disease activities of *T. impetiginosa* was performed using bibliographic databases. Keywords used for this study were 'anti-inflammatory,' 'T. impetiginosa,' 'Taheebo,' and other names synonymous with Taheebo. Research articles were chosen if they tested a compound isolated from *T. impetiginosa* and investigated the related pharmacological activity. Studies using in vitro assays included inhibition of nitric oxide, oxidative enzymes, or cytokines. In vivo trials were included if they used antigens to induce ear edema, arthritis, or colitis in inflammatory animal models. Websites, articles, and scientific papers were used as sources of information on historical uses, components, taxonomy, and morphology of *T. impetiginosa*. Other sites, including mapchart.net, were used to create a distribution map of *T. impetiginosa*.

3. Taxonomy and Botanical Traits

3.1. Taxonomy

T. impetiginosa is also known as *Handroanthus impetiginosus* (Mart. ex Dc.) Mattos as accepted on the website www.theplantlist.org [19]. There are 17 valid synonymous names for *Handroanthus impetiginosus* (Mart. ex Dc.) Mattos and one invalid synonymous name (*Tecoma impetiginosa* Mart.). Synonymous names for *Handroanthus impetiginosus* (Mart. ex DC.) Mattos within one confidence level are *T. ipe* var. *integra* (Sprague) Sandwith, *Tecoma avellanedae* var. *alba* Lillo, *Tecoma ipe* var. *integra* Sprague, *Tecoma ipe* var. *integrifolia* Hassl., and *Tecoma ipe f. leucotricha* Hassl. Synonymous names for *Handroanthus impetiginosus* (Mart. ex DC.) Mattos within three confidence levels are *Gelseminum avellanedae* (Lorentz ex Griseb.) Kuntze, *Handroanthus avellanedae* (Lorentz ex Griseb.) Mattos, *T. avellanedae* (Lorentz ex Griseb.), *T. dugandii* Standl., *T. impetiginosa* (Mart. ex DC.) Standl., *T. nicaraguensis* S.F. Blake, *T. palmeri* Rose, *T. schunkevigoi* D.R. Simpson, *Tecoma adenophylla* Bureau and K. Schum, *Tecoma avellanedae* (Lorentz ex Griseb.) Speg., *Tecoma impetiginosa* Mart. ex DC., and *Tecoma integra* (Sprague) Hassl (The Plant List, 2013) (Table 1). This paper will use the name *T. impetiginosa* (Mart. ex DC.) Standl and present it as *T. impetiginosa*. *T. impetiginosa* is a member of family Bignoniaceae, genus *Tabebuia*, and species *impetiginosa* as written in NCBI: txid429701. Its genus name is derived from a native language of Brazil, while the species name is derived from the Latin word impetigo, a common and highly contagious skin infection. It was so named because people believed that this plant could be used to treat impetigo [20].

Table 1. Synonymous names for *Tabebuia impetiginosa* from The Plant List, 2013.

Synonym Name	Remarks
Handroanthus impetiginosus (Mart. ex Dc.) Mattos	Accepted name
Tabebuia ipe var. *integra* (Sprague) Sandwith	One confidence level
Tecoma avellanedae var. *alba* Lillo	One confidence level
Tecoma ipe var. *integra* Sprague	One confidence level
Tecoma ipe var. *integrifolia* Hassl.	One confidence level
Tecoma ipe f. *leucotricha* Hassl.	One confidence level
Gelseminum avellanedae (Lorentz ex Griseb.) Kuntze	Three confidence levels
Handroanthus avellanedae (Lorentz ex Griseb.) Mattos	Three confidence levels
Tabebuia avellanedae Lorentz ex Griseb.	Three confidence levels
Tabebuia dugandii Standl.	Three confidence levels
Tabebuia impetiginosa (Mart. ex DC.) Standl.	Three confidence levels
Tabebuia nicaraguensis S.F. Blake	Three confidence levels
Tabebuia palmeri Rose	Three confidence levels
Tabebuia schunkevigoi D.R. Simpson	Three confidence levels
Tecoma adenophylla Bureau and K. Schum	Three confidence levels
Tecoma avellanedae (Lorentz ex Griseb.) Speg.	Three confidence levels
Tecoma impetiginosa Mart. ex DC.	Three confidence levels
Tecoma integra (Sprague) Hassl	Three confidence levels
Tecoma impetiginosa Mart	Invalid name

3.2. Botanical Traits

T. impetiginosa is also known as pink trumpet tree or purple trumpet tree due to its flower color [21]. In English, it is called Ipe, Taheebo (ant wood), and purple tabebuia. In French, it is known as Poui, while its Spanish names include Lapacho negro, lapacho, and quebracho. In German, the common name is Lapachobaum, Trompetenbaum, and Feenkraut. In Portuguese, this plant is recognized as Pau d'arco (bow tree), Ipe-roxo (red thick bark), and Ipe [19,20]. *T. impetiginosa* is well known due to its conspicuous appearance. This deciduous species can grow to a height of 30 m and sheds its leaves during the dry season. The palmately compound and serrated leaves are green and arranged in opposite or subopposite pairs. The leaf shape is elliptic or oblong with pinnate or banchidodrome venation. Showy purple, dark pink, or pink flowers appear in spring. The calyx is campanulate to tubular with five lobes and is trumpet shaped. Its fruit is contained in a pod and is comprised of an elongated cylindrical capsule with thin seeds [21,22].

3.3. Distribution

T. impetiginosa is a tree found in South and Central America and in some parts of North America. Information on the distribution of this species was obtained from www.tropicos.org [23] and a review paper on red lapacho [20]. Although it is best known for its presence in the Amazon rainforest, it is also found in Argentina, Bolivia, Brazil, Colombia, Costa Rica, Ecuador, El Salvador, French Guiana, Guatemala, Honduras, Mexico, Nicaragua, Panama, Paraguay, Peru, Suriname, Trinidad and Tobago, and Venezuela, as shown in Figure 1 and Table 2.

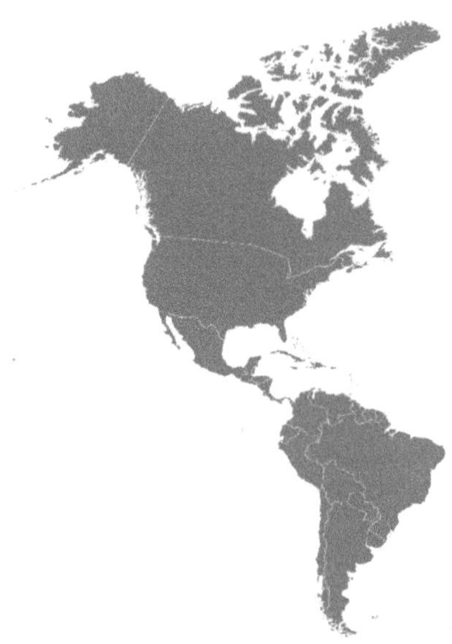

Figure 1. Distribution map of *Tabebuia impetiginosa*.

Table 2. Geographical distribution of *Tabebuia impetiginosa*.

Species	Distribution
Tabebuia avellanedae Lorentz ex Griseb.	Argentina
Handroanthus avellanedae (Lorentz ex Griseb.) Mattos	Bolivia
Bignonia heptaphylla Vell.	Brazil
Handroanthus impetiginosus (Mart. ex DC.) Mattos	Bolivia, Brazil, Mexico
Gelseminum avellanedae (Lorentz ex Griseb.) Kuntze	Bolivia
Tabebuia avellanedae var. *paulensis* Toledo	Brazil
Tabebuia dugandii Standl.	Colombia
Tabebuia eximia (Miq.) Sandwith	Bolivia, Panama
Tabebuia heptaphylla (Vell.) Toledo	Argentina, Bolivia, Brazil, Paraguay
Tabebuia hypodictyon (A. DC.) Standl.	Bolivia, Panama
* *Tabebuia ipe* (Mart.) Standl.	Panama
Tabebuia ipe var. *integra* (Sprague) Sandwith	Bolivia, Paraguay
Tabebuia nicaraguensis S.F. Blake	Nicaragua
Tabebuia palmeri Rose	Costa Rica, El Salvador, Guatemala, Honduras, Mexico, Nicaragua, Panama
Tabebuia schunkevigoi D.R. Simpson	Peru
Tecoma adenophylla Bureau ex K. Schum.	Brazil
Tecoma avellanedae (Lorentz ex Griseb.) Speg.	Honduras
Tecoma avellanedae var. *alba* Lillo	Argentina
Tecoma eximia Miq.	Brazil
Tecoma hassleri Sprague	Paraguay
! *Tecoma heptaphylla* (Vell.) Mart.	Panama
Tecoma hypodictyon A. DC.	Brazil
** *Tecoma impetiginosa* Mart.	Panama
!*Tecoma impetiginosa* Mart. ex DC.	Brazil
Tecoma impetiginosa var. *lepidota* Bureau	Brazil
Tecoma integra (Sprague) Chodat	Bolivia, Panama
Tecoma ipe fo. leucotricha Hassl.	Paraguay
** *Tecoma ipe* Mart.	Bolivia, Panama
Tecoma ipe var. *integra* Sprague	Paraguay
Tecoma ipe var. *integrifolia* Hassl.	Bolivia
Tecoma ochracea Cham.	Brazil

! = legitimate, * = illegitimate, ** = invalid.

4. Traditional Uses

T. impetiginosa has been used traditionally to treat cancer [24], obesity [25], depression [26], viral, fungal, and bacterial infections [27], and inflammatory symptoms such as pain [28], arthritis [15], colitis [29], and prostatitis since the Inca civilization. The Callaway Tribe makes a concentrated tea out of the tree's inner bark for treating skin inflammatory diseases [8]. Moreover, it can be used as an astringent and diuretic [30]. Caribbean folk healers utilize the bark and leaves of *T. impetiginosa* to cure toothaches, backaches, and sexually transmitted diseases [31]. Latino and Haitian populations were also reported to use this plant for the treatment of infectious disease [32]. Brazilian people have traditionally used this plant for anti-inflammatory, analgesic, and antiophidic purposes against snake venom [33]. Traditional healers in Brazil prescribed *T. impetiginosa* for cancer and tumor prevention or treatment; 69.05% for the treatment of tumors and cancer in general and 30.95% for specific tumors or cancers [34]. Such ethnomedicinal uses of *T. impetiginosa* led us to pay attention to it for a full understanding of its immunopharmacological properties for the future development of an effective drug against ethnopharmacologically targeted diseases with this plant.

5. Phytochemistry

Several categories of phytochemicals have been identified in the leaves, bark, and wood of *T. impetiginosa*. From *T. impetiginosa* bark, 19 glycosides comprised of four iridoid glycosides, two lignan glycosides, two isocoumarin glycosides, three phenylethanoid glycosides, and eight phenolic glycosides were methanol-extracted [35]. Major constituents of *T. impetiginosa* are furanonaphthoquinones, naphthoquinones, anthraquinones (e.g., anthraquinone-2-carboxylic acid (Compound **1** in Figure 2)), quinones, benzoic acid, flavonoids, cyclopentene dialdehydes, coumarins, iridoids, and phenolic glycosides [4,8,36]. The presence of naphthoquinones attracted scientific attention, with lapachol (**2**) and β-lapachone (**3**) especially piquing the interest of professionals in the medical field. Lapachol inhibits proliferation of tumor cells, while β-lapachone exhibits strong toxicity in murine and human cells. Lapachol has been shown to reduce the number of tumors caused by doxorubicin in *Drosophila melanogaster* heterozygous for the tumor suppressor gene. Lapachol can also decrease the invasion of HeLa cells, which could represent an interesting scaffold for the development of novel antimetastatic compounds [1].

Fatty acids, especially oleic acid (**4**), palmitic acid (**5**), and linoleic acid (**6**), are found in the bark of *T. impetiginosa*. Free sugars also were identified in the bark, with glucose being the most abundant, followed by fructose and sucrose. Organic acids, especially oxalic acid (**7**), are present, as well as the fat-soluble alcohols α-tocopherol (**8**) and γ-tocopherol (**9**). α-Tocopherol can reduce cardiovascular disease risk and neurodegenerative disorders [4]. In addition, *T. impetiginosa* has some volatile constituents that exhibit antioxidant activity. The major volatile constituents in *T. impetiginosa* include 4-methoxybenzaldehyde (**10**), 4-methoxyphenol (**11**), 5-allyl-1,2,3-trimethoxybenzene (**12**), 1-methoxy-4-(1*E*)-1-propenylbenzene (**13**), and 4-methoxybenzyl alcohol (**14**) [37].

Cyclopentene derivatives are secondary metabolites of plants, and this constituent from *T. impetiginosa* contained six known cyclopentenyl esters (avallaneine A–F (**15–20**)), two new cyclopentyl esters (avallaneine G (**21**) and H (**22**)), and two known cyclopentenyl esters. These cyclopentene derivatives may provide a significant anti-inflammatory effect on the lipopolysaccharide (LPS)-mediated inflammatory response by blocking the production of NO and PGE$_2$; therefore, it is important to determine the molecular mechanism whereby cyclopentenyl esters from *T. impetiginosa* inhibit inflammatory responses [16]. Moreover, Koyama et al. [38] isolated two cyclopentene dialdehydes, 2-formyl-5-(4′-methoxybenzoyloxy)-3-methyl-2-cyclopentene-1-acetaldehyde (**23**) and 2-formyl-5-(3′,4′-dimethoxybenzoyloxy)-3-methyl-2-cyclopentene-1-acetaldehyde (**24**), that exert anti-inflammatory activity in human leukocytes. Thus, it is necessary to further investigate their activities.

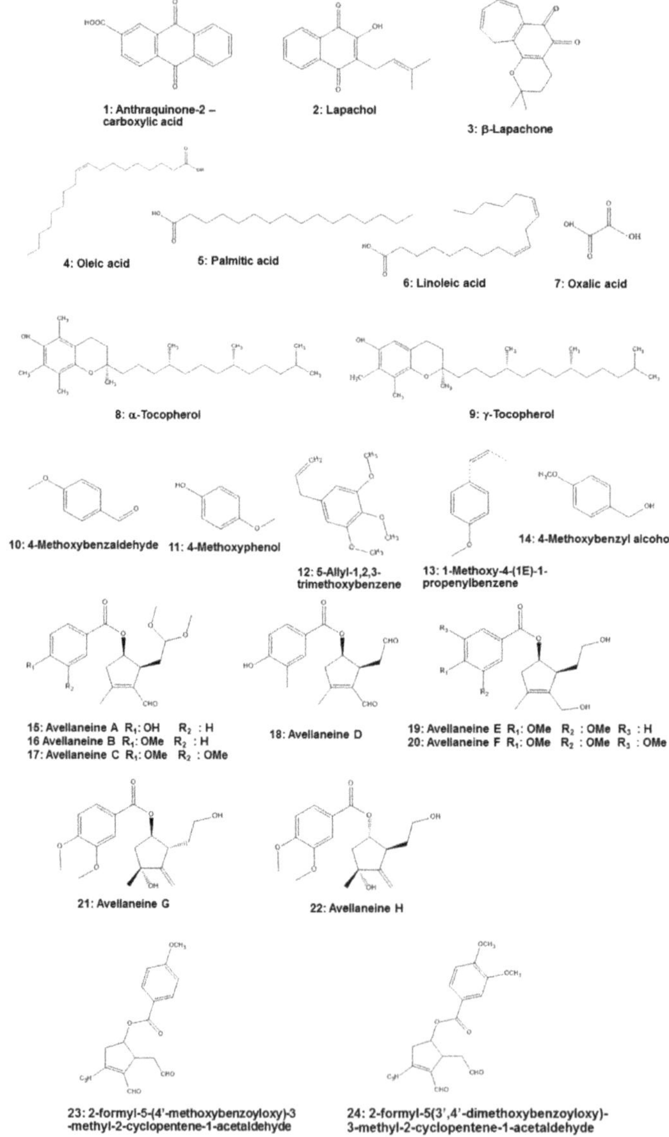

Figure 2. Chemical structures of *Tabebuia impetiginosa*-derived components.

6. Pharmacological Activities

Previous research has indicated various pharmacological effects of *T. impetiginosa* and its crude extracts and chemical compounds in a series of in vitro and animal models. It exhibits antibacterial, antioxidant, antifungal, antinociceptive, antidiabetic, anti-edema, anti-inflammatory, and anti-cancer activities at different concentrations or doses. The main pharmacological activities of extracts or compounds isolated from *T. impetiginosa* reported in in vitro and in vivo studies are briefly summarized in Table 3 and described in detail in the following subsections.

Table 3. Immunopharmacological effects of *Tabebuia impetiginosa*.

Pharmacological Activity	Extract/Isolated Compounds	Model	Concentration/Dose	Results	Ref.
Immunomodulatory	Water extract	RAW264.7 (murine macrophage cell), U937 (human promonocytic cell)	50, 100, 200, and 400 µg/mL	Maintained cluster formation of RAW264.7 cells even after lipopolysaccharide (LPS) treatment. Downregulated the phagocytic uptake of FITC-labeled dextran. Upregulated cell-cell interactions by decreasing migration of cells and enhancing CD-29-mediated cell-cell adhesion and the surface levels of adhesion molecules and costimulatory molecules linked to macrophage stimulation, as seen in upregulation of reaction oxygen species (ROS) release. Suppressed an alteration in the membrane level of macrophages (phagocytic uptake and morphological changes).	[39]
	Ethanol extract	IL-2-independent T-lymphocyte	0.25, 0.5, 0.75, 0.9, and 1.0, mg/mL	Inhibited activation and proliferation of IL-2-independent T-lymphocyte	[40]
Anti-inflammatory	Water extract	LPS-stimulated macrophages, arachidonic acid, or croton oil-induced mouse ear edema models	0–400 µg/mL, 100–400 mg/kg	Inhibited the production of NO and PGE_2 and suppressed the mRNA levels of COX-2 and iNOS. Curative effect in an in vivo PGE_2-based inflammatory symptoms model induced by arachidonic acid.	[8]
	Ethanol extract	TPA- or arachidonic acid-induced ear edema, hot plate, acetic acid-induced vascular permeability in rats	100, 200, or 400 mg/kg	Inhibited inflammation of paw edema, ear inflammation, and dye leakage in the vasculature using various animal models including acetic acid-induced vascular permeability, 12-*O*-tetradecanoylphorbol-13-acetate (TPA)-induced ear edema, arachidonic acid-induced mouse ear edema, and carrageenan-induced paw.	[28]
	Five novel compounds	Human myeloma THP-1 cells	25 µM	Showed inhibitory activity on production of the inflammatory cytokines, such as TNF-α and IL-1β.	[41]
	Cyclopentene derivatives	RAW264.7 cells	12.5, 25, 50 µg/mL	Suppressed the production of NO and PGE_2.	[16]
Anti-cancer	Naphthoquinones	MDA-BB-231, MCF7, and A549 cells	0–30 µM	Inhibited growth of cancer cell lines and STAT3 phosphorylation activity.	[14]
	Water extract	Estrogen receptor (ER)+ human mammary carcinoma MCF-7 cell line	0.05, 0.125, 0.25, 0.5, 0.75, 1.5 mg/mL	Exhibited dose-dependent growth inhibition of MCF-7 cells.	[24]
	β-lapachone	A549 human lung carcinoma cells		Inhibited growth of A549 cells and telomerase activity; induced apoptosis by reducing the expression of Bcl-2, increasing the expression of Bax, and activating caspase-3 and caspase-9.	[13]

Table 3. *Cont.*

Pharmacological Activity	Extract/Isolated Compounds	Model	Concentration/Dose	Results	Ref.
	β-lapachone	HepG2 hepatoma cell line		Inhibited the activity of HepG2 by inducing apoptosis; downregulation of Bcl-2 and Bcl-X_L, upregulation of Bax expression; induced apoptosis by activating caspase-3 and caspase-9 and degrading poly (ADP-ribose) polymerase protein.	[42]
	Methanol extract	Human tumor cell lines MCF-7, NCI-H460, HeLa, and HepG2; porcine liver primary cells (PLP2).	GI50 values: 110.76 ± 5.33 µg/mL (MCF-7), 76.67 ± 7.09 µg/mL (NCI-H460), 93.18 ± 1.46 µg/mL (HeLa), 83.61 ± 6.61 µg/mL (HepG2), and >400 µg/mL (PLP2).	Showed cytotoxic effects on MCF-7, NCI-H460, HeLa, and HepG2 cells.	[4]
Antinociceptive	Ethanol extract	Acetic acid-induced writhing response in rats	100, 200, or 400 mg/kg	Increased the pain threshold in a mouse model when assessed through the hot plate test and inhibited the number of writhes compared to controls in the acetic acid-induced writhing responses mouse model.	[28]
Osteoarthritis	Ethanol extract	RAW264.7 cells and chondrosarcoma cell line (SW1353); monoiodoacetate (MIA)-induced osteoarthritis in rats	75, 150, and 300 µg/mL	Showed a chondroprotective effect by preventing cartilage degradation through targeting of NF-κB and AP-1 signaling pathways in macrophage and chondrocyte cells. Downregulated MMP2, MMP9, and MMP13 in a PMA-induced, dose-dependent manner; no effect on the gene expression of COL2A1 and CHSY1.	[15]
Colitis	Water extract	RAW264.7 cells Dextran sulfate sodium (DSS)-induced colitis in mice	100, 300, 900, and 2700 µg/mL 2 mg/day, a total of 5 days	Activated DC to produce immunosuppressive IL10; upregulated anti-inflammatory Th2 and Foxp3$^+$ Treg cells in mesenteric lymph node (MLN) and downregulated pro-inflammatory Th1 and Th17 cells. By upregulating type II T-assisted immune response, weight loss and inflammation of colon tissue were downregulated in DSS-induced colitis mice.	[29]
Antioxidant	Methanol extract		EC50 values: 0.68 ± 0.03 (DPPH scavenging activity), 0.27 ± 0.01 (Reducing power), 0.23 ± 0.04 (β-carotene bleaching inhibition), 0.14 ± 0.01 (thiobarbituric acid Thiobarbituric acid reactive substances (TBARS) inhibition).	Showed the highest antioxidant activity, which may be related to its total phenol content.	[4]
	Methanol, butanol, and water extracts	H_2O_2-induced NIH3T3 cells	0–2 mg/mL	Regenerated superoxide dismutase (SOD), catalase, and glucose 6-phosphate dehydrogenase activities; enhanced the concentration of glutathione in the cell; protected proteins from oxidative attack of H_2O_2, reduced formation of malondialdehyde in the cell, and protected NIH3T3 cells from H_2O_2-induced oxidative stress.	[43]
	Volatile constituents		5, 10, 50, 100, and 500 µg/mL	Displayed dose-dependent activity in antioxidant assays	[37]
	Phenylpropanoid glycosides		Compound 5 had the highest antioxidant activity, with an IC_{50} of 0.12 µM	Had inhibitory effects on cytochrome CYP3A4 enzyme	[18]
Anti-obesity	*n*-butanol extract	Ovariectomized (OVX) mice. 3T3-L1 cells	A total of 16 weeks	Preventing the accumulation of adipocyte in mice, weight loss and fat mass ↓ in ovariectomized mice.	[17]
	Ethanol extract	Triton WR-1339-treated Wistar rats	A total of 24,700 kJ/kg energy	Decreased postprandial triglycerides in rats given a fatty meal.	[25]
Anti-allergic	Five novel compounds	RBL-2H3 cells	100 µM	Inhibited release of β-hexosaminidase of the allergy marker.	[41]
Antidepressant	Ethanol extract	Forced swimming test (FST) and tail suspension test (TST) in mice.	100 mg/kg, p.o. (in the FST) and 10–300 mg/kg, p.o. (in the TST)	Produced antidepressant effects in the tail suspension test and forced swimming test.	[26]
Antiplatelet	Methanol extract	Rabbit platelets and cultured rat aortic vascular smooth muscle cells (VSMCs)	10, 50, 100, and 200 µg/mL	Reduced platelet aggregation by inhibiting arachidonic acid release and ERK1/2 MAPK activation.	[30]

6.1. Anti-inflammatory Activity

6.1.1. Regulation of Inflammatory Mediators.

T. impetiginosa can alter the expression of signaling molecules involved in the inflammation process, including nitric oxide (NO), prostaglandin (PGE_2), and leukotriene B_4 (LTB_4) [8,15,28]. NO is essential for maintaining homeostasis and protecting human hosts and provides immunosuppressive effects as well as immunopathological and immunoprotective activities [44]. PGE_2 is a mediator of inflammation, especially in diseases such as rheumatoid arthritis and osteoarthritis, playing an important role in stimulating the inflammatory response, facilitating tissue regeneration, and maintaining homeostasis [45]. LTB_4, a pro-inflammatory lipid mediator, is synthesized from arachidonic acid, expressed on many inflammatory and immune cells, and is a powerful chemokine that promotes migration of macrophages and neutrophils to tissues [46]. *T. impetiginosa* can also inhibit the proinflammatory cytokines interleukin (IL)-1β and IL-6 [15,47]. IL-1β has an important homeostatic function; however, overproduction of IL-1β can result in pathophysiological changes related to pain and inflammation [48]. Likewise, IL-6 is a pro-inflammatory mediator with pleiotropic effects on immune response, inflammation, and hematopoiesis, but excessive production of IL-6 can cause various diseases [49]. In addition, the mRNA expressions of IL-1β and inflammatory genes inducible NO synthase (iNOS) and cyclooxygenase (COX)-2 were markedly decreased when treated with *T. impetiginosa* [8,15,28,47]. Information gained from in vitro and in vivo models provided insights to other researchers for further investigation. Some focused on macrophages, the main cells involved in inflammation, while others focused on neutrophils, the most abundant blood leukocytes, and their role in defense against pathogens [50,51]. Previously, Byeon et al. [8] discovered that suppression of PGE_2 production negatively regulated the macrophage-mediated inflammatory response. Similarly, Suzuki et al. [52] found that *T. impetiginosa* repressed neutrophil activation. Interestingly, *T. impetiginosa* did not inhibit the migration of neutrophils but instead inhibited the reactive oxygen species (ROS) produced by migrating neutrophils. The ROS produced from normal cellular metabolism play an important role in the signaling pathways of plant and animal cells in response to environmental changes [53], and future studies should investigate their mechanisms and active substances in the context of neutrophil functional modulation.

Our body has two protective effects against infections in the form of innate and adaptive immune cells. Adaptive immune cells include T and B cells, while innate immune cells include macrophages, dendritic cells, and other cell types. Dendritic cells are the most effective antigen presenting cells due to their ability to express high levels of major histocompatibility complex II (MHC II), cluster differentiation 80 (CD80), and CD86 that are required for antigen presentation. This expression allows dendritic cells to effectively trigger an immune response [54]. Dendritic cells are predominantly found in two forms, mature and immature. Mature dendritic cells are important for stimulating the T cell immune response, while immature dendritic cells support T cell tolerance [55]. Previous research has discovered that the water extract of *T. impetiginosa* impacted dendritic cells by upregulating the expression of MHC II and CD86, the markers of dendritic cell maturation, but had no effect on production of pro-inflammatory cytokines. On the other hand, dendritic cells can affect the differentiation of CD4$^+$ T cells, which are important for adaptive immunity, while treatment with *T. impetiginosa* can induce differentiation of CD4$^+$ T cells, resulting in induction of Th2 and differentiation of regulatory T cells. The expansion of regulatory T and Th2 cells may suppress the Th1 response, thereby preventing dextran sulfate sodium (DSS)-induced colitis in mice [29].

6.1.2. Effects on Inflammatory Signaling

When pattern recognition receptors (PRRs) interact with pathogen-associated molecular patterns (PAMPs) or damage-associated molecular patterns (DAMPs), intracellular signal transduction pathways are induced to activate and translocate transcription factors such as nuclear factor (NF)-κB, activator protein (AP)-1, signal transducer and activator of transcription 3 (STAT3), and interferon regulatory factor 3 (IRF3) into the nucleus to stimulate the expression of pro-inflammatory genes, thereby producing an inflammatory response [56]. NF-κB is one of the transcription factors that expresses pro-inflammatory genes and is involved in both innate and adaptive immune responses. NF-κB can be activated through canonical and non-canonical signaling pathways. The canonical NF-κB pathway is mostly involved in immune response, while the non-canonical NF-κB pathway is only involved in parts of the adaptive immune system [57].

Park et al. [15] used an immunoblotting technique to show that the ethanol extract of *T. impetiginosa* suppressed the activation of Src and spleen tyrosine kinase (Syk). Furthermore, to determine the direct molecular targets, they conducted kinase assays and found that both Syk and Src were suppressed by *T. impetiginosa* [46]. However, Byeon et al. [8] discovered that the water extract of *T. impetiginosa* did not function in the NF-κB pathway due to non-inhibition of phospho-IκB and the upstream molecules that activate phosphorylation of IκB and AKT. Results from Park et al. [15] showed inhibition of phospho-IκB, even though they did not assess AKT expression. However, phospho-Syk and phospho-Src upstream of AKT were inhibited by ethanol extracts of *T. impetiginosa*. These results could vary depending on the proportion of active components contained in extracts using different solvents [58].

Park et al. [59] investigated the effect of anthraquinone, a main component of *T. impetiginosa*. They specifically focused on anthraquinone-2-carboxlic acid (9,10-dihydro-9,10-dioxo-2-anthracenecarboxylic acid) (AQCA: **1**) and discovered through immunoblotting that an inhibitor of IκB (IKK) and IκBα decreased when treated with 100 μM of AQCA in LPS-induced RAW264.7 cells. They repeated the kinase assay and found that Syk and Src were inhibited by treatment with AQCA [59].

Another pathway, the mitogen-activated protein kinase (MAPK) pathway, activates the activator protein (AP)-1 transcription factor that can lead to expression of pro-inflammatory genes. The MAPK pathway consists of three families: extracellular-signal-regulated kinases (ERKs), c-Jun N-terminal kinases (JNKs)/stress-activated protein kinases (SAPKs), and p38s. ERKs can be divided into two subgroups: classic ERKs that include ERK1 and ERK2 and larger ERKs such as ERK5. Classic ERKs are mainly responsible for cell growth, survival, differentiation, and development. JNK family members, which include JNK1, JNK2, and JNK3, are stress-activated [60].

Anthraquinone-2-carboxlic acid (AQCA) was identified as one of the major anthraquinones in *T. impetiginosa*. Administration of AQCA to mice treated with HCl/EtOH and aspirin resulted in reduced expression of phospo-p38 and interleukin 1 receptor associated kinase 1 (IRAK1) [61]. Treatment with AQCA reduced the expression of phospo-p38, c-JNK, mitogen-activated protein kinase 3/6 (MKK3/6), and transforming growth factor β-activated kinase (TAK1) in RAW264.7 cells. However, the expression of ERK was not inhibited. The upstream level of TAK1 was inhibited, as evidenced by degradation of IRAK1. These findings were confirmed using a conventional kinase assay with purified enzyme, and results showed potent suppression of IRAK1 by AQCA. Transfection was performed using HEK293 cells with the IRAK1 gene to validate the results, and treatment with AQCA suppressed phosphorylation of p38 protein without altering FLAG and IRAK1 protein levels. Taken together, these findings suggest that downregulation of IRAK1 by AQCA contributes to an anti-inflammatory effect [59]. Results are summarized in a pathway chart (Figure 3).

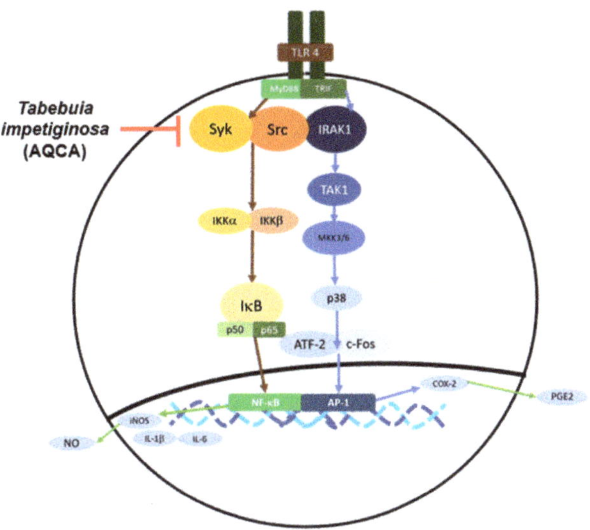

Figure 3. Inhibitory targets of *Tabebuia impetiginosa* in the NF-κB and AP-1 pathways.

6.2. Anti-Cancer Activity

T. impetiginosa exhibits inhibitory effects on the growth of several human tumor cell lines, such as breast carcinoma (MCF-7), lung carcinoma (NCI-H460), cervical carcinoma (HeLa), and hepatocellular carcinoma (HepG2), and the GI$_{50}$ values (corresponding to a sample concentration achieving 50% growth inhibition in human tumor cell lines) were 1.21, 1.03, 0.91, and 1.10 µg/mL, respectively [4]. Woo et al. [42] reported that β-lapachone isolated from *T. avellanedae* significantly inhibited the proliferation of human hepatoma cell line HepG2 by inducing apoptosis, which is associated with upregulation of pro-apoptotic Bax and downregulation of anti-apoptotic Bcl-2 and Bcl-X$_L$ expression, proteolytic activation of caspase 3 and 9, as well as degradation of poly (ADP-ribose) polymerase protein.

In a human breast carcinoma derived estrogen receptor (ER$^+$) MCF-7 cells model, Taheebo showed antiproliferative effects by upregulating xenobiotic metabolism-specific genes (dual specific phosphatase genes) and apoptosis-specific genes and by downregulating estrogen response and cell cycle regulatory genes [24]. Particularly, Taheebo treatment upregulated the dual specific phosphatase (DUSP) gene family and downregulated cyclin A and cdk2, indicating that Taheebo also inhibited the MAPK signaling pathway and phosphorylation of the ER *N*-terminal AF-1 domain [24]. Junior et al. [62] found that the anti-cancer activity of *T. impetiginosa* was correlated with the presence of lapachol and β-lapachone in its constitution. It is noteworthy that *T. impetiginosa* not only displayed growth inhibition against various tumor cell lines in vitro but also prolonged the duration of survival in a number of mouse models in vivo. For example, Queiroz et al. [63] examined the effects of *T. avellanedae* (30–500 mg/kg) and the naphtoquinone β-lapachone (1–5 mg/kg) in Ehrlich's ascites tumor-bearing mice. They observed that *T. avellanedae* administration prolonged the lifespan of tumor-bearing mice by increasing the number of bone marrow granulocyte-macrophage colony-forming units and reducing colony-stimulating activity levels; the optimal biologically active dose was 120 mg/kg. In addition, Tahara et al. [14] found that naphthoquinones isolated from *T. avellanedae* markedly blocked the STAT3 pathway while reducing hyperactivation of these signals as well as inhibited growth of cancer cell lines.

6.3. Anti-Autoimmune Diseases

Recent research has shown that *T. impetiginosa* has effects on various autoimmune diseases such as psoriasis, osteoarthritis, allergy, and inflammatory bowel disease. Suo et al. [41] found that five novel compounds isolated from the water extract of *Taheebo* had strong anti-inflammatory activity but displayed weak or no effect on anti-allergic and antioxidant activities. Muller et al. [64] reported that Lapacho, a common constituent in the inner bark of *T. impetiginosa*, suppressed growth of the human keratinocyte cell line (HaCaT) and could be promising as an effective anti-psoriatic agent. In addition, it has been reported that *T. impetiginosa* bark extracts significantly inhibited the growth of some bacterial species associated with gastrointestinal disease and diarrhea, implying their suitability for prophylactic therapeutic usage [7]. Park et al. [15] examined the effect of *T. avellanedae* on monoiodoacetate-induced osteoarthritis in a Sprague-Dawley rat model. They observed that *T. avellanedae* administration ameliorated osteoarthritis symptoms by decreasing the serum levels of proinflammatory cytokines and inflammatory mediators, such as PGE_2, LTB4, and IL-1β [15]. De Miranda et al. [5] further investigated its effects using animal models and described anti-edematogenic and antinociceptive effects of *T. impetiginosa* in rat paw edema induced by carrageenan. In this study, an aqueous extract containing a 200 mg/kg dose ameliorated rat paw edema in a way similar to indomethacin, the control drug. However, at a dose of 400 mg/kg, the edema was not reduced, suggesting that the edema-reducing compounds were competing with other constituents and nullifying any edema-reducing effect.

Lee et al. [28] investigated the analgesic and anti-inflammatory effects of *T. impetiginosa*, especially with regard to osteoarthritis. In this study, the analgesic effects were tested using pain threshold methods assessed by a hot plate test. A *T. impetiginosa* ethanol extract-treated group showed a significant analgesic effect at 200 mg/kg compared with a control group treated with diclofenac. Using an acetic acid-induced writhing response, they confirmed results from previous experiments that 100–400 mg/kg of *T. impetiginosa* ethanol extract significantly inhibited the number of writhes compared to the control group. This analgesic model used acetic acid because it causes inflammatory pain by increasing capillary permeability, and the hot plate-induced pain indicated narcotic involvement. Anti-inflammatory activity was assessed using acetic acid-induced vascular permeability, 12-*O*-tetradecanoylphorbol-13-acetate (TPA)-induced ear edema, arachidonic acid-induced mouse ear edema, and carrageenan-induced paw edema. Most of the group treated with *T. impetiginosa* exhibited reduced inflammation at a dose of 100–400 mg/kg, including suppression of ear weight and thickness, inhibition of ear inflammation, and reduction of edema in a TPA-induced ear edema test volume [28]. Byeon et al. [8] performed a similar study using a hot water extract and tested the edema model with different inducers. They found that prostaglandin E_2 (PGE_2) production was blocked and edema symptoms were reduced when treated with *T. impetiginosa*. However, in this study, *T. impetiginosa* only affected arachidonic acid-induced ear edema.

Park et al. [29] investigated the effect of *T. impetiginosa* on a DSS-induced colitis mouse model. They discovered that *T. impetiginosa* protected the colon from inflammation by reducing mucosal edema loss, epithelial crypts, and inflammatory cell infiltration. In addition, the use of *T. impetiginosa* in traditional arthritis medicines led researchers to perform experiments in an osteoarthritis model. Park et al. [46] used an ethanol extract of *T. impetiginosa* in the form of Tabetri™ (Ta-EE) in a monoiodoacetate-induced osteoarthritic mouse model. They compared the pain indicator of a mechanical paw withdrawal threshold to Von Frey stimuli and found that pain was significantly increased in osteoarthritic rats, which was suppressed by Ta-EE. Moreover, they also compared the results to those of methylsulfonylmethane (MSM) and Pc-LE and found that Ta-EE produced results comparable to those of these anti-inflammatory agents. Interestingly, results with Ta-EE were not dose-dependent, indicating that Ta-EE can be used in small doses. The osteoarthritic rats showed no weight loss, indicating no toxicity or side effects regarding weight loss or appetite caused by Ta-EE treatments. To investigate further, they measured the degradation of articular cartilage in rats administered Ta-EE and found it to be dramatically inhibited. Strangely, the chondroprotective effect of Ta-EE was better than that of MSM at 60 and 120 mg/kg doses in a dose-dependent manner.

7. Clinical Trials

In recent years, along with thorough research, some of the principal active components of *T. impetiginosa* have been used in clinical research. For example, β-lapachone, mainly distributed in heartwood of *T. impetiginosa,* has entered into phase 2 clinical trials for treatment of squamous cell carcinoma, and 2-acetylnaphtho (2,3-β) furan-4,9-dione, also referred to as STAT3 inhibitor BBI608 (Napabucacin), was developed by Boston Biomedical Inc [14].

8. Conclusions

In this paper, we summarized the traditional uses, botanical traits, phytochemistry, and pharmacological activities of *T. impetiginosa* with collation and analysis of relevant studies. *T. impetiginosa* has been used as a traditional medicine in Central and South America to treat edema, arthritis, diuretic, and infections. Based on its traditional use, in vivo and in vitro experiments examining its pharmacological potential have been conducted. In vivo experiments were conducted using edema, osteoarthritis, animal paw edema, and writhing (and other) models to screen effects of *T. impetiginosa*. Moreover, there are numerous studies confirming that extracts or compounds isolated from *T. impetiginosa* have various pharmacological activities such as anti-obesity, antibacterial, antifungal, antiviral, anti-psoriatic, antioxidant, anti-inflammatory, and anti-cancer activities.

Currently, substantial progress has been made in exploration of the phytochemistry and pharmacological activity of *T. impetiginosa*. Nonetheless, there are still challenges and gaps in published research papers that should be further explored to establish its clinical application value. Firstly, the extracts and compounds isolated from *T. impetiginosa* possess multiple pharmacological activities, though most functional mechanisms remain unclear and need to be further explored through in vivo and in vitro experiments. Furthermore, most studies on *T. impetiginosa* are still in the in vitro and in vivo mouse model stages. Toxicological research can be conducted on other animals such as rabbits in the future to evaluate its safety, which will pave the way for further clinical trials. In addition, further comprehensive experiments are needed to enrich the data and discover other pharmacological uses of *T. impetiginosa* and to find the exact mechanisms by which its extracts bind to target proteins.

Author Contributions: Original draft preparation, J.Z. and S.T.H.; conceptualization, Y.Y. and J.Y.C.; writing—review and editing, J.L. and J.Y.C.; funding acquisition, J.Y.C. All authors have read and agreed to the published version of the manuscript.

Funding: This research was supported by the Basic Science Research Program (2017R1A6A1A03015642) through the National Research Foundation of Korea (NRF) funded by the Ministry of Education, Korea.

Conflicts of Interest: The authors declare that they have no conflict of interest.

References

1. Ngo, L.T.; Okogun, J.I.; Folk, W.R. 21st century natural product research and drug development and traditional medicines. *Nat. Prod. Rep.* **2013**, *30*, 584–592. [CrossRef] [PubMed]
2. Itokawa, H.; Morris-Natschke, S.L.; Akiyama, T.; Lee, K.-H. Plant-derived natural product research aimed at new drug discovery. *J. Nat. Med.* **2008**, *62*, 263–280. [CrossRef]
3. Fabricant, D.S.; Farnsworth, N.R. The value of plants used in traditional medicine for drug discovery. *Environ. Health Perspect.* **2001**, *109*, 69–75.
4. Pires, T.C.S.P.; Dias, M.I.; Calhelha, R.C.; Carvalho, A.M.; Queiroz, M.-J.R.; Barros, L.; Ferreira, I.C. Bioactive Properties of *Tabebuia impetiginosa*-Based Phytopreparations and Phytoformulations: A Comparison between Extracts and Dietary Supplements. *Molecules* **2015**, *20*, 22863–22871. [CrossRef] [PubMed]
5. De Miranda, F.G.G.; Vilar, J.C.; Alves, I.A.N.; Cavalcanti, S.C.D.H.; Antoniolli, Â.R. Antinociceptive and antiedematogenic properties and acute toxicity of Tabebuia avellanedae Lor. ex Griseb. inner bark aqueous extract. *BMC Pharmacol.* **2001**, *1*, 6. [CrossRef]

6. Freitas, A.E.; Moretti, M.; Budni, J.; Balen, G.O.; Fernandes, S.C.; Veronezi, P.O.; Heller, M.; Micke, G.A.; Pizzolatti, M.G.; Rodrigues, A.L.S. NMDA Receptors and the L-Arginine-Nitric Oxide-Cyclic Guanosine Monophosphate Pathway Are Implicated in the Antidepressant-Like Action of the Ethanolic Extract fromTabebuia avellanedaein Mice. *J. Med. Food* **2013**, *16*, 1030–1038. [CrossRef]

7. Fernandez, A.; Cock, I.E. *Tabebuia impetiginosa* (Mart. Ex DC. Mattos) Bark Extracts Inhibit the Growth Gastrointestinal Bacterial Pathogens and Potentiate the Activity of some Conventional Antibiotics. *Pharmacogn. Commun.* **2020**, *10*, 75–82. [CrossRef]

8. Byeon, S.E.; Chung, J.Y.; Lee, Y.G.; Kim, B.H.; Kim, K.H.; Cho, J.Y. In vitro and in vivo anti-inflammatory effects of taheebo, a water extract from the inner bark of Tabebuia avellanedae. *J. Ethnopharmacol.* **2008**, *119*, 145–152. [CrossRef]

9. Sharma, P.K.; Khanna, R.N.; Rohatgi, B.K.; Thomson, R.H. Tecomaquinone-III: A new quinone from Tabebuia pentaphylla. *Phytochemistry* **1988**, *27*, 632–633. [CrossRef]

10. Manners, G.D.; Jurd, L. A new naphthaquinone from Tabebuia guayacan. *Phytochemistry* **1976**, *15*, 225–226. [CrossRef]

11. Blatt, C.T.; Salatino, A.; Salatino, M.L. Flavonoids of Tabebuia caraiba (Bignoniaceae). *Biochem. Syst. Ecol.* **1996**, *24*, 89. [CrossRef]

12. Wagner, H.; Kreher, B.; Lotter, H.; Hamburger, M.O.; Cordell, G.A. Structure Determination of New Isomeric Naphtho[2,3-b] furan-4,9-diones fromTabebuia avellanedae by the selective-INEPT technique. *Helvetica Chim. Acta* **1989**, *72*, 659–667. [CrossRef]

13. Woo, H.; Choi, Y. Growth inhibition of A549 human lung carcinoma cells by β-lapachone through induction of apoptosis and inhibition of telomerase activity. *Int. J. Oncol.* **2005**, *26*, 1017–1023. [CrossRef]

14. Tahara, T.; Watanabe, A.; Yutani, M.; Yamano, Y.; Sagara, M.; Nagai, S.; Saito, K.; Yamashita, M.; Ihara, M.; Iida, A. STAT3 inhibitory activity of naphthoquinones isolated from Tabebuia avellanedae. *Bioorganic Med. Chem.* **2020**, *28*, 115347. [CrossRef] [PubMed]

15. Park, J.G.; Yi, Y.-S.; Hong, Y.H.; Yoo, S.; Han, S.Y.; Kim, E.; Jeong, S.-G.; Aravinthan, A.; Baik, K.S.; Choi, S.Y.; et al. Tabetri™ (Tabebuia avellanedae Ethanol Extract) Ameliorates Osteoarthritis Symptoms Induced by Monoiodoacetate through Its Anti-Inflammatory and Chondroprotective Activities. *Mediat. Inflamm.* **2017**, *2017*, 1–14. [CrossRef] [PubMed]

16. Zhang, L.; Hasegawa, I.; Ohta, T. Anti-inflammatory cyclopentene derivatives from the inner bark of Tabebuia avellanedae. *Fitoterapia* **2016**, *109*, 217–223. [CrossRef] [PubMed]

17. Iwamoto, K.; Fukuda, Y.; Tokikura, C.; Noda, M.; Yamamoto, A.; Yamamoto, M.; Yamashita, M.; Zaima, N.; Iida, A.; Moriyama, T. The anti-obesity effect of Taheebo (Tabebuia avellanedae Lorentz ex Griseb) extract in ovariectomized mice and the identification of a potential anti-obesity compound. *Biochem. Biophys. Res. Commun.* **2016**, *478*, 1136–1140. [CrossRef] [PubMed]

18. Suo, M.; Ohta, T.; Takano, F.; Jin, S. Bioactive Phenylpropanoid Glycosides from Tabebuia avellanedae. *Molecules* **2013**, *18*, 7336–7345. [CrossRef] [PubMed]

19. The Plant List. 2013. Available online: http://www.theplantlist.org/ (accessed on 20 August 2020).

20. Castellanos, J.R.G.; Prieto, J.M.; Heinrich, M. Red Lapacho (*Tabebuia impetiginosa*)—A global ethnopharmacological commodity? *J. Ethnopharmacol.* **2009**, *121*, 1–13. [CrossRef]

21. University of Florida. 1994. University of Florida, Institute of Food and Agricultural Sciences, Environmental Horticulture Department. Available online: https://hort.ifas.ufl.edu/database/trees/trees_common.shtml/ (accessed on 17 September 2020).

22. The New York Botanical Garden. 1995. Available online: http://sweetgum.nybg.org/science/ (accessed on 16 September 2020).

23. Missouri Botanical Garden. 2018. Available online: http://www.tropicos.org/ (accessed on 20 August 2020).

24. Telang, N.; Mukherjee, B.; Wong, G.Y. Growth inhibition of estrogen receptor positive human breast cancer cells by Taheebo from the inner bark of Tabebuia avellandae tree. *Int. J. Mol. Med.* **2009**, *24*, 253–260. [CrossRef]

25. Kiage-Mokua, B.N.; Roos, N.; Schrezenmeir, J. Lapacho Tea (*Tabebuia impetiginosa*) Extract Inhibits Pancreatic Lipase and Delays Postprandial Triglyceride Increase in Rats. *Phytotherapy Res.* **2012**, *26*, 1878–1883. [CrossRef]

26. Freitas, A.E.; Budni, J.; Lobato, K.R.; Binfaré, R.W.; Machado, D.G.; Jacinto, J.; Veronezi, P.O.; Pizzolatti, M.G.; Rodrigues, A.L.S. Antidepressant-like action of the ethanolic extract from Tabebuia avellanedae in mice: Evidence for the involvement of the monoaminergic system. *Prog. Neuro-Psychopharmacology Biol. Psychiatry* **2010**, *34*, 335–343. [CrossRef] [PubMed]

27. Vasconcelos, C.M.; Vasconcelos, T.L.C.; Póvoas, F.T.X.; Santos, R.; Maynart, W.; Almeida, T.J.J.O.C.; Research, P. Antimicrobial, antioxidant and cytotoxic activity of extracts of *Tabebuia impetiginosa* (Mart. *ex DC.) Standl.* *J. Chem. Pharm. Res.* **2014**, *6*, 2673–2681.

28. Lee, M.H.; Choi, H.M.; Hahm, D.-H.; Her, E.; Yang, H.-I.; Yoo, M.-C.; Kim, K.S. Analgesic and anti-inflammatory effects in animal models of an ethanolic extract of Taheebo, the inner bark of Tabebuia avellanedae. *Mol. Med. Rep.* **2012**, *6*, 791–796. [CrossRef] [PubMed]

29. Park, H.J.; Lee, S.W.; Kwon, D.-J.; Heo, S.-I.; Park, S.-H.; Kim, S.Y.; Hong, S. Oral administration of taheebo (Tabebuia avellanedae Lorentz ex Griseb.) water extract prevents DSS-induced colitis in mice by up-regulating type II T helper immune responses. *BMC Complement. Altern. Med.* **2017**, *17*, 448. [CrossRef] [PubMed]

30. Son, D.J.; Lim, Y.; Park, Y.H.; Chang, S.K.; Yun, Y.P.; Hong, J.T.; Takeoka, G.R.; Lee, K.G.; Lee, S.E.; Kim, M.R.; et al. Inhibitory effects of *Tabebuia impetiginosa* inner bark extract on platelet aggregation and vascular smooth muscle cell proliferation through suppressions of arachidonic acid liberation and ERK1/2 MAPK activation. *J. Ethnopharmacol.* **2006**, *108*, 148–151. [CrossRef] [PubMed]

31. Mistrangelo, M.; Cornaglia, S.; Pizzio, M.; Rimonda, R.; Gavello, G.; Conte, I.D.; Mussa, A. Immunostimulation to reduce recurrence after surgery for anal condyloma acuminata: A prospective randomized controlled trial. *Color. Dis.* **2009**, *12*, 799–803. [CrossRef]

32. Camiel, L.D.; Whelan, J. Tropical American Plants in the Treatment of Infectious Diseases. *J. Diet. Suppl.* **2008**, *5*, 349–372. [CrossRef]

33. Malange, K.F.; Dos Santos, G.G.; Parada, C.A.; Kato, N.N.; Toffoli-Kadri, M.C.; Carollo, C.A.; Silva, D.B.; Portugal, L.C.; Alves, F.M.; Rita, P.H.S.; et al. Tabebuia aurea decreases hyperalgesia and neuronal injury induced by snake venom. *J. Ethnopharmacol.* **2019**, *233*, 131–140. [CrossRef]

34. De Melo, J.G.; Santos, A.G.; De Amorim, E.L.C.; Nascimento, S.C.D.; Albuquerque, U.P. Medicinal Plants Used as Antitumor Agents in Brazil: An Ethnobotanical Approach. *Evidence-Based Complement. Altern. Med.* **2011**, *2011*, 1–14. [CrossRef]

35. Warashina, T.; Nagatani, Y.; Noro, T. Constituents from the bark of *Tabebuia impetiginosa*. *Phytochemistry* **2004**, *65*, 2003–2011. [CrossRef] [PubMed]

36. Jin, Y.; Jeong, K.M.; Lee, J.; Zhao, J.; Choi, S.-Y.; Baek, K.-S. Development and Validation of an Analytical Method Readily Applicable for Quality Control of *Tabebuia impetiginosa* (Taheebo) Ethanolic Extract. *J. AOAC Int.* **2018**, *101*, 695–700. [CrossRef] [PubMed]

37. Park, B.-S.; Lee, K.-G.; Shibamoto, T.; Lee, S.-E.; Takeoka, G.R. Antioxidant Activity and Characterization of Volatile Constituents of Taheebo (*Tabebuia impetiginosa*Martius ex DC). *J. Agric. Food Chem.* **2003**, *51*, 295–300. [CrossRef] [PubMed]

38. Koyama, J.; Morita, I.; Tagahara, K.; Hirai, K.-I. Cyclopentene dialdehydes from *Tabebuia impetiginosa*. *Phytochemitry* **2000**, *53*, 869–872. [CrossRef]

39. Kim, B.H.; Lee, J.; Kim, K.H.; Cho, J.Y. Regulation of macrophage and monocyte immune responses by water extract from the inner bark of Tabebuia avellanedae. *JMPR* **2010**, *4*, 431–438.

40. Böhler, T.; Nolting, J.; Gurragchaa, P.; Lupescu, A.; Neumayer, H.-H.; Budde, K.; Kamar, N.; Klupp, J. Tabebuia avellanedae extracts inhibit IL-2-independent T-lymphocyte activation and proliferation. *Transpl. Immunol.* **2008**, *18*, 319–323. [CrossRef]

41. Suo, M.; Isao, H.; Kato, H.; Takano, F.; Ohta, T. Anti-inflammatory constituents from Tabebuia avellanedae. *Fitoterapia* **2012**, *83*, 1484–1488. [CrossRef]

42. Woo, H.J.; Park, K.-Y.; Rhu, C.-H.; Lee, W.H.; Choi, B.T.; Kim, G.Y.; Park, Y.-M.; Choi, Y.H. β-Lapachone, a Quinone Isolated from Tabebuia avellanedae, Induces Apoptosis in HepG2 Hepatoma Cell Line Through Induction of Bax and Activation of Caspase. *J. Med. Food* **2006**, *9*, 161–168. [CrossRef]

43. Eun, L.S.; Soo, P.B.; Jong, H.Y. Antioxidative activity of taheebo (*Tabebuia impetiginosa* Martius ex DC.) extracts on the H_2O_2-induced NIH3T3 cells. *J. Med. Plants Res.* **2012**, *6*, 5258–5265. [CrossRef]

44. Tripathi, P.; Tripathi, P.; Kashyap, L.; Singh, V. The role of nitric oxide in inflammatory reactions. *FEMS Immunol. Med. Microbiol.* **2007**, *51*, 443–452. [CrossRef]

45. Nakanishi, M.; Rosenberg, D.W. Multifaceted roles of PGE2 in inflammation and cancer. *Semin. Immunopathol.* **2012**, *35*, 123–137. [CrossRef] [PubMed]

46. Li, P.; Oh, D.Y.; Bandyopadhyay, G.; Lagakos, W.S.; Talukdar, S.; Osborn, O.; Johnson, A.; Chung, H.; Mayoral, R.; Maris, M.; et al. LTB4 promotes insulin resistance in obese mice by acting on macrophages, hepatocytes and myocytes. *Nat. Med.* **2015**, *21*, 239–247. [CrossRef] [PubMed]

47. Ma, S.; Yada, K.; Lee, H.; Fukuda, Y.; Iida, A.; Suzuki, K. Taheebo Polyphenols Attenuate Free Fatty Acid-Induced Inflammation in Murine and Human Macrophage Cell Lines as Inhibitor of Cyclooxygenase-2. *Front. Nutr.* **2017**, *4*, 4. [CrossRef]

48. Ren, K.; Torres, R. Role of interleukin-1β during pain and inflammation. *Brain Res. Rev.* **2009**, *60*, 57–64. [CrossRef] [PubMed]

49. Tanaka, T.; Narazaki, M.; Kishimoto, T. IL-6 in Inflammation, Immunity, and Disease. *Cold Spring Harb. Perspect. Biol.* **2014**, *6*, a016295. [CrossRef]

50. Rosales, C. Neutrophil: A Cell with Many Roles in Inflammation or Several Cell Types? *Front. Physiol.* **2018**, *9*, 113. [CrossRef]

51. Dunster, J. The macrophage and its role in inflammation and tissue repair: Mathematical and systems biology approaches. *Wiley Interdiscip. Rev. Syst. Biol. Med.* **2015**, *8*, 87–99. [CrossRef]

52. Ohno, S.; Ohno, Y.; Suzuki, Y.; Miura, S.; Yoshioka, H.; Mori, Y.; Suzuki, K. Ingestion of Tabebuia avellanedae (Tahee-bo) Inhibits Production of Reactive Oxygen Species from Human Pe-ripheral Blood Neutrophils. *Int. J. Food Sci. Nutr. Diet.* **2015**, *6*, 1–4.

53. Reuter, S.; Gupta, S.C.; Chaturvedi, M.M.; Aggarwal, B.B. Oxidative stress, inflammation, and cancer: How are they linked? *Free. Radic. Biol. Med.* **2010**, *49*, 1603–1616. [CrossRef]

54. Agrawal, A.; Agrawal, S.; Gupta, S. Role of Dendritic Cells in Inflammation and Loss of Tolerance in the Elderly. *Front. Immunol.* **2017**, *8*, 896. [CrossRef]

55. Morva, A.; Lemoine, S.; Achour, A.; Pers, J.-O.; Youinou, P.; Jamin, C. Maturation and function of human dendritic cells are regulated by B lymphocytes. *Blood* **2012**, *119*, 106–114. [CrossRef] [PubMed]

56. Hunto, S.T.; Shin, K.K.; Kim, H.G.; Park, S.H.; Oh, J.; Sung, G.-H.; Hossain, M.A.; Rho, H.S.; Lee, J.; Kim, J.-H.; et al. Phosphatidylinositide 3-Kinase Contributes to the Anti-Inflammatory Effect of Abutilon crispum L. Medik Methanol Extract. *Evidence-Based Complement. Altern. Med.* **2018**, *2018*, 1935902. [CrossRef] [PubMed]

57. Liu, T.; Zhang, L.; Joo, D.; Sun, S.-C. NF-κB signaling in inflammation. *Signal. Transduct. Target. Ther.* **2017**, *2*, 17023. [CrossRef] [PubMed]

58. Osadebe, P.O.; Okoye, F.B.C. Anti-inflammatory effects of crude methanolic extract and fractions of Alchornea cordifolia leaves. *J. Ethnopharmacol.* **2003**, *89*, 19–24. [CrossRef]

59. Park, J.G.; Son, Y.-J.; Kim, M.-Y.; Cho, J.Y. Syk and IRAK1 Contribute to Immunopharmacological Activities of Anthraquinone-2-carboxlic Acid. *Molecules* **2016**, *21*, 809. [CrossRef] [PubMed]

60. Morrison, D.K. MAP Kinase Pathways. *Cold Spring Harb. Perspect. Biol.* **2012**, *4*, a011254. [CrossRef]

61. Park, J.G.; Kim, S.C.; Kim, Y.H.; Yang, W.S.; Kim, Y.; Hong, S.; Kim, K.-H.; Yoo, B.C.; Kim, S.H.; Kim, J.-H.; et al. Anti-Inflammatory and Antinociceptive Activities of Anthraquinone-2-Carboxylic Acid. *Mediat. Inflamm.* **2016**, *2016*, 1–12. [CrossRef]

62. da Silva Junior, E.N.; de Souza, M.C.; Pinto, A.V.; Pinto Mdo, C.; Goulart, M.O.; Barros, F.W.; Pessoa, C.; Costa-Lotufo, L.V.; Montenegro, R.C.; de Moraes, M.O.; et al. Synthesis and potent antitumor activity of new arylamino derivatives of nor-beta-lapachone and nor-alpha-lapachone. *Bioorg. Med. Chem.* **2007**, *15*, 7035–7041. [CrossRef]

63. Queiroz, M.L.; Valadares, M.C.; Torello, C.O.; Ramos, A.L.; Oliveira, A.B.; Rocha, F.D.; Arruda, V.A.; Accorci, W.R. Comparative studies of the effects of Tabebuia avellanedae bark extract and β-lapachone on the hematopoietic response of tumour-bearing mice. *J. Ethnopharmacol.* **2008**, *117*, 228–235. [CrossRef]

64. Müller, K.; Sellmer, A.; Wiegrebe, W. Potential Antipsoriatic Agents: Lapacho Compounds as Potent Inhibitors of HaCaT Cell Growth. *J. Nat. Prod.* **1999**, *62*, 1134–1136. [CrossRef]

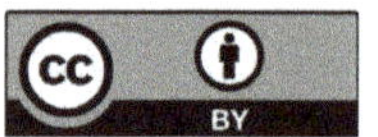

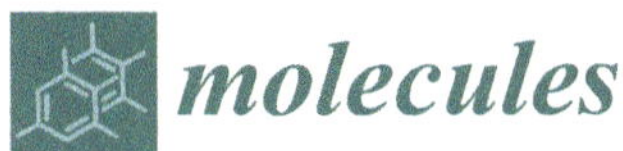 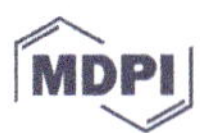

Review

Ethnopharmacology of Fruit Plants: A Literature Review on the Toxicological, Phytochemical, Cultural Aspects, and a Mechanistic Approach to the Pharmacological Effects of Four Widely Used Species

Aline T. de Carvalho [1], Marina M. Paes [1], Mila S. Cunha [1], Gustavo C. Brandão [2], Ana M. Mapeli [3], Vanessa C. Rescia [1], Silvia A. Oesterreich [4] and Gustavo R. Villas-Boas [1,*]

[1] Research Group on Development of Pharmaceutical Products (P&DProFar), Center for Biological and Health Sciences, Federal University of Western Bahia, Rua Bertioga, 892, Morada Nobre II, Barreiras-BA CEP 47810-059, Brazil; alineteixeiraufob@gmail.com (A.T.d.C.); marinameirelles@ymail.com (M.M.P.); milacunha035@gmail.com (M.S.C.); vanessa.rescia@ufob.edu.br (V.C.R.)

[2] Physical Education Course, Center for Health Studies and Research (NEPSAU), Univel University Center, Cascavel-PR, Av. Tito Muffato, 2317, Santa Cruz, Cascavel-PR CEP 85806-080, Brazil; gustavochavesbrandao@gmail.com

[3] Research Group on Biomolecules and Catalyze, Center for Biological and Health Sciences, Federal University of Western Bahia, Rua Bertioga, 892, Morada Nobre II, Barreiras-BA CEP 47810-059, Brazil; mmapeli@ufob.edu.br

[4] Faculty of Health Sciences, Federal University of Grande Dourados, Dourados, Rodovia Dourados, Itahum Km 12, Cidade Universitaria, Caixa. postal 364, Dourados-MS CEP 79804-970, Brazil; silviaoesterreich@gmail.com

* Correspondence: gustavo.villasboas@gmail.com; Tel.: +55-(77)-3614-3152

Academic Editors: Raffaele Pezzani and Sara Vitalini
Received: 22 July 2020; Accepted: 31 July 2020; Published: 26 August 2020

Abstract: Fruit plants have been widely used by the population as a source of food, income and in the treatment of various diseases due to their nutritional and pharmacological properties. The aim of this study was to review information from the most current research about the phytochemical composition, biological and toxicological properties of four fruit species widely used by the world population in order to support the safe medicinal use of these species and encourage further studies on their therapeutic properties. The reviewed species are: *Talisia esculenta, Brosimum gaudichaudii, Genipa americana,* and *Bromelia antiacantha.* The review presents the botanical description of these species, their geographical distribution, forms of use in popular medicine, phytochemical studies and molecules isolated from different plant organs. The description of the pharmacological mechanism of action of secondary metabolites isolated from these species was detailed and toxicity studies related to them were reviewed. The present study demonstrates the significant concentration of phenolic compounds in these species and their anti-inflammatory, anti-tumor, photosensitizing properties, among others. Such species provide important molecules with pharmacological activity that serve as raw materials for the development of new drugs, making further studies necessary to elucidate mechanisms of action not yet understood and prove the safety for use in humans.

Keywords: plant secondary metabolites; natural compounds; biological activity; phytochemistry; pharmacological activity; plant side effects; *Talisia esculenta*; *Brosimum gaudichaudii*; *Genipa americana*; *Bromelia antiacantha*

---

1. Introduction

The Cerrado is one of the most important and extensive Brazilian biomes, with a great richness of plant species that are used as food and therapeutic agents, highlighting their medicinal, sociocultural and nutritional importance, which make them attractive for research and commercialization [1].

The Brazilian population has great range of cultural knowledge about native plants, which are used in the treatment of diseases. These medicinal plants present molecules with pharmacological properties which expand the possibilities for the development of drugs and/or nutraceuticals. However, despite the great Brazilian biodiversity in species considered medicinal, research is still incipient, requiring active investigations on the phytochemical constituents present in these plants, as well as their pharmacological or nutritional properties [2].

Climatic factors directly affect the production of fruits and phytochemical constituents by plants, since water availability in the Cerrado is reduced over a period that can vary from two to five months. Some species adapt to reduced water availability in soil and increased temperature, being called sclerophyll plants. These plants make up the Cerrado vegetation, which is characterized by the presence of shrubs, grasses and trees with deep roots to facilitate water absorption; in the dry season, some species lose their leaves in an attempt to save water [3].

Given these environmental conditions to which Cerrado plants are exposed, another way to mitigate the damage caused by climate changes is the production of bioactive molecules that act in the defense of the plant against harmful agents. These compounds are alternative sources for the formulation of new products, not only in the pharmaceutical industry, but also in the food industry. In addition to climatic conditions associated with different geographic regions, factors such as cultivation, harvest time and growth stage of the collected plant can also change the concentration of these compounds [4].

Some Cerrado fruit species are used as functional foods, with fruits and seeds being the most used parts. The therapeutic and nutritional properties associated with these foods are constantly investigated through scientific studies, which highlight the high concentration of phenolic compounds found in these species, normally produced in response to water scarcity, intense exposure to solar radiation, attack of herbivores and infections by fungi, which are conditions common to Cerrado plants. The sale of parts of these plants for fresh consumption or therapeutic purposes has great prominence in the economy as source of livelihood for workers in regions covered by this biome [5].

Studies that have assessed the biological activity, toxicity and phytochemical composition of plants native to the Cerrado can contribute to ensuring the effectiveness and safety in the use of such species, favoring the healthy consumption of fruits and by-products, also encouraging further studies on the therapeutic properties of substances isolated from these plants, which are of great importance for popular medicine, nutrition and income in various regions of the world. In this sense, the aim of this study was to review the current literature to gather detailed and accurate information about the phytochemical, pharmacological and toxicological aspects of the following fruit plants: *Talisia esculenta, Brosimum gaudichaudii, Genipa americana, Bromelia antiacantha.*

2. Fruit Plants from the Brazilian Cerrado

Cerrado is considered the second largest Brazilian biome, only behind the Amazon, accounting for around 23% of the national territory and extending into 11 of the country's states. With abundant flora and fauna diversity, this biome has been annually targeted by deforestation caused by the expansion of agribusiness, livestock and urbanization, which already occupy 50% of the biome's extension [6].

The multiplicity of Cerrado plant species is superior to that found in other regions of the world, with shrub, liana and herbaceous plants, and the registered number reaches 12,669 species, of which, some stand out for their relevant pharmacological and nutritional properties, which play an important role in the commercial activities of regions where they are found. In addition, fruits of these plants also contribute to the promotion and development of family farming, generating income for communities through the preparation of sweets, ice cream, flavorings for alcoholic distillates and other by-products [7–9].

Fruits produced by Cerrado species are known not only for their flavor and aroma, which are generally striking, but also for their high concentrations of carotenoids, phenolic compounds, vitamins and minerals, whose antioxidant power is desired in the food and pharmaceutical industry. The identification and quantification of these components allow the assessment of their nutritional value and, consequently, the production and commercialization of by-products with guaranteed quality [10].

However, for the study of properties attributed to the phytochemical constituents found in fruits of these species, the correct identification of species must be performed by a botanist. Such species have their classification based on botanical nomenclatures, followed by norms created by an international commission of scientists, which are described in the International Botanical Nomenclature Code, which aims to guarantee the universality of names given to taxa. In this code, plants are categorized into Phylum, Class, Order, Family, Genus and species [11,12].

3. Sapindaceae Family

The Sapindaceae family belongs to the order of Sapindales angiosperm plants, has 141 genera and approximately 2000 identified species, 28 genera and about 418 species being native to Brazil. It is predominantly found in tropical and subtropical climates, with rare occurrence of some genera in countries with temperate climate [13]. This family is morphologically characterized by the presence of shrubs, lianas with tendrils and trees, whose leaves can be alternate or opposite, composed, trifoliate, unifoliated, pinnate or webbed, with present or absent stipules and unisexual and monoic flowers [14]. In addition, this plant family has species with edible fruits with industrial potential, for example, *Litchichinensis* Sonn. (lychee), *Melicoccus bijugatus* Jacq. (mamoncillo or Spanish lime), *Nephelium luppuceum* L. (rambutão) and *Talisia esculenta* (A. St. Hil) Radlk. (pitomba). Other species have known medicinal and ichthyotoxic properties, such as species of the genera *Paullinia* L. and *Serjania* Mill., and there are those that can be simply ornamental, such as *Paullinia pinnata* L. and *P. elegans* (cipó-timbó). The flowers of these species are usually tetrameric or pentameric, with an extra-stamen nectary, that is, located between the androceu and the perianth. Fruits can be dehiscent or indehiscent, ranging from berries and capsules to schizocarps [15–17].

3.1. Genus Talisia and Species Talisia esculenta

The genus *Talisia* was first described by Aublet in 1775. Soon after, in 1778, following up on Aublet's findings, Rodlkofer carried out several studies on this genus. About 10 species of the genus *Talisia* have nutritional properties, including *Talisia esculenta* (popularly known as "pitombeira", although the name is also used for other species of the same genus, such as *T. acutifolia* Raldk, *T. cerasina* (Benth). Radlk. and *T. cupularis* Radlk., all from the Amazon [14]).

The species has characteristics that help it adapt to areas along the margins of water courses, such as rapid growth and large seed production, which are dispersed with high water content, that is, recalcitrant seeds, which should be sown quickly, as they are only viable for a short time in the environment [18].

Fruits produced by this species are consumed by humans and birds, with economic importance attributed to their nutritional properties and characteristic flavor, desired in regional cuisine, being used in the manufacture of pulps, jams, sweets, and jellies. In addition, the wood derived from the trunks is used in the manufacture of furniture and decorative objects, while leaves and seeds have been investigated in several studies due to their reported therapeutic properties based on their popular use [19].

3.1.1. Geographic Distribution and Popular Use

T. esculenta although native to Brazil, has a cosmopolitan distribution and occurs in several other countries such as Bolivia, Paraguay, Colombia, Ecuador, Peru and Argentina, where the climate is favorable for its development [20]. It can be found in the native and wild state or cultivated and despite being a tropical climate plant, it adapts well to subtropical areas, with preference for alluvial soils in valley bottoms. Its flowering occurs from August to October and the fruit maturation occurs between January and March, which may vary according to the region in which the species is found [21,22].

The use of *T. esculenta* by the population is mainly for food and medicinal purposes. The fruit is commonly used for fresh consumption or in the form of by-products. The other plant parts are associated with therapeutic purposes, such as leaves, which are popularly used for back pain and rheumatism, seeds for diarrhea, dehydration and as astringents and barks for kidney problems [9,23].

The therapeutic use of teas made from the leaves can vary according to the region. An example was reported in an ethnobotanical study of species with medicinal use, which describes the use of *T. esculenta* leaves tea as antihypertensive, a property little mentioned by the inhabitants of other regions of the country [24]. Regarding the form of preparation, tea is usually obtained from freshly harvested or dried plant parts produced through the method of infusion or decoction, using leaves to prepare tea by infusion, while seeds and bark are used to prepare tea by decoction. Some studies point out a concern in relation to the hygiene of plant parts to be used and the way they are dried and stored, which can favor contamination or proliferation of deteriorating microorganisms [25,26].

In the preparation of teas using the infusion method, the popularly used solvent is boiling water, in which the vegetable is immersed for about 30 min. After this time, the tea is leached and cooled until it reaches an ideal temperature for consumption. Unlike infusion, in decoction, which is the most widely used form of tea preparation, the vegetable is in direct contact with water throughout the process, from heating to boiling; then the tea is leached and cooled to be consumed. A negative consequence associated with these methods is the degradation of some thermolabile compounds that do not resist exposure to intense heat [27].

3.1.2. Botanical Aspects

T. esculenta is an arboreal fruit plant of some 6–12 m in height, with terrestrial roots and aerial and erect cylindrical stems of dark and lenticelous in color; leaves are composite and alternate, with 2 to 4 pairs of leaflets, with petioles of 3–10 cm in length and a petiole of 1–5 mm and simple non-glandular trichomes on their surface. In addition, as to morphology, leaves are classified in oblong shape, acuminated apex, rounded or obtuse base and venation is of peninerval type [20,28].

Inflorescences are composed, of the thyrsus type, that is, forming racemes of crests. Flowers are white, aromatic, diclamid, with pedicels up to 4 mm in length, gamosepal, with five elliptical sepals and dialipetal, with five petals. Classification regarding sexual characteristics is not well defined, with monoclinous flowers, that is, hermaphrodites, or diclinous, which are unisexual male or female. They present about eight filiform and hairy stamens, oblong and apiculate anthers, trifid stigmas and ovoid ovary, tricarpellar and trilocular [14,20].

Fruit production occurs annually, about ten years after planting, and it is possible to harvest ten to twenty fruits in each raceme. Fruits are generally monospermic, globose, fleshy, drupe type and when ripe they have approximately 2.5 cm in diameter and the color of the epicarp changes from green to brown. The pulp of the ripe fruit has bittersweet flavor and its color varies from white to transparent [29].

Seeds are elongated, reddish in color immediately after harvest and dark after drying. They are surrounded by a pinkish-white aryl, which must be removed before planting, as it can harm germination. Regarding seed viability, it is about 15 days in the environment, but if stored in polyethylene package with 50% relative humidity under refrigeration (approx. 18 °C), they can remain viable for up to 25 days. Seed dispersion enables species maintenance; however, it is still not clear which agent is responsible for dissemination, since the fruits attract several animals [18,30,31].

3.1.3. Phytochemical Aspects

Table 1 presents a summary of phytochemical studies carried out with different *T. esculenta* organs, as well as the structures of isolated substances.

Table 1. Phytochemical analysis of *T. esculenta*.

Compounds	Molecular Structures	Chromatographic Methods for the Isolation and Identification	Solvent Used/Essential Oil	Plant Part Used	Collection Site	References
Myricetin (**1**, F)	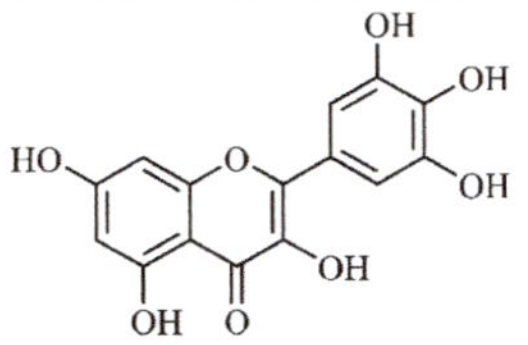	HPLC	Hydroalcoholic 5:95 (*v/v* water, ethanol)	Fruit	N.I.	[32]
Quercetin (**2**, F)	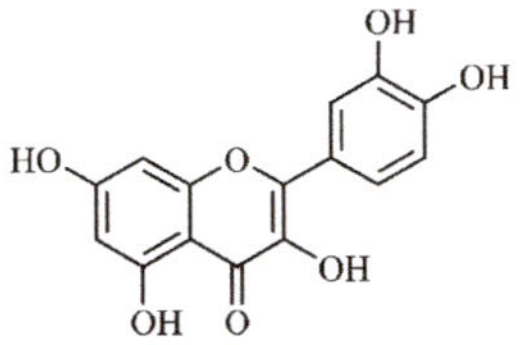					
Catechin (**3**, F)	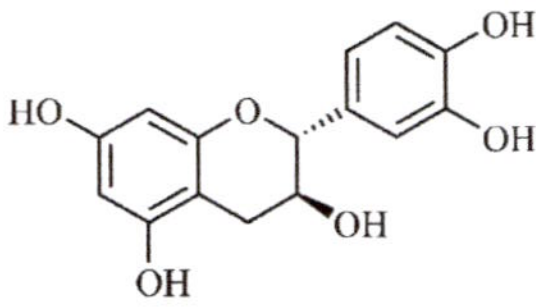	LC-MS	Acetone Methanol	Pulp Fruit peel Seed	Parintins, Amazonas-Brazil	[33]
Epicatechin (**4**, F)	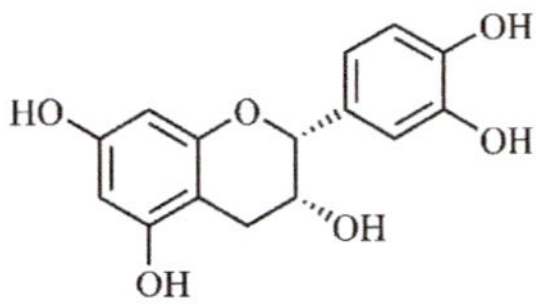		Acetone	Fruit peel Seed		

Table 1. *Cont.*

Compounds	Molecular Structures	Chromatographic Methods for the Isolation and Identification	Solvent Used/Essential Oil	Plant Part Used	Collection Site	References
Gallic acid (**5**, PA)	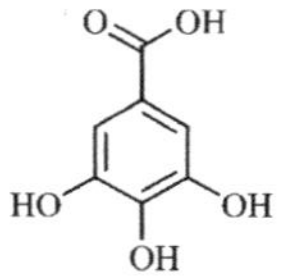		Acetone	Pulp		
Luteolin (**6**, F)	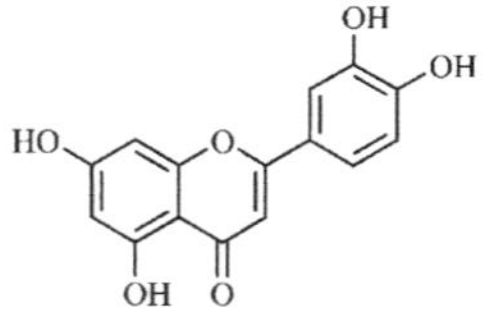		Acetone Methanol	Seed		
Naringenin (**7**, F)	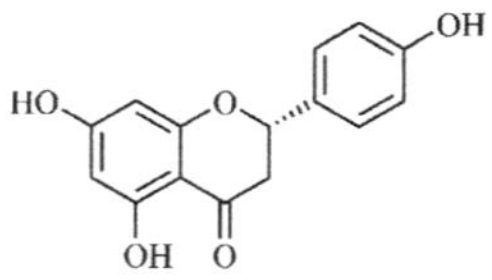		Acetone Methanol	Fruit peel Seed		
p-Coumaric acid (**8**, PA)	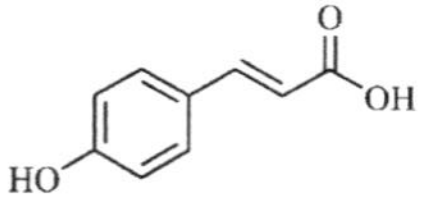		Acetone	Pulp		
Quinic acid (**9**, CL)	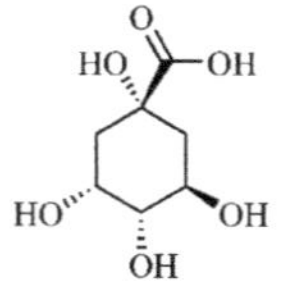		Acetone	Pulp		

Table 1. *Cont.*

Compounds	Molecular Structures	Chromatographic Methods for the Isolation and Identification	Solvent Used/Essential Oil	Plant Part Used	Collection Site	References
Rutin (**10**, F)	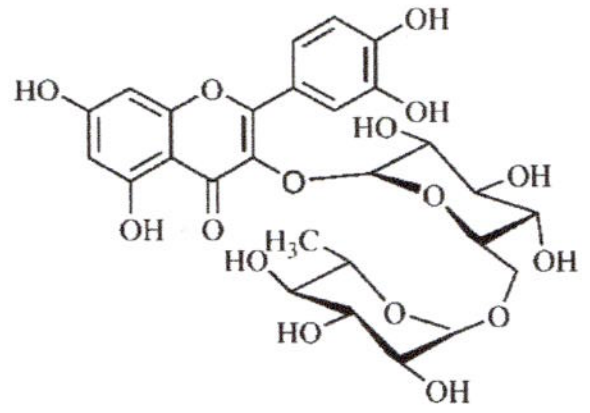		Acetone Methanol	Fruit peel		
Acacetin (**11**, F)	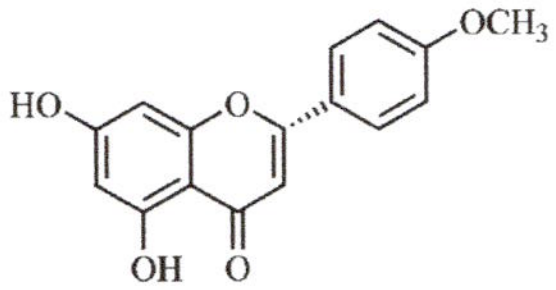					
Caffeic acid (**12**, PA)	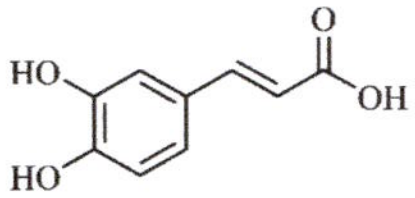	UHPLC–MS/MS	Methanol	Fruit	Manaus, Amazonas-Brazil	[34]
Catechin (**3**, F)	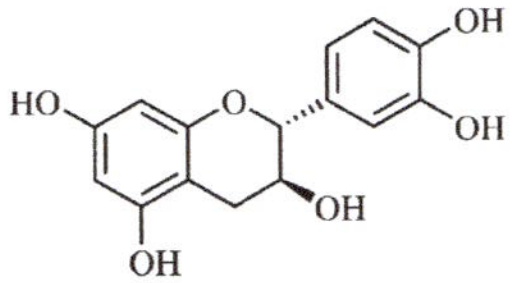					
Chlorogenic acid (**13**, PA)	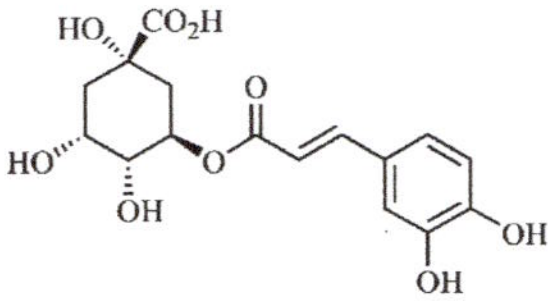					

Table 1. *Cont.*

Compounds	Molecular Structures	Chromatographic Methods for the Isolation and Identification	Solvent Used/Essential Oil	Plant Part Used	Collection Site	References
Epicatechin (**4**, F)						
Eriodictyol (**14**, F)						
Ferulic acid (**15**, PA)						
Gallic acid (**5**, PA)						
p-Coumaric acid (**8**, PA)						

Table 1. *Cont.*

Compounds	Molecular Structures	Chromatographic Methods for the Isolation and Identification	Solvent Used/Essential Oil	Plant Part Used	Collection Site	References
Quercetin (**2**, F)	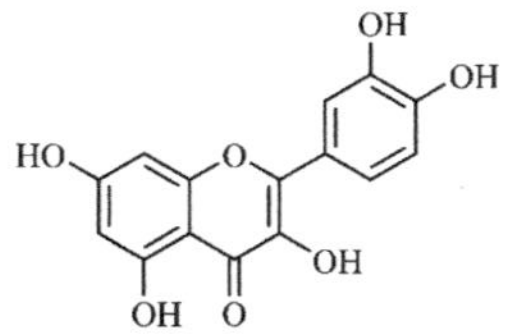					
Quinic acid (**9**, CL)	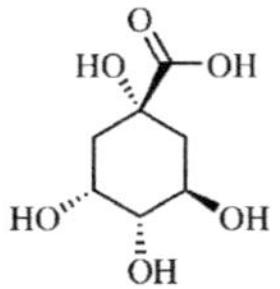					
Rutin (**10**, F)	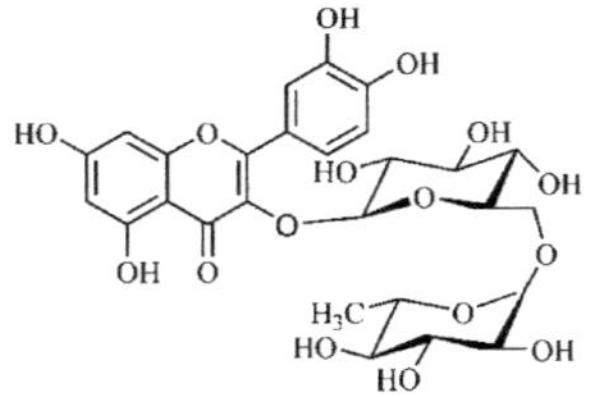					
Syringic acid (**16**, PA)	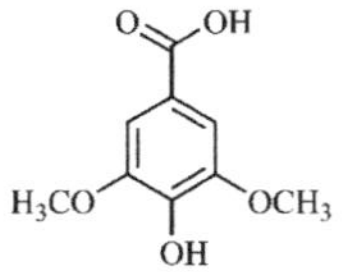					

Table 1. *Cont.*

Compounds	Molecular Structures	Chromatographic Methods for the Isolation and Identification	Solvent Used/Essential Oil	Plant Part Used	Collection Site	References
β-Bisabolene (**17**, T)		HS-SPME-GC-MS	DVB/CAR/PDMS			
Linalool (**18**, T)						
Dihydroxybenzoic acid hexoside (**19**, PA)	*					
Kaempferol-diglycoside (**20**, F)	*					
Methylquercetin-diglycoside (**21**, F)	*	UHPLC	Hydroalcoholic 1:1 (*v/v* methanol, water)	Leaf Stem	Dourados, Mato Grosso do Sul-Brazil	[35]
Quercetin-diglycoside (**22**, F)	*					
Quercetin-rhamnoside (**23**, F)	*					
Dicaffeoylquinic acid (**24**, PA)	*					
Acacetin (**11**, F)		UHPLC–MS/MS	Hydroalcoholic 1:4 (*m/v*, 70% ethanol)	Leaf	São Luís, Maranhão-Brazil	[36]
Caffeic acid (**12**, PA)						

Table 1. *Cont.*

Compounds	Molecular Structures	Chromatographic Methods for the Isolation and Identification	Solvent Used/Essential Oil	Plant Part Used	Collection Site	References
Catechin (**3**, F)						
Gallic acid (**5**, PA)						
Quercetin (**2**, F)						
Quinic acid (**9**, CL)						

Table 1. *Cont.*

Compounds	Molecular Structures	Chromatographic Methods for the Isolation and Identification	Solvent Used/Essential Oil	Plant Part Used	Collection Site	References
Rutin (**10**, F)	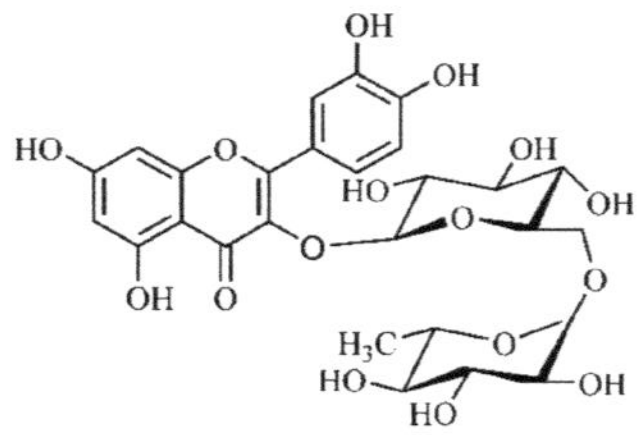					

N.I.: not identified; CL: cyclitol; F: flavonoid; PA: phenolic acid; T: terpenes; HPLC: High Performance Liquid Chromatography; HS-SPME-GC-MS: Headspace Solid Phase Microextraction/Gas Chromatography with Mass Spectrometry Detection; LC-MS: Liquid Chromatography Coupled to Mass Spectrometry; UHPLC: Ultra-High Performance Liquid Chromatography; UHPLC–MS/MS: Ultra-High Performance Liquid Chromatography associated with Mass Spectrometry; DVB/CAR/PDMS: Divinylbenzene/Carboxen/Polydimethylsiloxane. * Based on the lack of specificity in the indication of the substitution chemical groups it was not possible to design the structures once the article states that it was a tentative identification

Phytochemical investigations include the in-depth study of the target species, as well as extractive and separation methods, purification and structural determination of isolated chemical constituents [37]. Cerrado species are known to have significant amount of phenolic compounds in their composition, which are bioactive substances widely distributed in nature and derive from two biosynthetic routes, that of shikimic acid and that of acetyl-CoA, being divided into two large groups, phenolic acids and flavonoids, commonly found in fruits and vegetables [38].

To date, there is scarcity of studies on the bioactive compounds present in *T. esculenta*, mainly for roots and stems. [39] determined the centesimal composition of *T. esculenta* fruits. The average values found after triplicate analysis, were: 56.35 kcal/100 g of energy value, 83.16 g/100g of moisture, 1.15 g/100 g of proteins, 0.19 g/100 of lipids, 12.51 g/100 g of carbohydrates, 2.40 g/100 g dietary fiber and 0.61 g/100 g of fixed mineral residue. In addition, the analysis revealed 26.7 mg/100 g of calcium, 0.84 mg/100 g of zinc and 0.60 mg/100 g of iron, 0.0 mg/100 g of copper and 10.8 mg/100 g of magnesium. The phosphorus concentration was considered insignificant [40].

In a study on fruits and seeds in which extraction was performed using the technique of maceration in acetone and methanol, quinic (**9**), gallic (**5**) and *p*-coumaric (**8**) acids, in addition to epicatechin (**4**) and catechin (**3**), were identified in the ketone extract of the pulp, the latter being also found in the pulp methanolic extract. In the ketone extract of the fruit bark, naringenin (**7**), catechin (**3**) and epicatechin (**4**) were detected, not identified in the methanolic extract of the fruit bark. For seeds, epicatechin (**4**), catechin (**3**), naringenin (**7**) and luteolin (**6**) were found in the ketone extract (**6**) and in the methanolic naringenin extract (**7**) and luteolin (**6**) [33].

Other phytochemical findings of this species were analyzed using 5:95 hydroalcoholic extract (*v/v*, water, ethanol) from fruits, followed by evaporation and collection of the lipophilic fraction, which was homogenized in hexane. High mirecetin (**1**) and quercetin (**2**) concentrations were determined, approximately 89.90 mg/100 g and 30.20 mg/100 g, respectively, which are associated with possible antioxidant and antiproliferative properties [36].

Furthermore, the analysis of the methanolic extract of the pulp of *T. esculenta* fruits showed the presence of flavonoids and phenolic acids. The following 12 phenolic compounds were found: gallic acid (**5**), chlorogenic acid (**13**), catechin (**3**), epicatechin (**4**), caffeic acid (**12**), serum acid (**16**), *p*-coumaric acid (**8**), rutin (**10**), ferulic acid (**15**), quercetin (**2**), eriodicthiol (**14**) and acacetin (**11**); and the cyclitol quinic acid (**9**). This study identified 27 aromatic compounds, including esters, alcohols, aldehydes, hydrocarbons, fatty acids and terpenoids such as monoterpenolinalol (**18**) and the sesquiterpene β-bisabolene (**17**) [35].

In this sense, in order to investigate the phytochemical composition of *T. esculenta* leaves and stem, hydroalcoholic extract was produced, which, after analysis and characterization, allowed identifying derivatives of flavonoids, benzoic and cinnamic acids, fragments of aglycones, quercetin (**2**) and *dicaffeoylquinic* acid (**24**), which compounds being given the ability to influence renal hemodynamics and induce diuretic response in normotensive and spontaneously hypertensive Wistar rats [35].

Junior (2019) analyzed the hydroalcoholic extract of *T. esculenta* leaves and identified some compounds such as quinic acid (**9**), caffeic acid (**12**), gallic acid (**5**), which are classified as phenolic acids, in addition to flavonoids such as catechin (**3**), rutin (**10**), acacetin (**11**) and quercetin (**2**), which are associated with antioxidant and anti-inflammatory properties [36].

3.1.4. Pharmacological Studies

Flavonoids, phytochemicals present in different *T. esculenta* parts have pharmacological properties that are the focus of several studies, in which, among others, the anti-inflammatory, antioxidant and anti-tumor properties associated with these compounds are described. A study analyzed the anti-inflammatory activity of some flavonoids with a focus on the possible regulatory role in the activation of NLRP3 inflammasome. The mechanism proposed for inhibiting activation by flavonoids was based on the regulation of the expression of inflammasome components such as the amino-terminal pyrin domain (PYD), which interacts with the ASC pyrin domain (caspase recruitment domain) to initiate the assembly of the inflammasome; the central nucleotide binding and oligomerization domain (NACHT), which has the ATPase activity necessary for NLRP3 oligomerization after activation; and C-terminal leucine-rich repeat (LRR) domain, whose function has not yet been identified. These changes can prevent its assembly and lead to inhibition of caspase-1 activation and, consequently, maturation and secretion of pro-inflammatory cytokines [41,42].

Luteolin (**6**), a flavonoid found in *T. esculenta* seeds, has anti-inflammatory activity attributed to its ability to reduce the generation of reactive oxygen species (ROS) and inhibit the activation of NLRP3 inflammasome. Previous studies have described some Pattern-Recognition Receptors (PRR) located in the cytoplasm of cells, such as dendritic cells and macrophages, which are also involved in the induction of inflammatory responses [43]. Among these receivers, some belong to the family of NOD-like receptors (NRLs). NLRs are a large family of intracellular PRRs with similar structure [44,45]. Among the various types of NLRs, NLRP3 is recognized for responding to various stimuli, being responsible for the inflammasome activation (NLRP3 inflammasome), involved in the recruitment and activation of caspase-1 (pro-caspase 1) in association with the ASC adapter protein [46]. The role of activated caspase-1 is crucial for the conversion of pro-interleukin 1 beta (pro-IL-1β) and pro-interleukin 18 (pro-IL-18) into their mature and biologically active forms [47]. Thus, luteolin (**6**) is able to reduce the expression of interleukin-1 beta (IL-1β), a cytokine with a primary role in the inflammatory response, and interleukin-8 (IL-8), a chemokine that stimulates migration of immune cells. Another anti-inflammatory flavonoid found in *T. esculenta* seeds is rutin (**10**), which promotes the inhibition of the NLRP3 inflammasome activation through the negative regulation of the NLRP3, ASC and caspase-1 expression and reduced production of IL-1β and interleukin-18 (IL-18), which is also known as an interferon-γ inducing factor (IFN-γ) [41,48].

A previous study revealed the immunoregulatory properties of naringenin (**7**), a flavonoid also found in *T. esculenta* seeds. This compound promotes the inhibition of nuclear transcription factor kappa B (NF-κB), mitogen-activated protein kinase (MAPK) and reduces the production of tumor necrosis factor alpha (TNF-α) and interleukin-6 (IL-6), a pro-inflammatory cytokine [49].

Jhang et. al. [50] analyzed the therapeutic potential of catechin (**3**) and gallic acid (**5**), both found in *T. esculenta* fruits and possible anti-inflammatory properties were found. After subcutaneous injection in mice, whose inflammation was stimulated by the administration of monosodium urate (MSU), significant reduction in the production and secretion of IL-1β and IL-6 was observed. The secretion of IL-1β was modulated through two pathways that include the NF-κB pathway, which provides pro-IL-1β and the NLRP3 inflammasome pathway, which promotes the release of IL-1β from pro-IL-1β. The study demonstrated that catechin (**3**) and gallic acid (**5**) have potent activity to eliminate superoxide anions, consequently inhibiting MSU-induced IL-1β secretion and NLRP3 inflammasome activation. Catechin (**3**) also regulated the oxidative stress status in mitochondria through positive regulation of thioredoxin (TRX) and deglycase protein DJ-1 (DJ-1) and these effects prevented mitochondrial damage caused by MSU attack. These results suggest that catechin intake has potential to prevent acute gout attacks. In addition, researchers have demonstrated the role of these compounds on the intracellular calcium concentration, which is high during the inflammatory process, with significant reduction in calcium concentration by catechin (**3**), but not by gallic acid (**5**) (Figure 1a,b).

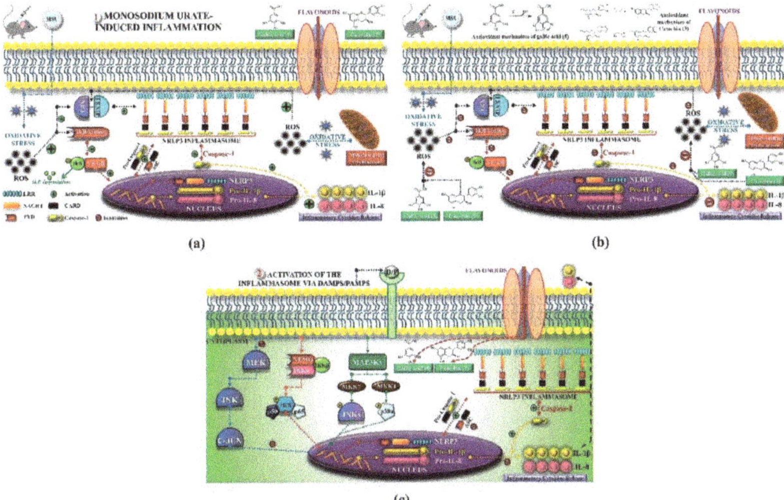

Figure 1. Molecular mechanism of flavonoids in inflammasome regulation: (**a**) Studies suggest that oxidative stress is an important mediator of monosodiumurate (MSU) induced inflammation [51]. The formation of reactive oxygen species (ROS) induces nuclear translocation of Nuclear Factor-kappa B (NF-kB) via phosphorylation by IkB kinase, which binds to target DNA that regulates Pro-IL-1β and Pro-IL-8 gene expression. In addition, ROS dissociates the thioredoxin (TRX) and thioredoxin interaction protein (TXNIP) conjugation [52], and released TXNIP further recruits and binds to NLRP3 inflammasome, leading to the release of IL-1β [53] and IL-8. NLRP3 inflammasome consists of NLRP3, caspase recruitment domain (ASC), and pro-caspase-1. Mitochondrial ROS (MtROS) is also associated with NLRP3 inflammasome activation [53]. In the process of NLRP3 inflammasome activation, activated caspase-1 transforms pro-IL-1b and pro-IL-18 into mature IL-1b and IL-18, resulting in the release of inflammatory cytokines; (**b**) Flavonoid uptake occurs either via passive diffusion through the cell membrane, or through membrane bound transport proteins. Cut circles indicate different points of flavonoid action, inhibiting the process of inflammasome formation with subsequent inhibition of inflammatory events [54]. Phenolic compounds block the inflammatory process by inhibiting ROS formation, thereby reducing the formation of pro-inflammatory cytokines. The nature and position of substituents in relation to the hydroxyl group affect the activity of polyphenols. The easily ionizable carboxylic group contributes to the efficient hydrogen donation tendency of phenolic acids [55]. Gallic acid has high antioxidant activity rate. This is due to a beneficial influence of carboxylate on the antioxidant activity of phenolic acids [56]. The tricyclic structure of flavonoids, such as catechin, determines their antioxidant effect. Phenolic quinoid tautomerism and the localization of electrons over the aromatic system eliminate reactive oxygen species. These aromatic rings directly neutralize free radicals and increase antioxidant defense [57]; (**c**) DAMPs/PAMPs bind to their receptor on the cell membrane and activate a signaling cascade. As a consequence, activation and formation of NRLP3 inflammasome occur, where the formation of active caspase-1 catalyzes the cleavage and secretion of mature IL-1β and IL-18, leading to propagate inflammation [54]. ASC, caspase recruitment domain; C-JUN/JNK, c-Jun N-terminal Kinase; CARD, caspase recruitment domain; DAMPs, damage-associated molecular patterns; IκB, inhibitor of κB; IKKα, IkBkinase α; IKKβ, IkBkinase β; IL-1β, Interleukin 1-beta; IL-8, Interleukin 8; LRR, leucine-rich repeats; MAP3Ks, mitogen-activated protein 3 kinases; MEK, mitogen-activated protein kinase; MKK4, mitogen-activated protein kinasekinase 4; MKK7, mitogen-activated protein kinase kinase 7; MtROS, Mitochondrial ROS; MSU, monosodiumurate; NACHT, central nucleotide-binding and oligomerization domain; NEMO, NF-kappa-B essential modulator; NF-KB, Nuclear Factor-kappa B; p38a, p38 kinase α; p50, NF-KB, Nuclear Factor-kappa B 1 (NF-KB1); p65, RelA; PAMPs, pathogen-associated molecular patterns; PYD, pyrin domain; ROS, reactive oxygen species; TXNIP, thioredoxin interaction protein; TRX, thioredoxin; TXNIP, thioredoxin interaction protein.

For the inflammasome activation, danger signals such as Damage-Associated Molecular Patterns (DAMPs) or Pathogen-Associated Molecular Patterns (PAMPs) bind to PRRs on the cell membrane and trigger the activation of a signaling cascade, which includes the activation of NF-κB, MAPK and MAPK activating protein kinase (MEK), leading to activation and assembly of the inflammasome, a protein complex where active caspase-1 catalyzes the cleavage and secretion of IL-1β and IL-18, important pro- inflammatory signaling gents. In this context, flavonoids cross the membrane through passive or facilitated diffusion using membrane-bound transport proteins. In the cell, different flavonoids act in the same pathway or in different pathways, blocking the formation of inflammasome and consequently inhibiting the inflammatory process (Figure 1c) [54].

The flavonoid quercetin (**2**), found in *T. esculenta* fruits, has anti-dyslipidemic activity, which is also associated with inflammation, since the accumulation of lipids is a factor that contributes to the inflammatory response and inflammasome formation. Quercetin (**2**) acts by suppressing the NLRP3 expression, inhibiting caspase-1 and the production of IL-1β, also reducing the levels of lipids, more specifically triacylglycerols [58].

In addition, quercetin (**2**) also has antioxidant activity, which is mainly mediated by its effects on glutathione (GSH), enzyme activity, signal transduction pathways and ROS. Increase in GSH levels in rats was observed after quercetin administration (**2**), which increases the antioxidant capacity of these animals, since GSH acts as hydrogen donor in the reaction of conversion of hydrogen peroxide into water, catalyzed by superoxide dismutase (SOD), reducing its toxicity. Quercetin (**2**) also acts by increasing the expression of endogenous antioxidant enzymes, including catalase (CAT) and glutathione peroxidase (GPx). In signal transduction pathways, quercetin (**2**) acts in the regulation of kinase protein activated by AMP (AMPK) and MAPK, stimulated by ROS, promoting antioxidant defense and maintaining the oxidative balance, since ROS lead to the activation of several pro-inflammatory and apoptotic signaling events mediated by p53, a cell cycle regulatory protein (Figure 2). Also, quercetin (**2**) inhibits the p38MAPK/inducible nitric oxide synthase (iNOS) signaling pathways, negative regulation of NF-κB levels and positive regulation of SOD activity to promote antioxidant activity [59].

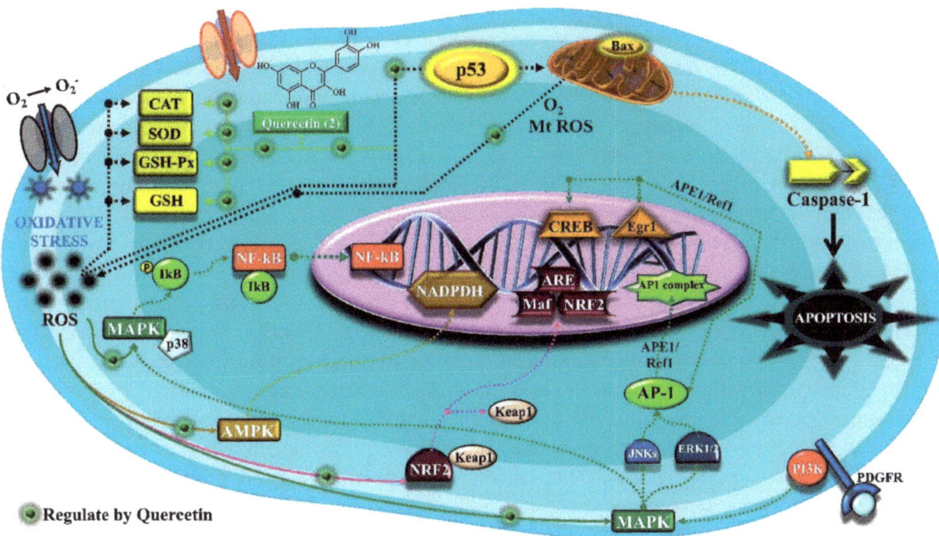

Figure 2. Antioxidant effect of quercetin on enzyme activity, signal transduction pathways and reactive oxygen species (ROS). Several conditions and environmental factors can increase ROS production. Besides, the mitochondrial electron transport chain is an important source of intracellular ROS generation. Flavonoid uptake occurs either via passive diffusion through cell membrane, or through membrane bound transport proteins [51]. After entering the cell, quercetin acts through the regulation of the enzyme-mediated antioxidant defense system and the non-enzymatic antioxidant defense system. Nuclear factor erythroid 2–related factor 2 (NRF2), AMP-activated protein kinase (AMPK), and mitogen-activated protein kinase (MAPK) pathways induced by ROS to promote the antioxidant defense system and maintain oxidative balance can also be regulated by phenolic compounds such as quercetin [59]. Through the neutralizing effect of ROS, quercetin can develop important anti-inflammatory effect due to inhibition of the Nuclear Factor-kappa B (NF-KB) pathway, preventing the activation of NRLP3 inflammasome (shown in Figure 1B). Through the p53 pathway, ROS induce apoptotic events. Therefore, quercetin can prevent apoptosis induced by excess ROS. In addition, it enhances the production of Apurinic/apyrimidinic Endonuclease 1/ Redox Effector Factor 1 (APE1/Ref1), activation of various signaling events and the NF-E2-related factor (NRF2)-mediated activation of genes, containing antioxidant response elements (ARE) and NF-κB [60–64]. AMPK, AMP-activated protein kinase; AP-1, activator protein 1; APE1, Apurinic/apyrimidinic endonuclease 1; ARE, antioxidant response element; Bax, BCL2 Associated X; CAT, catalase; CREB, cAMP-response element binding protein; EGR1, Early Growth Response 1; ERK, Extracellular signal-regulated kinase; GSH, glutathione; GSHPx, Glutathione peroxidase; IκB, κB inhibitor; JNK, c-Jun N-terminal Kinase; KEAP1, Kelch-like ECH-associated protein 1; Maf, musculoaponeurotic fibrosarcoma; MAPK, mitogen-activated protein kinase; MtROS, Mitochondrial ROS; NF-KB, Nuclear Factor-kappa B; Nrf2, nuclear factor erythroid 2–related factor 2; PDGFR, Platelet-derived growth factor receptors; PI3K, phosphatidylinositol-3-kinase; Ref-1, redox effector factor 1; ROS, reactive oxygen species; SOD, Superoxide dismutase.

p-Coumaric acid (**8**), identified in *T. esculenta* fruits, presents a phenyl hydroxyl group in its molecular structure, capable of promoting the neutralization of free radicals such as superoxide anion 2,2-diphenyl-1-picrylhydrazyl-hydrate (DPPH) and hydrogen peroxide (H2O2). This antioxidant property is intensified after conjugation with quinic acid (**9**), also found in *T. esculenta* fruits. In addition, *p*-coumaric acid (**8**) also has antimicrobial activity tested against three Gram-positive bacteria (*Streptococcus pneumonia*, *Staphylococcus aureus* and *Bacillus subtilis*) and three Gram-negative bacteria (*Escherichia coli*, *Shigelladys enteriae* and *Salmonella typhimurium*), by increasing the permeability of the bacterial membrane and binding to the phosphate anion of the DNA (deoxyribonucleic acid), altering the processes of bacterial transcription and replication [65].

In a previous study, researchers analyzed the antioxidant properties of *T. esculenta* fruits using two tests, the scavenging of DPPH radicals and the iron reduction capacity. Antioxidant activity was detected in the seed extract, in which naringenin (**7**), luteolin (**6**) and rutin (**10**) flavonoids were identified and also for pulp extracts, where phenolic compounds such as gallic acid (**5**), *p*-coumaric acid (**8**), rutin (**10**), catechin (**3**), epicatechin (**4**) were also found, as well the cyclitol quinic acid (**9**), to which antioxidant activity can be attributed [33].

Flavonoids mirecetin (**1**) and quercetin (**2**), also found in *T. esculenta* fruits, have significant antiproliferative activity, suggesting a chemopreventive and anti-tumor potential that should be investigated in the future [32]. [35] reported two other properties of *T. esculenta* phytochemicals, diuretic and antihypertensive. Studies have shown that the hydroalcoholic extract obtained from *T. esculenta* leaves and stem promotes significant increase in urinary volume, without changing urine pH and density, indicating a diuretic effect, and significant increase in renal potassium elimination, which are properties related to phenolic acids and flavonoids found in extracts.

Pinheiro et al. [66] analyzed the possible antifungal activity of lectin extracted from *T. esculenta* seeds. This activity was tested on *Microsporum canis*, a filamentous keratinophilic fungus that causes infections in skin, hair and nails in humans and animals. The results show the ability of lectin to inhibit the growth of the fungus, which may be associated with the interaction of lectin with carbohydrates on the surface of microorganism such as D-mannose and *N*-acetyl-glucosamine, since the addition of these carbohydrates caused inhibition of the antifungal effect, probably due to competition for the interaction of fungal carbohydrates with lectin. The ability of lectin to inhibit the adherence of microorganisms and exert antimicrobial effects was analyzed in another study, which tested such properties on bacteria *Streptococcus mutans* UA159, *Streptococcus sobrinus* 6715, *Streptococcus sanguinis* ATCC10556, *Streptococcus mitis* ATCC903 and *Streptococcus oralis* PB182. The results indicate that lectin was not able to inhibit the growth of bacteria at any of the applied concentrations and also did not inhibit the adherence of microorganisms, that is, it does not present antimicrobial activity and does not inhibit biofilm formation [67].

3.1.5. Toxicity Studies

So far, there are no records of human poisoning by *T. esculenta*, probably because seeds and leaves are not consumed in the fresh form, only the pulp; however, there are records of intoxication in some animals, such as sheep and cattle that ingest leaves and seeds without heat treatment, which may indicate that the toxic compound is affected by high temperatures [68].

The Northeastern region of Brazil presented an outbreak of spontaneous poisoning in sheep and cattle, which showed severe signs of nervous system damage, some irreversible. Thus, an experimental reproduction of the poisoning was carried out with 5 sheep by administering 30–60 g of leaves per kilogram of body weight, and two sheep with doses of 5–10 g of seeds per kilogram of body weight, with samples from different regions of Brazil. All sheep showed clinical signs of intoxication 72 h after exposure. The main signs and symptoms were mild to moderate tympanism, drowsiness, ataxia, depressive behavior and humeral hypomotility. The chemical compound present in leaves and seeds responsible for the toxic effect is still unknown. In addition, the minimum amount that exerted toxicity was lower for seeds than for leaves, indicating greater potential for seed toxicity [69].

In the same region, cattle spontaneously intoxicated with the same clinical signs, were analyzed 72 h after exposure. In autopsy exams, partially digested seeds and leaves were found in the rumen. Laboratory and histological exams showed no significant changes, either in spontaneous or experimental poisoning. However, the presence of seeds in the rumen content associated with clinical signs suggests that there is risk of human poisoning by both seeds and leaves [70]. Similar clinical signs were observed in a dog after ingestion of *T. esculenta* seeds. Although the substance responsible for the toxicity is unknown, the induction of inflammatory response by lectin found in seeds is the focus of a study that describes the recruitment of neutrophils and mononuclear cells caused by lectin. The proposed mechanism is related to the specific properties of lectin binding to carbohydrates in the cell membrane [71,72].

In contrast, Wistar rats treated with purified aqueous extract from *T. esculenta* leaves and stem at oral doses of 5, 50, 300 and 2000 mg did not show any sign of acute toxicity, and regardless of dose, there were no abnormal signs in comparison with control animals. Water intake and body weight did not change during the experimental period and the biochemical and hematological parameters showed no abnormalities. After euthanasia, heart, lung, spleen, kidney and liver samples were collected for pathological evaluation and also showed no signs of abnormality, which may be related to the lectin concentration, which is higher in seeds than in leaves and stem; therefore, the absence of toxicity may be due to the fact that seeds were not used in this study [35].

4. Moraceae Family

The Moraceae family has 53 genera and about 1500 identified species, with tropical prevalence, being more than 50% of the genera present in the Neotropical region, mainly in South America. Species of the Moraceae family are found in humid forests or in their vicinities. *Artocarpus, Brosimum, Ficus* and *Morus* are among the most widely known genera, which correspond to the widely known and consumed fruit-producing plants of great nutritional and economic importance such as jackfruit, walnut, fig, and blackberry. In addition, some species of this family provide wood and leaves, used as food for silkworm [11,73,74].

Belonging to the Rosales order, this family has members that stand out for their ornamental possibilities, such as the genus *Ficus, Maclura* and *Dorstenia* and medicinal possibilities such as *Brosimum gaudichaudii* Trécul. This family was classified as the most important in terms of number of species with phytotherapic potential, emphasizing the genus *Brosimum* [75,76].

Like other families characteristic of tropical climates, Moraceae members also present adaptations to water scarcity and intense solar radiation. An example of these adaptations is the development of a thick waxy layer, called cuticle, with significant photoprotective property, which due to its reflective capacity, prevents the intense and harmful absorption of excessive solar radiation [77].

4.1. Genus Brosimum and Species Brosimum gaudichaudii

The genus Brosimum is composed of 13 species: *Brosimuma cutifolium* Huber, *Brosimum alicastrum* Sw., *Brosimum gaudichaudii* Trécul, *Brosimum glaucum* Taub., *Brosimum glaziovii* Taub., *Brosimum guianense* (Aubl.) Huber, *Brosimum lactescens* (S. Moore) C.C. Berg, *Brosimum longifolium* Ducke, *Brosimum melanopotamicum* C.C. Berg, *Brosimum parinarioides* Ducke, *Brosimum potabile* Ducke, *Brosimum rubescens* Taub., and *Brosimu mutile* (Kunth) Pittier, with *B. gaudichaudii* being the only representative of the genus Brosimum found in the Cerrado vegetation [78,79].

There are several studies focused on the biological properties of *Brosimum gaudichaudii* Trécul, which has great economic importance due to the production of latex, in addition to the use of roots, stem bark and leaves in popular medicine, whose pharamacological activities are attributed to the high content of coumarins, its main class of active metabolites, which may represent about 3% of the dry root weight [80–82].

Popularly known as mama-cadela, mamica de cadela, conduru and inharé, this species has properties of agribusiness interest, contributing to the economic development of the country. Its wood is used in civil construction and paper-making industries, and although its fruit is edible, the use of roots, stems and leaves in popular medicine prevails [73].

4.1.1. Geographical Distribution and Popular Use

B. gaudichaudii is not endemic to Brazil, despite being widespread in the country, as it occurs in other countries, mainly in Paraguay, Bolivia, and Argentina. It is predominant in regions with typical Cerrado, Cerradão and Amazon savanna vegetation. However, it is under threat of extinction due to its occurrence in regions with constant change, such as the Brazilian cerrado, whose native vegetation is commonly subjected to burning and reduced by the expansion of the agricultural frontier, in addition to being affected by the indiscriminate extraction of latex [83,84].

Ribeiro et al. [85] conducted a survey on the popular use of several species, among them *B. gaudichaudii*, whose most used plant organs were roots, stem bark and latex, either in the fresh form or prepared by decoction, infusion, or maceration. The therapeutic indications reported in the research were: infections, venereal diseases, that is, those sexually transmitted, boils, superficial skin mycoses, cancer, anemia, cardiac arrhythmia, pneumonia, vitiligo, joint pain, inflammation, rheumatism, kidney disorders and wound healing.

For the treatment of vitiligo and other skin diseases, the extract, usually obtained by infusion or decoction of roots or stem bark, is used topically. In addition, it has also been described as a depurative, that is, it is used to eliminate toxins and improve blood circulation, and in this case, preparation is carried out by decoction or maceration of branches and leaves in dry wine. Its use against flu, colds and bronchitis occurs from the infusion of any plant part in wine or water [86].

Popularly known as bottleful, homemade preparations using dry wine as vehicle are produced by macerating the chosen vegetable organ in wine and honey for a period of at least 8 days. After this period, the liquid obtained is packed in capped bottles. Generally, extracts are orally administered and although they do not have a health record, they can be found available for purchase at street markets [87,88].

4.1.2. Botanical Aspects

B. gaudichaudii can be found as shrub, tree or bush, reaching up to 4 m in height. Roots are terrestrial and gemiferous, that is, with the ability to sprout and generate new plants, a strategy of survival to common fires that occur in the Cerrado region, they form a root system, composed of a main root to which longitudinal roots that grow in different directions are anchored. The stem is aerial, erect and of the trunk type, with sympodial growth; leaves are glabrous on the adaxial surface and may present glandular trichomes on the abaxial epidermis, phyllotaxis is alternate, with simple and petiolate leaves, with oblong, oblong-lanceolate or elliptical shape, obtuse to acuminate apex, oblique base, entire margins of the limb, wavy or serrated, with camptodrome-like peninerval venation, that is, secondary venation do not end at the margin [83].

It blooms between the months of June and October; inflorescences are monopodial, bisexual, ear-like, globose, composed of 30 to 100 flowers, which are pedunculated, aclamidic, diclinic, monoic, that is, they present unisexual female and male flowers in the same individual, and staminate flowers are protected by bracteole. They have green to yellowish color, with gamocarpelar gynoecium and unilocular ovary [89,90].

B. gaudichaudii fruits are edible, drupe type, fleshy, with about 2 to 4 cm in diameter, globose, monospermic, and should be harvested between the months of September and November. Each fruit contains an ellipsoid seed, whitish in color, considered recalcitrant, as it is not viable after drying. The embryo has two fleshy cotyledons and fills the entire seed volume. Regarding shape and size, these cotyledons have starch, protein, and lipid reserves. They have short and swollen hypocotyl located below the point of insertion of cotyledons [82].

4.1.3. Phytochemical Aspects

The summary of phytochemical studies carried out with different *B. gaudichaudii* plant organs and the structures of isolated substances are shown in Table 2.

Table 2. Phytochemical analysis of *B. gaudichaudii*.

Compounds	Molecular Structures	Chromatographic Methods for the Isolation and Identification	Solvent Used/Essential Oil	Plant Part Used	Collection Site	References
Psoralen (**25**, C)	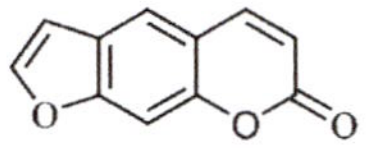	HPLC	Methanol	Root cortex Leaf Twigs Latex Heartwood of the root Root cortex	São Paulo-Brazil	[91]
Bergapten (**26**, C)	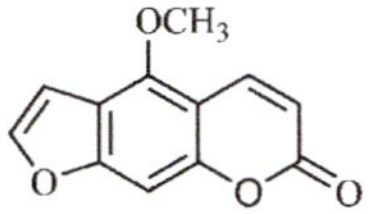					
5,7,3′,4′-Tetrahydroxy-6-*C*-glucopyranosylflavone (**27**, F)	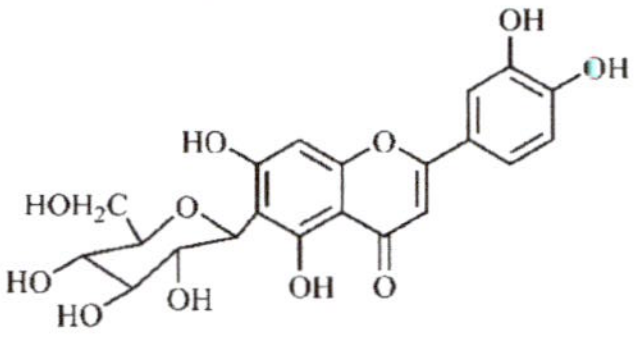		Water	Root cortex		
28 4 5,7,3′,4′-tetrahydroxy-3-*O*-β-D-galactopyranosylflavonol (F)	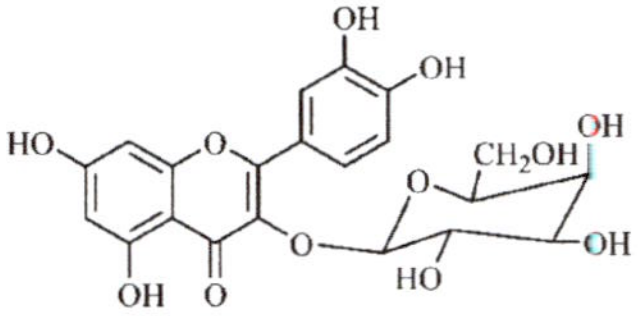					
Psoralen (**25**, C)	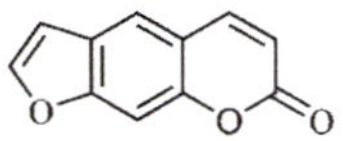					
Bergapten (**26**, C)	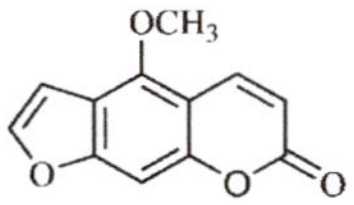					

Table 2. *Cont.*

Compounds	Molecular Structures	Chromatographic Methods for the Isolation and Identification	Solvent Used/Essential Oil	Plant Part Used	Collection Site	References
Psoralen (**25**, C)						
Bergapten (**26**, C)		HPLC	Ethanol (*v/v* 95%)	Root	Jussára, Goiás-Brazil	[92]
Gaudichaudine (**29**, C)						
Luvangetin (**30**, C)						
(+)-(2′*S*,3′*R*)-3′-hydroxymarmesin (**31**, C)		HPLC	Dichloromethane	Root bark	Araguari, Minas Gerais-Brazil	[93]
Xanthyletin (**32**, C)						
Psoralen (**25**, C)						

Table 2. *Cont.*

Compounds	Molecular Structures	Chromatographic Methods for the Isolation and Identification	Solvent Used/Essential Oil	Plant Part Used	Collection Site	References
Bergapten (**26**, C)	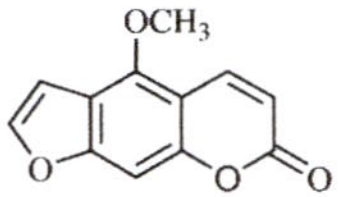					
Marmesin (**33**, C)	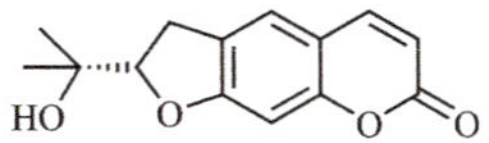	CC	Dichloromethane	Root bark	Araguari, Minas Gerais-Brazil	[94]
1′,2′-Dehydromarmesin (**34**, C)	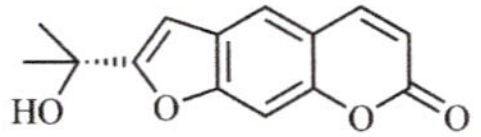					
8-Methoxymarmesin (**35**, C)	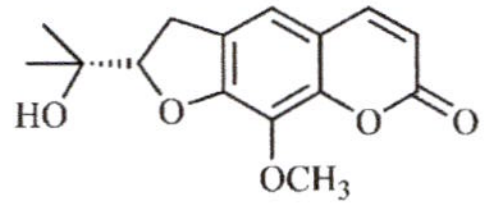					
1′-Hydroxy-3′-O-β-glucopyranosylmarmesin (**36**, C)	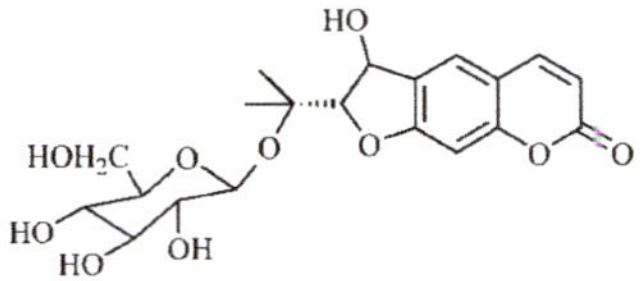					
2′,4′,4-Trihydroxy-3′3-diprenylchalcone (**37**, CH)	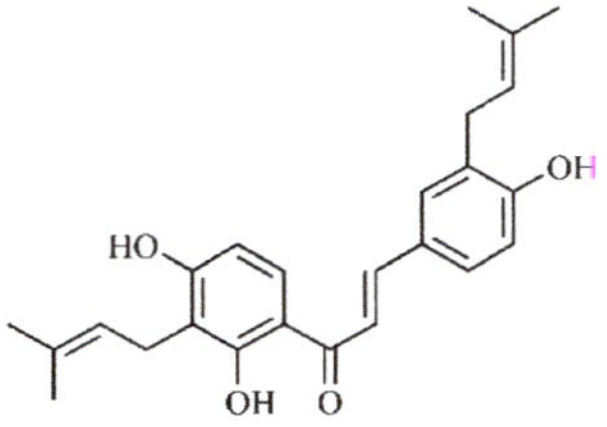					

Table 2. *Cont.*

Compounds	Molecular Structures	Chromatographic Methods for the Isolation and Identification	Solvent Used/Essential Oil	Plant Part Used	Collection Site	References
β-Amyrin (**38**, T)						

C: coumarin; CH: chalcone; F: flavonoid; T: terpene; CC: Column Chromatography; HPLC: High Performance Liquid Chromatography.

B. gaudichaudii is the target of some phytochemical screening studies, mainly qualitative, which show significant concentrations of coumarins, especially furanocoumarin psoralen (**25**) and bergaptene (**26**). The analysis of the proximate composition of the fresh ripe fruit with bark showed for every 100 g on a wet basis: 77.63 g of moisture, 1.63 g of proteins, 0.60 g of lipids, 13.35 g of carbohydrates, 5.11 g of dietary fiber, 0.82 g of ash content and 62.21 kcal of total energy value. In addition, 46.47 mgGAE (gallic acid equivalents) of phenolic compounds and 14.92 g of vitamins C were also quantified [95,96].

Lourenço, [91] identified and quantified the content of furanocoumarin psoralen (**25**) and bergaptene (**26**) in the lyophilized methanolic and aqueous extracts of the root cortex of *B. gaudichaudii*. For each 1 g of dry weight of the plant organ used, 27.6 mg of psoralen (**25**) and 32 mg of bergaptene (**26**) were found in the methanolic extract, which correspond, respectively, to 2.8% and 3% of the sample. For the aqueous extract, 7.1 mg/g of psoralen (**25**) were quantified, that is, 0.7% and 2.6 mg/g of baptapene (**26**). This study analyzed the composition of the methanolic extract of leaves, branches, latex, and heartwood of *B. gaudichaudii* roots. In leaves, glycosylated flavonoids 5,7,3′, 4′-tetrahydroxy-6-C-glucopyranosylflavone (**27**) and 5,7,3′,4′-tetrahydroxy-3-O-ß-D-galactopyranosyl-flavonol were detected (**28**), also in the extract of leaves, branches and heartwood in roots, psoralen (**25**) and bergaptene (**26**) were also isolated, but in less amount compared to that found in the root cortex, while furanocoumarins were not detected in the latex.

Other analyses using the hydroalcoholic extract of *B. gaudichaudii* roots also identified psoralen (**25**) and bergaptene (**26**). Two extraction techniques were compared, percolation and ultrasound-assisted extraction (UEA), and both showed satisfactory results, but UEA extraction technique was more quick [92].

Spectral analysis was carried out on an extract from *B. gaudichaudii* root bark, which led to the identification of a new coumarin called gaudichaudine (**29**), the coumarins psoralen (**25**), bergaptene (**26**), luvangetin (**30**) and (+)−(2′S, 3′R)-3′-hydroxyrmesin (**31**) and the pyranocoumarin xanthyletin (**32**). Subsequently, using the same type of extract and the same plant organ, the same researchers found the following secondary metabolites: coumarins marmesin (**33**), 1′,2′-dehydromarmesin (**34**), 8-methoxymarmesin (**35**) and 1′-hydroxy-3′-O-β-glucopyranosylmarmesin (**36**); the chalcone 2′,4′,4-trihydroxy-3′3-diprenylchalcone (**37**); and the triterpene β-amyrin (**38**) [93,94].

The determination of total tannins in the methanolic extract from *B. gaudichaudii* stem bark carried out by [97] revealed that for each 1 g of sample, there are approximately 17.50 mg of total tannins, which have not been isolated so far. Another study on the same species qualitatively identified in the alcoholic extract of leaves and stem bark, alkaloids, anthraquinones, phenols and tannins [98].

The qualitative analysis of the ethanolic extract from *B. gaudichaudii* root bark pointed out the presence of triterpenes, steroids, coumarins, alkaloids and anthraquinones, but tested negative for saponins and tannins [99]. To investigate the presence of these and other compounds in the ethanolic extract from *B. gaudichaudii* leaves, a previous study carried out a qualitative analysis of this extract, which was positive for alkaloids, coumarins, flavonoids and cardiotonic glycosides, and negative for anthraquinones, catechins and saponins [100].

4.1.4. Pharmacological Studies

The pharmacological use of *B. gaudichaudii* is widely explored due to its repigmentating property, clinically used for the treatment of vitiligo, a skin pigmentation anomaly. This property is attributed to the presence of furanocoumarins, molecules found mainly in the *B. gaudichaudii* root cortex, which have photosensitizing action, and associated with ultraviolet (UV) radiation, is used to treat not only vitiligo, but also other skin disorders such as psoriasis, systemic lupus erythematosus and mycoses [101] (Figure 3).

The mechanism of action of furanocoumarins for the UV phototherapy technique is not yet defined. However, previous studies have proposed that there is induction of apoptosis of cells that participate in the generation of disorders, such as T cells, mast cells and keratinocytes, in addition to increased proliferation of melanocytes and reduced histamine release by mast cells and basophils [102]. Lang et al. [103] reported an increase in CD8 + T lymphocytes specific for the skin in a patient with vitiligo and that this may be related to the etiology of the disease, since these cytotoxic T lymphocytes may participate in the reduction in the number of melanocytes observed in the disease (Figure 3).

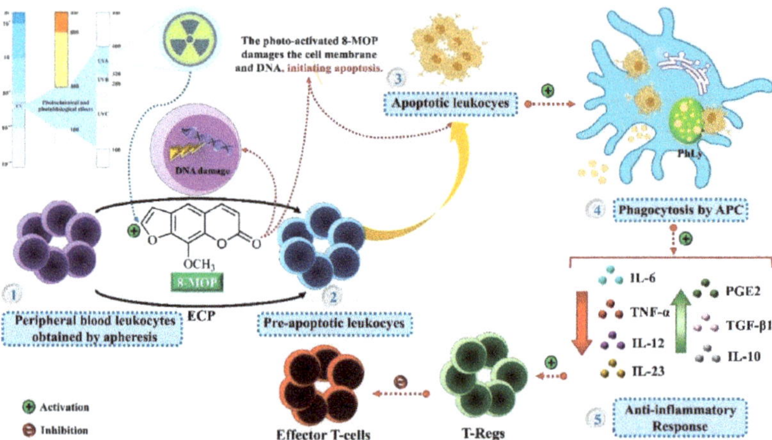

Figure 3. Use of furanocoumarins in the technique of extracorporeal photopheresis for the treatment of systemic or multifocal diseases: Leukocytes obtained by apheresis are exposed to 8-metoxipsoraleno (8-MOP), which is activated by UVA radiation and covalently binds to the DNA of these cells, causing damage and inducing apoptosis within 48 h. Pre-apoptotic leukocytes are reintroduced into the peripheral circulation, being recognized and phagocyted by antigen-presenting cells in phagolysosomes. This recognition induces tolerogenic anti-inflammatory response, which reduces the production of pro-inflammatory cytokines like IL-6, IL-12, IL-23, and TNF-α and increases the production of anti-inflammatory cytokines like IL-10, TGF-β1, and PGE2 [104]. 8-MOP, 8-metoxipsoraleno; IL-6, interleukin 6; IL-10, interleukin 10; IL-12, interleukin12; IL-23, interleukin 23; TGF-β1, Transforming growth factor beta 1; TNF-α, Tumor Necrosis Factor-Alpha. Another technique that uses furanocoumarins is extracorporeal photopheresis (ECP), which treats systemic or multifocal diseases such as Crohn's disease, type 1 diabetes mellitus, multiple sclerosis, and rheumatoid arthritis. In this technique, the most used furanocoumarin is 8-methoxypsoralen (8-MOP), to which leukocytes, obtained by apheresis, are exposed. 8-MOP is activated by radiation and covalently binds to leukocyte DNA, leading to apoptosis within 48 h. These pre-apoptotic leukocytes are reintroduced into the peripheral circulation, where are recognized and phagocyted by antigen-presenting cells in phagolysosomes. This recognition induces a tolerogenic anti-inflammatory response that leads to a reduction in the production of pro-inflammatory cytokines IL-6, interleukin-12 (IL-12), interleukin-23 (IL-23) and TNF-α and induces the production of anti-inflammatory cytokines such as interleukin-10 (IL-10), transforming growth factor beta 1 (TGF-β1) and prostaglandin E2 (PGE2) (Figure 3) [102,104].

Lourenço, [105] tested the possible antibacterial activity of the ethanolic extract of *B. gaudichaudii* leaves and stem bark against *S. aureus* from clinical samples, beta-hemolytic streptococci, *P. aeruginosa*, *E. coli*, *Citrobacter* sp. and *Proteus* sp. Both extracts showed antimicrobial activity against all bacterial strains, including multi-resistant strains, with variable percentage of bacterial growth inhibition. However, the bioactive compounds responsible for this activity have not yet been identified.

The ethanolic extract from *B. gaudichaudii* stem bark was analyzed for antifungal properties on *Candida albicans* and *Candida* sp. This activity was observed for *C. albicans* at concentration of 200 mg/mL and for *C. non albicans* at concentrations of 100 mg/mL and 200 mg/mL [96]. The hydroalcoholic extract from *B. gaudichaudii* leaves was also tested for trypanocidal activity. Mice previously infected with the blood form of *Trypanosoma cruzi* received the extract at different concentrations. The infection was assessed by counting parasites present in 10 μL of blood between the 5th and the 11th day after infection, showing reduction in the number of trypomastigotes at concentration of 100 mg/kg. Although the chemical compound responsible for this activity has not been identified, it is possible to associate it with furanocoumarins, which are the main components of the extract that may have acted through the production of oxide and superoxide radicals [106].

β-Amyrin (**38**), a triterpene found in *B. gaudichaudii* root bark promotes sleep modulation through the activation of the GABAergic system. For the analysis, a pentabarbital-induced sleep model was used in mice, and it was observed that, after the administration of 1, 3 or 10 mg/kg of β-amyrin (**38**), the time for the beginning of sleep was reduced and the sleep duration increased significantly, which effects were inhibited after administration of a type A gamma-aminobutyric acid antagonist receptor (GABA$_A$), demonstrating that this property is associated with the GABAergic system. In addition, the levels of gamma-aminobutyric acid (GABA) in the brain were analyzed, which increased after the administration of β-amyrin (**38**), which could be related to the blocking of GABA transaminase, inhibiting GABA degradation and, consequently, increasing its available concentration [107].

A study was carried out on the role of β-amyrin (**38**) in attenuating the neurodegeneration of Parkinson's disease using *Caenorhabditis elegans* strain. The analysis describes a protective effect of β-amyrin (**38**) against neurotoxicity induced by 6-hydroxydopamine (6-OHDA), which was related to the possible antioxidant role of β-amyrin (**38**). This study also investigated its anti-apoptotic activity on the expression of pro-apoptotic genes in *C. elegans*, which were not significantly altered after treatment with β-amyrin (**38**). The aggregation of α-synuclein protein is one of the mechanisms associated with Parkinson's disease. The effects of β-amyrin (**38**) on this mechanism were compared to the effect of the medicine clinically used to treat the disease, L-dopa and both substances significantly reduced the α-synuclein aggregation [108].

Sunil et al. [109] analyzed the antioxidant activity of β-amyrin (**38**) in Wistar rats with oxidative stress induced by carbon tetrachloride (CCl$_4$). The effect was positive in the elimination of DPPH radicals, hydroxyl, nitric oxide (NO), superoxide radicals and had strong reducing and suppressive power of lipid peroxidation. The increase in free radical levels also leads to elevated levels of hepatic enzymes serum glutamic oxalacetic transaminase (SGOT), serum glutamic pyruvic transaminase (SGPT) and LDH, which after administration of β-amyrin (**38**), had their levels reduced. In addition, the levels of the antioxidant enzymes SOD, CAT, GSH and GPx, were high.

A study analyzed the β-amyrin (**38**) activity on inflammation induced by lipopolysaccharide (LPS) and IFN-γ in the microglial cells of rats. β-amyrin (**38**) reduced the expression of pro-inflammatory factors such as TNF-α, IL-1β, IL-6, PGE-2 and cyclooxygenase-2 (COX-2) and increased the expression of arginase-1. The reduction of factors was attributed to the activation of the cannabinoid receptor, since antagonists of these receptors inhibit the anti-inflammatory effects of β-amyrin (**38**). Through another not yet identified mechanism, β-amyrin (**38**) reduces the activity of COX-2 and, consequently, the production of PGE-2, commonly inhibited by the action of non-steroidal anti-inflammatory drugs. Enzymes arginase-1 and NO synthase compete for the same substrate, L-arginine, with the overexpression of arginase-1, observed by the increase in its product, urea, NO production is compromised, since the availability of substrate for NO synthase is reduced [110].

Marmesin (**33**), a coumarin found in *B. gaudichaudii* root bark, is the target of several studies that investigate its medicinal properties, especially its anti-tumor properties. The in vitro and in vivo activity of marmesin (**33**) was evaluated on cells with human leukemia and healthy human monocytes. The results indicate that marmesin (**33**) exerts dose-dependent anti-tumor activity and that the cytotoxic effect on healthy monocytes was lower, which is essential for the safety of a probable treatment, since it predicts that the compound has action selectivity, reducing the possibility of adverse effects. Marmesin (**33**) increased the expression of pro-apoptotic protein Bax and reduced the expression of anti-apoptotic protein Bcl-2, increasing the Bax/Bcl-2 ratio, which promotes activation of caspase 3, leading to apoptosis, with mechanism of action similar to other chemotherapeutic drugs. Marmesin (**33**) also causes an increase in intracellular ROS and reduces the mitochondrial membrane potential

(MMP), which was related to the reduced migration of cells with leukemia, important in inhibiting metastases [111].

Another analysis of the same property associated with marmesin (**33**), but on lung cancer and tumor angiogenesis, reports anti-tumor activities of marmesin (**33**) mediated by the inactivation of mitogenic signaling pathways and negative regulation of proteins related to cell signaling, including vascular endothelial growth factor-2 receptor (VEGFR-2), integrin β1, integrin-linked kinase (ILK) and matrix metalloproteinases-2 (MMP-2), nullifying mitogen-stimulated proliferation and invasion in cells expressing p53 or not [112].

4.1.5. Toxicity Studies

Furanocoumarins, the major constituents of *B. gaudichaudii* roots, are phototoxic substances that the plant uses as a protection mechanism against phytopathogenic microorganisms and herbivores. The mechanism of action is intercalation in the double helix of the DNA structure and in molecular complexation, and when activated by light, they react with pyrimidine bases, mainly with thymine, which can promote toxic, mutagenic and carcinogenic effects [113].

The genotoxic activity of *B. gaudichaudii* was evaluated using aqueous and methanolic extracts on *Salmonella typhimurium* strains, which showed an increase in chromosomal aberrations in cultures submitted to the methanolic extract in the G1/S and S phases of the cell cycle. For the aqueous extract, results were not significant, which is due to the lower amount of furanocoumarins extracted by the aqueous extract compared to the methanolic extract [114].

Lourenço, [91] performed toxicity tests for the aqueous and methanolic extract from *B. gaudichaudii* root cortex and obtained through the MTT technique (3-[4,5-dimethylthiazol-2-yl]-2,5-diphenyl tetrazolium bromide), cytotoxicity indexes (IC_{50}) of 4.65 mg/mL and 1.31 mg/mL, for each extract, respectively. The mutagenicity assay was also performed with *Salmonella typhimurium*, which generated the mutagenicity ratio (MR) through the observation of revertants, that is, the number of individuals whose natural phenotype induced by mutation, was restored. The ratio is calculated using the average number of revertants in the test plate, spontaneous or induced, divided by the average number of revertants per negative control plate, that is, spontaneous, with the sample being considered positive with ratio greater than or equal to 2. MR was higher for the aqueous and methanolic extracts in the TA102 strain in the presence of microsomal fraction S9, which reveals whether the substance or sample is mutagenic in its original form or whether it needs to be metabolized or activated to become mutagenic, in this case, it has been metabolized.

A study determined the acute toxicity of the extract from *B. gaudichaudii* root bark orally and intraperitoneally administered in mice. Oral administration led some animals to death, and the median lethal oral dose (LD_{50}) was 3517.54 mg/kg and intraperitoneally, LD_{50} was 2871.76 mg/kg. Up to 2000 mg/kg, 40% of animals had diarrhea, and increasing the dose, some of them presented, in addition to diarrhea, dry eyes, eyelid occlusion, ocular hemorrhage, epistaxis, weight loss, tachypnea and death at the lethal dose. Dead animals were analyzed and showed dilation and hemorrhage, in addition to increase in the amount of hemosiderin in the spleen, indicating previous hemorrhage and destruction of erythrocytes [80].

Using dry *B. gaudichaudii* extract, the acute and subacute toxicities of this species were analyzed, with an estimated lethal dose (DLA) of 3800 mg/kg. In the acute study, 14 days after administration, leukopenia and hemosiderin accumulation were observed in the spleen, and in the subacute, after 30 days, changes in the levels of aspartate aminotransferase (AST), alanine aminotransferase (ALT), creatinine and total proteins were observed, indicating hepatotoxicity and nephrotoxicity for the dose of 100 mg/kg, in addition to leukopenia and renal hemorrhage [115].

These clinical signs of hemorrhage may be related to the anticoagulant property of some coumarins found in large amounts in this species. To exert such activity, coumarins act as competitive inhibitors of epoxide reductase, an enzyme that reduces vitamin K, oxidized by participating as co-factor in the synthesis of coagulation factors II, VII, IX and X. With the inhibition of epoxide reductase, this regeneration does not occur, depleting the levels of active vitamin K and consequently inhibiting the synthesis of coagulation factors (Figure 4) [116].

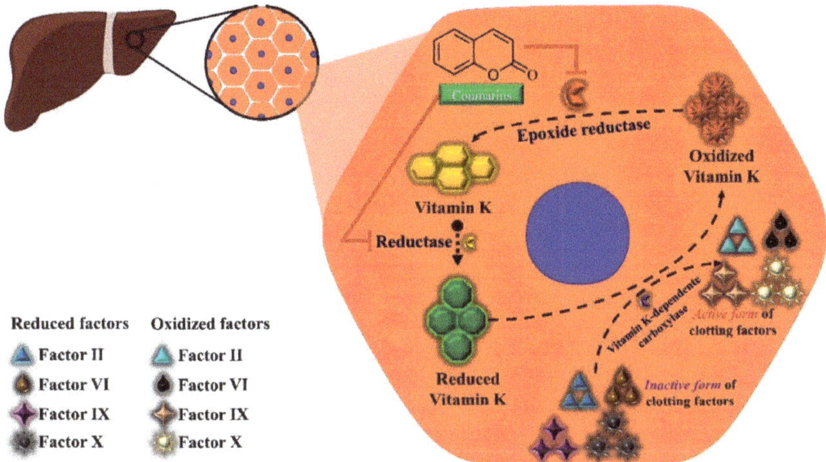

Figure 4. Proposed mechanism for inducing hemorrhage by coumarins: Coumarins act as competitive epoxide reductase inhibitors. This enzyme reduces oxidized vitamin K during its participation as co-factor in the synthesis of coagulation factors II, VII, IX, and X. With epoxide reductase inhibition, the reduction that occurs to regenerate vitamin K is blocked, depleting its levels and, consequently, inhibiting the synthesis of coagulation factors, causing hemorrhage.

5. Rubiaceae Family

The Rubiaceae family is the fourth largest family of angiosperms, composed of about 650 genera and more than 13,000 species. Belonging to the order Gentianales, it is a cosmopolitan and pantropical family distributed as herbs, shrubs, lianas, small and large trees. It has great biodiversity, being of paramount importance in floristic formation, in addition to the conservation of tropical vegetation [117].

This family includes important species for the economy of several countries, being widely used as food, such as *Coffea arabica*; in popular medicine such as *Cinchona* sp.; in civil construction such as species of the genera *Sarcomphalus, Mitragyna, Morindae Pausinystalia*; and in ornamentation such as *Gardenia* spp., *Ixora* spp. and *Mussaenda* spp. [118].

Most fruits produced by species of this family have high levels of iridoids, which act as plant defenders against the attack of herbivores. These substances make up pigments found in extracts of species of this family and which are used as cosmetics due to their pigmenting property for the dyeing of keratin fibers [119].

5.1. Genus Genipa L. and Species Genipa americana L.

Genipa L. is a neotropical genus with species distributed in several countries, mainly on the American continent. *Genipa americana* L. is a fruit species characterized by high survival rate against drastic environmental changes, such as floods, which can cause reduction in the growth of shoots and roots, reduction in biomass and changes in their partitioning, in addition to promoting plant senescence, which promotes a mechanism of tolerance in some species frequently exposed to these conditions [120,121].

This species has been used for the regeneration of reserve areas and environmental preservation. Due to its adaptive characteristics, it can be domesticated and used in urban afforestation and agriculture, since its wood and fruits have considerable commercial value. Although little consumed in the fresh form, fruits are used for the production of jams, candies, ice cream, soft drinks, wines and liqueurs [122].

Its seeds are of easy propagation, which can be sown soon after being removed from fruits and support up to 60 days of storage, which should be performed after drying or under freezing. In addition, *G. americana* can be grown not only from seeds, but also by budding or grafting of plant parts, which produces fruit about 6 years after planting [123,124].

5.1.1. Geographical Distribution and Popular Use

Genipa americana is widely distributed from South America to Central America. It has tropism for coastal regions and river banks, being found in the Cerrado vegetation and popularly known as jenipapo, janapabeiro, janipaba, janipapo, genipapeiro, jenipapinho, jenipá, jenipapeirol, genipapo, genipapeiro [125].

All plant organs of this species are used in folk medicine. Leaves, stem bark, fruits and roots are indicated for cough, anemia, bruises, dislocations, as depurative, cathartic, purgative, febrifuge, aphrodisiac, diuretic, for spleen and liver diseases, jaundice, and injuries. The pulp of the fresh fruit is indicated for diabetes and liver diseases, and the fruit juice is indicated for anemia [126–128].

For dermatitis, pulp and heated seeds are applied over the affected area. The use of tea from fruits and leaves produced by decoction for 1 h is described for the treatment of anemia, and tea from roots and stem bark is used as aphrodisiac. Tea from toasted stem bark obtained by decoction is applied in the form of poultice on bruises, fractures and twists [129–131].

Other forms of fruit use are reported for the treatment of anemia such as juice, bottleful, and dye. The juice is obtained after crushing the fresh vegetable organ and in its homemade preparation a pestle or blender is used, the former being more used for less juicy parts. The dye is a concentrated extract of medicinal plants and consists of an alcoholic or hydroalcoholic preparation in which the macerated plant is immersed in the extraction liquid for 8 to 10 days, and after that period the mixture is filtered, packed in a capped flask and used in the form of drops dissolved in water or used in ointments [132–134].

5.1.2. Botanical Aspects

G. americana is a tree with terrestrial, adventitious roots, aerial and erect stem of trunk and circular type and sympodial growth. Leaves are simple, petiolate, with opposite phyllotaxis with obovate, elliptical-obovate or oblanceolate shape, acuminated limb apex, cuneiform base and smooth margin, with gland trichomes on the abaxial epidermis and pinnate venation [120,135].

Flowering occurs between October and December; inflorescences are dichasium with about 16 flowers, which are hermaphroditic, white to yellowish in color, aromatic, pedunculated, pentamera, with bilocular ovary. Fruits are subglobous, polyspermic, indehiscent berries, with brown color when ripe and thin pericarp. Maturation usually occurs between the months of May and August [136,137].

Seeds have ovoid shape, flat, with rigid seed coat and dark brown in color and orthodox, that is, unlike recalcitrant seeds, the degree of humidity does not imply loss of viability and are resistant to low temperatures, so drying of seeds up to 10% does not compromise their germination [137,138].

5.1.3. Phytochemical Aspects

Table 3 presents a summary of phytochemical studies of *G. americana* extracts, as well as the structures of their phytochemical constituents.

Table 3. Phytochemical analysis of *G. americana*.

Compounds	Molecular Structures	Chromatographic Methods for the Isolation and Identification	Solvent Used/Essential Oil	Plant Part Used	Collection Site	References
Asystasioside D (**39**, T)	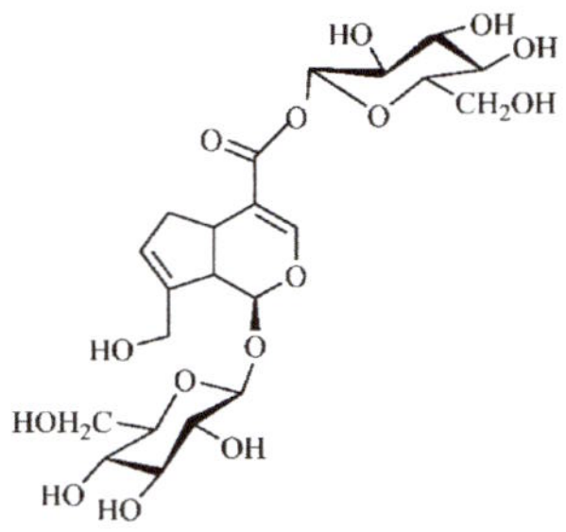					
Geniposidic acid (**40**, T)	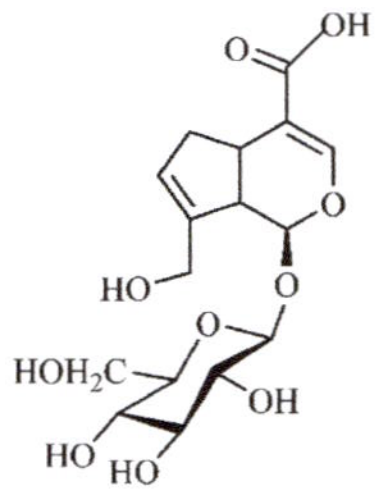	UHPLC	Hydroalcoholic 70:30 (*v/v* ethanol, water)	Leaf	Natal, Rio Grande do Norte-Brazil	[139]
Tarenoside (**41**, T)	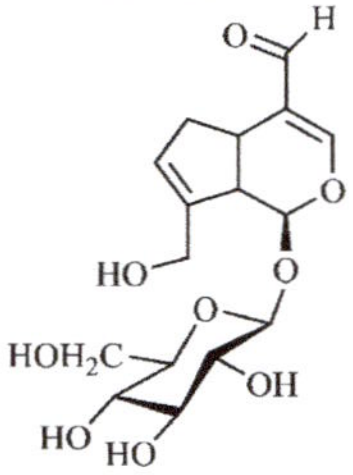					

Table 3. *Cont.*

Compounds	Molecular Structures	Chromatographic Methods for the Isolation and Identification	Solvent Used/Essential Oil	Plant Part Used	Collection Site	References
Teneoside A (**42**, T)	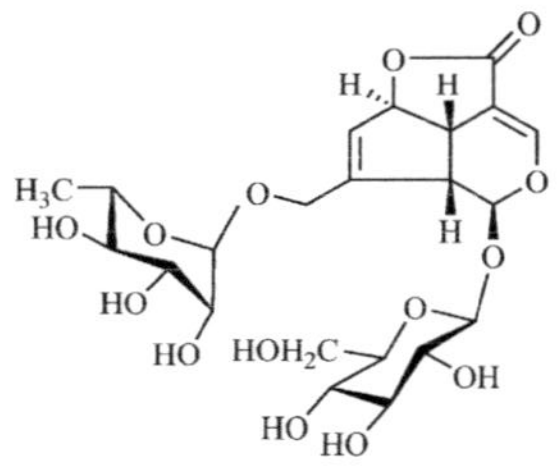					
Kaempferol-3-*O*-hexoside-deoxyhexoside-7-*O*-deoxyhexoside (**43**, F)	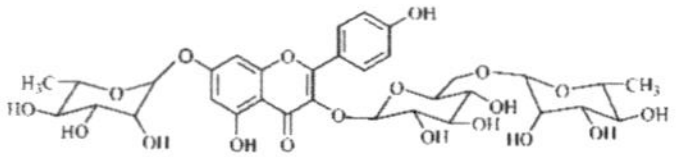					
Isorhamnetin-3-*O*-hexoside-deoxyhexoside-7-*O*-deoxyhexoside (**44**, F)	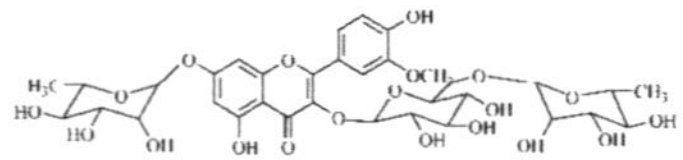					
Quercetin-3-*O*-hexoside-deoxyhexoside (**45**, F)	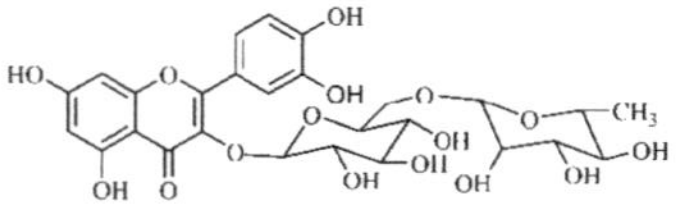					
Kaempferol-3-*O*-hexoside-deoxyhexoside (**46**, F)	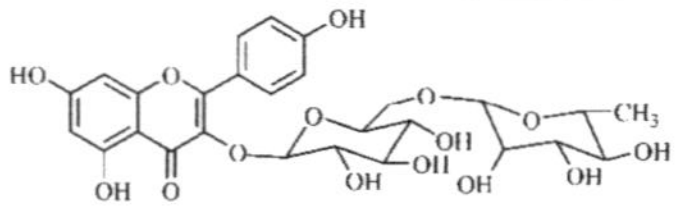					
Isorhamnetin-3-*O*-hexoside-deoxyhexoside (**47**, F)	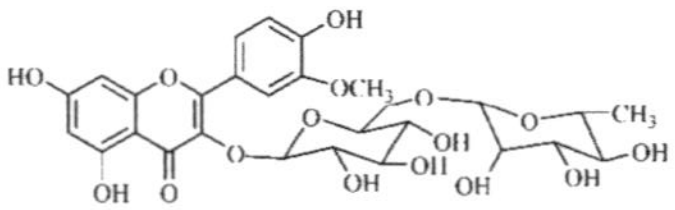					

Table 3. *Cont.*

Compounds	Molecular Structures	Chromatographic Methods for the Isolation and Identification	Solvent Used/Essential Oil	Plant Part Used	Collection Site	References
Geniposidic acid (**40**, T)	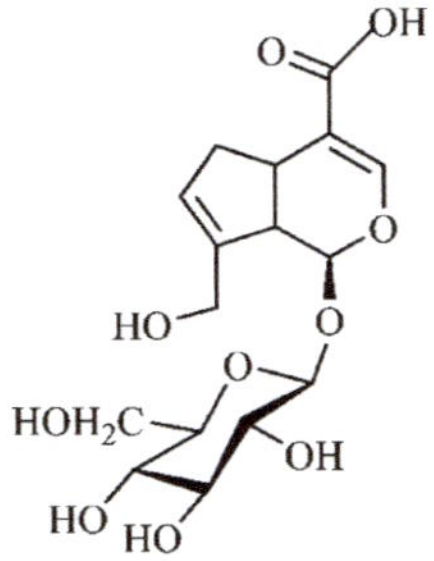					
Geniposide (**48**, T)	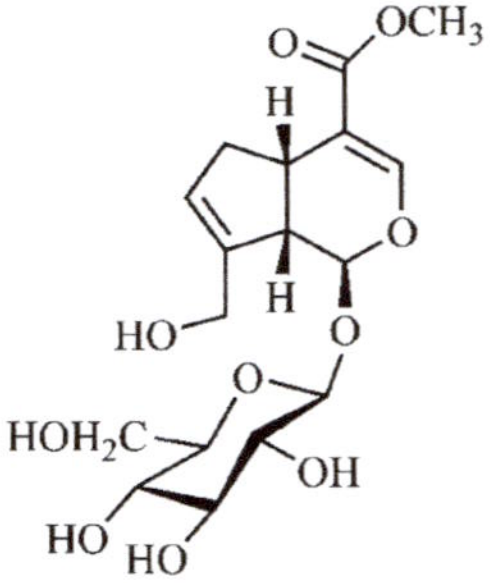					[140]

Table 3. *Cont.*

Compounds	Molecular Structures	Chromatographic Methods for the Isolation and Identification	Solvent Used/Essential Oil	Plant Part Used	Collection Site	References
Genipin-gentiobioside (**49**, T)						
Genameside A (**50**, T)						
Genameside B (**51**, T)						

Table 3. *Cont.*

Compounds	Molecular Structures	Chromatographic Methods for the Isolation and Identification	Solvent Used/Essential Oil	Plant Part Used	Collection Site	References
Genameside C (**52**, T)	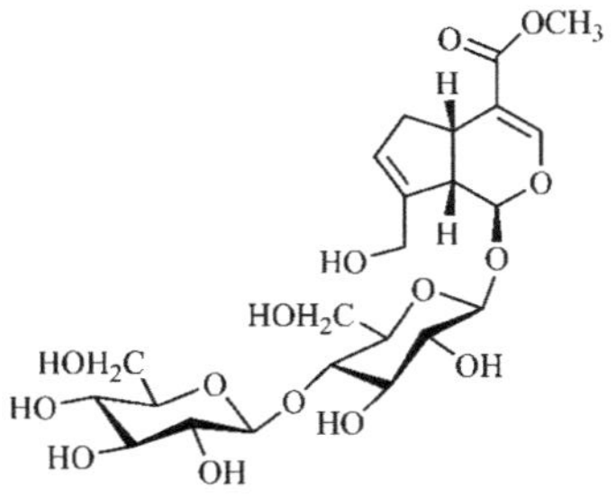					
Genameside D (**53**, T)	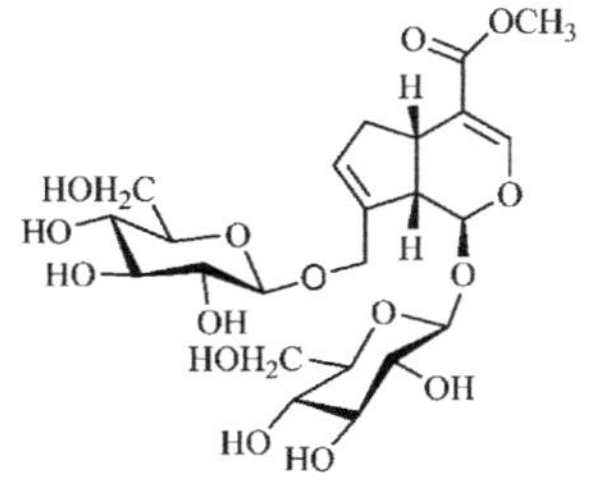					
Gardenoside (**54**, T)	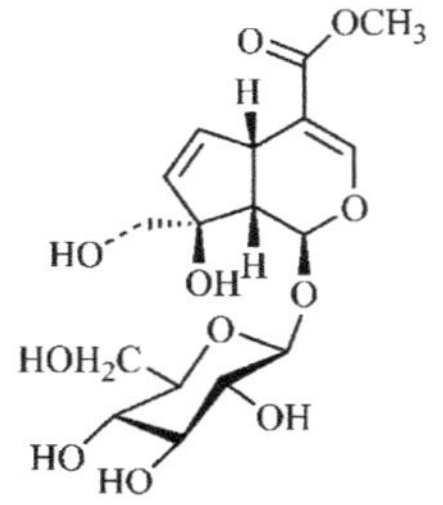					

Table 3. *Cont.*

Compounds	Molecular Structures	Chromatographic Methods for the Isolation and Identification	Solvent Used/Essential Oil	Plant Part Used	Collection Site	References
Genipin (**55**, T)		HPLC	Hydroalcoholic (*v/v*, 80% methanol, ultra-pure water)	Fruit	São Paulo-Brazil	[141]
1-Hydroxy-7-(hydroxymethyl)-1,4*aH*,5*H*,7*aH*-cyclopenta[*c*]pyran-4-carbaldehyde (**56**, T)		HPLC	Hydroalcoholic (*v/v*, 70 % ethanol, water)	Leaf	Natal, Rio Grande do Norte-Brazil	[142]
7-(Hydroxymethyl)-1-methoxy-1*H*,4*aH*,5*H*,7*aH*-cyclopenta[*c*]pyran-4-carbaldehyde (**57**, T)						
Geniposidic acid (**40**, T)		UHPLC	Methanol	Mesocarp Endocarp	Campinas, São Paulo-Brazil	[143]

Table 3. *Cont.*

Compounds	Molecular Structures	Chromatographic Methods for the Isolation and Identification	Solvent Used/Essential Oil	Plant Part Used	Collection Site	References
Gardenosid (**54**, T)	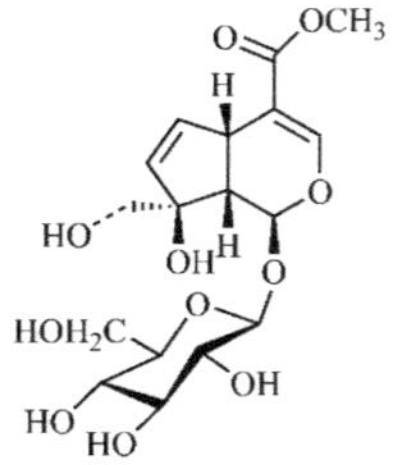					
Genipin-1-β-gentiobioside (**49**, T)	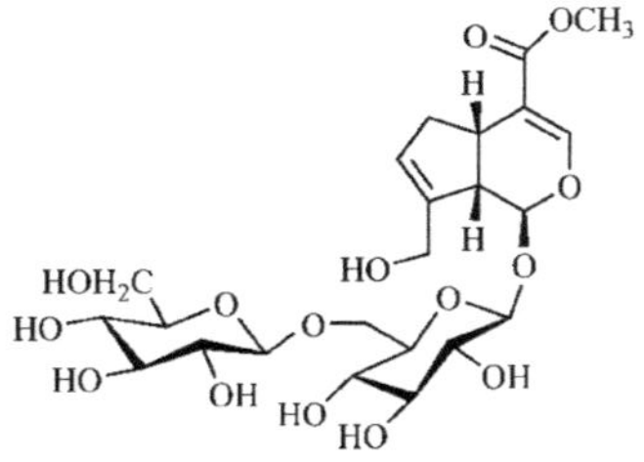					
Geniposide (**48**, T)	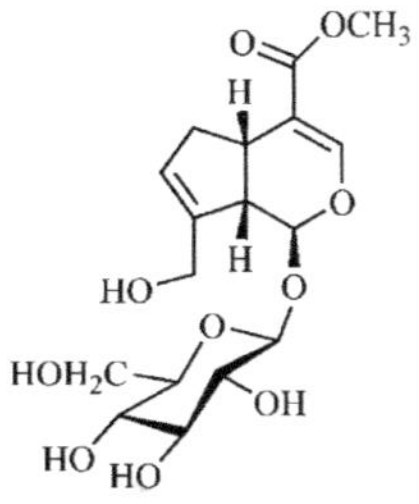					

Table 3. *Cont.*

Compounds	Molecular Structures	Chromatographic Methods for the Isolation and Identification	Solvent Used/Essential Oil	Plant Part Used	Collection Site	References
6″-*O*-*p*-Coumaroyl-1-β-gentiobiosyl geniposidic acid (**59**, T)	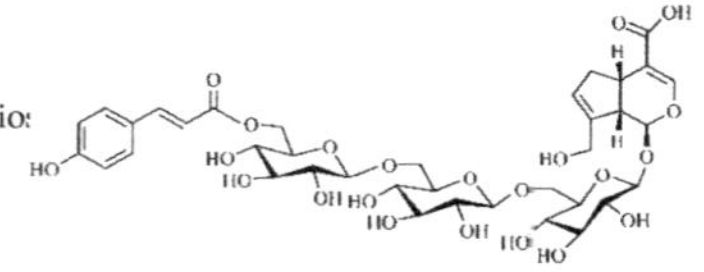					
6″-*O*-*p*-Coumaroylgenipin-gentiobioside (**60**, T)	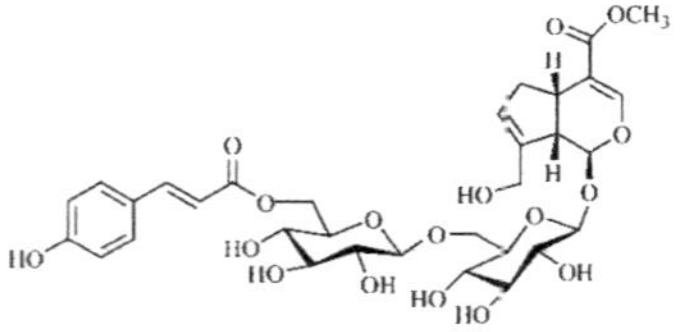					
Genipin (**55**, T)	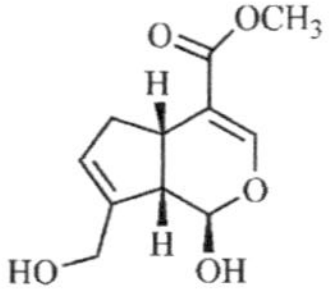					
6′-*O*-*p*-Coumaroyl-geniposidic acid (**61**, T)	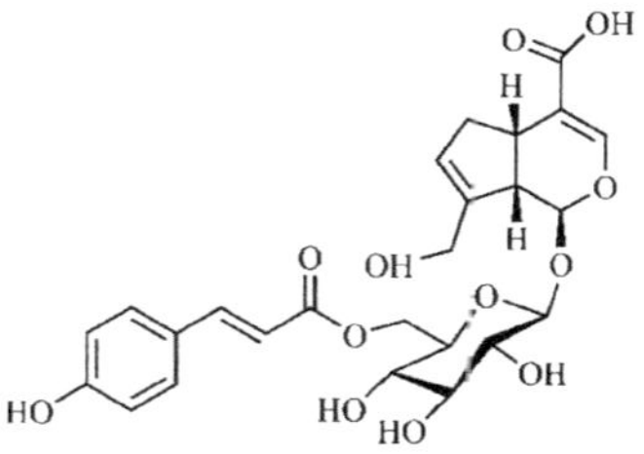					

Table 3. *Cont.*

Compounds	Molecular Structures	Chromatographic Methods for the Isolation and Identification	Solvent Used/Essential Oil	Plant Part Used	Collection Site	References
6′-*O*-Feruloyl-geniposidic acid (**62**, T)	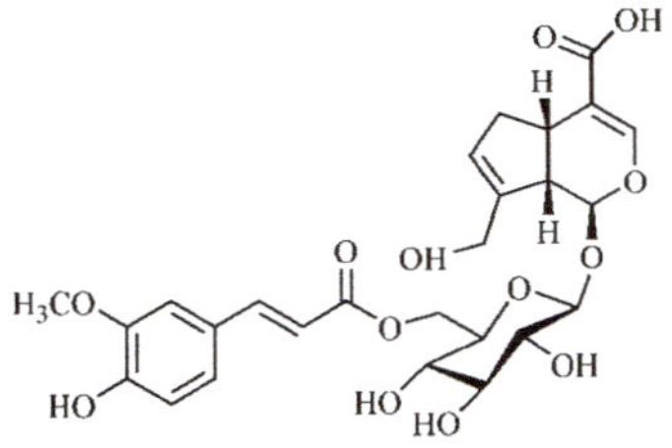					
Genipin (**55**, T)	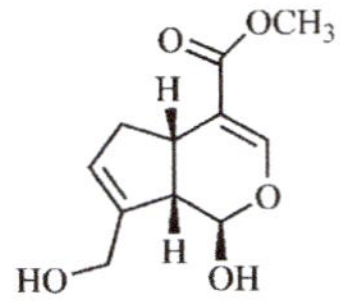	HPLC	Ethanol	Mesocarp Seeds Fruit peel Whole fruit Endocarp	Paraibuna, São Paulo-Brazil	[144]
Geniposide (**48**, T)	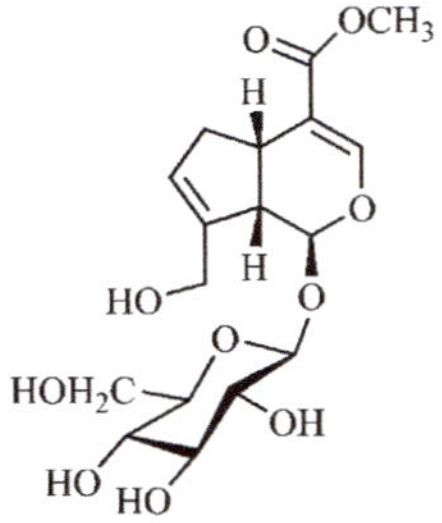					

F: flavonoid; T: terpene; HPLC: High Performance Liquid Chromatography; UHPLC: Ultra-High Performance Liquid Chromatography.5.1.4. Pharmacological Studies.

The chemical characterization of *G. americana* fruits and leaves presents iridoids as major constituents, belonging to the class of terpenes. Genipin (**55**) is the main iridoid found in *G. americana* fruits and has considerable economic potential due to its pigmentation property. The extraction of genipin (**55**) can occur by three different methods, enzymatic hydrolysis, extraction with solvents and ultrasound. A study performed the extraction of genipin (**55**) from *G. americana* fruits using the enzymatic method and quantified 7.85 mg/g of this phytochemical in the sample [119,145].

Pacheco et al. [146] carried out a study on the nutritional composition and energy value of the pulp of *G. americana* fruits. After triplicate analysis, 70% of moisture, 0.5% of proteins, 0.0% of lipids, 1.1% of ash, 22.1% of carbohydrates, 6.3% of dietary fiber, 0.0 mg/100g of beta-carotene, 22.5 mg/100g of vitamin C, 176 mg GAE/100g of phenolic compounds and 90.7 kcal/100g of total energy value were found.

In the methanolic extract of *G. americana* fruits, the following iridoid glycosides were identified, isolated and structurally elucidated: geniposidic acid (**40**), geniposide (**48**), gardenoside (**54**), genipin-gentiobioside (**49**) and 4 new iridoids not previously identified: genameside A (**50**), genameside B (**51**), genameside C (**52**) and genameside D (**53**) [140]. Also in *G. americana* fruits, iridoids geniposidic acid (**40**), gardenoside (**54**), genipin-1-β-gentiobioside (**49**), geniposide (**48**), 6″-*O*-*p*-coumaroyl-1-β-gentiobioside geniposidic acid (**59**), 6″-*O*-*p*-coumaroylgenipin gentiobioside (**60**), genipin (**55**), 6′-*O*-*p*-coumaroyl-geniposidic acid (**61**), 6′-*O*-feruloylgeniposidic acid (**62**) were found in the methanolic extract from the endocarp and mesocarp. In addition, possible antioxidant and antiproliferative properties have been attributed to the extract and, mainly, to genipin (**55**) [143].

After extraction by pressurized ethanol and analysis of the genipin (**55**) and geniposide (**48**) content in the whole fruit and its parts separately at 50 °C and pressure of 2 bars, 20.7 mg/g of genipin (**55**) and 59 mg/g of geniposide (**48**) were found in the mesocarp; 1.16 mg/g of genipin (**55**) and 0.06 mg/g of geniposide (**48**) were found in seeds; 7.5 mg/g of genipin (**55**) and 39.9 mg/g of geniposide (**48**) were found in fruit bark; 38.9 mg/g of genipin (**55**) and 0.01 mg/g of geniposide (**48**) were found in the endocarp; 22.9 mg/g of genipin (**55**) and 0.1 mg/g of geniposide (**48**) were found in the endocarp extract and seeds; and 37.2 mg/g of genipin (**55**) and 0.57 mg/g of geniposide (**48**) were found in the whole fruit [144].

For fruits, the presence of other classes of secondary metabolites was investigated in the hydroalcoholic extract. Mayer reagent was used to detect alkaloids; for tannins, reaction with ferric chloride; for anthraquinones, reaction with ammonia; for flavonoids, Shinoda's reaction; for steroids and triterpenes, the Libermann-Burchard reagent was used; the saponins test was carried out through agitation, observing the presence or absence of foam; and the coumarin test by fluorescence under UV light. The results for this qualitative analysis point to the presence of alkaloids, tannins, flavonoids, triterpenes, saponins and coumarins in the fruit pulp extract and absence of steroids and anthraquinones [147].

Silva et al. [139] identified 13 compounds in a hydroalcoholic extract of *G. americana* leaves. The following are among the isolated substances: (A) coniferin; (B) the iridoids asystasioside D (**39**), geniposidic acid (**40**), tarenoside (**41**) and teneoside A (**42**); (C) loganic, chlorogenic and 1,3-di-*O*-caffeoylquinic acids; and (D) flavonoids, first identified in this genus, kaempferol-3-*O*-hexoside-deoxyhexoside-7-*O*- deoxyhexoside (**43**), isorhamnetin-3-*O*-hexoside-deoxyhexoside-7-*O*-deoxy-hexoside (**44**), quercetin-3-*O*-hexoside-deoxyhexoside (**45**), kaempferol-3-*O*-hexoside-deoxyhexoside (**46**) and isorhamnetin-3-*O*-hexoside-deoxyhexoside (**47**). Other iridoids were also found in the hydroalcoholic extract of *G. americana* leaves such as genipin derivative (**55**), 1-hydroxy-7-(hydroxymethyl)-1*H*,4a*H*,5*H*, 7a*H*-cyclopenta[c]pyran-4-carbaldehyde (**56**) and 7-(hydroxymethyl)-1-methoxy-1*H*,4a*H*,5*H*,7a*H*-cyclopenta[c]pyran-4-carbaldehyde (**57**) [142].

There are few studies on phytochemical screening and characterization of compounds for *G. americana* stem, roots, and seeds. A qualitative study that analyzed the ethanolic extract of leaves and stem bark determined the presence of flavonoids, xanthones, saponins and triterpenes in the stem bark and saponins and triterpenes in leaves [148]. [149] isolated and characterized lectin present in *G. americana* stem bark, which was named GaBL and tested for hemagglutinating properties.

Neri-numa et al. [143] evaluated the antioxidant and antiproliferative activity of the methanolic extract from *G. americana* ripe and green fruits. The ability to eliminate DPPH radicals has been reported to be like that of ascorbic acid, and the extract from green fruits has higher concentration of iridoids and greater efficiency to eliminate radicals. The *in vitro* antiproliferative activity was also observed with efficiency in all tested cell lines, with greater activity for the extract from green fruits, which has high concentration of iridoid genipin (**55**), to which this property was attributed. In addition, the anticholinesterase activity of the ethanol extract from *G. americana* fruit bark, pulp and seeds was also observed and may be associated with the presence of chlorogenic acid, an acetylcholinesterase (AChE) inhibitor [139,150].

Genipin (**55**), a triterpene found in *G. americana* fruits was tested *in vitro* and *in vivo* for its anti-inflammatory property and its role on memory deficiencies induced by LPS. Microglia stimulation by LPS of gram-negative bacteria induces the production of inflammatory mediators, whose overproduction can cause neuronal damage. Genipin (**55**) inhibited the production of these mediators in the BV2 microglial cell line through the dose-dependent suppression of LPSe-induced NF-κB activation by activating the expression of erythroid nuclear factor 2 (Nrf2) and heme oxygenase-1 (HO-1). Active NF-κB induces the production of inflammatory mediators such as PGE2, TNF-α and IL-1β, while Nrf2 encodes antioxidant enzymes such as HO-1, which promote the elimination of ROS and, consequently, the inhibition of the NF-κB expression [151].

The anti-inflammatory role of genipin (**55**) is also associated to another mechanism, the inhibition of the activation of NLRP3 and NLRC4 inflammasomes by suppressing macrophage autophagy. Agonists of NLRP3 and NLRC4 inflammasomes promote the activation of autophagy in macrophages, which enhances the secretion of IL-1β and ASC oligomerization, while suppression of autophagy promoted by genipin (**55**) inhibits this effect [152].

The protective role of genipin (**55**) on LPS-induced acute lung injury has been investigated. Genipin (**55**) positively regulated the signaling of the phosphoinositide 3-kinase/phosphorylated protein kinase B (PI3K/p-AKT) pathway by increasing the levels of p-AKT. PI3K generates phosphatidylinositol-3,4,5-triphosphate (PIP3), which acts as a second messenger and facilitates the translocation of protein kinase B (AKT) to the plasma membrane, where it is activated by phosphorylation and can later be transported to the nucleus. AKT promotes the phosphorylation of some molecules, among them AMPc-responsive binding protein (CREB), whose activation is associated with increased Bcl-2 activity, which inhibits pro-apoptotic caspase-9, promoting a protective effect of cell survival [153,154].

In contrast, the action of genipin (**55**) on the PI3K/p-AKT pathway was also related to its inhibitory activity on the growth of human bladder cancer cells [155] and squamous cell carcinoma [156]. It was observed that genipin (**55**) induced the cell cycle to stop in G0/G1 phases, and promoted the apoptosis of cancer cells, with increase in the expression of pro-apoptotic protein Bax. Such cell growth suppressive effects have been associated with inactivation of the PI3K/p-AKT pathway, shown by the reduction of phosphorylated PI3K and AKT levels [155].

Zhao et al. [157] analyzed the protective role of genipin (**55**) against ischemia-reperfusion lesion associated with energy deficiency and oxidative stress, which are regulated by mitochondrial uncoupling protein 2 (UCP2) and NAD-dependent deacetylase sirtuin-3 (SIRT3), respectively. In this lesion, damage increases due to the increase in the ischemia duration, as well as the degree of energy deficiency and oxidative stress, with increase in UCP2 expression and SIRT3 activity. Genipin (**55**) acts as a specific inhibitor of UCP2. Therefore, in mice submitted to treatment with genipin (**55**), reduction in UCP2 expression and SIRT3 activity was observed, as well as a lower NAD +/NADH ratio and increased levels of adenosine triphosphate (ATP), reducing oxidative stress and energy deficiency and, consequently, mitigating damage.

The effects of genipin (**55**) on energy metabolism are also related to its anti-tumor property, capable of inhibiting the proliferation of several cancer cells in breast [158], colon [159], hepatocellular [160] cholangiocarcinoma [161] and gioblastoma [162]. UCP2 overexpression is observed in tumor cells, which gives genipin (**55**), a UCP2 inhibitor, a potential anti-tumor activity mechanism. UCP2 promotes the decoupling of the electron transport chain to oxidative phosphorylation, reducing energy availability and the production of O_2^-, a ROS.

Cancer cells are under oxidative stress and to protect themselves, they increase the UCP2 expression to reduce the formation of ROS. UCP2 inhibition by genipin (**55**) promotes an increase in ROS, triggers the nuclear translocation of glycolytic enzyme glyceraldehyde 3-phosphate dehydrogenase (GAPDH), formation of autophagosomes and expression of LC3-II autophagy marker, leading to cell death or growth inhibition, invasion and migration of tumor cells. In addition, genipin (**55**) enhances autophagic cell death induced by gemcitabine, a clinically used chemotherapeutic agent (Figure 5) [163,164].

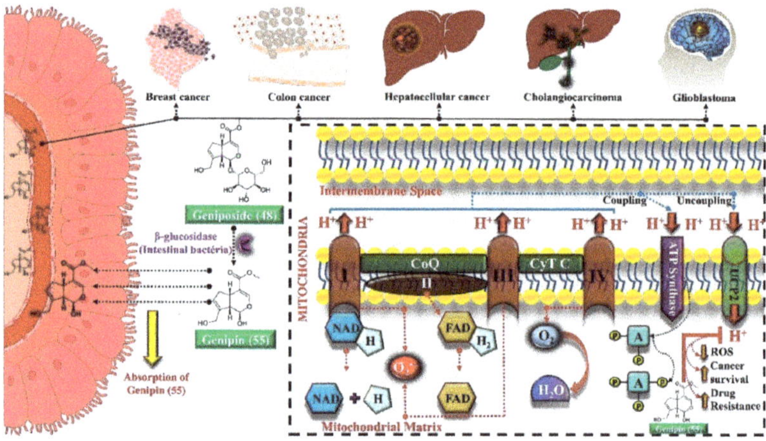

Figure 5. Effects of genipin on energy metabolism: anti-tumor property: Transport mechanisms of geniposide and genipin, which are abundantly present in extracts from plants such as *Genipa americana*, involve converting geniposide into genipin in the intestinal lumen through bacterial enzymes β-glucosidases. Uncoupling protein 2 (UCP2) is a genipin target in the treatment of cancer. In mitochondria, the respiratory chain, formed by complexes I to IV, transfers electrons from NADH through oxidation-reduction reactions. Complexes I, II, and III contribute to the production of H+ ion gradient. The electrochemical gradient generated is coupled to the ADP phosphorylation process via ATP synthase. Oxygen is the final electron acceptor and is reduced to water by the electron transfer of complex IV. However, its early reduction into complexes I and III leads to the formation of $O_2^{\bullet-}$. UCP2 is a protein widely expressed in tumor cells. Its function is to reduce ROS production and increase the survival of tumor cells by uncoupling the electrochemical gradient generated by the respiratory chain. For this purpose, UCP2 increases H^+ output from the intermembrane space to the mitochondrial matrix and reduces the mitochondrial membrane potential. This mechanism, present in tumor cells as a survival factor by reducing ROS generation, is the genipin target [165]. A, adenosine; CoQ, coenzyme Q; Cyt C, cytochrome C; FAD, flavin adenine dinucleotide; NAD, Nicotinamide adenine dinucleotide; ROS, reactive oxygen species; UCP2, uncoupling protein 2.

Another anti-tumor mechanism associated with genipin (**55**) occurs through negative regulation of the signal transducer and transcription activator (Stat)/cell differentiation protein of induced myeloid cell leukemia 1 (Mcl-1). Mcl-1 is a member of the Bcl-2 family and has anti-apoptotic activity, being associated with cell survival and is overexpressed in gastric cancer cells. The apoptotic mechanism of cancer cells promoted by genipin (**55**) is related to the negative regulation of Mcl-1, which can occur through the activation of the SHP-1 phosphatase and the suppressor of cytokine signaling 3 (SOCS3). In addition, this phytoconstituent inhibits the activity of JAK2 enzymes of the Janus kinase family (JAK), responsible for the activation of the Stat3 transcription factor, which regulates the expression of genes related to cell survival. Thus, inactivating JAK2 enzymes, there is no activation of Stat3 and expression of the MCL1 gene, which encodes the anti-apoptotic protein Mcl-1 (Figure 6a,b) [166].

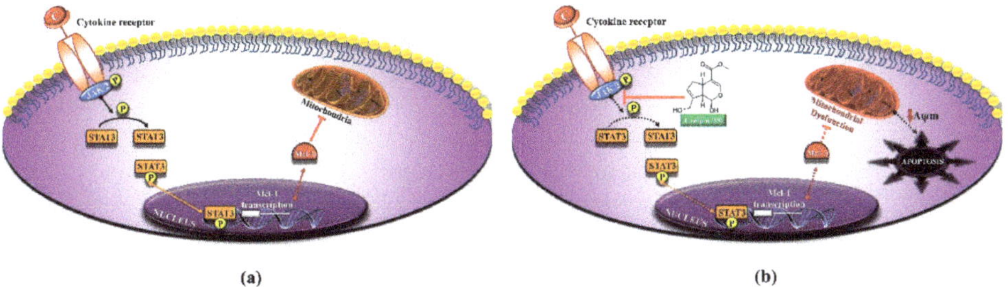

(a)   (b)

Figure 6. Apoptosis mediated by genipin through interference with myeloid cell leukemia-1 (Mcl-1) synthesis in gastric cancer cell lines: (**a**) Cytokine receptors without intrinsic protein kinase domain amplify extracellular signals through signal transduction via Janus Kinase (JAK) family (JAK1 to JAK3 and tyrosine kinase 2). After receptor activation, JAK2 phosphorylates the tyrosine residue of transcription factor Signal Transducer and Activator of Transcription 3 (STAT3), which enables its binding to the promoter of target genes related to survival and apoptosis. Subsequently, Mcl-1 is synthesized; (**b**) Genipin absorption by tumor cells induces mitochondrial dysfunction due to decreased Mcl-1 expression through the JAK2/STAT3 pathway. $\Delta\psi m$, mitochondrial membrane potential; JAK2, Janus Kinase 2; Mcl-1, myeloid cell leukemia-1; STA3, Signal transducer and activator of transcription 3 [166].

Inhibition of Sonic Hedgehog, one of three proteins in the signal family called hedgehog found in mammals by genipin (**55**), was also associated with its anti-tumor property. Genipin (**55**) binds to the protein of the Hedgehog Smoothened (SMO) signaling pathway through the drug-affinity-responsive target stability (DARTS), increasing the expression of p53 and NOXA, a protein of the Bcl-2 family that contributes to apoptosis promoted by p53. This mechanism occurs by inhibiting the expression of the GLI1 gene, a transcriptional activator of the Hedgehog pathway that reduces p53 expression. Thus, the binding of genipin (**55**) to SMO promoter induces a reduction in GLI1 activity and an increase in p53 expression [167].

Genipin (**55**) was used in cattle to increase corneal stiffness and induce corneal collagen cross-linking (CXL), which reduces the progression of ectasia, that is, corneal distention. Through a mechanism still unknown, genipin (**55**) induces CXL by up to 7%, a result superior to that induced by treatment with riboflavin and UV light applied in the control group, which presented only 5.6% cross-linking. To achieve 7% cross-linking, 140 μL of 0.5% genipin (**55**) was administered every 1 h for 2 h [168]. The role of genipin (**55**) investigated in cattle suggests further studies in humans. Furthermore, this cross-linking property of genipin (**55**) has also been used in the biotechnological production of hydrogels, gelatin biofilms and transdermal patches for the controlled release of drugs [169].

Also, for ophthalmic treatment, genipin (**55**) was used in posterior scleral contraction/reinforcement surgery (PSCR), which delays axial stretching of the eyeball, common in human myopia. However, despite the significant effect of the procedure, it was not sustained in the long term, which was related to the loss of sclera resistance to traction. The sclera is a layer of fibrous, opaque and dense tissue that lines the eye, on which the cross-linking capacity of genipin was tested (**55**), which doubled the sclera resistance and increased by 30 % resistance to enzymatic degradation, which could promote sclera weakening. The study points out the efficacy and safety of PSCR with sclera cross-linked with genipin (**55**) to restrict axial elongation of the eyeball [168].

Genipin (**55**) was tested for possible antiviral activity on Kaposi's sarcoma herpes virus (KSHV). Genipin (**55**) played a double and dose-dependent role. At lower concentration and administered for 48 h, the phytochemical significantly reduced the production of the nuclear antigen associated with KSHV latency (LANA) and increased the number of copies of the virus intracellular genome, favoring lytic replication of KSHV. Treatment with higher genipin (**55**) doses induced the activation of caspases 3 and 7 by reducing the expression of Bcl-2, promoting apoptosis, which is impaired, since the virus produces viral Bcl-2, approximately 60% identical to cellular Bcl-2, which makes the infected cell more resistant. New studies have been proposed to investigate the role of genipin (**55**) in modulating the KSHV life cycle and possibly prevent disorders associated with the virus [170].

Nonato et al. [171] evaluated the GABA-mediated anticonvulsant effect of the methanolic extract from *G. americana* leaves rich in polysaccharides. A heteropolysaccharide (PRE) with inhibitory and anticonvulsant effect on the central nervous system (CNS) was identified, which was reversed after the administration of the GABAergic flumazenil antagonist, indicating the participation of this receptor in the effect performed by PRE, which also reduced oxidative stress in the pre-frontal cortex, hippocampus and striated nucleus of animals that had induced seizures, observed by the increase of GSH levels and reduction of lipid peroxidation levels.

In *G. americana* leaves, a glycoconjugate rich in arabinogalactane and uronic acid was found, with anticoagulant, antiplatelet, and antithrombotic properties. Anticoagulant activity was observed in fraction containing uronic acid and occurs through the intrinsic and/or the common pathway of the coagulation cascade by a still unknown mechanism. Glycoconjugate inhibits platelet aggregation induced by adenosine diphosphate (ADP), but not collagen-induced aggregation. Antithrombotic action was observed in a model of rats with venous thrombosis and, similar to the antiplatelet activity, it was found in fraction rich in arabinogalactane [172].

The hydroalcoholic extract from *G. americana* stem bark was evaluated for its possible antimicrobial properties. Minimum Inhibitory Concentration (MIC) tests were carried out with *E. coli*, *S. aureus* and *P. aeruginosa* and MIC was ≥ 1024 µg/mL in all strains. Efficiency was not considered satisfactory, but the association of the extract with aminoglycoside drugs amikacin and gentamicin and the lincosamide clindamycin, increased the antimicrobial potential of these drugs. This property was attributed to tannins present in the extract with antimicrobial activity. The result of this association induced greater susceptibility of *P. aeruginosa* and *E. coli* to death by gentamicin and *S. aureus* by Amikacin in all strains submitted to this treatment [173].

The polysaccharide extract from *G. americana* leaves was tested against *Trypanosoma cruzi* epimastigotes, trypomastigotes and amastigotes. The results showed antiparasitic effect against the three forms of the protozoan with low toxicity to mammalian cells. In addition, it demonstrated potent activity even on amastigote forms, which are intracellular, suggesting that the compound responsible for this activity has access to the intracellular medium. After extract administration, ROS generation was observed, which causes damage to trypanothione reductase, an enzyme important for the oxidative balance of the protozoan. Morphological changes indicate cell death due to necrosis with rounding and shortening of the parasite, cytoplasmic leakage and membrane degradation [174].

5.1.4. Toxicity Studies

Studies focusing on the possible toxicological effects of *G. americana* extract and its chemical constituents are still scarce. A study carried out on the acute toxicological analysis of the hydroalcoholic extract from *G. americana* fruits reported that animals receiving the extract did not present any apparent behavioral or clinical changes; the microscopic study of organs also did not present any changes, there were no deaths by the end of the study, although it was estimated that the LD_{50} would be greater than 2000 mg/kg. In the analysis of the subchronic toxicity, macroscopic changes in kidneys were described, such as increased size, which may be related to renal hyperplasia or thrombosis at dose of 100 mg/kg [175].

The toxicological evaluation of the aqueous extract from *G. americana* leaves induced mortality in *Danio rerio* fish species at concentrations above 100 mg/L. No genetic mutations were observed; however, some nuclear abnormalities such as blebbed, lobed and notched nucleus and binucleated cells were rather observed [176].

6. Bromeliaceae Family

The Bromeliaceae family is composed of approximately 56 genera and 3086 species. Due to the great economic potential, extraction from natural environments and, mainly, due to the ornamental value among landscapers and gardeners, some species are threatened with extinction. Species are predominantly neotropical and can be found on the American and African continents. They present great ecological diversity, with terrestrial and epiphytic species, which are arboreal, shrub or cactaceae [175,177].

One species that stands out for its economic potential is *Ananas comosus* (L) Merr, known as pineapple which, in addition to its potential for fresh consumption, is also used as a raw material to produce numerous by-products. Many plants in this family are utilized in the automotive and textile industry, such as *Ananas lucidus* Miller and *Neoglaziovia variegata* Mez due to their important properties for the production of fibers [178].

In addition, some members of the Bromeliaceae family stand out for producing large amounts of proteins and enzymes that cleave peptide bonds between amino acids in proteins. The effect of these proteins on plant physiology is not yet known, but one hypothesis is that these enzymes play the role of protecting plants against pathogens and herbivores [179].

6.1. Genus Bromelia and Species Bromelia antiacantha

The genus *Bromelia* comprises about 46 species distributed throughout Americas and used in folk medicine against parasitic diseases, edema, respiratory and kidney problems, intestinal disorders, and diabetes. *B. antiacantha* Bertol. is popularly known as caraguatá, gravatá, carauatá or croatá and has properties that contribute on a large scale for the economic development of the region where it occurs or is cultivated [180–182].

The species adapts to different climatic conditions, being found in humid and flooded soils and even in the post-beach forest, which indicates tolerance to high salinity and soaked soils. In addition, it can also be found in xerophytic environments, in which there is scarcity of water and nutrients such as Cerrado soils submitted to drought periods, in these cases, the plant adapts with the presence of a structure for storing water and nutrients, the rhizome [183].

This species has great diversity of applications, and fruits are not only used as food in the production of jellies and ice cream, but the plant is also used for ornamental purposes. Proteolytic enzymes were detected in the crude extract from *B. antiacantha* fruits and the new protease Antiacanthain A, a molecule with interesting characteristics for biotechnological use, was recently isolated [179,184]. These enzymes are used in the chemical, pharmaceutical, food and textile industries and in the production of detergent for cleaning clothes due to their stain-removing property [185].

6.1.1. Geographical Distribution and Popular Use

Occurrences of *B. antiacantha* are recorded in several American countries, among them, Venezuela, Brazil, Mexico, Peru, Uruguay, and the Caribbean islands. The species has perennial germination cycle, its leaves are prickly and, due to the beauty of its flowers, attracts pollinators like hummingbirds, increasing the natural dispersion of the species [186,187].

In folk medicine, the fruits of this species are used for respiratory problems such as flu, asthma, and bronchitis through the administration of homemade syrup produced by decoction. For the production of this syrup, the pulp of 1 *B. antiacantha* fruit is submitted to heating together with one cup of solvent, which in this case is water, for about 5 min; then the mixture is filtered and sugar is added in the proportion of two cups of sugar for one cup of the mixture. Sugar must be mixed under heating until complete homogenization and acts not only as sweetener, but also as a preservative, which is used according to the dose of one tablespoon three times a day [188,189].

In some cases, vegetable organs of other species are added in the syrup preparation to enhance the expectorant action. The most added species are *Achillea millefolium*, *Mentha sativa* and *Zingiber officinale*. Other indications for the use of the fruit are purgative, diuretic, vermifuge and abortion. Leaves are used in the form of tea prepared by infusion or decoction, with drops of propolis, used in mouthwash for the treatment of thrush and other disorders of the oral mucosa and the extract produced by maceration is indicated as antipyretic and anthelmintic [182,190,191].

6.1.2. Botanical Aspects

B. antiacantha has stem with rhizomes about 1 m in length from which adventitious roots emerge. Rhizomes are covered by leaves and are responsible for the survival of the species under different climatic conditions. Leaves exhibit alternate and spiral phyllotaxis with 80 to 185 cm in length, arranged in non petiolated rosette without the cistern formation, with lanceolate and caniculate limb shape and aculeate limb margin [183,188].

Flowering is annual and occurs between the months of December and February. From the center of leaves, monopodial inflorescence emerges, which is composed of 150 to 350 meliophilous, ornithophilous and pedunculated flowers with oval sepals, entire margin of the sepal, oblong petal purple in color. During the flowering period, central leaves and bracts show intense red color. Fruits are polyspermic, fleshy, gaba type, yellow when ripe, with approximately 2 cm in diameter, pleasant odor, and edible pulp. Seeds are photoblastic, that is, they need sunlight to germinate, present 26% of moisture, with high germination rate at temperatures between 25 °C and 35 °C [78,183,191,192].

6.1.3. Phytochemical Aspects

Table 4 presents a summary of classes of secondary metabolites found in the respective extracts and plant organs of *B. antiacantha* species.

Table 4. Phytochemical analysis of *B. antiacantha*.

Compounds	Molecular Structures	Chromatographic Methods for the Isolation and Identification	Solvent Used/Essential Oil	Plant Part Used	Collection Site	References
Alkaloid	*					
Flavonoid	*					
Tannin	*			Fruit		
Terpene	*					
Anthraquinone	*					
Coumarin	*	–	Methanol		Rio Pomba, Minas Gerais-Brazil	[193]
Alkaloid	*					
Flavonoid	*					
Tannin	*			Leaf		
Terpene	*					
Coumarin	*					
Flavonoid	*			Fruit		
Tannin	*	–	Methanol	Leaf	Umuarama, Paraná-Brazil	[182]
Saponin	*					
Flavonoid	*	–	Water	Fruit	Vale do Itajaí, Santa Catarina-Brazil	[194]
Flavonoid	*			Leaf		
Anthocyanin	*	–	Hydroalcoholic		Viamão, Rio Grande do Sul-Brazil	[195]
Flavonoid	*			Bract		
Anthocyanin	*					
Daucosterol (**63**, S)		CC	Methanol	Leaf	Umuarama, Paraná-Brazil	[196]

S: saponin; CC: Column Chromatography. * Based on the lack of the isolation study of the chemical constituent, as it is a qualitative study, it was not possible to design the structures.

There are few studies on the chemical composition of *B. antiacantha*, and most of them only perform qualitative screening, without quantifying or isolating substances. The analysis of the proximate composition of ripe fruits showed 82.63% of moisture, 0.62% of protein, 2% of fiber, 8.75% of carbohydrates and 0.93% of ash. In addition, other compounds were quantified, which are associated with the antioxidant activity of fruits and are composed of 70.73 mg/100 g of phenolic compounds, 162.67 mg/100 g of total carotenoids and 60.01 mg/100 g of vitamin C [197].

A qualitative phytochemical analysis performed with the methanolic extract from *B. antiacantha* leaves and fruits detected, in the methanolic extract of fruits, the following groups of secondary metabolites: alkaloids, phenols, flavonoids, tannins, triterpenes, steroids, anthraquinones and coumarins. In the methanolic extract of leaves, the following groups of secondary metabolites were identified: alkaloids, phenols, flavonoids, tannins, triterpenes, steroids and coumarins [193]. The presence of flavonoids, tannins and saponins was confirmed by analyses from another study, which also used the methanolic extract from *B. antiacantha* leaves and [182]. With regard to *B. antiacantha* fruits, the presence of hydroxycinnamic acids and flavone derivative was detected in the aqueous extract, which was not structurally identified [194]. The characterization of secondary metabolites of *B. antiacantha* species using the ethanolic extract to quantify flavonoids and the hydromethanolic extract to quantify anthocyanins showed: (1) in leaf extracts, 1.68 mg/mL of flavonoids and 0.0 mg/mL of anthocyanins and; (2) in bract extracts, 0.43 mg/mL of flavonoids and 10.83 mg/mL of anthocyanins. The greater production of anthocyanins in bracts may indicate the effort in the allocation of energy by plants to attract pollinators, since the amount of flavonoids found in leaves, although larger than in bracts, is still insignificant compared to other species that are sources of flavonoids [195]. Analyzing *B. antiacantha* leaves, [196] detected the presence of saponins in the methanolic extract and isolated saponin daucosterol (**63**), which was attributed the hemolytic property of the extract.

6.1.4. Pharmacological Studies

The alcoholic extract from *B. antiacantha* fruits, and methanolic, hexanic, ethyl acetate and raw alcoholic extract from leaves were tested for antimicrobial, molluscicidal and antioxidant properties. All extracts were tested against clinically isolated *C. albicans* and *C. glabrata* strains and *C. albicans* (ATCC 90028), *E. coli* (ATCC 8739), *P. aeruginosa* (ATCC 9027) and *S. aureus* (ATCC 6538) reference strains. All strains tested were not affected by extracts, that is, none of the extracts showed antimicrobial or antifungal activity. The evaluated extracts were considered inactive in relation to the molluscicidal activity, since no significant effects were found at concentration of 400 μg/mL, a value above the maximum for this activity. To test the antioxidant activity, the performance of extracts against the DPPH radical was observed, showing unsatisfactory results, since only the extract from leaves with ethyl acetate obtained moderate performance, with 35% inhibition of radicals [182].

The methanolic (BAM), hexanic (BAH), dichloromethane (BAD), ethyl acetate (BAA) and hydromethanolic (BAHa) extracts from *B. antiacantha* leaves and fruits were submitted to antibacterial activity tests. Only BAM and BAD extracts from leaves and BAA extract from fruits inhibited the growth of *P. aeruginosa*, and the BAM extract from leaves showed activity on *E. coli* [193].

Daucosterol (**63**) is a saponin found in the methanolic extract from *B. antiacantha* leaves. This substance was the focus of a study that investigates its possible anti-inflammatory role on colitis induced by dextran sulfate sodium (DSS) in mice. Colitis is an inflammatory reaction in the large intestine, which source may be infectious or autoimmune. Pre or post-treatment with daucosterol (**63**) provided relief from the clinical symptoms of colitis, with reduction in the number of regulatory T cells, in the activity of Natural Killer (NK) cells and in the production of Immunoglobulin A (IgA), whose increase is characteristic of the disease. In addition, ROS inhibition and reduction in the expression of inflammatory cytokines such as TNF-α, IL-6, IL-1β and IFN-γ were observed, as well as increase in the anti-inflammatory cytokine IL-10 [198].

Induction of autophagic apoptosis in prostate cancer by daucosterol (**63**) was also analyzed, indicating anti-tumor activity. The action of this phytoconstituent on cancer cells promoted the interruption of the cell cycle by activating the mitochondrial-dependent apoptotic signaling pathway that leads to increased expression of the pro-apoptotic proteins caspase 3 and 9 and Bax, in addition to reducing the expression of Bcl-2. The administration of the 3-methyladenine (3-MA) autophagy inhibitor attenuated the apoptotic effect triggered by daucosterol (**63**), indicating that its mechanism of action is the induction of autophagic apoptosis. This mechanism may also be related to the action of JNK protein kinases, known for the regulatory role of cell proliferation, survival and death. Daucosterol (**63**) increased the level of JNK proteins active in cancer cells, while the specific JNK inhibitor (SP600125) inhibited its action, which indicates that this phytoconstituent has tumor suppressive effect through the induction of autophagic apoptosis dependent on the activation of the JNK signaling [199].

The apoptotic action promoted by daucosterol (**63**) has been investigated by several studies that correlate it with the anti-tumor action on breast [200] and prostate [201] cancers. Esmaeili et al. [202] investigated the anti-tumor mechanism of daucosterol (**63**) on human breast adenocarcinoma cells and concluded that the apoptotic mechanism is associated with the mitochondrial pathway, with loss of the mitochondria membrane potential and release of cytochrome C being observed after reduction of the Bcl-2/Bax ratio through the increase in the levels of intracellular ROS and decrease in the levels of antioxidant protein GSH and MMP. In addition, the PI3K/AKT pathway is inhibited by daucosterol (**63**) by reducing the AKT expression, whose levels are increased in some types of tumor. This reduction occurs by increasing the expression of the phosphatase and tensin homolog (PTEN), a negative regulator of the PI3K/AKT pathway. Thus, the inhibition of the PI3K/AKT pathway, the increase in Bax expression and the reduction of Bcl-2 levels, promote apoptosis mediated by the mitochondrial pathway and activation of caspases 3 and 9 (Figure 7) [202].

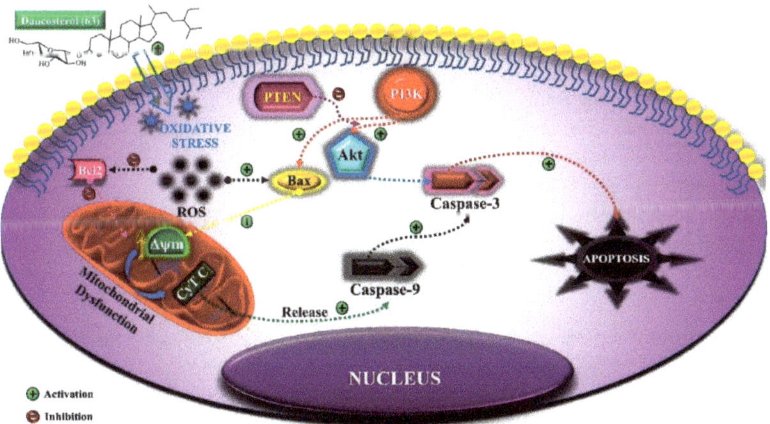

Figure 7. Daucosterol mechanism on human breast adenocarcinoma cells: After treatment of tumor cells (MCF-7) with daucusterol, a phytosterol abundantly present in *Bromelia antiacantha* extracts, the positive regulation of Phosphatase and Tensin Homologue (PTEN) blocks Protein Kinase B (Akt) activation through PI3K. Daucusterol induces reactive oxygen species (ROS) synthesis that leads to mitochondrial oxidative stress and, subsequently, release of cytochrome C. Subsequently, the activation of caspases causes cell apoptosis [202]. Δψm, mitochondrial membrane potential; Akt, Protein Kinase B; Bax, BCL2 Associated X; Bcl2, B-cell lymphoma 2; Cyt C, cytochrome C; PI3K, phosphatidylinositol-3-kinase; PTEN, phosphatase and tensin homologue; ROS, reactive oxygen species.

Another study also investigated the anti-tumor property of daucosterol (**63**), which inhibits the migration and invasion of hepatocellular carcinoma cells using another mechanism, the Wnt/β-catenin signaling pathway, which regulates various physiological processes such as cell proliferation, apoptosis, differentiation, transcription and translation. Daucosterol (**63**) acts by significantly inhibiting the expression of β-catenin, reducing the possibilities of cell proliferation, migration and invasion, which would occur through the Wnt/β-catenin pathway [203].

The neuroprotective effect of daucosterol (**63**) was also investigated in a study that reported the action of this compound as a modulator of the growth factor expression similar to insulin type 1 (IGF-1), which plays a neuroprotective role. Daucosterol (**63**) increased the level of AKT phosphorylation, resulting in more AKT in the active form and indicating that the AKT pathway was activated, resulting in protective effect on treated neurons, since the activation of the PI3K/AKT pathway favors cell survival, as it promotes the inactivation of GSK-3b, a pro-apoptotic protein, whose inhibition causes an increase in Mcl-1, which has the opposite effect, reducing the activity of caspase 3 [204].

6.1.5. Toxicity Studies

Regarding the toxic effects of extracts obtained from *B. antiacantha*, a cytotoxicity test was carried out using *Artemia salina* nauplii, on which the alcoholic extracts from fruits and methanolic and alcoholic extracts from leaves of this plant showed toxicity, with LD_{50} values of 618.3 μg/mL, 275.9 μg/mL and 362.1 μg/mL, respectively [182]. In another study, hexane extracts in dichloromethane and ethyl acetate from *B. antiacantha* leaves showed toxicity against *Artemia salina*, with LD_{50} values of 53.9 μg/mL, 112.4 μg/mL and 241.6 μg/mL, respectively. For fruits, extract in dichloromethane was the only one with cytototoxic activity, with an LD_{50} of 29.8 μg/mL [193].

The hemolysis index promoted by the aqueous extract from *B. antiacantha* leaves and fruits was stipulated after analyzing lamb blood, observing total hemolysis in 0.85% and 1.00% dilutions for fruits, and 0.90% and 1.00% for leaves, while partial hemolysis occurred at 0.70% dilution for fruits and leaves. This hemolytic action was associated with the presence of saponin compounds in extracts, such as daucosterol (**63**), which were isolated from this species [196].

Saponins have cytotoxic activity, and this activity can occur through the promotion of autophagic cell death or cytoskeleton disintegration. In the case of hemolysis promoted by saponins, this may occur due to their ability to complex with cholesterol of the erythrocyte cell membrane, which results in the formation of pores in the membrane, increasing its permeability. In addition, some saponins, such as daucosterol (**63**) can act through signaling pathways such as PI3K/AKT, Wnt/β-catenin, promoting apoptosis. Autophagy induction can also occur by increasing the levels of light chain protein 3 (LC3) induced by some saponins. LC3 is associated with microtubules and is a marker for autophagy, being related to the formation of autophagic vacuoles [205,206].

7. Clinical Trials

Finally, it is essential to note that medicinal plants are used to prevent and treat diseases by humans, being used by about 80% of the population for primary health care. The rich biodiversity of the Brazilian cerrado offers a unique and incomparable potential for discovering and developing bioactive agents. Therefore, clinical trials with metabolites isolated from these species are of fundamental importance.

Once the pharmacological effect and the absence of side and toxic effects are proven, the test substance goes on to the clinical trial phase. Clinical trials involve research conducted on humans to discover or confirm the clinical and pharmacological effects observed during preclinical research. Besides, they identify adverse events and study the process of absorption, distribution, biotransformation, and secretion of the test substance. In the present study, we list the phytochemicals from the four reviewed plants that stood out during pre-clinical research and reviewed the clinical studies involving these compounds in the current literature. Table 5 summarizes these clinical studies.

Table 5. Clinical trials with secondary metabolites of fruit plants belonging to the Brazilian cerrado.

Species	Compounds	Investigated Pathology	Search Result	References
Talisia esculenta	Catechin (3)	Hypercholesterolemia	Hypolipidemic and hepatoprotective effect	[207]
		Obesity and type 2 diabetes	Reduction of visceral fat, blood pressure and cholesterol	[208]
		Coronary artery disease	Reduction of oxidized LDL in plasma	[209]
		Child obesity	Reduction in waist circumference, systolic blood pressure and LDL levels	[210]
	Epicatechin (4)	Vascular dysfunction	Improved cardiovascular health	[211]
		Arterial hypertension	Ineffective on blood pressure, blood lipid profile and glucose control	[212]
		Cardiovascular diseases	Cardioprotective effect and improved insulin resistance	[213]
	Quercetin (2)	Arterial hypertension	Lowering blood pressure	[214]
		Increase in free radicals produced after eccentric exercises	Antioxidant and protective effect	[215]
		Hyperuricemia	Significant reduction in elevated plasma uric acid concentrations	[216]
		Rheumatoid arthritis	Significant improvement in clinical symptoms and reduced levels of TNF-α	[217]
		Gout and primary hypertension	Improvement of echocardiographic parameters, left ventricular diastolic function, purine metabolism, renal function, and normalization of blood pressure	[218]
		Overweight or obesity with polycystic ovary syndrome	Significant reduction in gene expression and plasma resistin concentration and considerable decrease in the level of luteinizing hormone and testosterone	[219]
		β-Thalassemia major	Reduced iron overload	[220]
	Chlorogenic acid (13)	Polycystic ovary syndrome	Improvement of insulin resistance and hormonal profile of women with the syndrome.	[221]
		Neuromuscular dysfunction	Improvement of neuromuscular performance	[222]
		Dyslipidemia	Decrease in cholesterol, triglycerides and LDL values, and increased HDL levels	[223]
		Sarcoidosis	Reduction of oxidative stress and inflammation	[224]
		Hypertension and fat accumulation	Reduction of blood pressure and body fat	[225]
		Cognitive dysfunction	Improvement of cognitive functions	[226]
		Arterial hypertension	Reduction of systolic and diastolic blood pressure	[227]

Table 5. *Cont.*

Species	Compounds	Investigated Pathology	Search Result	References
Brosimum gaudichaudii	Psoralen (**25**)	Fungal ringworm	Oral treatment with a low dose and low frequency of psoralen-UV-A, was safe and effective	[228]
		Chronic palmar eczema of the hand	Reduced severity of chronic palmar eczema of the hand	[229]
		Chronic moderate to severe plaque psoriasis	Psoralen plus ultraviolet A, are therapeutic options for chronic moderate to severe plaque psoriasis	[230]
		Cutaneous mastocytosis	Efficacy for the treatment of moderate to severe chronic psoriasis	[231]
		Vitiligo	Increased extent of skin repigmentation	[232]
	Bergaptene (**26**)	Psoriasis	Reduction of signs and symptoms of psoriasis	[233]
Genipa americana	Genipin (**55**)	Absence of clinical trials in the current literature	–	–
	Asystasioside D (**39**)			
	Geniposidic acid (**40**)			
	Tarenoside (**41**)			
Bromelia antiacantha	Daucosterol (**63**)	Anogenital warts	The treatment led to the elimination of injury	[234]
		Pulmonary Tuberculosis	Improvement in imaging tests and weight gain of the patient	[235]

All the species reviewed in the present study showed promising therapeutic potential due to the presence of phytochemicals. The species with the highest number of clinical trials found in the literature was *Talisia esculenta*. In general, clinical trials involving medicinal plants or their isolated secondary metabolites are scarce. However, studies like these are necessary for the development of more efficient pharmaceutical products for the treatment of various disorders that affect humans, in addition to being crucial for the health professional to be safe in prescribing these drugs.

8. Conclusions

The species under study reveal great economic importance not only in the consumption and marketing of fruits, but also as sources for the extraction of molecules with significant bioactive potential, which can be used as phytotherapeutic agents or as raw materials for the development of new drugs. *T. esculenta* has high concentration of phenolic acids, flavonoids, and terpenes, justifying its antioxidant, anti-tumor, anti-inflammatory and antimicrobial action reported by several studies, lacking studies that investigate toxicity associated with the ingestion of its seeds.

Future studies should perform quantitative analyses and isolation of substances from *B. gaudichaudii*, *G. americana* and *B. antiacantha*, favoring the understanding of the antiproliferative, antimicrobial, anti-inflammatory, neuroprotective, and photosensitizing effects associated with their extracts. Therefore, fruits of the Brazilian Cerrado offer an immeasurable richness of molecules with biological activity of great interest to the pharmaceutical and cosmetic industries, in addition to the possibility of marketing of fruits and their by-products. The knowledge of the mechanism of action of substances isolated in these extracts enables correlating concentration, effectiveness, desirable and side effects, which is fundamental for the establishment of a therapeutic planning and interventions in case of intoxication.

Author Contributions: The article was divided by topics and distributed to each researcher according to their affinity for the themes. All authors contributed equally to the writing and revision of the manuscript. G.R.V.-B.: General guidance for the development of the manuscript; Conceptualization; Investigation; Methodology; Project administration; Software (Making figures); Supervision; Validation; Visualization; Roles/Writing—original draft; Writing—review and editing. A.T.d.C., M.M.P., M.S.C., G.C.B., A.M.M., V.C.R., and S.A.O.: Investigation; Methodology; Validation; Visualization; Roles/Writing—original draft; Writing—review and editing. In addition to what was previously mentioned, all authors made due contributions to the conception or design of the work; or the acquisition, analysis, or interpretation of data; or the creation of new software used in the work; or have drafted the work or substantively revised it; has approved the submitted version and; agrees to be personally accountable for the author's own contributions and for ensuring that questions related to the accuracy or integrity of any part of the work, even ones in which the author was not personally involved, are appropriately investigated, resolved, and documented in the literature. All authors have read and agreed to the published version of the manuscript.

Funding: This research received no external funding.

Acknowledgments: We especially thank the Research Group on Development of Pharmaceutical Products (P&DProFar) for the partnership and support in the development of the manuscript.

Conflicts of Interest: The authors declare no conflict of interest.

References

1. Reis, A.F.; Schmiele, M. Características e potencialidades dos frutos do Cerrado na indústria de alimentos. *Brazilian J. Food Technol.* **2019**, *22*, e2017150. [CrossRef]
2. Mohanraj, K.; Karthikeyan, B.S.; Vivek-Ananth, R.P.; Chand, R.P.B.; Aparna, S.R.; Mangalapandi, P.; Samal, A. IMPPAT: A curated database of Indian Medicinal Plants, Phytochemistry And Therapeutics. *Sci. Rep.* **2018**, *8*, 4329. [CrossRef]
3. Souza, M.C.; Franco, A.C.; Haridasan, M.; Rossato, D.R.; de Araújo, J.F.; Morellato, L.P.C.; Habermann, G. The length of the dry season may be associated with leaf scleromorphism in cerrado plants. *Ann. Braz. Acad. Sci.* **2015**, *87*, 1691–1699. [CrossRef]
4. Petropoulos, S.A.; Karkanis, A.; Martins, N.; Ferreira, I.C.F.R. Halophytic herbs of the Mediterranean basin: An alternative approach to health. *Food Chem. Toxicol.* **2018**, *114*, 155–169. [CrossRef]

5. Bailão, E.; Devilla, I.; da Conceição, E.; Borges, L. Bioactive Compounds Found in Brazilian Cerrado Fruits. *Int. J. Mol. Sci.* **2015**, *16*, 23760–23783. [CrossRef]

6. Roa, F.; de Telles, M.P.C. The Cerrado (Brazil) plant cytogenetics database. *Comp. Cytogenet.* **2017**, *11*, 285–297. [CrossRef]

7. Klink, C.A.; Machado, R.B. Conservation of the Brazilian Cerrado. *Conserv. Biol.* **2005**, *19*, 707–713. [CrossRef]

8. Villas-Boas, G.R.; dos Santos, A.C.; Souza, R.I.C.; Araújo, F.H.S.; Traesel, G.K.; Marcelino, J.M.; Silveira, A.P.S.; Farinelli, B.C.F.; Cardoso, C.A.L.; de Lacerda, R.B.; et al. Preclinical safety evaluation of the ethanolic extract from guavira fruits (Campomanesia pubescens (D.C.) O. BERG) in experimental models of acute and short-term toxicity in rats. *Food Chem. Toxicol.* **2018**, *118*, 1–12. [CrossRef]

9. Zappi, D.C.; Filardi, F.L.R.; Leitman, P.; Souza, V.C.; Walter, B.M.T.; Pirani, J.R.; Morim, M.P.; Queiroz, L.P.; Cavalcanti, T.B.; Mansano, V.F.; et al. Growing knowledge: An overview of Seed Plant diversity in Brazil. *Rodriguésia* **2015**, *66*, 1085–1113. [CrossRef]

10. Schiassi, M.C.E.V.; de Souza, V.R.; Lago, A.M.T.; Campos, L.G.; Queiroz, F. Fruits from the Brazilian Cerrado region: Physico-chemical characterization, bioactive compounds, antioxidant activities, and sensory evaluation. *Food Chem.* **2018**, *245*, 305–311. [CrossRef]

11. Judd, W.S.; Campbell, C.S.; Kellogg, E.A.; Ste, P.F. *Sistemática Vegetal: Um Enfoque Filogenético*, 3rd ed.; Artmed: Porto Alegre, Brazil, 2009.

12. Turland, N.J.; Wiersema, J.H.; Barrie, F.R.; Greuter, W.; Knapp, S.; Kusber, W.-H.; Li, D.-Z.; Marhold, K.; May, T.W.; McNeill, J.; et al. *International Code of Nomenclature for Algae, fuNgi, and Plants*; Turland, N., Wiersema, J., Barrie, F., Greuter, W., Hawksworth, D., Herendeen, P., Knapp, S., Kusber, W.-H., Li, D.-Z., Marhold, K., et al., Eds.; Regnum Vegetabile; Koeltz Botanical Books: Glashütten, Germany, 2018; Volume 159, ISBN 9783946583165.

13. Miloski, J.; Somner, G.V.; Salimena, F.R.G.; Menini Neto, L. Sapindaceae na Serra Negra, Minas Gerais, Brasil. *Rodriguésia* **2017**, *68*, 671–690. [CrossRef]

14. Guarim, G.N.; Santana, S.R.; Silva, J.V.B. Repertório botânico da "Pitombeira" (*Talisia esculenta* (A. ST.-HIL.) Radlk. - Sapindaceae). *Acta Amaz.* **2003**, *33*, 237–242. [CrossRef]

15. Coutinho, D.J.G.; Ishiguro, M.A.; da Silva, T.G.; Mendes, L.C.A.; de Oliveira, A.F.M. Levantamento de espécies de Sapindaceae ocorrentes no estado de Pernambuco. *JEPEX* **2013**. Available online: http://www.eventosufrpe.com.br/2013/cd/resumos/R1350-3.pdf (accessed on 21 July 2020).

16. de Pereira, L.A.; Amorim, B.S.; Alves, M.; Somner, G.V.; de Barbosa, M.R.V. Flora da Usina São José, Igarassu, Pernambuco: Sapindaceae. *Rodriguésia* **2016**, *67*, 1047–1059. [CrossRef]

17. Urdampilleta, J.D. Estudo Citotaxonômico em Espécies de Paullinieae (Sapindaceae). Ph.D. Thesis, Universidade Estadual de Campinas, Campinas, Brazil, 2009.

18. De Sena, L.H.M.; Matos, V.P.; de Medeiros, J.É.; Santos, H.H.D.; Rocha, A.P.; Ferreira, R.L.C. Storage of pitombeira seeds [*Talisia esculenta* (A. St. Hil) Radlk - Sapindaceae] in different enviroments and packagings. *Rev. Árvore* **2016**, *40*, 435–445. [CrossRef]

19. Dos Santos, W.L.; Freire, M.D.G.M.; Bogorni, P.C.; Vendramim, J.D.; Macedo, M.L.R. Effect of the aqueous extracts of the seeds of *Talisia esculenta* and Sapindus saponaria on fall armyworm. *Brazilian Arch. Biol. Technol.* **2008**, *51*, 373–383. [CrossRef]

20. Dos Sena, L.H.M. Conservação de Sementes e Produção de Mudas de Pitombeira (*Talisia esculenta* (A. St. Hil.) Radlk.). Master's Thesis, Universidade Federal Rural de Pernambuco, Recife, Pernambuco, 2014.

21. Brasil. *Alimentos Regionais Brasileiros*, 2nd ed.; Ministério da Saúde: Brasília, Brazil, 2015; ISBN 8533404921.

22. Lorenzi, H. Árvores Brasileiras: Manual de Identificação e Cultivo de plAntas Arbóreas nativas do Brasil. *Plantarum* **2009**, *2*, 384.

23. Bieski, I.G.C.; Rios Santos, F.; de Oliveira, R.M.; Espinosa, M.M.; Macedo, M.; Albuquerque, U.P.; de Oliveira Martins, D.T. Ethnopharmacology of Medicinal Plants of the Pantanal Region (Mato Grosso, Brazil). *Evidence-Based Complement. Altern. Med.* **2012**. [CrossRef]

24. Vásquez, S.P.F.; de Mendonça, M.S.; do Noda, S.N. Etnobotânica de plantas medicinais em comunidades ribeirinhas do Município de Manacapuru, Amazonas, Brasil. *Acta Amaz.* **2014**, *44*, 457–472. [CrossRef]

25. Badke, M.R.; de Budó, M.L.D.; da Silva, F.M.; Ressel, L.B. Plantas medicinais na prática do cotidiano popular. *Esc. Anna Nery* **2011**, *15*, 132–139. [CrossRef]

26. De Nascimento, J.M.; da Conceição, G.M. Plantas medicinais e indicações terapêuticas da comunidade quilombola Olho d'água do Raposo, Caxias, Maranhão, Brasil. *Rev. Biol. e Farmácia* **2011**, *6*. [CrossRef]

27. Oliveira, V.B.; Zuchetto, M.; Oliveira, C.F.; Paula, C.S.; Duarte, A.F.S.; Miguel, M.D.; Miguel, O.G. Efeito de diferentes técnicas extrativas no rendimento, atividade antioxidante, doseamentos totais e no perfil por clae-dad de Dicksonia sellowiana (Presl.). Hook, dicksoniaceae. *Rev. Bras. Plantas Med.* **2016**, *18*, 230–239. [CrossRef]

28. Ribeiro, S.F. Influência de malhas fotoconversoras nos aspectos anatômicos e fisiológicos de mudas de *Talisia esculenta* (A. St.-Hil.) Radlk. Master's Thesis, Universidade Federal de Lavras, Lavras, Brazil, 2014.

29. Silva, M.L.M. Biologia reprodutiva e maturação de sementes de *Talisia esculenta* (Cambess.) Radlk. Ph.D. Thesis, Universidade Federal da Paraíba, Areia, Brazil, 2019.

30. Alves, E.U.; Silva, K.B.; Gonçalves, E.P.; Cardoso, E.D.A.; Alves, A.U. Germination and vigour of *Talisia esculenta* (St. Hil) Radlk seeds as a function of different fermentation periods. *Semin. Ciências Agrárias* **2009**, *30*, 761. [CrossRef]

31. Teixeira, N.; Melo, J.C.S.; Batista, L.F.; Paula-Souza, J.; Fronza, P.; Brandão, M.G.L. Edible fruits from Brazilian biodiversity: A review on their sensorial characteristics versus bioactivity as tool to select research. *Food Res. Int.* **2019**, *119*, 325–348. [CrossRef]

32. Neri-Numa, I.A.; de Carvalho-Silva, L.B.; Macedo Ferreira, J.E.; Tomazela Machado, A.R.; Malta, L.G.; Tasca Gois Ruiz, A.L.; de Carvalho, J.E.; Pastore, G.M. Preliminary evaluation of antioxidant, antiproliferative and antimutagenic activities of pitomba (*Talisia esculenta*). *LWT-Food Sci. Technol.* **2014**, *59*, 1233–1238. [CrossRef]

33. Souza, M.P. Caracterização química e avaliação do potencial antioxidante dos frutos mari-mari (*Cassia leiandra*), pajurá (*Couepia bracteosa*) e pitomba (*Talisia esculenta*). Master'sThesis, Universidade Federal do Amazonas, Manaus, Brazil, 2016.

34. De Souza, M.P.; Bataglion, G.A.; da Silva, F.M.A.; de Almeida, R.A.; Paz, W.H.P.; Nobre, T.A.; Marinho, J.V.N.; Salvador, M.J.; Fidelis, C.H.V.; Acho, L.D.R.; et al. Phenolic and aroma compositions of pitomba fruit (*Talisia esculenta* Radlk.) assessed by LC–MS/MS and HS-SPME/GC–MS. *Food Res. Int.* **2016**, *83*, 87–94. [CrossRef]

35. Tirloni, C.A.S.; Silva, A.O.; Palozi, R.A.C.; Vasconcelos, P.C.D.P.; Souza, R.I.C.; Dos Santos, A.C.; De Almeida, V.P.; Budel, J.M.; De Souza, L.M.; Gasparotto, A. Biological Characterization of an Edible Species from Brazilian Biodiversity: From Pharmacognostic Data to Ethnopharmacological Investigation. *J. Med. Food* **2018**, *21*, 1276–1287. [CrossRef]

36. Júnior, J.H.S. Avaliação da atividade antimicrobiana do extrato hidroetanólico de *Talisia esculenta* Radlk. Master's Thesis, Universidade Federal do Maranhão, São Luís, Brazil, 2019.

37. Sturm, S.; Seger, C. Liquid chromatography–nuclear magnetic resonance coupling as alternative to liquid chromatography–mass spectrometry hyphenations: Curious option or powerful and complementary routine tool? *J. Chromatogr. A* **2012**, *1259*, 50–61. [CrossRef]

38. Taiz, L.; Zeiger, E. *Fisiologia Vegetal*, 5th ed.; Artmed: Porto Alegre, Brazil, 2013.

39. Silva, M.R.; Lacerda, D.B.C.L.; Santos, G.G.; Martins, D.M.D.O. Caracterização química de frutos nativos do cerrado. *Ciência Rural* **2008**, *38*, 1790–1793. [CrossRef]

40. Marin, A.M.F.; Siqueira, E.M.A.; Arruda, S.F. Minerals, phytic acid and tannin contents of 18 fruits from the Brazilian savanna. *Int. J. Food Sci. Nutr.* **2009**, *60*, 177–187. [CrossRef]

41. Yi, Y.-S. Regulatory Roles of Flavonoids on Inflammasome Activation during Inflammatory Responses. *Mol. Nutr. Food Res.* **2018**, *62*, e1800147. [CrossRef] [PubMed]

42. Kelley, N.; Jeltema, D.; Duan, Y.; He, Y. The NLRP3 Inflammasome: An Overview of Mechanisms of Activation and Regulation. *Int.J. Mol. Sci.* **2019**, *20*, 3328. [CrossRef] [PubMed]

43. Kumar, H.; Kawai, T.; Akira, S. Pathogen Recognition by the Innate Immune. *Int. Rev. Immunol.* **2011**, *30*, 16–34. [CrossRef] [PubMed]

44. Franchi, L.; Warner, N.; Viani, K.; Nuñez, G. Function of Nod-like Receptors in Microbial Recognition and Host Defense. *Immunol. Rev.* **2009**, *227*, 106–128. [CrossRef]

45. Davis, B.K.; Wen, H.; Ting, J.P. The Inflammasome NLRs in Immunity, Inflammation, and Associated Diseases. *Annu. Rev. Immunol.* **2011**, *29*, 707–735. [CrossRef]

46. Martinon, F.; Mayor, A.; Tschopp, J. The Inflammasomes: Guardians of the Body. *Annu. Rev. Immunol.* **2009**, *27*, 229–265. [CrossRef]

47. Dinarello, C.A. Immunological and Inflammatory Functions of the Interleukin-1 Family. *Annu. Rev. Immunol.* **2009**, *27*, 519–550. [CrossRef]

48. Turner, M.D.; Nedjai, B.; Hurst, T.; Pennington, D.J. Cytokines and chemokines: At the crossroads of cell signalling and inflammatory disease. *Biochim. Biophys. Acta J.* **2014**, *1843*, 2563–2582. [CrossRef]

49. Shuang, L.; Wen-Qing, Y.; TAO Ye-Zheng, M.L.; Xing, L. Serotonergic neurons in the median raphe nucleus mediate anxiety- and depression- like behavior. *Acta Physiol. Sin.* **2018**, *70*, 228–236. [CrossRef]

50. Jhang, J.-J.; Lu, C.-C.; Ho, C.-Y.; Cheng, Y.-T.; Yen, G.-C. Protective Effects of Catechin against Monosodium Urate-Induced Inflammation through the Modulation of NLRP3 Inflammasome Activation. *J. Agric. Food Chem.* **2015**, *63*, 7343–7352. [CrossRef]

51. Zhang, Y.; Liu, L.; Sun, D.; He, Y.; Jiang, Y.; Cheng, K.W.; Chen, F. DHA protects against monosodium urate-induced inflammation through modulation of oxidative stress. *Food Funct.* **2019**, *10*, 4010–4021. [CrossRef] [PubMed]

52. Zhou, R.; Tardivel, A.; Thorens, B.; Choi, I.; Tschopp, J. Thioredoxin-interacting protein links oxidative stress to inflammasome activation. *Nat. Immunol.* **2009**, *11*, 136–140. [CrossRef] [PubMed]

53. Zhou, R.; Yazdi, A.S.; Menu, P. A role for mitochondria in NLRP3 inflammasome activation. *Nature* **2011**, *469*, 221–225. [CrossRef] [PubMed]

54. Owona, B.A.; Abia, W.A.; Moundipa, P.F. Natural compounds flavonoids as modulators of inflammasomes in chronic diseases. *Int. Immunopharmacol.* **2020**, *84*, 106498. [CrossRef] [PubMed]

55. Leopoldini, M.; Marino, T.; Russo, N.; Toscano, M. Antioxidant Properties of Phenolic Compounds: H-Atom versus Electron Transfer Mechanism. *J. Phys. Chem.* **2004**, *108*, 4916–4922. [CrossRef]

56. Badhani, B.; Sharma, N.; Kakkar, R. Gallic acid: A versatile antioxidant with promising therapeutic and industrial applications. *RSC Adv.* **2015**, *5*, 27540–27557. [CrossRef]

57. Katz, D.L.; Doughty, K.; Ali, A. Cocoa and Chocolate in Human Health and Disease. *Antioxid. ad Redos Sinaling* **2011**, *15*, 2779–2811. [CrossRef]

58. Wang, C.; Pan, Y.; Zhang, Q.-Y.; Wang, F.-M.; Kong, L.-D. Quercetin and Allopurinol Ameliorate Kidney Injury in STZ-Treated Rats with Regulation of Renal NLRP3 Inflammasome Activation and Lipid Accumulation. *PLoS ONE* **2012**, *7*. [CrossRef]

59. Xu, D.; Hu, M.; Wang, Y.; Cui, Y. Antioxidant Activities of Quercetin and Its Complexes for Medicinal Application. *Molecules* **2019**, *24*, 1123. [CrossRef]

60. Kawamura, K.; Qi, F.; Kobayashi, J. Potential relationship between the biological effects of low-dose irradiation and mitochondrial ROS production. *J. Radiat. Res.* **2018**, 1–7. [CrossRef]

61. Zhao, Y.; Hu, X.; Liu, Y.; Dong, S.; Wen, Z.; He, W.; Zhang, S.; Huang, Q. ROS signaling under metabolic stress: Cross-talk between AMPK and AKT pathway. *Mol. Cancer* **2017**, *16*, 1–12. [CrossRef] [PubMed]

62. Jalmi, S.K.; Sinha, A.K. ROS mediated MAPK signaling in abiotic and biotic stress- striking similarities and differences. *Front. Plant Sci.* **2015**, *6*, 1–9. [CrossRef] [PubMed]

63. Stoiber, W.; Obermayer, A.; Steinbacher, P.; Krautgartner, W. The Role of Reactive Oxygen Species (ROS) in the Formation of Extracellular Traps (ETs) in Humans. *Biomolecules* **2015**, *5*, 702–723. [CrossRef] [PubMed]

64. Vurusaner, B.; Poli, G.; Basaga, H. Tumor suppressor genes and ROS: Complex networks of interactions. *Free Radic. Biol. Med.* **2012**, *52*, 7–18. [CrossRef]

65. Pei, K.; Ou, J.; Huang, J.; Ou, S. p-Coumaric acid and its conjugates: Dietary sources, pharmacokinetic properties and biological activities. *J. Sci. Food Agric.* **2016**, *96*, 2952–2962. [CrossRef]

66. Pinheiro, A.Q.; Melo, D.F.; Macedo, L.M.; Freire, M.G.M.; Rocha, M.F.G.; Sidrim, J.J.C.; Brilhante, R.S.N.; Teixeira, E.H.; Campello, C.C.; Pinheiro, D.C.S.N.; et al. Antifungal and marker effects of *Talisia esculenta* lectin on Microsporum canis in vitro. *J. Appl. Microbiol.* **2009**, *107*, 2063–2069. [CrossRef]

67. Oliveira, M.R.T.R.; Napimoga, M.H.; Cogo, K.; Gonçalves, R.B.; Macedo, M.L.R.; Freire, M.G.M.; Groppo, F.C. Inhibition of bacterial adherence to saliva-coated through plant lectins. *J. Oral Sci.* **2007**, *49*, 141–145. [CrossRef]

68. Riet-Correa, F.; Medeiros, R.M.T.; Pfister, J.A.; Mendonça, F.S. Toxic plants affecting the nervous system of ruminants and horses in Brazil. *Pesqui. Veterinária Bras.* **2017**, *37*, 1357–1368. [CrossRef]

69. Riet-Correa, F.; Bezerra, C.W.; Medeiros, M.A.; da Silva, T.R.; Neto, E.G.M.; Medeiros, R.M.T. Poisoning by *Talisia esculenta* (A. St.-Hil.) Radlk in sheep and cattle. *J. Vet. Diagnostic Investig.* **2014**, *26*, 412–417. [CrossRef]

70. Melo, J.K.A.; Soares, G.S.L.; Ramos, T.R.R.; Almeida, V.M.; Nascimento, A.L.O.; Silva Filho, G.B.; Chaves, H.A.S.; Mendonça, F.S. Spontaneous poisoning by *Talisia esculenta* in cattle. *Pesqui. Veterinária Bras.* **2019**, *39*, 949–953. [CrossRef]

71. Freire, M.G.; Desouza, I.; Silva, A.C.; Macedo, M.L.; Lima, M.; Tamashiro, W.M.S.; Antunes, E.; Marangoni, S. Inflammatory responses induced in mice by lectin from *Talisia esculenta* seeds. *Toxicon* **2003**, *42*, 275–280. [CrossRef]

72. Da Mota, T.M.; Silva, A.E.V.N.; de Melo Filho, E.V.; de Siqueira, J.O.; Ferreira, D.R.C.; Groschke, H.M.; da Braz, R.S.; Teixeira, M.W. Intoxicação por sementes de pitombeira (*Talisia esculenta*) em um cão—Relato de caso. *Clín. Vet.* **2016**, *21*, 78–84.

73. De Castro, R.M. Flora da Bahia–Moraceae. Master's Thesis, Universidade Estadual de Feira de Santana, Florianópolis, Brazil, 2006.

74. Leite, V.G.; Mansano, V.F.; Pádua Teixeira, S. Floral development of Moraceae species with emphasis on the perianth and androecium. *Flora* **2018**, *240*, 116–132. [CrossRef]

75. De Filho, A.B.L.; da Silva, J.M.; dos de Santana, M.A.; de Melo, E.M. Espécies da família moraceae com potencial fitoterápico em dois fragmento de floresta urbana no município de camaragibe. *JEPEX-UFRPE* **2013**. Available online: http://www.eventosufrpe.com.br/2013/cd/resumos/R0533-1.pdf (accessed on 21 July 2020).

76. Jacomassi, E.; Moscheta, I.S.; Machado, S.R. Morfoanatomia e histoquímica de órgãos reprodutivos de *Brosimum gaudichaudii* (Moraceae). *Rev. Bras. Botânica* **2010**, *33*, 115–129. [CrossRef]

77. Mitsuko Aoyama, E.; Mazzoni-Viveiros, C. ADAPTAÇÕES ESTRUTURAIS DAS PLANTAS AO AMBIENTE 2006. Available online: http://www.biodiversidade.pgibt.ibot.sp.gov.br/Web/pdf/Adaptacoes_estruturais_das_Plantas_ao_Ambiente_Elisa_Aoyama.pdf (accessed on 21 July 2020).

78. Ribeiro, J.E.L.S.; Pederneiras, L.C. Brosimum in Flora do Brasil 2020 em construção. Jardim Botânico do Rio de Janeiro. Available online: http://floradobrasil.jbrj.gov.br/ (accessed on 26 June 2020).

79. Palhares, D.; de Paula, J.E.; dos Santos Silveira, C.E. Morphology of stem and subterranean system of *Brosimum gaudichaudii* (Moraceae). *Acta Botanica Hungarica*. **2006**, *48*, 89–101. [CrossRef]

80. Da Cunha, L.C.; de Paula, J.R.; de Sá, V.A.; da e Amorim, M.E.P.; Barros, I.C.M.; Brito, L.A.B.; da Silveira, N. Acute toxicity of *Brosimum gaudichaudii* Trécul. root extract in mice: Determination of both approximate and median lethal doses. *Rev. Bras. Farmacogn.* **2008**, *18*, 532–538. [CrossRef]

81. De Faria, R.A.P.G.; de Coelho, M.F.B.; de Albuquerque, M.C.F.; de Azevedo, R.A.B. Fenologia de *Brosimum gaudichaudii* TRÉCUL. (Moraceae) no cerrado de Mato Grosso. *Ciência Florest.* **2015**, *25*, 67–75. [CrossRef]

82. Jacomassi, E.; Moscheta, I.S.; Machado, S.R. Morfoanatomia e histoquímica de *Brosimum gaudichaudii* Trécul (Moraceae). *Acta Bot. Brasilica* **2007**, *21*, 575–597. [CrossRef]

83. Jacomassi, E. Morfoanatomia e histoquímica de orgãos vegetativos reprodutivos de *Brosimum gaudichaudii* Trécul (Moraceae). *Inst. Biociências – Dep. Botânica* **2006**.

84. Faria, R.A.P.G.; Silva, A.N.; Albuquerque, M.C.F.; Coelho, M.F.B. Características biométricas e emergência de plântulas de *Brosimum gaudichaudii* Tréc. oriundas de diferentes procedências do cerrado mato-grossense. *Rev. Bras. Plantas Med.* **2009**, *11*, 414–421. [CrossRef]

85. Ribeiro, R.V.; Bieski, I.G.C.; Balogun, S.O.; de Martins, D.T.O. Ethnobotanical study of medicinal plants used by Ribeirinhos in the North Araguaia microregion, Mato Grosso, Brazil. *J. Ethnopharmacol.* **2017**, *205*, 69–102. [CrossRef] [PubMed]

86. Rodrigues, V.E.G.; Carvalho, D.A. Levantamento etnobotânico de plantas medicinais no domínio dos cerrados na região do Alto Rio Grande - Minas Gerais. *Rev. Bras. Plantas Med.* **2007**, *9*, 17–35.

87. de Braga, C.M. *Histórico da Utilização de Plantas Medicinais*; Monography; Universidade de Brasília/Universidade Federal de Gioás: Brasília, Brazil, 2011.

88. dos Passos, M.M.B.; da Albino, R.C.; Feitoza-Silva, M.; de Oliveira, D.R. A disseminação cultural das garrafadas no Brasil: Um paralelo entre medicina popular e legislação sanitária. *Saúde em Debate* **2018**, *42*, 248–262. [CrossRef]

89. Da Borges, J.C. Atividade antimicrobiana de extrato de *Brosimum gaudichaudii* trécul. contra bactérias isoladas de lesões de pés diabéticos. Master's Thesis, Universidade Federal de Tocantins, Palmas, Brazil, 2016.

90. Martins, D. Morfologia e Anatomia do caule e do sistema subterrâneo de *Brosimum gaudichaudii* Tréc. (Moraceae). Master's Thesis, Universidade de Brasília, Brasília, Brazil, 2004.

91. Lourenço, M.V. Estudo comparativo dos constituintes químicos de *Brosimum gaudichaudii* Trécul e do medicamento "V.". Ph.D. Thesis, Universidade Estadual Paulista, Araraquara, Brazil, 2001.

92. Martins, F.S.; Pascoa, H.; De Paula, J.R.; Da Conceição, E.C. Technical aspects on production of fluid extract from *Brosimum gaudichaudii* Trécul roots. *Pharmacogn. Mag.* **2015**, *11*, 226–231. [CrossRef]

93. Vieira, I.J.C.; Mathias, L.; Monteiro, V.D.F.F.; Braz-Filho, R.; Rodrigues-Filho, E. A New Coumarln from *Brosimum gaudichaudii* Trecul. *Nat. Prod. Lett.* **1999**, *13*, 47–52. [CrossRef]

94. De Monteiro, V.F.F.; Mathias, L.; Vieira, I.J.C.; Schripsema, J.; Braz-Filho, R. Prenylated Coumarins, Chalcone and New Cinnamic Acid and Dihydrocinnamic Acid Derivatives from *Brosimum gaudichaudii*. *J. Braz. Chem. Soc.* **2002**, *13*, 281–287. [CrossRef]

95. Land, L.R.B.; Borges, F.M.; Borges, D.O.; Pascoal, G.B. Composição centesimal, compostos bioativos e parâmetros físico-químicos da mama-cadela (*Brosimum gaudichaudii* Tréc) proveniente do Cerrado Mineiro. *DEMETRA Aliment. Nutr. Saúde* **2017**, *12*, 509–518. [CrossRef]

96. Silva, S.M.F.Q.; Pinheiro, S.M.B.; Queiroz, M.V.F.; Pranchevicius, M.C.; Castro, J.G.D.; Perim, M.C.; Carreiro, S.C. Atividade in vitro de extratos brutos de duas espécies vegetais do cerrado sobre leveduras do gênero Candida. *Cien. Saude Colet.* **2012**, *17*, 1649–1656. [CrossRef]

97. Monteiro, J.M.; de Souza, J.S.N.; Neto, E.M.F.L.; Scopel, K.; Trindade, E.F. Does total tannin content explain the use value of spontaneous medicinal plants from the Brazilian semi-arid region? *Rev. Bras. Farmacogn.* **2014**, *24*, 116–123. [CrossRef]

98. De Moreira, C.C.S. *Atividade Antimicrobiana da Casca e Folha do Brosimum gaudichaudii Trécul*; Monography; Centro Universitário Luterano de Palmas: Palmas, Brazil, 2019.

99. De Quintão, W.S.C. Desenvolvimento, caracterização e avaliação in vitro de nanoemulsões O/A a partir de extratos de *Brosimum gaudichaudii* (mama cadela) como alternativa parao tratamento tópico de vitiligo. Master's Thesis, Universidade de Brasília, Brasília, Brazil, 2018.

100. De Filho, A.C.P.M.; de Castro, C.F.S. Identificação das classes de metabólitos secundários nos extratos etanólicos foliares de *Brosimum gaudichaudii*, Qualea grandiflora, Rollinia laurifolia e Solanum cernuum. *Rev. Multitexto* **2019**, *7*, 22–32.

101. Leão, A.R.; da Cunha, L.C.; Parente, L.M.L.; Castro, L.C.M.; Chaul, A.; Carvalho, H.E.; Rodrigues, V.B.; Bastos, M.A. Avaliação clínica toxicólogica preliminar do Viticromin em pacientes com vitiligo. *Rev. Eletrônica Farmácia* **2007**, *2*, 15–23. [CrossRef]

102. Del Río, J.A.; Díaz, L.; García-Bernal, D.; Blanquer, M.; Ortuño, A.; Correal, E.; Moraleda, J.M. Furanocoumarins: Biomolecules of therapeutic interest. *Stud. Nat. Prod. Chem.* **2014**, *43*, 145–195.

103. Lang, K.S.; Muhm, A.; Moris, A.; Stevanovic, S.; Rammensee, H.-G.; Caroli, C.C.; Wernet, D.; Schittek, B.; Knauss-Scherwitz, E.; Garbe, C. HLA-A2 Restricted, Melanocyte-Specific CD8+ T Lymphocytes Detected in Vitiligo Patients are Related to Disease Activity and are Predominantly Directed Against MelanA/MART1. *J. Investig. Dermatol.* **2001**, *116*, 891–897. [CrossRef] [PubMed]

104. Mankarious, M.; Matthews, N.C.; Snowden, J.A.; Alfred, A. Extracorporeal Photopheresis (ECP) and the Potential of Novel Biomarkers in Optimizing Management of Acute and Chronic Graft vs. Host Disease (GvHD). *Front. Immunol.* **2020**, *11*, 1–14. [CrossRef] [PubMed]

105. Da Borges, J.C.; Perim, M.C.; de Castro, R.O.; de Araújo, T.A.S.; da Peixoto Sobrinho, T.J.S.; da Silva, A.C.O.; Mariano, S.M.B.; Carreiro, S.C.; da Pranchevicius, M.C.S. Evaluation of antibacterial activity of the bark and leaf extracts of *Brosimum gaudichaudii* Trécul against multidrug resistant strains. *Nat. Prod. Res.* **2017**, *31*, 2931–2935. [CrossRef]

106. Ferreira, P.C. Toxicidade e Atividade Tripanocida do Extrato Bruto de *Brosimum gaudichaudii* trécul (Moraceae) (Mama-cadela) no Pré-tratamento e tratamento de Camundongos Infectados por Trypanosoma cruzi. Master's Thesis, Universidade Federal de Uberlândia, Uberlândia, Brazil, 2008.

107. Jeon, S.J.; Park, H.J.; Gao, Q.; Lee, H.E.; Park, S.J.; Hong, E.; Jang, D.S.; Shin, C.Y.; Cheong, J.H.; Ryu, J.H. Positive effects of β-amyrin on pentobarbital-induced sleep in mice via GABAergic neurotransmitter system. *Behav. Brain Res.* **2015**, *291*, 232–236. [CrossRef]

108. Wei, C.-C.; Chang, C.-H.; Liao, V.H.-C. Anti-Parkinsonian effects of β-amyrin are regulated via LGG-1 involved autophagy pathway in Caenorhabditis elegans. *Phytomedicine* **2017**, *36*, 118–125. [CrossRef]

109. Sunil, C.; Irudayaraj, S.S.; Duraipandiyan, V.; Al-Dhabi, N.A.; Agastian, P.; Ignacimuthu, S. Antioxidant and free radical scavenging effects of β-amyrin isolated from S. cochinchinensis Moore. leaves. *Ind. Crops Prod.* **2014**, *61*, 510–516. [CrossRef]

110. Askari, V.R.; Fereydouni, N.; Baradaran Rahimi, V.; Askari, N.; Sahebkar, A.H.; Rahmanian-Devin, P.; Samzadeh-Kermani, A. β-Amyrin, the cannabinoid receptors agonist, abrogates mice brain microglial cells inflammation induced by lipopolysaccharide/interferon-γ and regulates Mφ1/Mφ2 balances. *Biomed. Pharmacother.* **2018**, *101*, 438–446. [CrossRef]

111. Dong, L.; Xu, W.-W.; Li, H.; Bi, K.-H. In vitro and in vivo anticancer effects of marmesin in U937 human leukemia cells are mediated via mitochondrial-mediated apoptosis, cell cycle arrest, and inhibition of cancer cell migration. *Oncol. Rep.* **2018**, *39*, 597–602. [CrossRef] [PubMed]

112. Kim, Y.-K.; Jeon, S.W. Neuroinflammation and the Immune-Kynurenine Pathway in Anxiety Disorders. *Curr. Neuropharmacol.* **2018**, *16*, 574–582. [CrossRef] [PubMed]

113. Marques, G.; Gutiérrez, A.; Del Río, J.C. Chemical characterization of lignin and lipophilic fractions from leaf fibers of curaua (Ananas erectifolius). *J. Agric. Food Chem.* **2007**, *55*, 1327–1336. [CrossRef]

114. Varanda, E.A.; Pozetti, G.L.; Lourenço, M.V.; Vilegas, W.; Raddi, M.S.G. Genotoxicity of *Brosimum gaudichaudii* measured by the Salmonella/microsome assay and chromosomal aberrations in CHO cells. *J. Ethnopharmacol.* **2002**, *81*, 257–264. [CrossRef]

115. e Amorim, M.E.P.; da Cunha, L.C.; da Silveira, N.A. Estudo Da Toxicidade Aguda E Subaguda De *Brosimum gaudichaudii* Trécul (Mamacadela) Em Ratos (Rattus Norvergicus) P.O. *Rev. Eletrônica Farmácia* **2004**, *1*, 52. [CrossRef]

116. Orme, M.L.; Breckenridge, A.M. Coumarin anticoagulants. In *Meyler's Side Effects of Drugs*; Elsevier: Dordrecht, The Netherlands, 2016; Volume 58, pp. 702–737.

117. Delprete, P.G.; Jardim, J.G. Systematics, taxonomy and floristics of Brazilian Rubiaceae: An overview about the current status and future challenges. *Rodriguésia* **2012**, *63*, 101–128. [CrossRef]

118. Baldin, T. Anatomia do Lenho do Genero Calycophyllum A. DC. (Rubiaceae). Master's Thesis, Universidade Federal de Santa Maria, Santa Maria, Brazil, 2015.

119. Bellé, A.S. Extração de Genipina a Partir do Jenipapo (*Genipa americana* Linnaeus) para Imobilização de Enzimas. Master's Thesis, Universidade Federal do Rio Grande do Sul, Proto Alegre, Brazil, 2017.

120. Erbano, M.; Duarte, M.R. Morfoanatomia de folha e caule de *Genipa americana* L., Rubiaceae. *Rev. Bras. Farmacogn.* **2010**, *20*, 825–832. [CrossRef]

121. Mielke, M.S.; de Almeida, A.-A.F.; Gomes, F.P.; Aguilar, M.A.G.; Mangabeira, P.A.O. Leaf gas exchange, chlorophyll fluorescence and growth responses of *Genipa americana* seedlings to soil flooding. *Environ. Exp. Bot.* **2003**, *50*, 221–231. [CrossRef]

122. Luzia, D.M.M. Propriedades funcionais de óleos extraídos de sementes de frutos do cerrado brasileiro. Master's Thesis, Universidade Estadual Paulista, São José do Rio Preto, Brazil, 2012.

123. Ferreira, W.R.; Ranal, M.; Dorneles, M.C.; Santana, D.G. Crescimento de mudas de *Genipa americana* L. submetidas a condições de pré-semeadura. *Braz. J. Bioc.* **2007**, *5*, 1026–1028.

124. Da Santos, W.C. Germinação e Vigor de Sementes de *Genipa americana* L. em Função do Estresse Hídrico em *Diferentes Temperaturas*; Monography; Universidade Federal da Paraíba: Areia, Brazil, 2018.

125. De Barbosa, D.A. Avaliação Fitoquímica e Farmacológica de *Genipa americana* L. (Rubiaceae). Master's Thesis, Universidade Federal do Rio de Janeiro, Rio de Janeiro, Brazil, 2008.

126. Santos, L.; Salles, M.; Pinto, C.; Pinto, O.; Rodrigues, I. O saber etnobotânico sobre plantas medicinais na comunidade da Brenha, Redenção, CE. *Agrar. Acad.* **2018**, *5*, 127–145. [CrossRef]

127. Souza, R.K.D.; Mendonça, A.C.A.M.; da Silva, M.A.P. Ethnobotanical, phytochemical and pharmacological aspects Rubiaceae species in Brazil. *Rev. Cuba. Plantas Med.* **2013**, *18*, 140–156.

128. Bieski, I.G.C.; Leonti, M.; Arnason, J.T.; Ferrier, J.; Rapinski, M.; Violante, I.M.P.; Balogun, S.O.; Pereira, J.F.C.A.; Figueiredo, R.D.C.F.; Lopes, C.R.A.S.; et al. Ethnobotanical study of medicinal plants by population of Valley of Juruena Region, Legal Amazon, Mato Grosso, Brazil. *J. Ethnopharmacol.* **2015**, *173*, 383–423. [CrossRef] [PubMed]

129. Cartaxo, S.L.; de Almeida Souza, M.M.; de Albuquerque, U.P. Medicinal plants with bioprospecting potential used in semi-arid northeastern Brazil. *J. Ethnopharmacol.* **2010**, *131*, 326–342. [CrossRef] [PubMed]

130. Yazbek, P.B.; Tezoto, J.; Cassas, F.; Rodrigues, E. Plants used during maternity, menstrual cycle and other women's health conditions among Brazilian cultures. *J. Ethnopharmacol.* **2016**, *179*, 310–331. [CrossRef]

131. Odonne, G.; Valadeau, C.; Alban-Castillo, J.; Stien, D.; Sauvain, M.; Bourdy, G. Medical ethnobotany of the Chayahuita of the Paranapura basin (Peruvian Amazon). *J. Ethnopharmacol.* **2013**, *146*, 127–153. [CrossRef]

132. De Carvalho, T.L.G.S. Etnofarmacologia e fisiologia de plantas medicinais do quilombo Tiningú, Santarém, Pará. Master's Thesis, Universidade Federal do Oeste do Pará, Santarém, Brazil.

133. Bueno, M.J.A.; Martínez, B.B.; Bueno, J.C. *Manual de Plantas Medicinais e Fitoterápicos: Utilizados na Cicatrização de Feridas*; UNIVÁS: Pouso Alegre, Brazil, 2016; ISBN 9788533415973.

134. Rodrigues, V.G.S. *Cultivo, Uso e Manipulação de Plantas Medicinais*; Embrapa-Empres: Rondônia, Brazil, 2004; Volume 1, pp. 1–25.

135. Santiago, E.F.; Paoli, A.A.S. Respostas morfológicas em Guibourtia hymenifolia (Moric.) J. Leonard (Fabaceae) e *Genipa americana* L. (Rubiaceae), submetidas ao estresse por deficiência nutricional e alagamento do substrato. *Rev. Bras. Botânica* **2007**, *30*, 131–140. [CrossRef]

136. De Crestana, C.S.M. Ecologia e polinização de *Genipa americana* L. (Rubiaceae) na estação ecológica de Moji-guaçu, estado de São Paulo. *Rev. Inst. Flor* **1995**, *7*, 169–195.

137. Carvalho, P.E.R. *Jenipapeiro*; Embrapa-Bol: Colombo, Brazil, 2003; Volume 14, pp. 2–14. ISSN 1517-5278.

138. De Carvalho, J.E.U.; do Nascimento, W.M.O. Sensibilidade de sementes de jenipapo (*Genipa americana* L.) ao dessecamento e ao congelamento. *Rev. Bras. Frutic.* **2000**, *22*, 53–56.

139. Silva, L.; Alves, J.; da Silva Siqueira, E.; de Souza Neto, M.; Abreu, L.; Tavares, J.; Porto, D.; de Santis Ferreira, L.; Demarque, D.; Lopes, N.; et al. Isolation and Identification of the Five Novel Flavonoids from *Genipa americana* Leaves. *Molecules* **2018**, *23*, 2521. [CrossRef]

140. Ono, M.; Ueno, M.; Masuoka, C.; Ikeda, T.; Nohara, T. Iridoid Glucosides from the Fruit of *Genipa americana*. *Chem. Pharm. Bull. (Tokyo)* **2005**, *53*, 1342–1344. [CrossRef]

141. Bellé, A.S.; Hackenhaar, C.R.; Spolidoro, L.S.; Rodrigues, E.; Klein, M.P.; Hertz, P.F. Efficient enzyme-assisted extraction of genipin from genipap (*Genipa americana* L.) and its application as a crosslinker for chitosan gels. *Food Chem.* **2018**, *246*, 266–274. [CrossRef] [PubMed]

142. Alves, J.S.F.; de Medeiros, L.A.; de Fernandes-Pedrosa, M.F.; Araújo, R.M.; Zucolotto, S.M. Iridoids from leaf extract of *Genipa americana*. *Rev. Bras. Farmacogn.* **2017**, *27*, 641–644. [CrossRef]

143. Neri-Numa, I.A.; Pessôa, M.G.; Arruda, H.S.; Pereira, G.A.; Paulino, B.N.; Angolini, C.F.F.; Ruiz, A.L.T.G.; Pastore, G.M. Genipap (*Genipa americana* L.) fruit extract as a source of antioxidant and antiproliferative iridoids. *Food Res. Int.* **2020**, *134*, 109252. [CrossRef] [PubMed]

144. Náthia-Neves, G.; Tarone, A.G.; Tosi, M.M.; Maróstica Júnior, M.R.; Meireles, M.A.A. Extraction of bioactive compounds from genipap (*Genipa americana* L.) by pressurized ethanol: Iridoids, phenolic content and antioxidant activity. *Food Res. Int.* **2017**, *102*, 595–604. [CrossRef] [PubMed]

145. Ramos-de-la-Peña, A.M.; Renard, C.M.G.C.; Wicker, L.; Montañez, J.C.; García-Cerda, L.A.; Contreras-Esquivel, J.C. Environmental friendly cold-mechanical/sonic enzymatic assisted extraction of genipin from genipap (*Genipa americana*). *Ultrason. Sonochem.* **2014**, *21*, 43–49. [CrossRef]

146. Pacheco, P.; Da Paz, J.G.; Da Silva, C.O.; Pascoal, G.B. Composição centesimal, compostos bioativos e parâmetros físico-químicos do jenipapo (*Genipa americana* L.) in natura. *DEMETRA Aliment. Nutr. Saúde* **2014**, *9*, 1041–1054. [CrossRef]

147. Costa, R.G.; Da Silva, D.A.; Alves, S.F. Obtenção e caracterização do extrato fluido de *Genipa americana* Linnaeus. *Rev. Eletrônica Farmácia* **2019**, *16*, 1–7. [CrossRef]

148. Mendes, W.B.S.; Andrade, T.O.; Moraes, S.M. Estudo Fitoquímico e Avaliação da Atividade Antiacetilcolinestersásica da Folha e Casca do Jenipapaeiro (*Genipa americana* L.). 57° Congresso Brasileiro de Química, 2017. Available online: http://www.abq.org.br/cbq/2017/trabalhos/7/11151-24611.html (accessed on 21 July 2020).

149. Costa, R.B.; Campana, P.T.; Chambergo, F.S.; Napoleão, T.H.; Paiva, P.M.G.; Pereira, H.J.V.; Oliva, M.L.V.; Gomes, F.S. Purification and characterization of a lectin with refolding ability from *Genipa americana* bark. *Int. J. Biol. Macromol.* **2018**, *119*, 517–523. [CrossRef]

150. Kwon, S.-H.; Lee, H.-K.; Kim, J.-A.; Hong, S.-I.; Kim, H.-C.; Jo, T.-H.; Park, Y.-I.; Lee, C.-K.; Kim, Y.-B.; Lee, S.-Y.; et al. Neuroprotective effects of chlorogenic acid on scopolamine-induced amnesia via anti-acetylcholinesterase and anti-oxidative activities in mice. *Eur. J. Pharmacol.* **2010**, *649*, 210–217. [CrossRef]

151. Wang, J.; Chen, L.; Liang, Z.; Li, Y.; Yuan, F.; Liu, J.; Tian, Y.; Hao, Z.; Zhou, F.; Liu, X.; et al. Genipin Inhibits LPS-Induced Inflammatory Response in BV2 Microglial Cells. *Neurochem. Res.* **2017**, *42*, 2769–2776. [CrossRef]

152. Yu, S.X.; Du, C.T.; Chen, W.; Lei, Q.Q.; Li, N.; Qi, S.; Zhang, X.J.; Hu, G.Q.; Deng, X.M.; Han, W.Y.; et al. Genipin inhibits NLRP3 and NLRC4 inflammasome activation via autophagy suppression. *Sci. Rep.* **2016**, *5*, 17935. [CrossRef] [PubMed]

153. Luo, X.; Lin, B.; Gao, Y.; Lei, X.; Wang, X.; Li, Y.; Li, T. International Immunopharmacology Genipin attenuates mitochondrial-dependent apoptosis, endoplasmic reticulum stress, and in fl ammation via the PI3K/AKT pathway in acute lung injury. *Int. Immunopharmacol.* **2019**, *76*, 105842. [CrossRef] [PubMed]

154. Pugazhenthi, S.; Nesterova, A.; Sable, C.; Heidenreich, K.A.; Boxer, L.M.; Heasley, L.E.; Reusch, J.E. Akt/Protein Kinase B Up-regulates Bcl-2 Expression through cAMP-response Element-binding Protein. *J. Biol. Chem.* **2000**, *275*, 10761–10766. [CrossRef] [PubMed]

155. Li, Z.; Zhang, T.; Jia, D.; Sun, W.; Wang, C.; Gu, A.; Yang, X. Genipin inhibits the growth of human bladder cancer cells via inactivation of PI3K/Akt signaling. *Oncol. Lett.* **2017**, *15*, 2619–2624. [CrossRef]

156. Wei, M.; Wu, Y.; Liu, H.; Xie, C. Genipin Induces Autophagy and Suppresses Cell Growth of Oral Squamous Cell Carcinoma via PI3K/AKT/MTOR Pathway. *Drug Des. Devel. Ther.* **2020**, *14*, 395–405. [CrossRef]

157. Zhao, B.; Lian-kun, S.; Jiang, X.; Zhang, Y.; Kang, J.; Meng, H.; Li, H.; Jing, S. Genipin protects against cerebral ischemia- reperfusion injury by regulating the UCP2-SIRT3 signaling pathway. *Eur. J. Pharmacol.* **2018**, *845*, 56–64. [CrossRef]

158. Ayyasamy, V.; Owens, K.M.; Desouki, M.M.; Liang, P.; Bakin, A.; Thangaraj, K.; Buchsbaum, D.J.; LoBuglio, A.F.; Singh, K.K. Cellular Model of Warburg Effect Identifies Tumor Promoting Function of UCP2 in Breast Cancer and Its Suppression by Genipin. *PLoS ONE* **2011**, *6*, e24792. [CrossRef]

159. Wang, R.; MoYung, K.; Zhao, Y.; Poon, K. A Mechanism for the Temporal Potentiation of Genipin to the Cytotoxicity of Cisplatin in Colon Cancer Cells. *Int. J. Med. Sci.* **2016**, *13*, 507–516. [CrossRef]

160. Lou, J.; Wang, Y.; Wang, X.; Jiang, Y. Uncoupling Protein 2 Regulates Palmitic Acid-Induced Hepatoma Cell Autophagy. *Biomed Res. Int.* **2014**, *2014*, 1–14. [CrossRef]

161. Yu, J.; Shi, L.; Shen, X.; Zhao, Y. UCP2 regulates cholangiocarcinoma cell plasticity via mitochondria-to-AMPK signals. *Biochem. Pharmacol.* **2019**, *166*, 174–184. [CrossRef]

162. Ahani, N.; Sangtarash, M.H.; Houshmand, M.; Eskandani, M.A. Genipin induces cell death via intrinsic apoptosis pathways in human glioblastoma cells. *J. Cell. Biochem.* **2019**, *120*, 2047–2057. [CrossRef] [PubMed]

163. Shanmugam, M.K.; Shen, H.; Tang, F.R.; Arfuso, F.; Rajesh, M.; Wang, L.; Kumar, A.P.; Bian, J.; Goh, B.C.; Bishayee, A.; et al. Potential role of genipin in cancer therapy. *Pharmacol. Res.* **2018**, *133*, 195–200. [CrossRef] [PubMed]

164. Dando, I.; Fiorini, C.; Pozza, E.D.; Padroni, C.; Costanzo, C.; Palmieri, M.; Donadelli, M. UCP2 inhibition triggers ROS-dependent nuclear translocation of GAPDH and autophagic cell death in pancreatic adenocarcinoma cells. *Biochim. Biophys. Acta Mol. Cell Res.* **2013**, *1833*, 672–679. [CrossRef] [PubMed]

165. Habtemariam, S.; Lentini, G. Plant-derived anticancer agents: Lessons from the pharmacology of geniposide and its aglycone, genipin. *Biomedicines* **2018**, *6*, 39. [CrossRef] [PubMed]

166. Jo, M.J.; Jeong, S.; Yun, H.K.; Kim, D.Y.; Kim, B.R.; Kim, J.L.; Na, Y.J.; Park, S.H.; Jeong, Y.A.; Kim, B.G.; et al. Genipin induces mitochondrial dysfunction and apoptosis via downregulation of Stat3/mcl-1 pathway in gastric cancer. *BMC Cancer* **2019**, *19*, 739. [CrossRef] [PubMed]

167. Kim, B.R.; Jeong, Y.A.; Na, Y.J.; Park, S.H.; Jo, M.J.; Kim, J.L.; Jeong, S.; Lee, S.-Y.; Kim, H.J.; Oh, S.C.; et al. Genipin suppresses colorectal cancer cells by inhibiting the Sonic Hedgehog pathway. *Oncotarget* **2017**, *8*, 101952–101964. [CrossRef]

168. Xue, A.; Zheng, L.; Tan, G.; Wu, S.; Wu, Y.; Cheng, L.; Qu, J. Genipin-Crosslinked Donor Sclera for Posterior Scleral Contraction/Reinforcement to Fight Progressive Myopia. *Investig. Opthalmology Vis. Sci.* **2018**, *59*, 3564. [CrossRef]

169. Manickam, B.; Sreedharan, R.; Elumalai, M. 'Genipin' – The Natural Water Soluble Cross-linking Agent and Its Importance in the Modified Drug Delivery Systems: An Overview. *Curr. Drug Deliv.* **2014**, *11*, 139–145. [CrossRef]

170. Cho, M.; Jung, S.W.; Lee, S.; Son, K.; Park, G.H.; Jung, J.-W.; Shin, Y.S.; Seo, T.; Hyosun, C.; Kang, H. Genipin Enhances Kaposi's Sarcoma-Associated Herpesvirus Genome Maintenance. *PLoS ONE* **2016**, *11*, e0163693. [CrossRef]

171. Nonato, D.T.T.; Vasconcelos, S.M.M.; Mota, M.R.L.; de Barros Silva, P.G.; Cunha, A.P.; Ricardo, N.M.P.S.; Pereira, M.G.; Assreuy, A.M.S.; Chaves, E.M.C. The anticonvulsant effect of a polysaccharide-rich extract from *Genipa americana* leaves is mediated by GABA receptor. *Biomed. Pharmacother.* **2018**, *101*, 181–187. [CrossRef]

172. Madeira, J.C.; da Silva, G.V.L.; Batista, J.J.; Saraiva, G.D.; Santos, G.R.C.; Assreuy, A.M.S.; Mourão, P.A.S.; Pereira, M.G. An arabinogalactan-glycoconjugate from *Genipa americana* leaves present anticoagulant, antiplatelet and antithrombotic effects. *Carbohydr. Polym.* **2018**, *202*, 554–562. [CrossRef] [PubMed]

173. De Júnior, D.L.S.; da Silva, Í.M.; Benjamim, L.E.; Teotônio, O.; Gonçalves, F.J.; Tôrres, C.M.; Salviano, R.C.; Leandro; Lopes, M.J.P.; de Aquino, P.E.A.; et al. Efeito antimicrobiano e modulador do extrato hidroalcoólico de *Genipa americana* (Jenipapo). *Rev. Saúde (Sta. Maria)* **2019**, *45*.

174. Da Souza, R.O.S.; Sousa, P.L.; de Menezes, R.R.P.P.B.; Sampaio, T.L.; Tessarolo, L.D.; Silva, F.C.O.; Pereira, M.G.; Martins, A.M.C. Trypanocidal activity of polysaccharide extract from *Genipa americana* leaves. *J. Ethnopharmacol.* **2018**, *210*, 311–317. [CrossRef] [PubMed]

175. Moura, M.N. Hipóteses Filogenéticas Baseadas em Caracteres Moleculares e Estudos do Tamanho do Genoma em Dyckia Schult. & Schult.f. E Encholirium Mart. ex Schult. & Schult.f. (Bromeliaceae). Master's Thesis, Universidade Federal de Viçosa, Viçosa, Brazil, 2014.

176. Pacchioni, F.V.T.L.; Oliveira, R.; Matias, R.; Wendt, C.L.G.R. Perfil toxicológico da planta *Genipa americana* L. com potencial farmacológico em Danio rerio. *9° Semin. Inic. Cient.* **2018**. Available online: https://repositorio.pgsskroton.com.br/bitstream/123456789/22514/1/UNIDERP%20-%20Felipe%20Villar%20Telles%20Lunardelli.pdf (accessed on 21 July 2020).

177. Manetti, L.M.; Delaporte, R.H.; Laverde, A., Jr. Metabólitos secundários da família bromeliaceae. *Quim. Nova* **2009**, *32*, 1885–1897. [CrossRef]

178. Souza, C.P.F. Caracterização de Variedades de Abacaxi e Sua Potencial Utilização Como Fonte de Fibras. Master's Thesis, Universidade Federal do Recôncavo da Bahia, Cruz das Almas, Brazil, 2015.

179. Vallés, D.; Cantera, A.M.B. Antiacanthain A: New proteases isolated from *Bromelia antiacantha* Bertol. (Bromeliaceae). *Int. J. Biol. Macromol.* **2018**, *113*, 916–923. [CrossRef]

180. Da Cruz, M.P. Estudo fitoquímico e avaliação da atividade antimicrobiana de Bromelia laciniosa Mart. ex Schult. f. (Bromeliaceae). Master's Thesis, Universidade Federal do Vale do São Francisco, Petrolina, Brazil, 2017.

181. Filippon, S.; Fernandes, C.D.; Ferreira, D.K.; da Silva, D.L.S.; Altrak, G.; Duarte, A.S.; dos Reis, M.S. *Bromelia antiacantha* Bertol.(Bromeliaceae): Caracterização demográfica e potencial de manejo em uma população no Planalto Norte Catarinense. *Biodiversidade Bras.* **2012**, *2*, 83–91.

182. Manetti, L.M.; Turra, A.F.; Takemura, O.S.; Svidzinski, T.I.E.; Laverde Junior, A. Avaliação das atividades antimicrobiana, citotóxica, moluscicida e antioxidante de *Bromelia antiacantha* Bertol. (Bromeliaceae). *Rev. Bras. Plantas Med.* **2010**, *12*, 406–413. [CrossRef]

183. Dettke, G.A.; Milaneze-Gutierre, M.A. Anatomia vegetativa de *Bromelia antiacantha* Bertol. (Bromeliaceae, Bromelioideae). *Balduinia* **2014**, *13*, 1–14. [CrossRef]

184. Vallés, D.; Furtado, S.; Cantera, A.M.B. Characterization of news proteolytic enzymes from ripe fruits of *Bromelia antiacantha* Bertol. (Bromeliaceae). *Enzyme Microb. Technol.* **2007**, *40*, 409–413. [CrossRef]

185. Bersi, G.; Vallés, D.; Penna, F.; Cantera, A.M.; Barberis, S. Valorization of fruit by-products of *Bromelia antiacantha* Bertol.: Protease obtaining and its potential as additive for laundry detergents. *Biocatal. Agric. Biotechnol.* **2019**, *18*, 101099. [CrossRef]

186. Nogueira, A.C.; Côrtes, I.M.R.; Verçoza, F.C. A família Bromeliaceae na Área de Proteção Ambiental de Grumari, Rio de Janeiro, RJ, Brasil. *Nat. Line* **2011**, *9*, 91–95.

187. Monteiro, R.F.; Mantovani, A.; Forzza, R.C. Morphological Phylogenetic Analysis of Two Early-Diverging Genera of Bromelioideae (Bromeliaceae). *Rodriguésia* **2015**, *66*, 505–521. [CrossRef]

188. Grandi, T.S.M. *Tratado de Plantas Medicinais Mineiras, Nativas e Cultivadas*, 1st ed.; Adequatio Estúdio: Belo Horizonte, Brazil, 2014; ISBN 978-85-68322-00-0.

189. Yazbek, P.B.; Matta, P.; Passero, L.F.; Santos, G.; Braga, S.; Assunção, L.; Sauini, T.; Cassas, F.; Garcia, R.J.F.; Honda, S.; et al. Plants utilized as medicines by residents of Quilombo da Fazenda, Núcleo Picinguaba, Ubatuba, São Paulo, Brazil: A participatory survey. *J. Ethnopharmacol.* **2019**, *244*, 112123. [CrossRef] [PubMed]

190. Carvalho, F.H.; Martins, G.V.; Oliveira, C.; Contrera, M.G.D.; Ferro, D.; Regrado, S.C.H.; Lopes, R.A.; Sala, M.A. Hepatotoxicidade de plantas medicinais na preparação fitoterápica usada popularmente como vermífugo contendo Mentha villosa L., *Bromelia antiacantha* Bertol, *Chenopodium ambrosioides* L., *Citrus sinensis* L., *Punica granatum* L. e *Curcubita pepo* L. em camund. *Rev. Científica da Univ. Fr.* **2005**, *5*, 215–222.

191. Filippon, S. Aspectos da demografia, fenologia e uso tradicionaldo Caraguatá (*Bromelia antiacantha* Bertol.) no Planalto Norte Catarinense. Master's Thesis, Universidade Federal de Santa Catarina, Florianópolis, Brazil, 2009.

192. Nasser, N.P.A.; Scheeren, N.B.; Ramos, R.F.; Bellé, C.; Nora, D.D.; Betemps, D.L. Germinação de sementes de *Bromelia antiacantha* em diferentes fotoperíodos. *Rev. Eletrônica Científica UERGS* **2019**, *5*, 296–301. [CrossRef]

193. Fabri, R.L.; da Costa, J.A.B.M. Perfil farmacognóstico e avaliação das atividades citotóxica e antibacteriana de *Bromelia antiacantha* Bertol. *Rev. Electron. Farmácia* **2012**, *9*, 37–48. [CrossRef]

194. Santos, V.N.C.; de Freitas, R.A.; Deschamps, F.C.; Biavatti, M.W. Ripe fruits of *Bromelia antiacantha*: Investigations on the chemical and bioactivity profile. *Rev. Bras. Farmacogn.* **2009**, *19*, 358–365. [CrossRef]

195. Zanella, C.M. Caracterização genética, morfológica e fitoquímica de populações de *Bromelia antiacantha* (Bertol.) do Rio Grande do Sul. Master's Thesis, Universidade Federal do Rio Grande do Sul, Porto Alegre, Brazil, 2009.

196. Manetti, L.M.; Turra, A.F.; Takemura, O.S.; Júnior, A.L. Avaliação da atividade hemolítica de *Bromelia antiacantha* Bertol. (Bromeliaceae). *Arq. Ciênc. Saúde UNIPAR* **2010**, *14*, 43–47.

197. Krumreich, F.D.; Corrêa, A.P.A.; da Silva, S.D.S.; Zambiazi, R.C. Composição físico-química e de compostos bioativos em frutos de *Bromelia antiacantha* Bertol. *Rev. Bras. Frutic.* **2015**, *37*, 450–456. [CrossRef]

198. Jang, J.; Kim, S.-M.; Yee, S.-M.; Kim, E.-M.; Lee, E.-H.; Choi, H.-R.; Lee, Y.-S.; Yang, W.-K.; Kim, H.-Y.; Kim, K.-H.; et al. Daucosterol suppresses dextran sulfate sodium (DSS)-induced colitis in mice. *Int. Immunopharmacol.* **2019**, *72*, 124–130. [CrossRef] [PubMed]

199. Gao, P.; Huang, X.; Liao, T.; Li, G.; Yu, X.; You, Y.; Huang, Y. Daucosterol induces autophagic-dependent apoptosis in prostate cancer *via* JNK activation. *Biosci. Trends* **2019**, *13*, 160–167. [CrossRef] [PubMed]

200. Han, B.; Jiang, P.; Liu, W.; Xu, H.; Li, Y.; Li, Z.; Ma, H.; Yu, Y.; Li, X.; Ye, X. Role of Daucosterol Linoleate on Breast Cancer: Studies on Apoptosis and Metastasis. *J. Agric. Food Chem.* **2018**, *66*, 6031–6041. [CrossRef] [PubMed]

201. Zingue, S.; Gbaweng Yaya, A.J.; Michel, T.; Ndinteh, D.T.; Rutz, J.; Auberon, F.; Maxeiner, S.; Chun, F.K.II.; Tchinda, A.T.; Njamen, D.; et al. Bioguided identification of daucosterol, a compound that contributes to the cytotoxicity effects of Crateva adansonii DC (capparaceae) to prostate cancer cells. *J. Ethnopharmacol.* **2020**, *247*, 112251. [CrossRef] [PubMed]

202. Esmaeili, M.A.; Farimani, M.M. Inactivation of PI3K/Akt pathway and upregulation of PTEN gene are involved in daucosterol, isolated from Salvia sahendica, induced apoptosis in human breast adenocarcinoma cells. *South African J. Bot.* **2014**, *93*, 37–47. [CrossRef]

203. Zeng, J.; Liu, X.; Li, X.; Zheng, Y.; Liu, B.; Xiao, Y. Daucosterol Inhibits the Proliferation, Migration, and Invasion of Hepatocellular Carcinoma Cells via Wnt/β-Catenin Signaling. *Molecules* **2017**, *22*, 862. [CrossRef]

204. Jiang, L.; Yuan, X.; Yang, N.; Ren, L.; Zhao, F.; Luo, B.; Bian, Y.; Xu, J.; Lu, D.; Zheng, Y.; et al. Daucosterol protects neurons against oxygen–glucose deprivation/reperfusion-mediated injury by activating IGF1 signaling pathway. *J. Steroid Biochem. Mol. Biol.* **2015**, *152*, 45–52. [CrossRef]

205. Podolak, I.; Galanty, A.; Sobolewska, D. Saponins as cytotoxic agents: A review. *Phytochem. Rev.* **2010**, *9*, 425–474. [CrossRef]

206. Ellington, A.A. Induction of macroautophagy in human colon cancer cells by soybean B-group triterpenoid saponins. *Carcinogenesis* **2004**, *26*, 159–167. [CrossRef]

207. Venkatakrishnan, K.; Chiu, H.-F.; Cheng, J.-C.; Chang, Y.-H.; Lu, Y.-Y.; Han, Y.-C.; Shen, Y.-C.; Tsai, K.-S.; Wang, C.-K. Comparative studies on the hypolipidemic, antioxidant and hepatoprotective activities of catechin-enriched green and oolong tea in a double-blind clinical trial. *Food Funct.* **2018**. [CrossRef]

208. Nagao, T.; Meguro, S.; Hase, T.; Otsuka, K.; Komikado, M.; Tokimitsu, I.; Yamamoto, T.; Yamamoto, K. A Catechin-rich Beverage Improves Obesity and Blood Glucose Control in Patients With Type 2 Diabetes. *Obesity* **2009**, *17*, 310–317. [CrossRef] [PubMed]

209. Inami, S.; Takano, M.; Yamamoto, M.; Murakami, D.; Tajika, K.; Yodogawa, K.; Yokoyama, S.; Ohno, N.; Ohba, T.; Sano, J.; et al. Tea Catechin Consumption Reduces Circulating Oxidized Low-Density Lipoprotein. *Int. Heart J.* **2007**, *48*. [CrossRef] [PubMed]

210. Matsuyama, T.; Tanaka, Y.; Kamimaki, I.; Nagao, T.; Tokimitsu, I. Catechin Safely Improved Higher Levels of Fatness, Blood Pressure, and Cholesterol in Children. *Obesity* **2008**, *16*. [CrossRef] [PubMed]

211. Alañón, M.E.; Castle, S.M.; Serra, G.; Lévèques, A.; Poquet, L.; Actis-Goretta, L.; Spencer, J.P.E. Acute study of dose-dependent effects of (−)-epicatechin on vascular function in healthy male volunteers: A randomized controlled trial. *Clin. Nutr.* **2020**. [CrossRef] [PubMed]

212. Hollands, W.J.; Tapp, H.; Defernez, M.; Perez Moral, N.; Winterbone, M.S.; Philo, M.; Lucey, A.J.; Kiely, M.E.; Kroon, P.A. Lack of acute or chronic effects of epicatechin-rich and procyanidin-rich apple extracts on blood pressure and cardiometabolic biomarkers in adults with moderately elevated blood pressure: A randomized, placebo-controlled crossover trial. *Am. J. Clin. Nutr.* **2018**, *108*, 1006–1014. [CrossRef] [PubMed]

213. Dower, J.I.; Geleijnse, J.M.; Gijsbers, L.; Zock, P.L.; Kromhout, D.; Hollman, P.C.H. Effects of the pure flavonoids epicatechin and quercetin on vascular function and cardiometabolic health: A randomized, double-blind, placebo-controlled, crossover trial. *Am. J. Clin. Nutr.* **2015**. [CrossRef]

214. Edwards, R.L.; Lyon, T.; Litwin, S.E.; Rabovsky, A.; Symons, J.D.; Jalili, T. Quercetin Reduces Blood Pressure in Hypertensive Subjects. *J. Nutr.* **2007**. [CrossRef]

215. Duranti, G.; Ceci, R.; Patrizio, F.; Sgrò, P.; Di Luigi, L.; Sabatini, S.; Felici, F.; Bazzucchi, I. Chronic consumption of quercetin reduces erythrocytes oxidative damage: Evaluation at resting and after eccentric exercise in humans. *Nutr. Res.* **2018**. [CrossRef]

216. Shi, Y.; Williamson, G. Quercetin lowers plasma uric acid in pre-hyperuricaemic males: A randomised, double-blinded, placebo-controlled, cross-over trial. *Br. J. Nutr.* **2016**, *115*, 800–806. [CrossRef]

217. Javadi, F.; Ahmadzadeh, A.; Eghtesadi, S.; Aryaeian, N.; Zabihiyeganeh, M.; Rahimi Foroushani, A.; Jazayeri, S. The Effect of Quercetin on Inflammatory Factors and Clinical Symptoms in Women with Rheumatoid Arthritis: A Double-Blind, Randomized Controlled Trial. *J. Am. Coll. Nutr.* **2017**. [CrossRef]

218. Kondratiuk, V.E.; Synytsia, Y.P. Effect of quercetin on the echocardiographic parameters of left ventricular diastolic function in patients with gout and essential hypertension. *Wiad. Lek.* **2018**, *71*, 1554–1559. [PubMed]

219. Khorshidi, M.; Moini, A.; Alipoor, E.; Rezvan, N.; Gorgani-Firuzjaee, S.; Yaseri, M.; Hosseinzadeh-Attar, M.J. The effects of quercetin supplementation on metabolic and hormonal parameters as well as plasma concentration and gene expression of resistin in overweight or obese women with polycystic ovary syndrome. *Phyther. Res.* **2018**, 1–8. [CrossRef] [PubMed]

220. Sajadi Hezaveh, Z.; Azarkeivan, A.; Janani, L.; Hosseini, S.; Shidfar, F. The effect of quercetin on iron overload and inflammation in β-thalassemia major patients: A double-blind randomized clinical trial. *Complement. Ther. Med.* **2019**, *46*. [CrossRef] [PubMed]

221. Rezvan, N.; Moini, A.; Janani, L.; Mohammad, K.; Saedisomeolia, A.; Nourbakhsh, M.; Gorgani-Firuzjaee, S.; Mazaherioun, M.; Hosseinzadeh-Attar, M. Effects of Quercetin on Adiponectin-Mediated Insulin Sensitivity in Polycystic Ovary Syndrome: A Randomized Placebo-Controlled Double-Blind Clinical Trial. *Horm. Metab. Res.* **2016**. [CrossRef]

222. Patrizio, F.; Ditroilo, M.; Felici, F.; Duranti, G.; De Vito, G.; Sabatini, S.; Sacchetti, M.; Bazzucchi, I. The acute effect of Quercetin on muscle performance following a single resistance training session. *Eur. J. Appl. Physiol.* **2018**. [CrossRef]

223. Talirevic, E.; Sehovic, J. Quercetin in the Treatment of Dyslipidemia. *Med. Arch.* **2012**, *66*, 87–88. [CrossRef]

224. Boots, A.W.; Drent, M.; de Boer, V.C.J.; Bast, A.; Haenen, G.R.M.M. Quercetin reduces markers of oxidative stress and inflammation in sarcoidosis. *Clin. Nutr.* **2011**, *30*, 506–512. [CrossRef]

225. Katada, S.; Watanabe, T.; Mizuno, T.; Kobayashi, S.; Takeshita, M.; Osaki, N.; Kobayashi, S.; Katsuragi, Y. Effects of Chlorogenic Acid-Enriched and Hydroxyhydroquinone-Reduced Coffee on Postprandial Fat Oxidation and Antioxidative Capacity in Healthy Men: A Randomized, Double-Blind, Placebo-Controlled, Crossover Trial. *Nutrients* **2018**, *10*, 525. [CrossRef]

226. Saitou, K.; Ochiai, R.; Kozuma, K.; Sato, H.; Koikeda, T.; Osaki, N.; Katsuragi, Y. Effect of Chlorogenic Acids on Cognitive Function: A Randomized, Double-Blind, Placebo-Controlled Trial. *Nutrients* **2018**, *10*, 1337. [CrossRef]

227. Mubarak, A.; Bondonno, C.P.; Liu, A.H.; Considine, M.J.; Mas, E.; Croft, K.D.; Hodgson, J.M. Acute effects of chlorogenic acid on nitric oxide status, endothelial function and blood pressure in healthy volunteers: A randomised trial. *J. Agric. Food Chem.* **2012**, *53*, S191–S192. [CrossRef]

228. Vieyra-Garcia, P.; Fink-Puches, R.; Porkert, S.; Lang, R.; Pöchlauer, S.; Ratzinger, G.; Tanew, A.; Selhofer, S.; Paul-Gunther, S.; Hofer, A.; et al. Evaluation of Low-Dose, Low-Frequency Oral Psoralen–UV-A Treatment With or Without Maintenance on Early-Stage Mycosis Fungoides. *JAMA Dermatol.* **2019**. [CrossRef] [PubMed]

229. Brass, D.; Fouweather, T.; Stocken, D.D.; Macdonald, C.; Wilkinson, J.; Lloyd, J.; Farr, P.M.; Reynolds, N.J.; Hampton, P.J. An observer-blinded randomized controlled pilot trial comparing localized immersion psoralen-ultraviolet A with localized narrowband ultraviolet B for the treatment of palmar hand eczema. *Br. J. Dermatol.* **2018**, *179*, 8–9. [CrossRef] [PubMed]

230. Khanna, N.; Nazli, T.; Siddiqui, K.; Kalaivani, M. Rais-ur-Rahman A non-inferiority randomized controlled clinical trial comparing Unani formulation & psoralen plus ultraviolet A sol in chronic plaque psoriasis. *Indian J. Med. Res.* **2018**, 66–72. [CrossRef]

231. Brazzelli, V.; Grassi, S.; Merante, S.; Grasso, V.; Ciccocioppo, R.; Bossi, G.; Borroni, G. Narrow-band UVB phototherapy and psoralen-ultraviolet A photochemotherapy in the treatment of cutaneous mastocytosis: A study in 20 patients. *Photodermatol. Photoimmunol. Photomed.* **2016**, *32*, 238–246. [CrossRef]

232. Bansal, S.; Sahoo, B.; Garg, V. Psoralen-narrowband UVB phototherapy for the treatment of vitiligo in comparison to narrowband UVB alone. *Photodermatol. Photoimmunol. Photomed.* **2013**. [CrossRef]

233. Calzavara-Pinton, P.; Ortel, B.; Carlino, A.; Honigsmann, H.; Panfilis, G. A reappraisal of the use of 5-methoxypsoralen in the therapy of psoriasis. *Exp. Dermatol.* **1992**. [CrossRef]

234. Stefanaki, C.; Fasoulaki, X.; Kouris, A.; Caroni, C.; Papagianaki, K.; Mavrogianni, P.; Nicolaidou, E.; Gregoriou, S.; Antoniou, C. A randomized trial of efficacy of beta-sitosterol and its glucoside as adjuvant to cryotherapy in the treatment of anogenital warts. *J. Dermatolog. Treat.* **2015**, 1–4. [CrossRef]

235. Donald, P.R.; Lamprecht, J.H.; Freeston, M.; Al, E. A randomised placebo-controlled trial of the efficacy of beta-sitosterol and its glucoside as adjuvants in the treatment of pulmonary tuberculosis. *Int. J. Tuberc. Lung. Dis.* **1997**, *1*, 518–522.

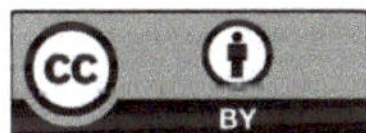

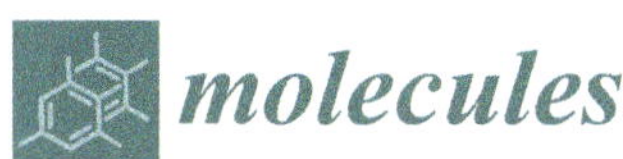 *molecules*

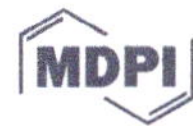

Review

Preclinical Activities of Epigallocatechin Gallate in Signaling Pathways in Cancer

Mehdi Sharifi-Rad [1,†], Raffaele Pezzani [2,3,*,†], Marco Redaelli [3,4], Maira Zorzan [2,4], Muhammad Imran [5], Anees Ahmed Khalil [5], Bahare Salehi [6,*], Farukh Sharopov [7,*], William C. Cho [8,*] and Javad Sharifi-Rad [9,*]

1. Department of Medical Parasitology, Kerman University of Medical Sciences, Kerman 7616913555, Iran; mehdi_sharifirad@yahoo.com
2. Endocrinology Unit, Department of Medicine (DIMED), University of Padova, via Ospedale 105, 35128 Padova, Italy; maira.zorzan@vimset.it
3. AIROB, Associazione Italiana per la Ricerca Oncologica di Base, 35046 Padova, Italy; marcoredaelli@email.it
4. Venetian Institute for Molecular Science and Experimental Technologies, VIMSET, Pz. Milani 4, Liettoli di Campolongo Maggiore (VE), 30010 Venice, Italy
5. University Institute of Diet and Nutritional Sciences, Faculty of Allied Health Sciences, The University of Lahore, Lahore 54590, Pakistan; mic_1661@yahoo.com (M.I.); aneesahmedkhalil@gmail.com (A.A.K.)
6. Student Research Committee, School of Medicine, Bam University of Medical Sciences, Bam 44340847, Iran
7. Department of Pharmaceutical Technology, Avicenna Tajik State Medical University, Rudaki 139, Dushanbe 734003, Tajikistan
8. Department of Clinical Oncology, Queen Elizabeth Hospital, Hong Kong, China
9. Phytochemistry Research Center, Shahid Beheshti University of Medical Sciences, Tehran 1991953381, Iran
* Correspondence: raffaele.pezzani@unipd.it (R.P.); bahar.salehi007@gmail.com (B.S.); shfarukh@mail.ru (F.S.); williamcscho@gmail.com (W.C.C.); javad.sharifirad@gmail.com (J.S.-R.)
† These authors contributed equally to this work.

Academic Editor: Saverio Bettuzzi

Received: 27 December 2019; Accepted: 19 January 2020; Published: 22 January 2020

Abstract: Epigallocatechin gallate (EGCG) is the main bioactive component of catechins predominantly present in various types of tea. EGCG is well known for a wide spectrum of biological activities as an anti-oxidative, anti-inflammatory, and anti-tumor agent. The effect of EGCG on cell death mechanisms via the induction of apoptosis, necrosis, and autophagy has been documented. Moreover, its anti-proliferative action has been demonstrated in many cancer cell lines. It was also involved in the modulation of cyclooxygenase-2, oxidative stress and inflammation of different cellular processes. EGCG has been reported as a promising agent target for plasma membrane proteins, such as epidermal growth factor receptor. In addition, it has been demonstrated a mechanism of action relying on the inhibition of ERK1/2, p38 MAPK, NF-κB, and vascular endothelial growth factor. Furthermore, EGCG and its derivatives were used in proteasome inhibition and they were involved in epigenetic mechanisms. In summary, EGCG is the most predominant and bioactive constituent of tea and may play a role in cancer prevention.

Keywords: epigallocatechin-3-gallate; EGCG; catechin; green tea; cancer preventive; pharmacological activities

---

1. Introduction

Tea has been known to be the world most renowned non alcoholic beverage since ancient times and it is currently being utilized by two-thirds population of the world, owing to its taste, stimulating effects, unique aroma, and associated health perspectives [1,2]. Various types of tea like green, black and oolong tea are derived from the *Camellia sinensis* (L.) plant containing variety of components among which polyphenols are most significant ones. Basic differences among all of these teas depends upon the stage of fermentation processes from which they are produced. Purposely, green tea is not fermented while black tea and oolong tea are completely and partially fermented, respectively. Amongst all of the investigated teas around the globe, green tea is well studied, owing to its health promoting benefits. In general, tea based phenolics possess protective action against numerous metabolic syndromes.

Several nutraceutical aspects of green tea extracts depends upon the concentration of phenolics and their associated derivatives. The major biologically active moiety present in leaves of green tea are classified as catechins that nearly account for 25–35% on dry weight basis. This catechin group comprises eight phenolic flavonoid constituents, specifically, catechin, epicatechin, gallocatechin, epigallocatechin, catechin gallate, epicatechin gallate, gallocatechin gallate, and epigallocatechin gallate (EGCG) [3,4]. Among above mentioned polyphenols, EGCG is the most vital tea based catechin which is considered to be the main reason for bioactivity of green tea [5–8].

Catechins are plant secondary metabolites [9,10]. They possess numerous functions in plant survival, growth, and metabolism, but they can also interact with other living organisms if ingested or came into direct contact. Catechins or flavanols probably constitute the most abundant subclass of flavonoids and they are essentially represented by (–)-epigallocatechin-3-gallate (EGCG), (–)-epigallocatechin (EGC), (–)-epicatechin-3-gallate (ECG), and (–)-epicatechin (EC) [11]. These last four bioactive compounds are found in large amount in green tea (leaves of *Camellia sinensis*) and cocoa/chocolate, but they are also present in many fruits or seeds, such apples, blueberries (*Vaccinium myrtillus*) and grapes (red wine and beer) and peanuts [12]. This review focuses on catechins that are derived from green tea and in particular on EGCG, which represents 50% to 80% of all *Camellia sinensis* catechins (200–300 mg/brewed cup of green tea) [13]. Moreover, we analyzed preclinical works examining its pharmacological and biomolecular mechanism of action.

Epigallocatechin gallate is the most bioactive catechin that is predominantly present in tea. Among all of the tea types, it is found at maximum comncentration in green tea leaves. EGCG molecule (Figure 1) comprises two aromatic structures that are co-joined by three carbon bridge structure (C6-C3-C6) along with hydroxyl group (OH) at simultaneous carbons i.e., 3′, 4′, 5′ of ring-B. Carbon-3 of ring-C is esterified with a gallate molecule (features of catechins originated from tea are responsible for bioactivity due to position and number of OH-group on the rings. They regulate their capability to interact with biological matter via hydrogen bonding, a hydrogen and electron transferring process contained by their antioxidative potentials. The presence and absence of a galloyl molecule differentiates EGCG from remaining three catechins [14].

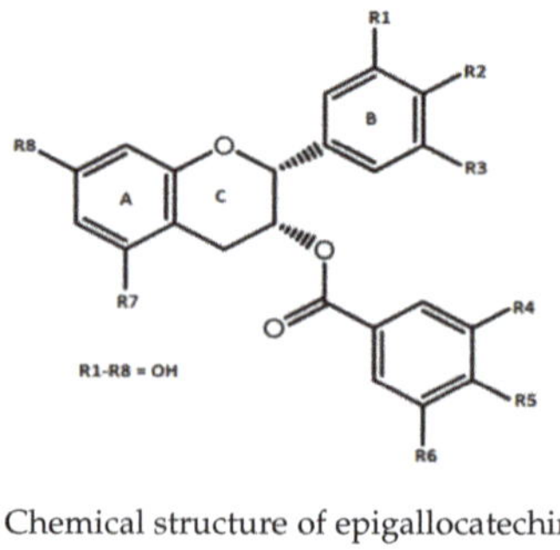

Figure 1. Chemical structure of epigallocatechin gallate.

Pure epigallocatechin gallate is classified as an odourless crystal and/or powder available in white, pink, or cream colour. It is considered to be soluble in water as a colorless and clear solution (5 mg mL^{-1}). It is also soluble in methanol, tetrahydrofuran, acetone, pyridine, and ethanol. EGCG have a melting point at 218 °C [15].

Even though EGCG is found to be the most predominant and bioactive constituent present in tea, it is considered to be poorly stable in aqueous solutions and poorly soluble in oils and fats [16–19]. This poor stability and solubility restricts its direct addition in food products. Numerous delivery systems are, in practice, to preserve its structural integrity and shield EGCG from degradation [18,20–24]. Additionally, structural modification in EGCG has also aided in elevating its lipophilicity [25,26].

Numerous physical aspects like pH, light, oxidants contents, oxygen, temperature, and concentration of EGCG, influence the stability of epigallocatechin gallate [17,26–29]. Epimerization and auto-oxidation are two most important reactions that result in instability of EGCG and loss of its health promoting properties [30]. EGCG is oxidized at low concentration and temperature i.e., 20 to 100 µM & < 44 °C, respectively. On the other hand, it is epimerized to gallocatechin gallate at elevated temperature (greater than 44 °C) and acidic conditions (pH 2 to 5.5) [30–33]. EGCG at a concentration of 300 mg per litre has been found to be stable at 25 °C (24 h) in a pH range of 3 to 6, nonetheless if kept at 4 °C & 25 °C for 24 h (pH 7), a loss of 25 & 83%, respectively, was observed [29].

EGCG is an abundant source of phenolic OH-groups that leads to its health escalating properties. Various scientific studies (in vivo and in vitro) have been carried out to authenticate the potential of EGCG as an anti-oxidative, antiinflammatory, and anti-cancerous agent [34,35].

Wei and co-authors have reported that EGCG exerts an anti-tumor effect through the inhibition of key enzymes that participate in the glycolytic pathway and the suppression of glucose metabolism [36]. Shang and coworkers proposed that tea catechins in combination with anticancer drugs are being evaluated as a new cancer treatment strategy [37]. It has a potential role as adjuvant in cancer therapy and it could enhance the effect of conventional cancer therapies through additive or synergistic effects, as well as through the amelioration of deleterious side effects [38]. EGCG interacts with catalase and highlighted as an anticancer drug [39]. Green tea polyphenols are reported as a translational perspective of chemoprevention and treatment for cancer with concrete influence on signaling pathways [2]. EGCG as a powerful antioxidant, antiangiogenic, and antitumor agent, and as a modulator of tumor cell has the potential to impact in variety of human diseases [40].

This review was prepared systematically searching for articles, papers, books from different sources, such as Embase-Elsevier, Google Scholar, Ovid, PubMed, Science Direct, Scopus, and Web of Science. The search strategy was based on the combination of different keywords, such as EGCG, cancer, tumor, mechanism of action, preclinical, and clinical data, while considering any time of publication. Only sources written in English were included.

2. Occurrence of Epigallocatechin-3-Gallate in Different Foods

The close relationship between food and disease is well known [41], thus EGCG consumed in food could be a natural potential source of health benefits, even in complex and intricated disorder as cancer.

Principal catechin in tea is EGCG, which is also known to be responsible for various health modulating perspectives tht are related to utilization of tea. According to Wu et al., (2012), a cup of green tea prepared by adding 2500 mg leaves in 0.2 L of water contains 90 mg of EGCG [42]. The content of EGCG in black tea is less when compared to green tea, mainly due to polymerization of catechins [43]. EGCG that are derived from tea possess various bioactive properties and, therefore, have attained attention as potent functional and nutraceutical ingredient in food and pharmaceutical industry. Table 1 lists EGCG contents in some selected foods.

Table 1. Occurrence of epigallocatechin-3-gallate in different food.

Description	Content	Reference
Japanese green tea	18.1–23.1 mg/g	
Long-jing tea	32.9–35.5 mg/g	
Jasmine tea	29.8–31.0 mg/g	
Pu-erh tea	16.9–19.19.1 mg/g	[44]
Iron Buddha tea	0.12–0.30 mg/g	
Oolong tea	11.8–12.2 mg/g	
Ceylon tea	7.4–8.9 mg/g	
Green tea	4.62 mg/100 mL	[45]
Black tea	1.35 mg/100 mL	
Ban-cha (tea leaves)	12.2–27.3 mg/g DM	
Fukamushi-cha (tea leaves)	13.8–18.6 mg/g DM	
Yame-cha (tea leaves)	19.7–32.9 mg/g DM	
Uji-cha tea leaves)	22.2–35.9 mg/g DM	[46]
Sayama-cha (tea leaves)	21.5–37.2 mg/g DM	
Uji-matt-cha (Powder tea)	20.1–29.6 mg/g DM	
Gyokuro-cha (Powder tea)	29.9–37.2 mg/g DM	
Sen-cha (tea bags)	12.9–23.6 mg/g DM	
Green tea (Bagged leave form)	54.3–153.0 mg/g dry tea	
Green tea (Loose leave form)	56.5–205.0 mg/g dry tea	[47]
White tea (Bagged leave form)	46.0–154.0 mg/g dry tea	
White tea (Loose leave form)	38.9–144.0 mg/g dry tea	
Green tea (Infusions)	117 to 442 mg/l	[48]
Typhoo,	7.9 mg/230 mL (mg/serving)	
Tesco standard blend,	4.7 mg/230 mL (mg/serving)	
Tesco premium blend,	5.6 mg/230 mL (mg/serving)	
Sainsbury red blend,	8.5 mg/230 mL (mg/serving)	[49]
Sainsbury gold blend,	11.8 mg/230 mL (mg/serving)	
PG Tips,	7.1 mg/230 mL (mg/serving)	
Tetley	5.7 mg/230 mL (mg/serving)	
Apples, Fuji, raw, with skin	1.93 mg/100 g edible portion	
Apples, Golden Delicious, raw, with skin	0.19 mg/100 g edible portion	
Apples, Granny Smith, raw, with skin	0.24 mg/100 g edible portion	
Apples, Red Delicious, raw, without skin	0.46 mg/100 g edible portion	
Apples, Red Delicious, raw. with skin	0.13 mg/100 g edible portion	
Avocados, raw,	0.15 mg/100 g edible portion	
Blackberries, raw (Rubus spp.)	0.68 mg/100 g edible portion	
Cranberries, raw	0.97 mg/100 g edible portion	
Peaches, raw	0.30 mg/100 g edible portion	
Pears, raw	0.17 mg/100 g edible portion	
Plums, black diamond, with peel, raw	0.48 mg/100 g edible portion	
Raspberries, raw	0.54 mg/100 g edible portion	
Nuts, hazelnuts or filberts	1.06 mg/100 g edible portion	[50]
Nuts, pecans	2.30 mg/100 g edible portion	
Nuts, pistachio nuts, raw	0.40 mg/100 g edible portion	
Tea, black, brewed, prepared with tap water	9.36 mg/100 g edible portion	
Tea, black, brewed, prepared with tap water, decaffeinated	1.01 mg/100 g edible portion	
Tea, fruit, dry	415.0 mg/100 g edible portion	
Tea, green, brewed	64.0 mg/100 g edible portion	
Tea, green, brewed, decaffeinated	26.0 mg/100 g edible portion	
Tea, green, large leaf, Quingmao, dry leaves	7380 mg/100 g edible portion	
Tea, oolong, brewed	34.48 mg/100 g edible portion	
Tea, white, brewed	46.0 mg/100 g edible portion	
Tea, white, dry leaves	4245 mg/100 g edible portion	
Carob flour	109.46 mg/100 g edible portion	

3. Signaling Pathways Involving EGCG: Proliferation, Differentiation, Apoptosis, Inflammation, Angiogenesis and Metastasis

A plethora of biomolecular mechanisms has been demonstrated and proposed to be involved in the use of this catechin in preclinical models. These can include, but are not limited to, the induction of apoptosis, cell cycle changes, antioxidant activity, modulation of drug metabolism enzymes, etc. EGCG possesses multiple pharmacological activities, depending on cancer cell type, thus reflecting different protein expression and epigenetic mechanisms. Every cell model can express and modulate at convenience its genetic background, and this is at the basis of the diverse biomolecular targets triggered by EGCG. More consistently, EGCG has been analyzed in different tumor cell lines and less frequently in animal models: this paragraph investigates the association of EGCG with proliferation, differentiation, apoptosis, inflammation, angiogenesis, and metastasis, i.e., the main signaling pathways and processes of living cells (Figure 2).

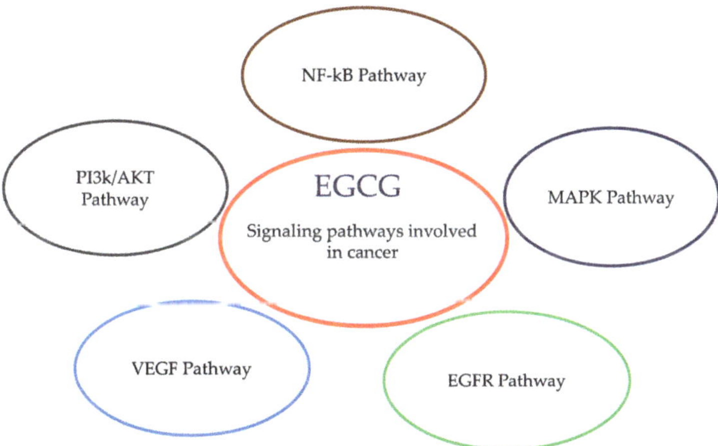

Figure 2. Epigallocatechin gallate (EGCG) involved in the signaling pathways in cancer.

3.1. Cell Death Induction (Apoptosis, Necrosis, Autophagy)

The effects of EGCG on cell death induction, including apoptosis and autophagy, have been investigated in several preclinical studies. Jian and colleagues demonstrated that EGCG induced apoptosis of human liver hepatocellular carcinoma HepG2 cells and rat pheochromocytoma PC12 cells by decreasing the Bcl-2 protein and up-regulating Bax, when used at >20 μM [51]. The proposed mechanism of action of EGCG was related to Human antigen R (HuR, also known as ELAVL1), which can control amyloid protein precursor (APP) via HuR-Erk1/2-APP pathway. APP is implicated in Alzheimer's disease and cancer, blocking ATP with EGCG might be useful in the treatment.

A combination of clofarabine (640 nM and 50 nM in MCF7 and MDA-MB-231 cells, respectively) and EGCG (10 μM) also induced apoptosis in human breast cancer cells, followed by hypomethylation of the tumor suppressor gene RARβ (retinoic acid receptor β) and the upregulation of RARβ, PTEN, and CDKN1A genes [52]. Clofarfabine can inhibit DNA methylation reaction and, thus, its combination with EGCG can have a role in blocking breast cancer development.

The effects of EGCG (>80 μM) on tongue squamous cell carcinoma were recently investigated, showing that it reduced proliferation while promoting apoptosis in CAL27 and SCC 15 cells via the Hippo-TAZ signaling pathway [53]. Similar to other tumor cell models, EGCG (10 200 μM) induced apoptosis in a dose-dependent manner in human thyroid carcinoma cell lines by increasing the Bax/Bcl-2 ratio, thus pointing to an increase of mitochondrial-mediated apoptosis and the involvement of EGFR/RAS/RAF/MEK/ERK signaling pathway [54]. In addition to apoptosis, cell treated with

EGCG has been associated with autophagy regulation. The treatment of human embryonic kidney cell line (HEK293T cells) with EGCG increased cell viability by promoting autophagy through mTOR pathway [55]. In hepatocellular carcinoma cells, EGCG induced autophagy via direct interaction with LC3-I protein and, consequently, led to the degradation of α-fetal protein (AFP); an effect that suggests a potential therapeutic application for the treatment of this type of tumor [56]. EGCG-induced autophagy is also involved in the regulation of ectopic lipid accumulation in vascular endothelial cells, which indicates a potential beneficial effect in preventing cardiovascular diseases [57]. Thus, EGCG is involved in autophagy, even in different tumor cell lines, but with concentration dependent on cell tissue origin. The effect of EGCG on cell death mechanisms is well documented. EGCG has been also proposed as protective agent against necrosis induction because of its demonstrated action on reduction of oxidative stress and inflammatory responses [58].

3.2. Cell Cycle Arrest (Cyclin, CDK)

The effect of EGCG on cell proliferation and cycle has been investigated in various cancers. EGCG in a early work has been demonstrated to play an effective role as an anti-proliferative and chemopreventive agent breast cancer, colon cancer, and skin cancers, such as melanoma in experiments while using MCF-7, HT-29, and UACC-375 cell lines [59]. Specific effects on cell cycle modulation were also investigated in a liver cancer model in which EGCG inhibited the proliferation of liver cancer cells in G2 phase and induced apoptosis after the blocking of the cell cycle progression in the G1 phase [60]. Similar effects were supported in a study on skin cancer, in which the benefits of using polyphenols, such as EGCG, in the treatment and prevention of skin cancer were extensively presented [61]. The effect of EGCG treatment has been also investigated on different cancer types in which cell cycle modulation was demonstrated through the alteration of the pattern of cell cycle proteins with specific reference to CDKs. EGCG increased the expression of CDK1 proteins and inhibited the expression of Cyclin D1 and the phosphorylation of retinoblastoma proteins. Moreover, EGCG treatment has been associated to cell cycle arrest affecting upregulation/downregulation balance in which p1/p21, Kip1/p27, p16/INK4A, cyclin D1, cyclin E, CDK2, and CDK4 proteins are involved. This effect was demonstrated to be the first step of the apoptosis cascade induction via ROS and subsequent caspase-3 and caspase-9 action [62]. These conclusions were then supported by additional in vitro and in vivo experiments in melanoma cancer cells. EGCG treatment of melanoma cells results in the modulation of cyclin-dependent kinases inhibitor network and Bcl2 family proteins with a consequent inhibition of viability and growth, cell cycle blocking, and apoptosis induction [63]. Nevertheless, it was also demonstrated that EGCG can enhance the therapeutic effect if used in synergy with IFN in both in vitro and in vivo models of melanoma, which could be an important advantage in reducing the concentration of IFN and the toxicity of the treatment [64]. The reliability of the treatment or the synergic use of EGCG is additionally supported by a large number of in vitro and in vivo scientific reports on the effects of EGCG on cell cycle modulation and apoptosis induction without affecting normal cells [65]. The studies that are presented in this paragraph point to the usefulness of EGCG in treatment against malignancies by cell cycle modulation and cell death induction, both as therapeutic agent and synergic adjuvant [13,66].

3.3. COX-2

Cyclooxygenase-2 (COX-2) is involved in the modulation of different cell processes, such as oxidative stress and inflammation. COX-2 interaction was considered to be part of the mechanism since EGCG was associated with cell cycle modulation and cell death induction in different cancer models. Dysregulated activity of COX-2 were described in many cancers and pathologic conditions. EGCG was demonstrated to inhibit COX-2 both in terms of transcription and translation in human prostate carcinoma cells (androgen-sensitive LNCaP and androgen-insensitive PC-3), without interfering with COX-1 regulation, and this is an important issue in cancer research. These findings point to the use of EGCG >10 μM in the treatment or prevention of prostate cancer [67]. Furthermore, the EGCG inhibition of COX-2 was investigated on a colon cancer model, in which a significant decrease of COX-2 activity in the cells of the colon of rats treated with green tea extract pointing to a prevention in the formation of preneoplastic foci [68]. The authors fed the animals with freshly prepared an aqueous solution of green tea extract, reconstituted from the lyophilisate, at a concentration of 0.02% (wt/vol) in which EGCG was at 14% dry weight. COX-2 inhibition was also studied on the potential antitumor activity of EGCG in skin cancer [69]. EGCG was administred to mice by gavage at a dose of either 20 or 50 mg/kg body weight 1 h before topical application of the tumor promoter 12-*O*-tetradecanoylphorbol-13-acetate to the shaved back. In this paper, the inhibitor mechanism of COX-2 by EGCG was described as the cascade effect of EGCG inhibition of the catalytic activity of ERK and p38 MAPK that are the upstream enzymes that regulate COX-2 expression [69]. From another point of view, the interaction between EGCG and COX-2 were investigated in arthritis. A solution of 0.2% green tea polyphenols in the water was prepared and given *ad libitum* (the sole source of drinking water for mice). Treatment with this preparation in a collagen II-induced arthritis mouse model demonstrated to reduce the pathological picture of arthritis, with decrease of TNF-α, IFN-γ, and Cox-2 especially in mice arthritic joints [70]. Thus, it was demonstrated that the treatment of human chondrocytes with EGCG at concentration >100 μM was related to the inhibition of COX-2 and iNOS activity indicating a possible involvement of this treatment in the inhibition of cartilage resorption in arthritis [71].

3.4. EGFR Pathway

EGFR (epidermal growth factor receptor) is a plasma membrane protein that is characterized by an intracellular region acting as tyrosine kinase and an extracellular receptor domain. The dysregulation of EGFR expression has been associated with cellular neoplastic transformation. EGCG interaction with EGFR was demonstrated and described in its mechanism. EGCG binds to a specific laminin receptor whose expression is reported in a variety of tumor cells: this connection can interfere with the activity of the kinase-phosphatase cascades [72]. The laminin receptor has been recently related to MAPK signaling in human melanoma metastasis mechanism [73]. EGCG inhibition of EGFR and HER2 was demonstrated in colon cancer cells line (HT29), in which these proteins are overexpressed in comparison with normal tissue. EGCG at 20 μg/mL resulted in cell growth reduction, cell cycle arrest in G1 phase, and apotosis induction by the activation of caspase-3 and -9, with critical impact on EGFR/ERK and EGFR/Akt signaling pathways [74]. The adjuvant effect of EGFR in breast cancer treatment was demonstrated in different cell lines (MCF-7, MCF-7TAM, and MDA-MB-231). The combined treatment of EGCG with IIF (6-OH-11-O-hydroxyphenanthrene) reduced the invasive phenotype and up-regulated the expression of molecules that are involved in the invasion process, again acting on EGFR/Akt pathway and their regulated targets, such as CD44, extracellular matrix metalloproteinases inducer (EMMPRIN), matrix metalloproteinases, and tissue inhibitor of metalloproteinases (TIMPs) [75]. Similarly EGCG activity was also investigated in MCF-7tam (a breast carcinoma cell line resistant to the chemoagent tamoxifen), where EGCG was demonstrated to reduce the resistance to Tamoxifen and block cell growth and invasion [76]. In this last work, the EGFR/ERK pathway was downregulated, with effects on matrix metalloproteinase-2 and -9, EMMPRIN. It emerges as the effects EGCG on EGFR pathway depend on cancer cell type and suggest as EGCG can have an adjuvant role in EGFR targeted therapy approach.

3.5. MAPK Pathway

The MAPK pathway (or extensively "Ras-Raf-MEK-ERK pathway") is a key signaling pathway frequently dysregulated in human cancer and can control multiple cell functions, such as proliferation and growth [77]. For these reasons, different chemotherapeutic drugs have been already clinically evaluated or are currently undergoing to specific clinical trials, for example, most promising are the MEK1/2 and Raf inhibitors [78]. In mammalian cells, three major types of MAP kinases are present; ERK, p38 MAP kinase, and JNK, and they can activate c-JNK and ELK [79]. These were the main actors studied and they were associated with EGCG interaction in the MAPK pathway. A recent work studied EGCG and candesartan (anti-hypertensive drug) in a rat model of gentamicin-induced nephrotoxicity [80]. EGCG was administred at 25 mg/kg, intraperitoneally, alone or combined with the above drugs for 21 days. While renal disease revealed increased levels of NF-κB, p38-MAPK, caspase 3, TNF-α, and interleukin-1 β, the pre-treatments with EGCG and candesartan (co-treatment had the best results if compared to compounds alone) reduced such key factors, which impacted the MAPK pathway. On the same line, a work with mice of Wang et al. showed that, in animals with artificial unilateral ureteral obstruction, the intraperitoneally administration of EGCG (5 mg/kg) for 14 days inhibited phosphorylation of ERK, JNK and p38 MAPK [81]. The effect of EGCG on mastitis in rats were evaluated by injecting lipopolysaccharide (LPS) into the duct of mammary gland. EGCG was orally given at 25 or 100 mg/kg/day in the morning for 14 days. MAPKs, NFκB-p65 and hypoxia-inducible factor-1α (HIF-1α) were decreased after the treatment with EGCG at both concentrations. The results showed that EGCG suppressed MAPK related oxidative stress and inflammatory responses [82]. In another rat disease model, EGCG exhibited cardioprotective effects in myocardial ischemia/reperfusion (I/R) injuries [83]. The authors showed that EGCG 10mg/kg intravenously administered alone or with wortmannin (PI3K inhibitor) 5 min. before the onset of reperfusion reduced p38 and JNK phosphorylation while enhancing AKT and GSK-3β, but not ERK1/2. Additionally, in artificial induced hypertensive rats, ERK, p38, and JNK phosphorylation were decreased, when the rats were treated with 50 mg/kg EGCG per day, intraperitoneally for 21 days [84]. Previously in human umbilical vein endothelial cell (HUVEC) model, EGCG induced cell proliferation inhibition during ischemia/reperfusion, but, in contrast with previous work, JNK1/2 (and c-Jun) phosphorylation was increased [85]. These data could be imputable to the different model and time of incubation proposed. Also, EGCG >50 μM inhibited angiotensin II- induced phosphorylation of ERK and p38 in HUVEC cells, influencing vascular cell adhesion molecules (VCAMs) and intercellular adhesion molecules (ICAMs) expression [86,87]. In addition, EGCG impacted AKT phosphorylation and its downstream substrates Foxo1, Foxo3a, and ERK1/2. In a prostate cancer mouse model (TRAMP mice: Transgenic Adenocarcinoma Mouse Prostate), Harper and collaborators demonstrated that EGCG given *ad libitum* as 0.06% in water reduced ERK phosphorylation, together with androgen receptor (AR), insulin-like growth factor-1 (IGF-1), IGF-1 receptor (IGF-1R), COX-2, and inducible nitric oxide synthase (iNOS) [88]. The authors claimed that the EGCG dose should mimic a human consumption of six cups of green tea and that the catechin, through the decrease of MAPK signaling, could modulate inflammation biomarkers, reduce cell proliferation, and induce apoptosis. In the same mouse TRAMP model, another work showed a key role for IGF-I/IGFBP-3 signaling pathway, with the modulation of ERK [89]. However, the authors used a solution of 0.1% green tea polyphenols (in which EGCG represented 62%) to experimental animals [89]. The two works are very similar in EGCG dose, but analyzed and demonstrated the implaction of different key factors: they are probably the two sides of the same coin, but more research is needed to confirm this hyphothesis. Moreover, in a NOD mouse, a model for Sjogren's syndrome, oral administration of 0.2% green tea extract in *ad libitum* water for 21 days (in which EGCG represented 40%) reduced the total autoantibody levels in the serum and lymphocytic infiltration of submandibular glands (a key point of Sjogren's syndrome) [90]. The research was also expanded in normal human keratinocytes and immortalized normal human salivary acinar cells, where EGCG was able to protect the cells by specific phosphorylation of p38 MAPK [90–93], contrary to most of works in which there is a de-phosphorylation/deactivation of MAPK pathway. Again, these apparently inconsistent results should be ascribed to different models used and the different human-derived tissue.

In SKH-1 hairless mouse model, the topical application of green tea polyphenols (in which EGCG represented 18.8%) showed a decrease in UVB-induced thickness, skin edem, a and infiltration of leukocytes, processes mediated by inhibition of ERK, c-JUN, and p38, as well as NF-kB [94]. Before the animal model, the authors demonstrated the same results in cell models in which EGCG was used at 10–40 μM [92,95]. In addition, EGCG diminished the negative effects of ultraviolet irradiation in human dermal fibroblasts, reducing the phosphorylation of MAPK, JNK, p38 MAPK, and ERK1/2 [95,96]. Collagen destruction was reduced by inhibiting matrix metalloproteinases (MMP-1, MMP-8, and

MMP-13). In human AC16 cardiomyocytes, EGCG was examined for alleviating cigarette smoke medium (CSM)-induced inflammation: EGCG protected from oxidative stress, inflammation, and apoptosis, modifying interleukin (IL)-8 productions via the inhibition of ERK1/2, p38 MAPK, and NF-κB pathways [97]. In the human retinal endothelial cell (HREC) line, a preclinical model for diabetic retinopathy, EGCG was able to decrease phosphorylated p38, ERK, VEGF, and the expression of inflammatory markers, such as TNF-α, IL-6, and ICAM-1 [98]. In addition, EGCG amended the negative effect of high glucose concentrations acting on the MAPK pathway. Furthermore, EGCG in chronic myeloid leukaemia cells inhibited cell growth and induced apoptosis through the inhibition of Bcr/Abl oncoprotein and regulation of its downstream signals, such as p38-MAPK and JNK (in addition to involvement of JAK2/STAT3/AKT pathway) [99]. In a different cellular context, JB6 mouse epidermal cell line, it has been shown that EGCG could inhibit AP-1(activating protein-1)-dependent transcriptional activity through the inhibition of a c-JUN, but not ERK [100]. AP-1 is a transcription factor involved that can be stimulated by cytokines, growth factors, stress, and, consequently, implicated in proliferation and apoptosis, with overlapping role to MAPK pathway. Successively, another work remarked the importance of AP-1 (and MAPK), with the inhibition of c-JUN, and also ERK by EGCG, differently from previous research [101]. Of note that a different cell line was used (human gastric AGS cells). EGCG also impacted endothelial cell activation, where the catechin could downregulate endothelial inflammation by acting on MAPK signaling through a caveolae-regulated cell mechanism [102]. Endothelial cells are fundamental in atherosclerosis: EGCG demonstrated antiatherogenic effect in reducing oxidized LDL upregulated by c-Jun phosphorylation and blocking oxidized LDL-induced endothelial apoptosis [103]. In the pancreatic alpha TC1-6 (αTC1-6) cell line, EGCG confirmed its anti-hyperglycemia and antioxidant potential [104]. Indeed, EGCG re-established glucagon secretion and reduced ROS, while inhibiting JNK and p38 and activating AKT signaling. It is of note that a higher concentration of EGCG (100 μM) was used, if compared to previous studies, and this can potentially reduce EGCG efficacy when moved to clinical trials. Moreover, in a cell model of insulin-stimulated mitogenesis (3T3-L1 preadipocytes), it has been shown that EGCG inhibited the insulin effects, switching off signaling through both insulin receptor-β, insulin receptor substrates 1 and 2 (IRS1 and IRS2) and RAF1, MEK1/2, and ERK1/2, but not JNK [105].

Interestingly, EGCG was associated with sunitinib, which is a multi-target receptor tyrosine kinase inhibitor approved for renal carcinoma and gastrointestinal stromal tumor, in MCF-7 (breast cancer) and H460 (lung cancer) mouse xenograft tumors [106]. The authors found that synergize with sunitinib due to its ability to suppress both insulin receptor substrate-1 pathway and MAPK signaling induced by sunitinib. In another breast cancer cell line T47D, EGCG induced the phosphorylation of JNK/SAPK and p38 and modulated cyclin A, cyclin B1, and cdk proteins, triggering G2 arrest [107]. In a human colon cancer cell line (HT-29), it was found that EGCG activated phospho-AKT, phospho-ERK, phospho-JNK, and phospho-p38α/γ/δ and, consequently, induced cell death, a potential mechanism for anti-cancer effect of EGCG [108]. Previously with same cell line, Chen et al. showed the activation of caspase-3 and -9, cytochrome *c*, mitochondria, c-Jun, and MAPK pathway after treatment with EGCG, with the end result of apoptosis induction [109]. In another colon cancer cell line (SW480), EGCG induced the phosphorylation of p38, which mediated the phosphorylation of EGFR at Ser1046/1047, leading to a downregulation of the EGFR/MAPK pathway [110]. The author claimed that this phosphorylation could play a pivotal role in EGFR downregulation that is induced by EGCG. Furthermore, in HCT116 colorectal carcinoma cells, EGCG triggered the phosphorylation of ERK, JNK, and p38, which, in turn, conducted to apoptosis [111]. In human lung cancer cell line PC-9, EGCG was associated with celecoxib (a cyclooxygenase-2 selective inhibitor) provoking an activation of ERK1/2 and p38 regulated by GADD153 (DNA damage-inducible 153) expression [112]. EGCG induced apoptosis and the authors suggested that GADD153 could be a new molecular target for cancer prevention in combination with EGCG. Similarly, EGCG was found to suppress cell proliferation by upregulating BTG2 (B-cell translocation gene 2) expression via MAPK pathway in oral squamous cell carcinoma (OSCC), in particular with the phosphorylation of p38, JNK, and ERK [113].

Moreover, in anaplastic thyroid cell carcinoma (ARO cells), EGCG 50 μM showed anti-proliferative and pro-apoptotic effects, being mediated by the suppression of phosphorylated EGFR, ERK1/2, JNK, and p38 and p21, caspase-3, and cleaved PARP increase and cyclin B1/CDK1 expression decline [114]. In a previous work, human hepatoma HepG2-C8 cells and human cervical squamous carcinoma HeLa cells were used to evaluate EGCG [115]. The results indicated that catechin induced the activation of ERK, JNK, and p38 in a dose- and time-dependent manner, with stimulation of apoptosis (mediated by caspase-3) and antioxidant response element (ARE). In DU-145 prostate cancer cells, EGCG associated with ibuprofen reduced >90% tumor cell growth through the activation of both MAPK and caspases [116]. Similarly, human prostate cancer androgen-unresponsive and responsive cells (DU145 and LNCaP, respectively) that were treated with EGCG showed an increase of ERK1/2 with concomitant decrease of phosphorylated AKT and the level of PI3K, again underlining the anticancer effect of the catechin [117].

3.6. NF-kB Pathway

NF-κB (Nuclear factor-κB) is involved in a variety of cellular mechanisms, such as death, growth, inflammation, and immune response. NF-κB mainly acts as a regulator of gene transcription in response to oxidative stress. The interaction with EGCG was described in a variety of cell models, both in vivo and in vitro [64]. NF-κB is one of the most investigated targets in cancer research and the interaction with this pathway should be considered to be a relevant topic in cancer treatment design. The inhibitory activity of EGCG on NF-κB has been demonstrated in a large number of independent studies. Studies that were performed in normal human epidermal keratinocytes in which EGCG was used at different concentration to modulate NF-κB activity, leading to a protective effect towards the negative cascade that was induced by UV radiation. This is considered the proof of the mechanism of action of green tea as a photoprotective agent [92]. Moreover EGCG has been shown to reduce significantly the gut mucosa inflammation in response to injury, thus inhibiting the production of inflammatory factors via the modulation of NF-κB expression and other involved genes [118]. The authors showed that, in ulcerative colitis (a refractory inflammatory disease of the large intestine) rat model, EGCG intraperitoneally administered at 50 mg/kg/d could reduce the severity of the disease, through the TLR4/MyD88/NF-κB signaling pathway. Moving on cancer research, EGCG was able to activate caspases in epidermoid carcinoma cells, and this has been demonstrated to play a relevant role in the inhibition of NF-κB and induction of apoptosis [119]. Nevertheless, EGCG has been demonstrated to play a potential role in human colon cancer prevention inhibiting AP-1, c-fos, cyclin D1 promoters, and NF-κB activity in four different human colon cancer cell lines, with an IC_{50} value of about 20 μg/mL [74].

3.7. PI3k/AKT Pathway

Numerous studies on diseases that involve PI3K/AKT signaling investigated the possible effect of green tea administration [120]. Since green tea role in asthma treatment or occurrence need to be better clarified [121,122], the effect on molecular pathways at the basis of pathological processes has been explored. Recently, a possible mechanism of action has been proposed in brochial asthma. EGCG, being administered in drinking water 0.5 mg/mL, was demonstrated to reduce inflammation and the subsequent cellular infiltration in lung tissue of ovalbumin-challenged asthmatic mouse, inhibiting EMT via PI3/AKT pathway modulation in vivo and in vitro models [123]. On the other hand, EGCG modulation on the PI3K/AKT signaling pathway was associated to lung cancer prevention and suppression. EGCG activation/inhibition of PI3K/AKT was found to be a key switch in H1299 cells growth inhibition ad apoptosis induction [124]. Another interesting research has been carried on the neuroprotective action of EGCG in a middle cerebral artery occlusion model (MCAO), acting as a modulating agent PI3K/AKT/eNOS signaling pathway [125]. The rats were treated with 20 mg/kg EGCG, injecting it with an arterial pump and the expressions of PI3K, p-AKT, and eNOS were detected by both immunohistochemistry and Western blot. Similarly, in unilateral chronic constriction injury to the sciatic nerve, EGCG role as neuroprotective agent was confirmed in rats [126]. 50 mg/kg EGCG was intraperitoneally administered daily for three days after nerve crush injury.

3.8. VEGF Pathway

Angiogenesis is known to play a major role in the pathogenesis of many cancer types [127]. Given its involvement in metastasis and growth of tumor cells, angiogenesis possesses a key player in vascular endothelial growth factor (VEGF, also known as VEGF-A) and it has been intensively studied as a therapeutic target [128]. Consequently, EGCG has been investigated in the VEGF pathway, discovering its capacity to modulate angiogenesis, with stimutating effects in nervous tissue and inhibiting effects in tumor tissue. For example, in a mouse model of transient middle cerebral artery occlusion (MCAO), the authors showed that EGCG injected intraperitoneally daily for seven days could stimulate angiogenesis. EGCG had a neuroprotective effect, indeed treated mice had better neurologic outcome, a decreased infarct volume, greater vascular density, with the modulation of VEGF signaling pathway and increased Nrf2 expression (fundamental role in against ischemic stroke) [129]. Similarly, hepatic tissue from mice that were treated with EGCG showed increased heme oxygenase-1 (HO-1) and decreased vascular cell adhesion molecule (VCAM)-1 expression, with an increased expression of Nrf-2 (mediated by p38) that drives the expression of HO-1, as also demonstrated in human aortic endothelial cells (HAEC) [130]. Another group used the same mouse model (MCAO) and demonstrated the involvement of the PI3K/AKT/eNOS signaling pathway with a concomitant reduction of apoptotic rate and caspase-3 in neurons, while Bcl-2 increased in the ECGC treated set (EGCG intraperitoneally injected at 20 mg/kg for 24 h) [125]. Similarly, it was studied on the effects of EGCG on murine dendritic cells (DC), with a reduction of ERK1/2, p38, JNK, and blockade of NF-κB p65 translocation [131]. EGCG was given to cells at different doses, but 100 μM was the most effective with suppression of the phenotypic and functional maturation of DC. Differently in tumor tissue EGCG acted in a opposite way. For example, in human gastric cancer SGC7901 cells (in hypoxic state) EGCG (5, 10, 20, 40 μM), reduced expressions of HIF-1α (a subunit of a heterodimeric transcription factor hypoxia-inducible factor 1-HIF1) and VEGF with a concentration-dependent effect. In addition, in SGC-7901 mouse xenografts, 1.5 mg/day EGCG intraperitoneally injected reduced VEGF, tumor microvessel density, endothelial cell proliferation, migration, and tube formation, substantially blocking tumor growth [132]. Similarly, in gastric cancer 5-fluorouracil (5-FU) resistant cells (MGC803/FU treated with 100 μg/mL and SGC7901/FU treated with 20 μM), EGCG inhibited VEGF and HIF-1 expression, reversing 5-FU resistance that is mediated by VEGF pathway [133,134]. HIF-1 is a master regulator of cell homeostatic response to hypoxia by activating the transcription of numerous genes that are implicated in growth, apoptosis, angiogenesis, and metabolism [135]. HIF-1 is strictly connected with VEGF (it is a primary target of HIF-1) and, thus, understanding the regulation of HIF-1 will offer new insight into VEGF pathway and new potential therapeutic targets. In human gastric cancer cells (AGS) EGCG >10 μM reduce dose-dependently VEGF expression and secretion mediated by signal transducer and activator of transcription 3 (Stat3) activity [136]. In colon cancer cells (Caco2, HCT116, HT29, SW480, and SW837 lines) and SW837 mouse xenograft, EGCG impacted on VEGF/VEGFR axis suppressing VEGFR2 (a primary responder to VEGF signal), together with HIF-1α, ERK, and AKT [137]. Moreover in a different human colon cancer cell line (HT29) and derived mouse xenografts, EGCG lessened VEGF expression and its promoter activity, while decreasing the tumour growth and microvessel density in mice (treated daily intraperitoneally with 1.5 mg EGCG), and modulating cell proliferation and apoptosis in HT29 cells [138]. In breast cancer cells (MCF-7), HIF-1α and VEGF was decreased by EGCG in a dose-dependent manner (25, 50, 100 mg/L) [139], similarly to non-small lung cancer cells (A549), in which the catechin (25, 50, 100 μM) was able both to inhibit HIF-1α protein expression (stimulated by IGF-I, insulin growth factor-1, a growth hormone mediating cell growth) and the formation of capillary tube-like structures on a model of extracellular matrix [140]. In head and neck squamous cell carcinoma (YCU-H891) and breast carcinoma cell lines (MDA-MB-231), EGCG blocked VEGF activity, thanks to the inhibition of constitutive activation of Stat3 and NF-κB [141]. The results showed that EGCG could modulate a plethora a key factors, such as TNF-α, Rantes, monocyte chemotactic protein-1 (MCP-1), intercellular adhesion molecule-1 (ICAM-1), nitric oxide (NO), VEGF, and MMP-2, through the inhibition of NF-κB and MAPK signaling pathways (downregulation of p-IκBα, p65, p-p65, p-p38, p-ERK1/2, and p-AKT). EGCG repressed hypoxia- and serum-induced HIF-1α and VEGF, through MAPK and PI3K/AKT pathways, in another hepatoma cell line (HepG2) and in human cervical carcinoma cell line (HeLa) [142]. In a group of acute myeloid leukemia (AML) cell lines harboring FLT3 mutation (FLT3 is a commonly mutated gene in AML), EGCG 60 μM (and (−)-epigallocatechin (EGC), (−)-epicatechin-3-gallate (ECG), and (+)-Catechin (C)) showed reduced levels of FLT3 and the suppression of phosphorylated MAPK, AKT, and STAT5 [143]. Moreover, in B-cell chronic lymphocytic leukemia (B-CLL), EGCG 3–25 μM reduced VEGF-R1 and VEGF-R2 phosphorylation (fundamental in B-CLL survival and growth) and induced apoptosis by caspase-3 activation, poly-adenosine diphosphate ribose polymerase (PARP) cleavage, and B-cell leukemia/lymphoma-2 protein (Bcl-2) [144,145].

Additionally, in non-tumoral cell lines, EGCG demonstrated a concrete role. In human microvascular endothelial cells (HMVEC) used as a model of angiogenesis, EGCG inhibited VEGF-induced tube formation through the suppression of vascular endothelial-cadherin phosphorylation and AKT activation [146]. In normal human keratinocytes (NHK) that were stimulated by TNFα, EGCG at different concentrations (0.1 to 10 μM) decreased VEGF and interleukin-8 (proinflammatory cytokine involved in skin inflammation) [147]. Similarly, in human umbilical vein endothelial cells (HUVEC), EGCG inhibited VEGF in a concentration dependent manner and reduced cell proliferation [148]. On the same line, two works from the same research group used HUVEC cells (and MDA-MB231 breast cancer cell) and found that EGCG decreased VEGF production in a concentration-dependent manner (6.25, 25, 100 μM) [149,150]. They also demonstrated that, in HUVEC and MDA-MB231 mouse xenografts, in addition to cell line, green tea extract reduced the proliferation, tumor size, and tumor vessel density [150]. Mice fed with green tea extract in water *ad libitum* with a concentration of 0.62, 1.25, and 2.5 g/L (in which EGCG represented 46.8% weight). The effects were both time and concetration dependent. In human vascular smooth muscle cells (hVSMCs), EGCG was investigated after cell stimulation with platelet-derived growth factor (PDGF), which is known to induce VEGF expression [151]. EGCG blocked dose-dependently VEGF expression and PDGF receptor activation, in addition to ERK1/2 and AP-1. Additionally, in livestock ovarian cell model (swine granulosa cells), EGCG was evaluated as a food supplement. The catechin reduced VEGF production independently of oxygen condition and decreased cell growth, which suggested a role in angiogenic process, fundamental for follicle development [152].

3.9. Proteasome

The proteasome is a protein complex that is dedicated to degrade damaged or useless proteins that are unusable to cell [153]. It is strictly dependent on ubiquitins, molecules that tag unwanted proteins and continues with the degradation process mediated by proteases [154]. The proteasome has been investigated as a key target for multiple diseases, given its importance in cell physiology. Effectively, three approved drugs are available, bortezomib (for multiple myeloma and mantle cell lymphoma), carfilzomib and ixazomib (for relapsed or refractory multiple myeloma), and many others are in development [155]. Different cell types were tested with EGCG: human Jurkat T, prostate cancer (LNCaP, PC-3), breast cancer (MCF-7), normal (WI-38), and SV40-transformed (VA-13) human fibroblast cells [156,157]. The works showed that EGCG specifically blocked proteasome activity in LNCaP, PC-3, and MCF-7 cell extracts with a range of IC$_{50}$ from 86 to 194 nm. In addition, in cell models, EGCG 1–10 μM induced the accumulation of two natural proteasome substrates, p27(Kip1) and IkappaB-alpha, an inhibitor of transcription factor NF-κB, together with G1 cell cycle phase arrest. Moreover, EGCG derivatives were studied both to understand the biochemical role of such molecules in proteasome inhibition and to find novel potent or stabilized alternatives to EGCG [158]. For example, a work of Kazi and collaborators revealed that the A-ring and gallate ester/amide bond are necessary for the blockade of proteasome [159]. Similarly, EGCG modified with peracetate presented higher proteasome-inhibitory activity if compared to EGCG, with increased cell death mechanism in Jurkat T cells [160]. Again, other EGCG analogs were tested and showed that B-ring/D-ring peracetate-protected EGCG derivatives could induce cell death [161,162]. Additionally, peracetate-protected EGCG in breast carcinoma cell line (MDA-MB-231) and in MDA-MB-231 mouse xenografts (daily *sub cute* injection with 50 mg/kg) was tested, showing tumor growth decrement, with concomitant proteasome inhibition and apoptosis activation [163]. Later, different fluoro-substituted EGCG analogs were generated and, among these, Pro-F-EGCG4 ((-)-(2R,3R)-5,7-Diacetoxy-2-(3,4,5-triacetoxyphenyl)chroman-3-yl3,4-difluorobenzoate) had potent effects than peracetate EGCG inducing apoptosis and decreasing cell proliferation (concentration-dependent effects from 10 to 50 μM) in the Jurkat and MDA-MB-231 cell lines, in addition to reducing tumor size in MDA-MB-231 mouse xenografts (daily *subcutaneous* injection with 50 mg/kg) [164,165]. In the same cell line (MDA-MB-231), EGCG was tested with catechol-σ-methyltransferase (COMT), an human enzyme that degrades catecholamines [166]. COMT can methylate EGCG, reducing its biological activity. The work reported that decreasing COMT activity could augment EGCG efficacy through apoptosis induction and proteasome inhibition. In YT (human natural killer) and Jurkat cell lines, EGCG (and other proteasome inhibitors) produced cell cycle modulation (subG0/G1 phase increase in Jurkat cells and G2/M phase arrest in YT cells), apoptosis with caspase-3 activation, and with mitochondrial membrane potential decrement [167]. Moreover, in Caco-2 cells, EGCG inhibited 20S proteasomes activity with antioxidant and proteasome blocking properties in cell lysates [168]. In the human neuroblastoma cell line (SH-SY5Y), EGCG at low concentration (1 μM) impacted on BCL2 associated agonist of cell death (Bad) levels, while the protein kinase C (PKC) inhibitor GF109203X impeded Bad degradation [169]. The authors claimed that EGCG promoted neuronal survival through the rapid removal of Bad (PKC-mediated) by proteasome, while using low doses, whereas most of works showed general EGCG inhibitory effects at 50 μM. This difference could probably reside in the specific cell model used. In a mouse model of experimental autoimmune encephalomyelitis (EAE), EGCG administered by gavage 300 μL per mouse twice daily was able to decrease clinical severity, as suggested by reduced brain inflammation and neuronal damage [170]. In addition, in the same work with human myelin-specific CD4+ T cells, EGCG impacted cyclin-dependent kinase 4 expression (with cell cycle arrest) and on 20S/26S proteasome complex activity (with subsequent NF-κB inhibition), demonstrating anti-inflammatory and neuronal protective capacities. In skin cancer cells (SCC-13 and A431), EGCG alone or associated to 3-deazaneplanocin A (a potent inhibitor of S-adenosylhomocysteine hydrolase, enzyme that is involved in homocysteine metabolism) suppressed cell cycle progression and increased apoptosis, through proteasome-dependent degradation of the polycomb group proteins, molecules that are involved in development, differentiation, and survival [171]. A study investigated the effects of extremely low frequency electromagnetic fields (ELFEF) on 20S proteasome while using EGCG in Caco-2 cells [172]. It is known that ELFEF can modulate intracellular ROS levels and the cell cycle progression, indeed EGCG was able to reduce the pro-oxidant effects, regulate cell cycle, and proteasome functionality. However, EGCG did not alter cell viability as measured by MTT assay.

Though numerous works demonstrated a positive interaction of EGCG in proteasome function, others showed a deleterious activity of EGCG. For example, in HepG2 cells, EGCG 50 μM exerted anti-cholesterolemic activity, reducing apolipoprotein B-100 (apoB) production and lipid assembly, thorough a proteasome-independent pathway, as demonstrated by a lack of response to N-acetyl-leucyl-leucyl-norleucinal, a proteasome inhibitor [173]. Moreover, the association of EGCG and bortezomib (proteasome inhibitor for multiple myeloma) should not be suggested, as their experimentation in human multiple myeloma cells (RPMI/8226 and U266) showed strong antagonism, with EGCG blocking proteasome inhibition being produced by bortezomib and, thus, stopping tumor cell death [174,175]. Similarly, in prostate cancer cells (PC3), bortezomib anti-tumor effects was counteracted by EGCG which induced autophagy while decreasing endoplasmic reticulum stress [176]. These data underline in a different cell model, as EGCG can antagonize bortezomib, blocking prostate cancer cells death, and thus negatively supporting tumor pro-survival.

3.10. Senescence

Senescence is defined the condition or process of deterioration with age [177]. Senescence plays a role in multiple biological events, such as embryogenesis, tissue regeneration and repair, ageing, cardiovascular, renal, liver diseases, and cancer [178,179]. EGCG has been implicated in senescence in different works. For example human mesenchymal stem cells (hMSCs) show the peculiar behavior of producing abundant ROS during culturing and this issue has been exploited with a natural anti-oxidant as EGCG [180]. The work explored the anti-senescent effect of EGCG in H_2O_2-exposed hMSCs and proved that EGCG reversed oxidative stress by downregulating the p53–p21 signaling pathway and upregulating Nrf2 expression. Similarly, in primary cells, including rat vascular smooth muscle cells (RVSMCs), human dermal fibroblasts (HDFs) and human articular chondrocytes (HACs), the same concentrations of EGCG (50 or 100 μM) could prevent senescence and recover cell cycle progression, again impacting on the p53 pathway at least in HDFs cells [181]. Furthermore, in 3T3-L1 preadipocytes, EGCG could inhibit stress-induced senescence (H_2O_2-induced) by countering DNA damage and cell cycle arrest [182]. In this work, EGCG (same concentrations as above, 50 or 100 μM) modulated PI3K/Akt/mTOR and AMPK pathways by blocking ROS, iNOS, Cox-2, NF-kB, and p53, and increasing apoptosis by suppressing antiapoptotic protein Bcl-2. Moreover, in WI-38 fibroblasts at late-stage (population doubling > 25) used as model of oxidative stress and inflammation, EGCG (25, 50, 100 μM) reduced TNF-α, IL-6, ROS, again acting on p53 [183]. ECGC also decreased retinoblastoma expressions, while enhancing E2F2 expressions and superoxide dismutase (SOD) 1 and 2, all being implicated in oxidation processes. EGCG has been shown to affect the development and severity of cellular senescence, but from a therapeutic perspective more work is needed. Senolytic attributes of EGCG are interesting, especially for attenuating age-associated disorders, though clinical trails and health consequence still need to be proposed and discovered.

3.11. Epigenetics and Mirnas

Epigenetics refers to heritable phenotype changes, in which DNA sequence alteration are not included. The most known epigenetic mechanisms involve DNA methylation and histone modification [184]. Extensively, epigenetics concerns all events "outside" DNA sequence modification; indeed, this paragraph wants to describe those mechanisms characteristic of DNA methylation and histone modification involving EGCG. Numerous works have been reported the significant impact of EGCG in epigenetic mechanism. For example, in 2003, EGCG was first studied as an inhibitor of DNA hypermethylation of CpG islands by acting on 5-cytosine DNA methyltransferase (DNMT). EGCG was used at 20 and 50 μM with concentration-dependent effects in human esophageal cancer cells (KYSE 510), colon cancer HT-29, and prostate cancer PC3 cells [185]. The authors showed that EGCG could block DMNT and reactivate methylated-silenced genes, as p16(INK4a), retinoic acid receptor β (RARβ), O-(6)-methylguanine methyltransferase (MGMT), and human mutL homologue 1 (hMLH1). Similar results were obtained in human breast cancer cell lines (MCF-7 and MDA-MB-231), whereas EGCG was able to block prokaryotic SssI DNA methyltransferase (DNMT) and human DNMT1 [186]. A recent work used the same cell lines (MCF-7 and MDA-MB-231) investigating RARβ expression and methylation, as mentioned in the first paragraph [52]. EGCG combined with 2-chloro-2′-fluoro-2′-deoxyarabinosyladenine (a deoxyadenosine analogue) reduced RARβ methylation with consequent increase of its expression, together with PTEN and CDKN1A, and with apoptosis induction and cell proliferation inhibition. EGCG acted on inhibitor of matrix metalloproteinases (TIMPs) and MMPs, being highly involved in tumorigenesis, in human prostate cancer cells (DUPRO and LNCaP) [187]. The authors showed that EGCG restored TIMP-3 expression and concomitantly increased histone H3K9/18 acetylation and decreased class I histone deacetylase, impacting on cell invasion and migration. Interestingly in serum of patients undergoing prostatectomy consuming 800 mg EGCG up to 6 weeks (participating to clinical trial NCT01340599), TIMP-3 levels were increased, suggesting a potential mechanism of action of EGCG in prostate cancer [187]. However, the trial failed to show a significant benefit of EGCG-treated prostate cancer patients [188].

Moreover, in a SKH-1 hairless mouse model, EGCG added to a hydrophilic cream and applied to approximately 1 mg/cm^2 skin area could protect against photocarcinogenesis through the reduction of tumor incidence, tumor multiplicity, and tumor size [189]. Mechanisms at the basis of these results are related to the inhibition of DNA hypomethylation induced by ultraviolet B treatment. Likewise, in human skin cancer cells (A431) and squamous cell carcinoma (SCC 13) cells, EGCG could reactivate p16INK4a and Cip1/p21, impacting not only on DNA methylation and DNMT activity, but also on histone deacetylase (HDAC) activity and acetylated histones [190]. Again, in CD4+ Jurkat T cells, EGCG 50 μM could inhibit DNMT and induce a concomitant Foxp3 (a factor regulating the development and function of regulatory T cells) and IL-10 expression. Moreover, in mice that were treated with EGCG (injected intraperitoneally daily per mouse 50 mg/kg), there was an increase of regulatory T cells frequencies and numbers [191]. In human malignant lymphoma cells (CA46), EGCG alone (6 μg/mL) or combined with trichostatin A (inhibitor of HDACs) diminished p16INK4a gene methylation (thus increasing its expression) and provoked a cell proliferation decrement [192]. The effects were more evident with the combination of the compounds, rather than EGCG alone, being suggestive an additive or synergist effect. In human breast tumor tissues, expression of DNMTs was found increased by Mirza et al., consequently MCF-7 and MDA MB 231 cells were used as models for testing EGCG and other compounds [193]. The authors showed that EGCG decreased DNMT1, HDAC1, and methyl-CpG binding protein 2 (MeCP2 essential for nerve function), with a reversal of epigenetic changes present in cancer cells. On the same line, another work investigated a co-treatment of 5-aza-2'-deoxycytidine and EGCG in breast cancer cells (MCF-10A) and confirmed the effects on DNA methylation and histone modifications [194]. In a mouse lung tumor model that was induced by the tobacco-specific carcinogen 4-(Methylnitrosamino)-1-(3-pyridyl)-1-butanone (NNK), EGCG (0.5% in diet *ad libitum*) was implicated in DMNT1 reduction with simultaneous decrease of p-AKT, phospho-histone H2AX and tumor growth, again emphasizing the epigenetic effects of the catechin, potentially due the antioxidant activity of EGCG, as suggested by the authors. [195]. Furthermore EGCG was studied in the methylation status of the reversion-inducing cysteine-rich protein with Kazal motifs (RECK) gene, a tumour suppressor gene downregulating matrix metalloproteinases and blocking metastatic potential [196]. It has been shown in a salivary adenoid cystic carcinoma cells (SACC83) that the catechin was able to demethylate RACK gene and thus impact on invasion, migration, and metastasis. EGCG has been also implicated in autophagic process, as seen in Paragraph 3.1. It is known that in macrophages from aged mice Atg5 and LC3B genes are normally hypermethylated (genes regulating autophagy). The use of EGCG (probably a high dose, even if the authors did not report any cell viability change) in macrophages restored these genes expressions both in vivo and in vitro [197]. Similarly, in macrophages cells of cystic fibrosis (CF) mice, EGCG (administered intratracheally for three days with 25 mg/kg) restored Atg12 gene expression, improving autophagy in such a disease, where autophagic process highly impaired [198]. EGCG (10 μM given diabetic pregnant mice at embryonic day 5.5 in drinking water) inhibited DNA hypermethylation in maternal diabetes-induced neural tube defects, decreasing the congenital defects and opposing the high glucose levels in embryo [199]. In another animal models, C57BL/6J male mice thatwere fed with high-fat diet (HFD) or control diet (CD), EGCG administered *ad libitum* at 25 mg/kg body weight per day in water modulated DNMT1 and MutL homologue 1 genes methylation, ameliorating inflammatory status in HFD mice [200]. In addition, EGCG enhanced gut microbiota, as evidenced by DNA damage in the *Firmicutes/Bacteroidetes* ratio and the total number of bacteria in the same work. In HeLa cells, EGCG abrogated DNMT3B and HDAC1 activity, while only the expression of DNMT3B was reduced, also affecting expression of retinoic acid receptor-β, cadherin 1, and death-associated protein kinase-1 [201]. A genome-wide study of DNA methylation reported the effects of EGCG in oral squamous cell carcinoma (CAL-27) [202]. The results showed that the main differentially expressed genes that were derived from MAPK, Wnt, and cell cycle signaling pathways, cell processes that are strongly associated cancer proliferation.

MicroRNA (miRNA) is a small non-coding RNA molecule that contains about 22 nucleotides that can post-transcriptionally regulate gene expression [203]. miRNAs are involved in numerous cell processes, including growth, proliferation, apoptosis, autophagy, metabolism, etc., and play a fundamental part in cancer. In prostate cancer cells (PC3) and PC3 mouse xenografts, EGCG blocked nuclear translocation and protein expression of androgen receptor (implicated in prostate cancer etiology), and these effects were associated with the down-regulation of androgen-regulated miRNA-21 and up-regulation of miRNA-330, a tumor suppressor [204]. Another target of EGCG was miRNA-210, being upregulated by the catechin in lung cancer cell lines (CL13, H1299, H460, A549), with induced accumulation of HIF-1α, which is a known miRNA-210 activator [205]. Moreover, in tobacco carcinogen-induced lung tumors in A/J mice, miRNAs profile was analysed after EGCG treatment (mice fed with purified diet containing 0.4% EGCG) [206]. It has been revealed that these miRNAs were strictly connected with MAPK, AKT, NF-κB pathways, and cell cycle regulation. Rat hepatoma cell line (FAO) were used to test different extracts and polyphenols, including EGCG [207]. The catechin reduced miR-33a and miR-122 levels (both being involved in dyslipidemia, cholesterol homeostasis, insulin resistance), with direct binding to miRNAs, as demonstrated by ^{1}H NMR spectroscopy and, thus, could potentially impact cell metabolism. In non-small cell lung cancer cells (A549) mouse xenografts, EGCG that was associated with cisplatin was able to reduce tumor size, while in NCI-H460 cells (another non-small cell lung cancer cell line) was not [208]. This difference was imputable to different expression of miRNA-98-5p and miRNA-125a-3p after EGCG treatment, consequently, the authors suggested that EGCG and cisplatin could have a therapeutic role in some subtype of non-small cell lung cancer and could conveniently be associated. In nasopharyngeal carcinoma cell line (CNE2) differential miRNAs expression was observed, in particular 16 miRNAs with 20 μM EGCG-treated and 32 miRNAs with 40 μM EGCG-treated were modulated (>2-fold expression changes when compared with the control) [209]. Furthermore, while using an in vitro subarachnoid hemorrhage model (oxyhemoglobin added to PC12 cells), EGCG at 1 and 50 μM altered miRNAs expression and mainly impacted on the MAPK pathway (p38, Ca^{2+}, autophagic activation), suggesting that the differential expression of miRNAs could be at the basis of the therapeutic efficacy of different concentrations of EGCG [210]. EGCG in a dose- and time-dependent manner inhibited the proliferation and regulated miRNAs expression of miR-210, miR-29a, miR-203, and miR-125b in different cervical carcinoma cells in multiple human cervical cancer cell lines (HeLa (HPV16/18+), SiHa (HPV16+), CaSki (HPV16+), and C33A (HPV-)) [211]. In osteosarcoma cell lines (MG-63 and U-2OS), EGCG induced miRNA-1 upregulation and inhibited c-MET expression, while its combination with c-MET inhibitor enhanced inhibitory effects on tumor cell growth, heading to cell proliferation reduction, cell cycle arrest, and apoptosis induction [212]. EGCG downregulated Ca^{2+} (CRAC) channel (Orai1), its regulator stromal cell-interaction molecule 2 (STIM2), and store operated Ca^{2+} entry (SOCE), all being implicated in Ca^{2+} regulation, in murine CD4+ T cells and human Jurkat T cells. The work showed that EGCG repressed Ca^{2+} entry by up-regulation of miR-15b, which ruled STIM2, Orai1, SOCE, and acted on AKT/PTEN pathway [213]. In anaplastic thyroid carcinoma cells (SW1736 and 8505C), EGCG and other natural compounds had heterogeneous effects, with curcumin being the most effective [214]. Nonetheless, EGCG provoked a significant reduction of miRNA-221 only, even if five important miRNAs that were implicated in thyroid cancer progression were studied (miRNA-221, miRNA-222, miRNA-21, miRNA-146b, and miRNA-204). In multiple myeloma cells (MM1.s), EGCG (1 and 5 μM) was shown to inhibit miRNA-25, miRNA-92, miRNA-141, and miRNA-200a, all being implicated in p53 targeting reduction, a hallmark of multiple myeloma [215]. The suppression of these miRNAs could have a potential effect in the treatment of such disease, as the authors claimed that the EGCG doses were physiologically relevant and within the range of human consumption. In pancreatic ductal adenocarcinoma cell lines (BxPc-3, MIA-PaCa2, and CRL-1097), EGCG and other catechins (also associated with quercetin and sulforaphane) were used and showed to reduce apoptosis, migration, and the matrix metalloproteinases MMP-9 and MMP-2, with the activation of miR-let-7 leading to the inhibition of its target gene K-Ras [216]. Of note that EGCG was not among the most effective compounds, whereas the combination of sulforaphane, quercetin, and catechins extract seemed to have a strong therapeutic action.

3.12. Other Mechanisms

The effects of EGCG have been also reported in many other signaling pathways and other diseases other than cancer could be involved in the benefit of the catechin. For example, EGCG treatment inhibited VEGF signaling, leading to a reduction in mitogenesis of human umbelical arterial cells [217]. Mitogenesis is key process for cell energy and its modulation can impact the survival, growth, and replication. As already reported in paragraphs 3.8 and 3.10, the inhibition of some components of MMP family by EGCG could reduce tumor invasion and metastasis. For instance, MMP-2 and MMP-9 are both inhibited by EGCG in the prostate of transgenic adenocarcinoma of mouse prostate (TRAMP) model, as mentioned before [89], as well in endothelial cells [218]. In addition, the anticancer properties of EGCG may be dependent on the inhibition of the protease urokinase-plasminogen activator (uPA), which is often overexpressed in human tumors and whose activity is involved in the regulation of apoptosis, cell replication, migration, and adhesion [219]. EGCG was also studied in the amyloid aggregation and neurotoxicity model. The catechin effects were examined in relation to misfolded or misassembled proteins in human islet amyloid polypeptide (hIAPP) transgenic mice, an animal model for investigating the formation of amyloid fibrils and, thus, pancreas dysfunction and diabetes [220]. EGCG was administered at 60 mg/kg in drinking water for three weeks and revealed potential benefit in reducing amyloid fibril formation. Another work explored the effect of EGCG on the aggregation process and toxicity of the expanded ataxin-3 (AT3), the polyglutamine (polyQ) containing protein responsible for spinocerebellar ataxia type 3 (SCA3) [221]. EGCG interfered with fibril aggregation and blocked mature fibrils formation of both the cell and animal model. Indeed, in fibroblast-like cells (COS-7), co-incubation of EGCG and AT3 diminished the toxicity of protein aggregates, as also demonstrated in in vivo model (*Caenorhabditis elegans* simplified SCA3), whereas EGCG increased motility of affected worms. In Alzheimer disease, amyloid β (Aβ) accumulates in the brain, leading to neuronal cell death. EGCG reduced the inflammation and neurotoxicity in EOC 13.31 mouse cell line, with a mechanism suppressing TNFα, IL-1β, IL-6, iNOS, NF-κB, JNK, p38, ERK, and restoring Nrf2/HO-1 antioxidant signaling in neuroinflammatory responses of Aβ -stimulated microglia [222]. Moreover, the effect of EGCG on cAMP activated protein kinase (PKA) is currently under investigation: pioneeristic studies were considering a possible role of EGCG in the regulation of glucose homeostasis via PKA inhibition downregulation of FoxO1. The proposed model needs further confirmation, but opens a new door for EGCG [223].

4. Conclusions

EGCG is responsible for a wide variety of biological activities, including cancer prevention. The preclinical activities of EGCG are associated with proliferation, differentiation, apoptosis, inflammation, angiogenesis, and metastasis. More efforts are needed to translate the plethora of preclinical data in effective human therapeutic options.

Author Contributions: All authors contributed to the manuscript. Conceptualization, R.P. and J.S.-R.; validation investigation, resources, data curation, writing—all authors; review and editing, J.S.-R., R.P., F.S., B.S., and W.C.C., All authors have read and agreed to the published version of the manuscript.

Funding: This research received no external funding.

Conflicts of Interest: The authors declare no conflict of interest.

Abbreviations

EGCG:	(−)-epigallocatechin-3-gallate
ELK:	Eph-related tyrosine kinase
ERK:	extracellular signal–regulated kinase
JNK:	c-Jun N-terminal kinase
MAPK:	mitogen-activated protein kinase
MEK:	mitogen-activated protein kinase kinase
PIK3:	phosphoinositide 3-kinases
PTEN:	phosphatase and tensin homolog
SAPK:	stress-activated protein kinase
VEGF:	vascular endothelial growth factor
VEGFR:	vascular endothelial growth factor receptor
Wnt:	Wingless-related integration site

References

1. Gupta, S.; Saha, B.; Giri, A.K. Comparative antimutagenic and anticlastogenic effects of green tea and black tea: A review. *Mutat. Res. Rev. Mutat. Res.* **2002**, *512*, 37–65. [CrossRef]
2. Hu, G.; Zhang, L.; Rong, Y.; Ni, X.; Sun, Y. Downstream carcinogenesis signaling pathways by green tea polyphenols: A translational perspective of chemoprevention and treatment for cancers. *Curr. Drug Metab.* **2014**, *15*, 14–22. [CrossRef] [PubMed]
3. Sang, S.; Lambert, J.D.; Ho, C.-T.; Yang, C.S. The chemistry and biotransformation of tea constituents. *Pharmacol. Res.* **2011**, *64*, 87–99. [CrossRef] [PubMed]
4. Min, K.; Kwon, T.K. Anticancer effects and molecular mechanisms of epigallocatechin-3-gallate. *Integr. Med. Res.* **2014**, *3*, 16–24. [CrossRef]
5. Nagle, D.G.; Ferreira, D.; Zhou, Y.-D. Epigallocatechin-3-gallate (EGCG): Chemical and biomedical perspectives. *Phytochemistry* **2006**, *67*, 1849–1855. [CrossRef]
6. Sutherland, B.A.; Rahman, R.M.; Appleton, I. Mechanisms of action of green tea catechins, with a focus on ischemia-induced neurodegeneration. *J. Nutr. Biochem.* **2006**, *17*, 291–306. [CrossRef]
7. Mereles, D.; Hunstein, W. Epigallocatechin-3-gallate (EGCG) for Clinical Trials: More Pitfalls than Promises? *Int. J. Mol. Sci.* **2011**, *12*, 5592–5603. [CrossRef]
8. Das, S.; Tanwar, J.; Hameed, S.; Fatima, Z. Antimicrobial potential of epigallocatechin-3-gallate (EGCG): A green tea polyphenol. *J. Biochem. Pharmacol. Res.* **2014**, *2*, 167–174.
9. Wink, M. *Functions and Biotechnology of Plant Secondary Metabolites*, 2nd ed.; Wiley-Blackwell: Chichester, UK, 2010; p. xiii.
10. Cechinel-Filho, V. *Plant Bioactives and Drug Discovery: Principles, Practice, and Perspectives*; John Wiley & Sons: Hoboken, NJ, USA, 2012; p. vii.
11. Grotewold, E. *The Science of Flavonoids*; Springer: New York, NY, USA, 2008; p. vii.
12. Fraga, C.G. *Plant Phenolics and Human Health: Biochemistry, Nutrition, and Pharmacology*; Wiley: Hoboken, NJ, USA, 2010.
13. Khan, N.; Afaq, F.; Saleem, M.; Ahmad, N.; Mukhtar, H. Targeting Multiple Signaling Pathways by Green Tea Polyphenol (−)-Epigallocatechin-3-Gallate. *Cancer Res.* **2006**, *66*, 2500–2505. [CrossRef]
14. Botten, D.; Fugallo, G.; Fraternali, F.; Molteni, C. Structural Properties of Green Tea Catechins. *J. Phys. Chem. B* **2015**, *119*, 12860–12867. [CrossRef]
15. James, K.; Whitesell, B. *An Encyclopedia of Chemicals, Drugs & Biologicals*, 5nd ed.; Chapman & Hall: New York, NY, USA, 1997.
16. Istenič, K.; Korošec, R.C.; Ulrih, N.P. Encapsulation of (−)-epigallocatechin gallate into liposomes and into alginate or chitosan microparticles reinforced with liposomes. *J. Sci. Food Agric.* **2016**, *96*, 4623–4632. [CrossRef] [PubMed]
17. Li, N.; Taylor, L.S.; Ferruzzi, M.G.; Mauer, L.J. Kinetic Study of Catechin Stability: Effects of pH, Concentration, and Temperature. *J. Agric. Food Chem.* **2012**, *60*, 12531–12539. [CrossRef] [PubMed]
18. Puligundla, P.; Mok, C.; Ko, S.; Liang, J.; Recharla, N. Nanotechnological approaches to enhance the bioavailability and therapeutic efficacy of green tea polyphenols. *J. Funct. Foods* **2017**, *34*, 139–151. [CrossRef]

19. Zhong, Y.; Shahidi, F. Lipophilized Epigallocatechin Gallate (EGCG) Derivatives as Novel Antioxidants. *J. Agric. Food Chem.* **2011**, *59*, 6526–6533. [CrossRef]

20. Bhushani, J.A.; Karthik, P.; Anandharamakrishnan, C. Nanoemulsion based delivery system for improved bioaccessibility and Caco-2 cell monolayer permeability of green tea catechins. *Food Hydrocoll.* **2016**, *56*, 372–382. [CrossRef]

21. Du, L.-L.; Fu, Q.-Y.; Xiang, L.-P.; Zheng, X.-Q.; Lu, J.-L.; Ye, J.-H.; Li, Q.-S.; Polito, C.A.; Liang, Y.-R. Tea Polysaccharides and Their Bioactivities. *Molecules* **2016**, *21*, 1449. [CrossRef]

22. Liang, R.; Chen, L.; Yokoyama, W.; Williams, P.A.; Zhong, F. Niosomes Consisting of Tween-60 and Cholesterol Improve the Chemical Stability and Antioxidant Activity of (−)-Epigallocatechin Gallate under Intestinal Tract Conditions. *J. Agric. Food Chem.* **2016**, *64*, 9180–9188. [CrossRef]

23. Paximada, P.; Echegoyen, Y.; Koutinas, A.A.; Mandala, I.G.; Lagaron, J.M. Encapsulation of hydrophilic and lipophilized catechin into nanoparticles through emulsion electrospraying. *Food Hydrocoll.* **2017**, *64*, 123–132. [CrossRef]

24. Wang, X.; Xie, Y.; Ge, H.; Chen, L.; Wang, J.; Zhang, S.; Guo, Y.; Li, Z.; Feng, X. Physical properties and antioxidant capacity of chitosan/epigallocatechin-3-gallate films reinforced with nano-bacterial cellulose. *Carbohydr. Polym.* **2018**, *179*, 207–220. [CrossRef]

25. Zhong, Y.; Ma, C.-M.; Shahidi, F. Antioxidant and antiviral activities of lipophilic epigallocatechin gallate (EGCG) derivatives. *J. Funct. Foods* **2012**, *4*, 87–93. [CrossRef]

26. Zhu, Q.Y.; Zhang, A.; Tsang, D.; Huang, Y.; Chen, Z.-Y. Stability of Green Tea Catechins. *J. Agric. Food Chem.* **1997**, *45*, 4624–4628. [CrossRef]

27. Wang, R.; Zhou, W.; Wen, R.-A.H. Kinetic Study of the Thermal Stability of Tea Catechins in Aqueous Systems Using a Microwave Reactor. *J. Agric. Food Chem.* **2006**, *54*, 5924–5932. [CrossRef] [PubMed]

28. Zeng, L.M.J.; Li, C.; Luo, L.Y. Stability of tea polyphenols solution with different pH at different temperatures. *Int. J. Food Prop.* **2017**, *20*, 1–18. [CrossRef]

29. Fan, F.-Y.; Shi, M.; Nie, Y.; Zhao, Y.; Ye, J.-H.; Liang, Y.-R. Differential behaviors of tea catechins under thermal processing: Formation of non-enzymatic oligomers. *Food Chem.* **2016**, *196*, 347–354. [CrossRef] [PubMed]

30. Sang, S.; Lee, M.-J.; Hou, Z.; Ho, C.-T.; Yang, C.S. Stability of Tea Polyphenol (−)-Epigallocatechin-3-gallate and Formation of Dimers and Epimers under Common Experimental Conditions. *J. Agric. Food Chem.* **2005**, *53*, 9478–9484. [CrossRef] [PubMed]

31. Krupkova, O.; Ferguson, S.J.; Wuertz-Kozak, K. Stability of (−)-epigallocatechin gallate and its activity in liquid formulations and delivery systems. *J. Nutr. Biochem.* **2016**, *37*, 1–12. [CrossRef] [PubMed]

32. Wang, R.; Zhou, W.; Jiang, X. Reaction Kinetics of Degradation and Epimerization of Epigallocatechin Gallate (EGCG) in Aqueous System over a Wide Temperature Range. *J. Agric. Food Chem.* **2008**, *56*, 2694–2701. [CrossRef]

33. Suzuki, M.; Sano, M.; Yoshida, R.; Degawa, M.; Miyase, T.; Maeda-Yamamoto, M. Epimerization of Tea Catechins and O-Methylated Derivatives of (−)-Epigallocatechin-3-O-gallate: Relationship between Epimerization and Chemical Structure. *J. Agric. Food Chem.* **2003**, *51*, 510–514. [CrossRef]

34. Cai, Y.; Zhang, J.; Chen, N.G.; Shi, Z.; Qiu, J.; He, C.; Chen, M. Recent advances in anticancer activities and drug delivery systems of tannins. *Med. Res. Rev.* **2017**, *37*, 665–701. [CrossRef]

35. Thangapandiyan, S.; Miltonprabu, S. Epigallocatechin gallate effectively ameliorates fluoride-induced oxidative stress and DNA damage in the liver of rats. *Can. J. Physiol. Pharmacol.* **2013**, *91*, 528–537. [CrossRef]

36. Wei, R.; Mao, L.; Xu, P.; Zheng, X.; Hackman, R.M.; MacKenzie, G.G.; Wang, Y. Suppressing glucose metabolism with epigallocatechin-3-gallate (EGCG) reduces breast cancer cell growth in preclinical models. *Food Funct.* **2018**, *9*, 5682–5696. [CrossRef] [PubMed]

37. Shang, W.; Lu, W.; Han, M.; Qiao, J. The interactions of anticancer agents with tea catechins: Current evidence from preclinical studies. *Anti-Cancer Agents Med. Chem.* **2014**, *14*, 1343–1350. [CrossRef] [PubMed]

38. Lecumberri, E.; Dupertuis, Y.M.; Miralbell, R.; Pichard, C. Green tea polyphenol epigallocatechin-3-gallate (EGCG) as adjuvant in cancer therapy. *Clin. Nutr.* **2013**, *32*, 894–903. [CrossRef]

39. Pal, S.; Dey, S.K.; Saha, C. Inhibition of Catalase by Tea Catechins in Free and Cellular State: A Biophysical Approach. *PLoS ONE* **2014**, *9*, e102460. [CrossRef] [PubMed]

40. Singh, B.N.; Shankar, S.; Srivastava, R.K. Green tea catechin, epigallocatechin-3-gallate (EGCG): Mechanisms, perspectives and clinical applications. *Biochem. Pharmacol.* **2011**, *82*, 1807–1821. [CrossRef] [PubMed]

41. Ross, S.A. Evidence for the relationship between diet and cancer. *Exp. Oncol.* **2010**, *32*, 137–142. [PubMed]

42. Wu, F.; Sun, H.; Kluz, T.; Clancy, H.A.; Kiok, K.; Costa, M. Epigallocatechin-3-gallate (EGCG) protects against chromate-induced toxicity in vitro. *Toxicol. Appl. Pharmacol.* **2012**, *258*, 166–175. [CrossRef] [PubMed]

43. Cabrera, C.; Artacho, R.; Giménez, R. Beneficial Effects of Green Tea—A Review. *J. Am. Coll. Nutr.* **2006**, *25*, 79–99. [CrossRef] [PubMed]

44. Lee, B.-L.; Ong, C.-N. Comparative analysis of tea catechins and theaflavins by high-performance liquid chromatography and capillary electrophoresis. *J. Chromatogr. A* **2000**, *881*, 439–447. [CrossRef]

45. De Pascual-Teresa, S.; Santos-Buelga, C.; Rivas-Gonzalo, J.C. Quantitative analysis of flavan-3-ols in Spanish foodstuffs and beverages. *J. Agric. Food Chem.* **2000**, *48*, 5331–5337. [CrossRef]

46. Shishikura, Y.; Khokhar, S. Factors affecting the levels of catechins and caffeine in tea beverage: Estimated daily intakes and antioxidant activity. *J. Sci. Food Agric.* **2005**, *85*, 2125–2133. [CrossRef]

47. Rusak, G.; Komes, D.; Likić, S.; Horžić, D.; Kovač, M. Phenolic content and antioxidative capacity of green and white tea extracts depending on extraction conditions and the solvent used. *Food Chem.* **2008**, *110*, 852–858. [CrossRef] [PubMed]

48. Reto, M.; Figueira, M.E.; Filipe, H.M.; Almeida, C.M.M. Chemical Composition of Green Tea (*Camellia sinensis*) Infusions Commercialized in Portugal. *Plant Foods Hum. Nutr.* **2007**, *62*, 139–144. [CrossRef] [PubMed]

49. Rechner, A.; Wagner, E.; Van Buren, L.; Van De Put, F.; Wiseman, S.; Rice-Evans, C. Black tea represents a major source of dietary phenolics among regular tea drinkers. *Free Radic. Res.* **2002**, *36*, 1127–1135. [CrossRef]

50. Bhagwat, S.; Haytowitz, D.B.; Holden, J.M. *USDA Database for the Flavonoid Content of Selected Foods*; US Department of Agriculture: Beltsville, MD, USA, 2011.

51. Jian, W.; Fang, S.; Chen, T.; Fang, J.; Mo, Y.; Li, D.; Xiong, S.; Liu, W.; Song, L.; Shen, J.; et al. A novel role of HuR in-Epigallocatechin-3-gallate (EGCG) induces tumour cells apoptosis. *J. Cell. Mol. Med.* **2019**, *23*, 3767–3771. [CrossRef] [PubMed]

52. Lubecka, K.; Kaufman-Szymczyk, A.; Cebula-Obrzut, B.; Smolewski, P.; Szemraj, J.; Fabianowska-Majewska, K. Novel Clofarabine-Based Combinations with Polyphenols Epigenetically Reactivate Retinoic Acid Receptor Beta, Inhibit Cell Growth, and Induce Apoptosis of Breast Cancer Cells. *Int. J. Mol. Sci.* **2018**, *19*, 3970. [CrossRef]

53. Li, A.; Gu, K.; Wang, Q.; Chen, X.; Fu, X.; Wang, Y.; Wen, Y. Epigallocatechin-3-gallate affects the proliferation, apoptosis, migration and invasion of tongue squamous cell carcinoma through the hippo-TAZ signaling pathway. *Int. J. Mol. Med.* **2018**, *42*, 2615–2627. [CrossRef]

54. Wu, D.; Liu, Z.; Li, J.; Zhang, Q.; Zhong, P.; Teng, T.; Chen, M.; Xie, Z.; Ji, A.; Li, Y. Epigallocatechin-3-gallate inhibits the growth and increases the apoptosis of human thyroid carcinoma cells through suppression of EGFR/RAS/RAF/MEK/ERK signaling pathway. *Cancer Cell Int.* **2019**, *19*, 43. [CrossRef]

55. Holczer, M.; Besze, B.; Zámbó, V.; Csala, M.; Bánhegyi, G.; Kapuy, O. Epigallocatechin-3-Gallate (EGCG) Promotes Autophagy-Dependent Survival via Influencing the Balance of mTOR-AMPK Pathways upon Endoplasmic Reticulum Stress. *Oxidative Med. Cell. Longev.* **2018**, *2018*, 1–15. [CrossRef]

56. Zhao, L.; Liu, S.; Xu, J.; Li, W.; Duan, G.; Wang, H.; Yang, H.; Yang, Z.; Zhou, R. A new molecular mechanism underlying the EGCG-mediated autophagic modulation of AFP in HepG2 cells. *Cell Death Dis.* **2017**, *8*, e3160. [CrossRef]

57. Kim, H.S.; Montana, V.; Jang, H.J.; Parpura, V.; Kim, J.A. Epigallocatechin gallate (EGCG) stimulates autophagy in vascular endothelial cells: A potential role for reducing lipid accumulation. *J. Biol. Chem.* **2013**, *288*, 22693–22705. [CrossRef] [PubMed]

58. Basiricò, L.; Morera, P.; DiPasquale, D.; Bernini, R.; Santi, L.; Romani, A.; Lacetera, N.; Bernabucci, U. (−)-Epigallocatechin-3-gallate and hydroxytyrosol improved antioxidative and anti-inflammatory responses in bovine mammary epithelial cells. *Animal* **2019**, *13*, 2847–2856. [CrossRef] [PubMed]

59. Valcic, S.; Timmermann, B.N.; Alberts, D.S.; Wächter, G.A.; Krutzsch, M.; Wymer, J.; Guillén, J.M. Inhibitory effect of six green tea catechins and caffeine on the growth of four selected human tumor cell lines. *Anti-Cancer Drugs* **1996**, *7*, 461–468. [CrossRef] [PubMed]

60. Kuo, P.-L.; Lin, C.-C. Green tea constituent (−)-Epigallocatechin-3-gallate inhibits hep G2 cell proliferation and induces apoptosis through p53-dependent and fas-mediated pathways. *J. Biomed. Sci.* **2003**, *10*, 219–227. [PubMed]

61. Mukhtar, H.; Agarwal, R. Skin cancer chemoprevention. *J. Investig. Dermatol. Symp. Proc.* **1996**, *1*, 209–214. [PubMed]

62. Gupta, S.; Ahmad, N.; Nieminen, A.-L.; Mukhtar, H. Growth Inhibition, Cell-Cycle Dysregulation, and Induction of Apoptosis by Green Tea Constituent (–)-Epigallocatechin-3-gallate in Androgen-Sensitive and Androgen-Insensitive Human Prostate Carcinoma Cells. *Toxicol. Appl. Pharmacol.* **2000**, *164*, 82–90. [CrossRef]

63. Nihal, M.; Ahmad, N.; Mukhtar, H.; Wood, G.S. Anti-proliferative and proapoptotic effects of (?)-epigallocatechin-3-gallate on human melanoma: Possible implications for the chemoprevention of melanoma. *Int. J. Cancer* **2005**, *114*, 513–521. [CrossRef]

64. Nihal, M.; Ahsan, H.; Siddiqui, I.A.; Mukhtar, H.; Ahmad, N.; Wood, G.S. (–)-Epigallocatechin-3-gallate (EGCG) sensitizes melanoma cells to interferon induced growth inhibition in a mouse model of human melanoma. *Cell Cycle* **2009**, *8*, 2057–2063. [CrossRef]

65. Ahmad, N.; Feyes, D.K.; Agarwal, R.; Mukhtar, H.; Nieminen, A.-L.; Wynder, E.L.; Cohen, L.A. Green Tea Constituent Epigallocatechin-3-Gallate and Induction of Apoptosis and Cell Cycle Arrest in Human Carcinoma Cells. *J. Natl. Cancer Inst.* **1997**, *89*, 1881–1886. [CrossRef]

66. Yusuf, N.; Irby, C.; Katiyar, S.K.; Elmets, C.A. Photoprotective effects of green tea polyphenols. *Photodermatol. Photoimmunol. Photomed.* **2007**, *23*, 48–56. [CrossRef]

67. Hussain, T.; Gupta, S.; Adhami, V.M.; Mukhtar, H. Green tea constituent epigallocatechin-3-gallate selectively inhibits COX-2 without affecting COX-1 expression in human prostate carcinoma cells. *Int. J. Cancer* **2005**, *113*, 660–669. [CrossRef] [PubMed]

68. Metz, N.; Lobstein, A.; Schneider, Y.; Gossé, F.; Schleiffer, R.; Anton, R.; Raul, F. Suppression of Azoxymethane-Induced Preneoplastic Lesions and Inhibition of Cyclooxygenase-2 Activity in the Colonic Mucosa of Rats Drinking a Crude Green Tea Extract. *Nutr. Cancer* **2000**, *38*, 60–64. [CrossRef] [PubMed]

69. Kundu, J.K.; Na, H.-K.; Chun, K.-S.; Kim, Y.-K.; Lee, S.J.; Lee, S.S.; Lee, O.-S.; Sim, Y.-C.; Surh, Y.-J. Inhibition of phorbol ester-induced COX-2 expression by epigallocatechin gallate in mouse skin and cultured human mammary epithelial cells. *J. Nutr.* **2003**, *133*, 3805S–3810S. [CrossRef] [PubMed]

70. Haqqi, T.M.; Anthony, N.D.; Gupta, S.; Ahmad, N.; Lee, M.-S.; Kumar, G.K.; Mukhtar, H. Prevention of collagen-induced arthritis in mice by a polyphenolic fraction from green tea. *Proc. Natl. Acad. Sci. USA* **1999**, *96*, 4524–4529. [CrossRef]

71. Ahmed, S.; Rahman, A.; Hasnain, A.; LaLonde, M.; Goldberg, V.M.; Haqqi, T.M. Green tea polyphenol epigallocatechin-3-gallate inhibits the IL-1 beta-induced activity and expression of cyclooxygenase-2 and nitric oxide synthase-2 in human chondrocytes. *Free. Radic. Biol. Med.* **2002**, *33*, 1097–1105. [CrossRef]

72. Tachibana, H.; Koga, K.; Fujimura, Y.; Yamada, K. A receptor for green tea polyphenol EGCG. *Nat. Struct. Mol. Biol.* **2004**, *11*, 380–381. [CrossRef]

73. Givant-Horwitz, V. Laminin-Induced Signaling in Tumor Cells: The Role of the Mr 67,000 Laminin Receptor. *Cancer Res.* **2004**, *64*, 3572–3579. [CrossRef]

74. Shimizu, M.; Deguchi, A.; Lim, J.T.; Moriwaki, H.; Kopelovich, L.; Weinstein, I.B. (–)-Epigallocatechin Gallate and Polyphenon E Inhibit Growth and Activation of the Epidermal Growth Factor Receptor and Human Epidermal Growth Factor Receptor-2 Signaling Pathways in Human Colon Cancer Cells. *Clin. Cancer Res.* **2005**, *11*, 2735–2746. [CrossRef]

75. Farabegoli, F.; Govoni, M.; Spisni, E.; Papi, A. EGFR inhibition by (–)-epigallocatechin-3-gallate and IIF treatments reduces breast cancer cell invasion. *Biosci. Rep.* **2017**, *37*, BSR20170168. [CrossRef]

76. Farabegoli, F.; Papi, A.; Orlandi, M. (–)-Epigallocatechin-3-gallate down-regulates EGFR, MMP-2, MMP-9 and EMMPRIN and inhibits the invasion of MCF-7 tamoxifen-resistant cells. *Biosci. Rep.* **2011**, *31*, 99–108. [CrossRef]

77. Burotto, M.; Chiou, V.L.; Lee, J.-M.; Kohn, E.C. The MAPK pathway across different malignancies: A new perspective. *Cancer* **2014**, *120*, 3446–3456. [CrossRef] [PubMed]

78. Liu, F.; Yang, X.; Geng, M.; Huang, M. Targeting ERK, an Achilles' Heel of the MAPK pathway, in cancer therapy. *Acta Pharm. Sin. B* **2018**, *8*, 552–562. [CrossRef] [PubMed]

79. Aggarwal, B.B.; Shishodia, S. Molecular targets of dietary agents for prevention and therapy of cancer. *Biochem. Pharmacol.* **2006**, *71*, 1397–1421. [CrossRef] [PubMed]

80. Ahmed, H.I.; Mohamed, E.A. Candesartan and epigallocatechin-3-gallate ameliorate gentamicin-induced renal damage in rats through p38-MAPK and NF-kappaB pathways. *J. Biochem. Mol. Toxicol.* **2019**, *33*, e22254. [CrossRef] [PubMed]

81. Wang, Y.; Liu, N.; Bian, X.; Sun, G.; Du, F.; Wang, B.; Su, X.; Li, D. Epigallocatechin-3-gallate reduces tubular cell apoptosis in mice with ureteral obstruction. *J. Surg. Res.* **2015**, *197*, 145–154. [CrossRef] [PubMed]

82. Chen, J.; Xu, J.; Li, J.; Du, L.; Chen, T.; Liu, P.; Peng, S.; Wang, M.; Song, H. Epigallocatechin-3-gallate attenuates lipopolysaccharide-induced mastitis in rats via suppressing MAPK mediated inflammatory responses and oxidative stress. *Int. Immunopharmacol.* **2015**, *26*, 147–152. [CrossRef] [PubMed]

83. Kim, S.J.; Li, M.; Jeong, C.W.; Bae, H.B.; Kwak, S.H.; Lee, S.H.; Lee, H.J.; Heo, B.H.; Yook, K.B.; Yoo, K.Y. Epigallocatechin-3-gallate, a green tea catechin, protects the heart against regional ischemia-reperfusion injuries through activation of RISK survival pathways in rats. *Arch. Pharmacal Res.* **2014**, *37*, 1079–1085. [CrossRef]

84. Chen, D.-D.; Dong, Y.-G.; Liu, D.; He, J.-G. Epigallocatechin-3-Gallate Attenuates Cardiac Hypertrophy in Hypertensive Rats in Part by Modulation of Mitogen-Activated Protein Kinase Signals. *Clin. Exp. Pharmacol. Physiol.* **2009**, *36*, 925–932. [CrossRef]

85. Zhang, T.; Yang, D.; Fan, Y.; Xie, P.; Li, H. Epigallocatechin-3-gallate enhances ischemia/reperfusion-induced apoptosis in human umbilical vein endothelial cells via AKT and MAPK pathways. *Apoptosis* **2009**, *14*, 1245–1254. [CrossRef]

86. Chae, Y.J.; Kim, C.H.; Ha, T.S.; Hescheler, J.; Ahn, H.Y.; Sachinidis, A. Epigallocatechin-3-O-Gallate Inhibits the Angiotensin II-Induced Adhesion Molecule Expression in Human Umbilical Vein Endothelial Cell Via Inhibition of MAPK Pathways. *Cell. Physiol. Biochem.* **2007**, *20*, 859–866. [CrossRef]

87. Won, S.-M.; Park, Y.-H.; Kim, H.-J.; Park, K.-M.; Lee, W.-J. Catechins inhibit angiotensin II-induced vascular smooth muscle cell proliferation via mitogen-activated protein kinase pathway. *Exp. Mol. Med.* **2006**, *38*, 525–534. [CrossRef] [PubMed]

88. Harper, C.E.; Patel, B.B.; Wang, J.; Eltoum, I.A.; Lamartiniere, C.A. Epigallocatechin-3-Gallate suppresses early stage, but not late stage prostate cancer in TRAMP mice: Mechanisms of action. *Prostate* **2007**, *67*, 1576–1589. [CrossRef] [PubMed]

89. Adhami, V.M. Oral Consumption of Green Tea Polyphenols Inhibits Insulin-Like Growth Factor-I-Induced Signaling in an Autochthonous Mouse Model of Prostate Cancer. *Cancer Res.* **2004**, *64*, 8715–8722. [CrossRef] [PubMed]

90. Hsu, S.D.; Dickinson, U.P.; Qin, H.; Borke, J.; Ogbureke, K.U.E.; Winger, J.N.; Camba, A.M.; Bollag, W.B.; Stöppler, H.J.; Sharawy, M.M.; et al. Green tea polyphenols reduce autoimmune symptoms in a murine model for human Sjogren's syndrome and protect human salivary acinar cells from TNF-α-induced cytotoxicity. *Autoimmunity* **2007**, *40*, 138–147. [CrossRef] [PubMed]

91. Hsu, S.; Dickinson, U.P.; Qin, H.; Lapp, C.; Lapp, D.; Borke, J.; Walsh, U.S.; Bollag, W.B.; Stöppler, H.; Yamamoto, T.; et al. Inhibition of Autoantigen Expression by (−)-Epigallocatechin-3-gallate (the Major Constituent of Green Tea) in Normal Human Cells. *J. Pharmacol. Exp. Ther.* **2005**, *315*, 805–811. [CrossRef] [PubMed]

92. Afaq, F.; Adhami, V.M.; Ahmad, N.; Mukhtar, H. Inhibition of ultraviolet B-mediated activation of nuclear factor kappaB in normal human epidermal keratinocytes by green tea Constituent (−)-epigallocatechin-3-gallate. *Oncogene* **2003**, *22*, 1035–1044. [CrossRef]

93. Balasubramanian, S.; Efimova, T.; Eckert, R.L. Green tea polyphenol stimulates a Ras, MEKK1, MEK3, and p38 cascade to increase activator protein 1 factor-dependent involucrin gene expression in normal human keratinocytes. *J. Biol. Chem.* **2002**, *277*, 1828–1836. [CrossRef] [PubMed]

94. Afaq, F.; Ahmad, N.; Mukhtar, H. Suppression of UVB-induced phosphorylation of mitogen-activated protein kinases and nuclear factor kappa B by green tea polyphenol in SKH-1 hairless mice. *Oncogene* **2003**, *22*, 9254–9264. [CrossRef]

95. Katiyar, S.K.; Afaq, F.; Azizuddin, K.; Mukhtar, H. Inhibition of UVB-Induced Oxidative Stress-Mediated Phosphorylation of Mitogen-Activated Protein Kinase Signaling Pathways in Cultured Human Epidermal Keratinocytes by Green Tea Polyphenol (−)-Epigallocatechin-3-gallate. *Toxicol. Appl. Pharmacol.* **2001**, *176*, 110–117. [CrossRef]

96. Bae, J.-Y.; Choi, J.-S.; Choi, Y.-J.; Shin, S.-Y.; Kang, S.-W.; Han, S.J.; Kang, Y.-H. (−)Epigallocatechin gallate hampers collagen destruction and collagenase activation in ultraviolet-B-irradiated human dermal fibroblasts: Involvement of mitogen-activated protein kinase. *Food Chem. Toxicol.* **2008**, *46*, 1298–1307. [CrossRef]

97. Liang, Y.; Ip, M.S.M.; Mak, J.C.W. (−)-Epigallocatechin-3-gallate suppresses cigarette smoke-induced inflammation in human cardiomyocytes via ROS-mediated MAPK and NF-kappaB pathways. *Phytomed. Int. J. Phytother. Phytopharm.* **2019**, *58*, 152768. [CrossRef]

98. Zhang, L.; Zhang, Z.; Liang, S. Epigallocatechin-3-gallate protects retinal vascular endothelial cells from high glucose stress in vitro via the MAPK/ERK-VEGF pathway. *Genet. Mol. Res.* **2016**, *15*, 15027874. [CrossRef] [PubMed]

99. Xiao, X.; Jiang, K.; Xu, Y.; Peng, H.; Wang, Z.; Liu, S.; Zhang, G. (−)-Epigallocatechin-3-gallate induces cell apoptosis in chronic myeloid leukaemia by regulating Bcr/Abl-mediated p38-MAPK/JNK and JAK2/STAT3/AKT signalling pathways. *Clin. Exp. Pharmacol. Physiol.* **2019**, *46*, 126–136. [CrossRef] [PubMed]

100. Dong, Z.; Ma, W.; Huang, C.; Yang, C.S. Inhibition of tumor promoter-induced activator protein 1 activation and cell transformation by tea polyphenols, (−)-epigallocatechin gallate, and theaflavins. *Cancer Res.* **1997**, *57*, 4414–4419. [PubMed]

101. Kim, H.S.; Kim, M.H.; Jeong, M.; Hwang, Y.S.; Lim, S.H.; Shin, B.A.; Ahn, B.W.; Jung, Y.D. EGCG blocks tumor promoter-induced MMP-9 expression via suppression of MAPK and AP-1 activation in human gastric AGS cells. *Anticancer Res.* **2004**, *24*, 747–753. [PubMed]

102. Zheng, Y.; Lim, E.J.; Wang, L.; Smart, E.J.; Toborek, M.; Hennig, B. Role of caveolin-1 in EGCG-mediated protection against linoleic-acid-induced endothelial cell activation. *J. Nutr. Biochem.* **2009**, *20*, 202–209. [CrossRef] [PubMed]

103. Choi, J.-S.; Choi, Y.-J.; Shin, S.-Y.; Li, J.; Kang, S.-W.; Bae, J.-Y.; Kim, D.S.; Ji, G.-E.; Kang, J.-S.; Kang, Y.-H. Dietary flavonoids differentially reduce oxidized LDL-induced apoptosis in human endothelial cells: Role of MAPK and JAK/STAT signaling. *J. Nutr.* **2008**, *138*, 983–990. [CrossRef] [PubMed]

104. Cao, T.; Zhang, X.; Yang, D.; Wang, Y.-Q.; Qiao, Z.-D.; Huang, J.-M.; Zhang, P. Antioxidant effects of epigallocatechin-3-gallate on the aTC1-6 pancreatic alpha cell line. *Biochem. Biophys. Res. Commun.* **2018**, *495*, 693–699. [CrossRef]

105. Ku, H.-C.; Chang, H.-H.; Liu, H.-C.; Hsiao, C.-H.; Lee, M.-J.; Hu, Y.-J.; Hung, P.-F.; Liu, C.-W.; Kao, Y.-H. Green tea (−)-epigallocatechin gallate inhibits insulin stimulation of 3T3-L1 preadipocyte mitogenesis via the 67-kDa laminin receptor pathway. *Am. J. Physiol. Physiol.* **2009**, *297*, C121–C132. [CrossRef]

106. Zhou, Y.; Tang, J.; Du, Y.; Ding, J.; Liu, J.-Y. The green tea polyphenol EGCG potentiates the antiproliferative activity of sunitinib in human cancer cells. *Tumor Biol.* **2016**, *37*, 8555–8566. [CrossRef]

107. Deguchi, H.; Fujii, T.; Nakagawa, S.; Koga, T.; Shirouzu, K. Analysis of cell growth inhibitory effects of catechin through MAPK in human breast cancer cell line T47D. *Int. J. Oncol.* **2002**, *21*, 1301–1305. [CrossRef]

108. Cerezo-Guisado, M.I.; Zur, R.; Lorenzo, M.J.; Risco, A.; Martín-Serrano, M.A.; Álvarez-Barrientos, A.; Cuenda, A.; Centeno, F. Implication of Akt, ERK1/2 and alternative p38MAPK signalling pathways in human colon cancer cell apoptosis induced by green tea EGCG. *Food Chem. Toxicol.* **2015**, *84*, 125–132. [CrossRef] [PubMed]

109. Chen, C.; Shen, G.; Hebbar, V.; Hu, R.; Owuor, E.D.; Kong, A.-N. Epigallocatechin-3-gallate-induced stress signals in HT-29 human colon adenocarcinoma cells. *Carcinogenesis* **2003**, *24*, 1369–1378. [CrossRef]

110. Adachi, S.; Shimizu, M.; Shirakami, Y.; Yamauchi, J.; Natsume, H.; Matsushima-Nishiwaki, R.; To, S.; Weinstein, I.; Moriwaki, H.; Kozawa, O. (−)-Epigallocatechin gallate downregulates EGF receptor via phosphorylation at Ser1046/1047 by p38 MAPK in colon cancer cells. *Carcinogenesis* **2009**, *30*, 1544–1552. [CrossRef] [PubMed]

111. Inaba, H.; Nagaoka, Y.; Kushima, Y.; Kumagai, A.; Matsumoto, Y.; Sakaguchi, M.; Baba, K.; Uesato, S. Comparative Examination of Anti-proliferative Activities of (−)-Epigallocatechin Gallate and (−)-Epigallocatechin against HCT116 Colorectal Carcinoma Cells. *Biol. Pharm. Bull.* **2008**, *31*, 79–84. [CrossRef] [PubMed]

112. Suganuma, M.; Kurusu, M.; Suzuki, K.; Tasaki, E.; Fujiki, H. Green tea polyphenol stimulates cancer preventive effects of celecoxib in human lung cancer cells by upregulation ofGADD153 gene. *Int. J. Cancer* **2006**, *119*, 33–40. [CrossRef]

113. Lee, J.-C.; Chung, L.-C.; Chen, Y.-J.; Feng, T.-H.; Chen, W.-T.; Juang, H.-H. Upregulation of B-cell translocation gene 2 by epigallocatechin-3-gallate via p38 and ERK signaling blocks cell proliferation in human oral squamous cell carcinoma cells. *Cancer Lett.* **2015**, *360*, 310–318. [CrossRef]

114. Lim, Y.C.; Cha, Y.Y. Epigallocatechin-3-gallate induces growth inhibition and apoptosis of human anaplastic thyroid carcinoma cells through suppression of EGFR/ERK pathway and cyclin B1/CDK1 complex. *J. Surg. Oncol.* **2011**, *104*, 776–780. [CrossRef]

115. Chen, C.; Yu, R.; Owuor, E.D.; Kong, A.-N.T. Activation of antioxidant-response element (ARE), mitogen-activated protein kinases (MAPKs) and caspases by major green tea polyphenol components during cell survival and death. *Arch. Pharmacal Res.* **2000**, *23*, 605–612. [CrossRef]

116. Kim, M.H.; Chung, J. Synergistic cell death by EGCG and ibuprofen in DU-145 prostate cancer cell line. *Anticancer Res.* **2007**, *27*, 3947–3956.

117. Siddiqui, I.A.; Adhami, V.M.; Ahmad, N.; Afaq, F.; Mukhtar, H. Modulation of phosphatidylinositol-3-kinase/ protein kinase B- and mitogen-activated protein kinase-pathways by tea polyphenols in human prostate cancer cells. *J. Cell. Biochem.* **2004**, *91*, 232–242. [CrossRef] [PubMed]

118. Bing, X.; Xuelei, L.; Wanwei, D.; Linlang, L.; Keyan, C. EGCG Maintains Th1/Th2 Balance and Mitigates Ulcerative Colitis Induced by Dextran Sulfate Sodium through TLR4/MyD88/NF-κB Signaling Pathway in Rats. *Can. J. Gastroenterol. Hepatol.* **2017**, *2017*, 1–9. [CrossRef] [PubMed]

119. Afzal, M.; Gupta, J.; Siddique, Y.; Bég, T.; Ara, G. A Review on the Beneficial Effects of Tea Polyphenols on Human Health. *Int. J. Pharmacol.* **2008**, *4*, 314–338. [CrossRef]

120. Vasudevan, K.M.; Garraway, L.A. AKT Signaling in Physiology and Disease. *Measles* **2010**, *347*, 105–133.

121. Shirai, T.; Sato, A.; Hara, Y. Epigallocatechin gallate. The major causative agent of green tea-induced asthma. *Chest* **1994**, *106*, 1801–1805. [CrossRef]

122. Yang, N.; Shang, Y.-X. Epigallocatechin gallate ameliorates airway inflammation by regulating Treg/Th17 imbalance in an asthmatic mouse model. *Int. Immunopharmacol.* **2019**, *72*, 422–428. [CrossRef]

123. Yang, N.; Zhang, H.; Cai, X.; Shang, Y. Epigallocatechin-3-gallate inhibits inflammation and epithelialmesenchymal transition through the PI3K/AKT pathway via upregulation of PTEN in asthma. *Int. J. Mol. Med.* **2018**, *41*, 818–828. [CrossRef]

124. Gu, J.-J.; Qiao, K.-S.; Sun, P.; Chen, P.; Li, Q. Study of EGCG induced apoptosis in lung cancer cells by inhibiting PI3K/Akt signaling pathway. *Eur. Rev. Med Pharmacol. Sci.* **2018**, *22*, 4557–4563.

125. Nan, W.; Zhonghang, X.; Keyan, C.; Tongtong, L.; Wanshu, G.; Zhongxin, X. Epigallocatechin-3-Gallate Reduces Neuronal Apoptosis in Rats after Middle Cerebral Artery Occlusion Injury via PI3K/AKT/eNOS Signaling Pathway. *BioMed Res. Int.* **2018**, *2018*, 1–9. [CrossRef]

126. Renno, W.M.; Al-Maghrebi, M.; Alshammari, A.; George, P. (−)-Epigallocatechin-3-gallate (EGCG) attenuates peripheral nerve degeneration in rat sciatic nerve crush injury. *Neurochem. Int.* **2013**, *62*, 221. [CrossRef]

127. Kieran, M.W.; Kalluri, R.; Cho, Y.-J. The VEGF Pathway in Cancer and Disease: Responses, Resistance, and the Path Forward. *Cold Spring Harb. Perspect. Med.* **2012**, *2*, a006593. [CrossRef] [PubMed]

128. Nilsson, M.; Heymach, J.V. Vascular endothelial growth factor (VEGF) pathway. *J. Thorac. Oncol.* **2006**, *1*, 768–770. [CrossRef] [PubMed]

129. Bai, Q.; Lyu, Z.; Yang, X.; Pan, Z.; Lou, J.; Dong, T. Epigallocatechin-3-gallate promotes angiogenesis via up-regulation of Nfr2 signaling pathway in a mouse model of ischemic stroke. *Behav. Brain Res.* **2017**, *321*, 79–86. [CrossRef] [PubMed]

130. Pullikotil, P.; Chen, H.; Muniyappa, R.; Greenberg, C.C.; Yang, S.; Reiter, C.E.; Lee, J.W.; Chung, J.H.; Quon, M.J. Epigallocatechin gallate induces expression of heme oxygenase-1 in endothelial cells via p38 MAPK and Nrf-2 that suppresses proinflammatory actions of TNF-alpha. *J. Nutr. Biochem.* **2012**, *23*, 1134–1145. [CrossRef] [PubMed]

131. Ahn, S.-C.; Kim, G.-Y.; Kim, J.-H.; Baik, S.-W.; Han, M.-K.; Lee, H.-J.; Moon, N.-O.; Lee, C.-M.; Kang, J.-H.; Kim, B.-H.; et al. Epigallocatechin-3-gallate, constituent of green tea, suppresses the LPS-induced phenotypic and functional maturation of murine dendritic cells through inhibition of mitogen-activated protein kinases and NF-κB. *Biochem. Biophys. Res. Commun.* **2004**, *313*, 148–155. [CrossRef] [PubMed]

132. Zhu, B.-H.; Zhan, W.-H.; Li, Z.-R.; Wang, Z.; He, Y.-L.; Peng, J.-S.; Cai, S.-R.; Ma, J.-P.; Zhang, C.-H. (−)-Epigallocatechin-3-gallate inhibits growth of gastric cancer by reducing VEGF production and angiogenesis. *World J. Gastroenterol.* **2007**, *13*, 1162–1169. [CrossRef] [PubMed]

133. Fu, J.D.; Yao, J.J.; Wang, H.; Cui, W.G.; Leng, J.; Ding, L.Y.; Fan, K.Y. Effects of EGCG on proliferation and apoptosis of gastric cancer SGC7901 cells via down-regulation of HIF-1alpha and VEGF under a hypoxic state. *Eur. Rev. Med. Pharmacol. Sci.* **2019**, *23*, 155–161. [CrossRef]

134. Tang, H.; Zeng, L.; Wang, J.; Zhang, X.; Ruan, Q.; Wang, J.; Cui, S.; Yang, D. Reversal of 5-fluorouracil resistance by EGCG is mediate by inactivation of TFAP2A/VEGF signaling pathway and down-regulation of MDR-1 and P-gp expression in gastric cancer. *Oncotarget* **2017**, *8*, 82842–82853. [CrossRef]

135. Sitkovsky, M.; Lukashev, D. Regulation of immune cells by local-tissue oxygen tension: HIF1α and adenosine receptors. *Nat. Rev. Immunol.* **2005**, *5*, 712–721. [CrossRef]

136. Zhu, B.-H.; Chen, H.-Y.; Zhan, W.-H.; Wang, C.-Y.; Cai, S.-R.; Wang, Z.; Zhang, C.-H.; He, Y.-L. (−)-Epigallocatechin-3-gallate inhibits VEGF expression induced by IL-6 via Stat3 in gastric cancer. *World J. Gastroenterol.* **2011**, *17*, 2315–2325. [CrossRef]

137. Shimizu, M.; Shirakami, Y.; Sakai, H.; Yasuda, Y.; Kubota, M.; Adachi, S.; Tsurumi, H.; Hara, Y.; Moriwaki, H. (−)-Epigallocatechin gallate inhibits growth and activation of the VEGF/VEGFR axis in human colorectal cancer cells. *Chem. Interact.* **2010**, *185*, 247–252. [CrossRef] [PubMed]

138. Jung, Y.D.; Kim, M.S.; Shin, B.A.; Chay, K.O.; Ahn, B.W.; Liu, W.; Bucana, C.D.; Gallick, G.E.; Ellis, L.M. EGCG, a major component of green tea, inhibits tumour growth by inhibiting VEGF induction in human colon carcinoma cells. *Br. J. Cancer* **2001**, *84*, 844–850. [CrossRef] [PubMed]

139. Luo, H.Q.; Xu, M.; Zhong, W.T.; Cui, Z.Y.; Liu, F.M.; Zhou, K.Y.; Li, X.Y. EGCG decreases the expression of HIF-1alpha and VEGF and cell growth in MCF-7 breast cancer cells. *J. BU ON Off. J. Balk. Union Oncol.* **2014**, *19*, 435–439.

140. Li, X.; Feng, Y.; Liu, J.; Feng, X.; Zhou, K.; Tang, X. Epigallocatechin-3-Gallate Inhibits IGF-I-Stimulated Lung Cancer Angiogenesis through Downregulation of HIF-1a and VEGF Expression. *J. Nutr. Nutr.* **2013**, *6*, 169–178. [CrossRef]

141. Masuda, M.; Suzui, M.; Lim, J.T.E.; Deguchi, A.; Soh, J.-W.; Weinstein, I.B. Epigallocatechin-3-gallate decreases VEGF production in head and neck and breast carcinoma cells by inhibiting EGFR-related pathways of signal transduction. *J. Exp. Ther. Oncol.* **2002**, *2*, 350–359. [CrossRef]

142. Zhang, Q.; Tang, X.; Lu, Q.; Zhang, Z.; Rao, J.; Le, A.D. Green tea extract and (−)-epigallocatechin-3-gallate inhibit hypoxia and serum-induced HIF-1α protein accumulation and VEGF expression in human cervical carcinoma and hepatoma cells. *Mol. Cancer Ther.* **2006**, *5*, 1227–1238. [CrossRef]

143. Ly, B.T.K.; Chi, H.T.; Yamagishi, M.; Kano, Y.; Hara, Y.; Nakano, K.; Sato, Y.; Watanabe, T. Inhibition of FLT3 Expression by Green Tea Catechins in FLT3 Mutated-AML Cells. *PLoS ONE* **2013**, *8*, e66378. [CrossRef]

144. Chen, H.; Treweeke, A.T.; West, D.C.; Till, K.J.; Cawley, J.C.; Zuzel, M.; Toh, C.H. In vitro and in vivo production of vascular endothelial growth factor by chronic lymphocytic leukemia cells. *Blood* **2000**, *96*, 3181–3187. [CrossRef]

145. Lee, Y.K.; Bone, N.D.; Strege, A.K.; Shanafelt, T.D.; Jelinek, D.F.; Kay, N.E. VEGF receptor phosphorylation status and apoptosis is modulated by a green tea component, epigallocatechin-3-gallate (EGCG), in B-cell chronic lymphocytic leukemia. *Blood* **2004**, *104*, 788–794. [CrossRef]

146. Tang, F.-Y.; Nguyen, N.; Meydani, M. Green tea catechins inhibit VEGF-induced angiogenesisin vitro through suppression of VE-cadherin phosphorylation and inactivation of Akt molecule. *Int. J. Cancer* **2003**, *106*, 871–878. [CrossRef]

147. Trompezinski, S.; Denis, A.; Schmitt, D.; Viac, J. Comparative effects of polyphenols from green tea (EGCG) and soybean (genistein) on VEGF and IL-8 release from normal human keratinocytes stimulated with the proinflammatory cytokine TNF? *Arch. Dermatol. Res.* **2003**, *295*, 112–116. [CrossRef] [PubMed]

148. Kondo, T.; Ohta, T.; Igura, K.; Hara, Y.; Kaji, K. Tea catechins inhibit angiogenesis in vitro, measured by human endothelial cell growth, migration and tube formation, through inhibition of VEGF receptor binding. *Cancer Lett.* **2002**, *180*, 139–144. [CrossRef]

149. Sartippour, M.R.; Shao, Z.-M.; Heber, D.; Beatty, P.; Zhang, L.; Liu, C.; Ellis, L.; Liu, W.; Go, V.L.; Brooks, M.N. Green tea inhibits vascular endothelial growth factor (VEGF) induction in human breast cancer cells. *J. Nutr.* **2002**, *132*, 2307–2311. [CrossRef] [PubMed]

150. Sartippour, M.R.; Heber, D.; Ma, J.; Lu, Q.; Go, V.L.; Nguyen, M. Green Tea and Its Catechins Inhibit Breast Cancer Xenografts. *Nutr. Cancer* **2001**, *40*, 149–156. [CrossRef]

151. Park, J.S.; Kim, M.H.; Chang, H.J.; Kim, K.M.; Kim, S.M.; Shin, B.A.; Ahn, B.W.; Jung, Y.D. Epigallocatechin-3-gallate inhibits the PDGF-induced VEGF expression in human vascular smooth muscle cells via blocking PDGF receptor and Erk-1/2. *Int. J. Oncol.* **2006**, *29*, 1247–1252. [CrossRef]

152. Basini, G.; Bianco, F.; Grasselli, F. EGCG, a major component of green tea, inhibits VEGF production by swine granulosa cells. *BioFactors* **2005**, *23*, 25–33. [CrossRef]

153. Tanaka, K. The proteasome: Overview of structure and functions. *Proc. Jpn. Acad. Ser. B* **2009**, *85*, 12–36. [CrossRef]

154. Schwartz, A.L.; Ciechanover, A. The Ubiquitin-Proteasome Pathway and Pathogenesis of Human Diseases. *Annu. Rev. Med.* **1999**, *50*, 57–74. [CrossRef]

155. Nunes, A.T.; Annunziata, C.M. Proteasome inhibitors: Structure and function. *Semin. Oncol.* **2017**, *44*, 377–380. [CrossRef]

156. Nam, S. Ester Bond-containing Tea Polyphenols Potently Inhibit Proteasome Activity In Vitro and In Vivo. *J. Biol. Chem.* **2001**, *276*, 13322–13330. [CrossRef]

157. Smith, D.M.; Wang, Z.; Kazi, A.; Li, L.-H.; Chan, T.-H.; Dou, Q.P. Synthetic analogs of green tea polyphenols as proteasome inhibitors. *Mol. Med.* **2002**, *8*, 382–392. [CrossRef]

158. Chen, D.; Wan, S.B.; Yang, H.; Yuan, J.; Chan, T.H.; Dou, Q.P. EGCG, green tea polyphenols and their synthetic analogs and prodrugs for human cancer prevention and treatment. *Adv. Clin. Chem.* **2011**, *53*, 155–177. [PubMed]

159. Kazi, A.; Wang, Z.; Kumar, N.; Falsetti, S.C.; Chan, T.-H.; Dou, Q.P. Structure-activity relationships of synthetic analogs of (−)-epigallocatechin-3-gallate as proteasome inhibitors. *Anticancer Res.* **2004**, *24*, 943–954. [PubMed]

160. Lam, W.H.; Kazi, A.; Kuhn, D.J.; Chow, L.M.; Chan, A.S.; Dou, Q.P.; Chan, T.H. A potential prodrug for a green tea polyphenol proteasome inhibitor: Evaluation of the peracetate ester of (−)-epigallocatechin gallate [(−)-EGCG]. *Bioorg. Med. Chem.* **2004**, *12*, 5587–5593. [CrossRef] [PubMed]

161. Landis-Piwowar, K.R.; Kuhn, D.J.; Wan, S.B.; Chen, D.; Chan, T.H.; Dou, Q.P. Evaluation of proteasome-inhibitory and apoptosis-inducing potencies of novel (−)-EGCG analogs and their prodrugs. *Int. J. Mol. Med.* **2005**, *15*, 735–742. [CrossRef]

162. Kuhn, D.; Lam, W.H.; Kazi, A.; Daniel, K.G.; Song, S.; Chow, L.M.C.; Chan, T.H.; Dou, Q.P. Synthetic peracetate tea polyphenols as potent proteasome inhibitors and apoptosis inducers in human cancer cells. *Front. Biosci.* **2005**, *10*, 1010–1023. [CrossRef]

163. Landis-Piwowar, K.R.; Huo, C.; Chen, D.; Milacic, V.; Shi, G.; Chan, T.H.; Dou, Q.P. A Novel Prodrug of the Green Tea Polyphenol (−)-Epigallocatechin-3-Gallate as a Potential Anticancer Agent. *Cancer Res.* **2007**, *67*, 4303–4310. [CrossRef]

164. Yu, Z.; Qin, X.L.; Gu, Y.Y.; Chen, D.; Cui, Q.C.; Jiang, T.; Wan, S.B.; Dou, Q.P. Prodrugs of Fluoro-Substituted Benzoates of EGC as Tumor Cellular Proteasome Inhibitors and Apoptosis Inducers. *Int. J. Mol. Sci.* **2008**, *9*, 951–961. [CrossRef]

165. Yang, H.; Sun, D.K.; Chen, D.; Cui, Q.C.; Gu, Y.Y.; Jiang, T.; Chen, W.; Wan, S.B.; Dou, Q.P. Antitumor activity of novel fluoro-substituted (−)-epigallocatechin-3-gallate analogs. *Cancer Lett.* **2010**, *292*, 48–53. [CrossRef]

166. Landis-Piwowar, K.; Chen, D.; Chan, T.H.; Dou, Q.P. Inhibition of catechol-O-methyltransferase activity in human breast cancer cells enhances the biological effect of the green tea polyphenol (−)-EGCG. *Oncol. Rep.* **2010**, *24*, 563–569.

167. Lu, M.; Dou, Q.P.; Kitson, R.P.; Smith, D.M.; Goldfarb, R.H. Differential effects of proteasome inhibitors on cell cycle and apoptotic pathways in human YT and Jurkat cells. *J. Cell. Biochem.* **2006**, *97*, 122–134. [CrossRef] [PubMed]

168. Pettinari, A.; Amici, M.; Cuccioloni, M.; Angeletti, M.; Fioretti, E.; Eleuteri, A.M. Effect of Polyphenolic Compounds on the Proteolytic Activities of Constitutive and Immuno-Proteasomes. *Antioxid. Redox Signal.* **2006**, *8*, 121–129. [CrossRef]

169. Kalfon, L.; Youdim, M.B.H.; Mandel, S.A. Green tea polyphenol (−)-epigallocatechin-3-gallate promotes the rapid protein kinase C- and proteasome-mediated degradation of Bad: Implications for neuroprotection. *J. Neurochem.* **2007**, *100*, 992–1002. [CrossRef] [PubMed]

170. Aktas, O.; Prozorovski, T.; Smorodchenko, A.; Savaskan, N.E.; Lauster, R.; Kloetzel, P.-M.; Infante-Duarte, C.; Brocke, S.; Zipp, F. Green Tea Epigallocatechin-3-Gallate Mediates T Cellular NF-κB Inhibition and Exerts Neuroprotection in Autoimmune Encephalomyelitis. *J. Immunol.* **2004**, *173*, 5794–5800. [CrossRef] [PubMed]

171. Choudhury, S.R.; Balasubramanian, S.; Chew, Y.C.; Han, B.; Marquez, V.E.; Eckert, R.L. (−)-Epigallocatechin-3-gallate and DZNep reduce polycomb protein level via a proteasome-dependent mechanism in skin cancer cells. *Carcinogenesis* **2011**, *32*, 1525–1532. [CrossRef]

172. Eleuteri, A.M.; Amici, M.; Bonfili, L.; Cecarini, V.; Cuccioloni, M.; Grimaldi, S.; Giuliani, L.; Angeletti, M.; Fioretti, E. 50 Hz Extremely Low Frequency Electromagnetic Fields Enhance Protein Carbonyl Groups Content in Cancer Cells: Effects on Proteasomal Systems. *J. Biomed. Biotechnol.* **2009**, *2009*, 1–10. [CrossRef]

173. Yee, W.L.; Wang, Q.; Agdinaoay, T.; Dang, K.; Chang, H.; Grandinetti, A.; Franke, A.A.; Theriault, A. Green tea catechins decrease apolipoprotein B-100 secretion from HepG2 cells. *Mol. Cell. Biochem.* **2002**, *229*, 85–92. [CrossRef]

174. Golden, E.B.; Lam, P.Y.; Kardosh, A.; Gaffney, K.J.; Cadenas, E.; Louie, S.G.; Petasis, N.A.; Chen, T.C.; Schönthal, A.H. Green tea polyphenols block the anticancer effects of bortezomib and other boronic acid–based proteasome inhibitors. *Blood* **2009**, *113*, 5927–5937. [CrossRef]

175. Glynn, S.J.; Gaffney, K.J.; Sainz, M.A.; Louie, S.G.; Petasis, N.A. Molecular characterization of the boron adducts of the proteasome inhibitor bortezomib with epigallocatechin-3-gallate and related polyphenols. *Org. Biomol. Chem.* **2015**, *13*, 3887–3899. [CrossRef]

176. Modernelli, A.; Naponelli, V.; Troglio, M.G.; Bonacini, M.; Ramazzina, I.; Bettuzzi, S.; Rizzi, F. EGCG antagonizes Bortezomib cytotoxicity in prostate cancer cells by an autophagic mechanism. *Sci. Rep.* **2015**, *5*, 15270. [CrossRef]

177. Falandry, C.; Bonnefoy, M.; Freyer, G.; Gilson, E. Biology of Cancer and Aging: A Complex Association With Cellular Senescence. *J. Clin. Oncol.* **2014**, *32*, 2604–2610. [CrossRef] [PubMed]

178. Calcinotto, A.; Kohli, J.; Zagato, E.; Pellegrini, L.; DeMaria, M.; Alimonti, A. Cellular Senescence: Aging, Cancer, and Injury. *Physiol. Rev.* **2019**, *99*, 1047–1078. [CrossRef] [PubMed]

179. Capasso, S.; Alessio, N.; Squillaro, T.; Di Bernardo, G.; Melone, M.A.; Cipollaro, M.; Peluso, G.; Galderisi, U. Changes in autophagy, proteasome activity and metabolism to determine a specific signature for acute and chronic senescent mesenchymal stromal cells. *Oncotarget* **2015**, *6*, 39457–39468. [CrossRef] [PubMed]

180. Shin, J.-H.; Jeon, H.-J.; Park, J.; Chang, M.-S. Epigallocatechin-3-gallate prevents oxidative stress-induced cellular senescence in human mesenchymal stem cells via Nrf2. *Int. J. Mol. Med.* **2016**, *38*, 1075–1082. [CrossRef]

181. Han, D.-W.; Lee, M.H.; Kim, B.; Lee, J.J.; Hyon, S.-H.; Park, J.-C. Preventive Effects of Epigallocatechin-3-O-Gallate against Replicative Senescence Associated with p53 Acetylation in Human Dermal Fibroblasts. *Oxidative Med. Cell. Longev.* **2012**, *2012*, 1–13. [CrossRef]

182. Kumar, R.; Sharma, A.; Kumari, A.; Gulati, A.; Padwad, Y.; Sharma, R. Epigallocatechin gallate suppresses premature senescence of preadipocytes by inhibition of PI3K/Akt/mTOR pathway and induces senescent cell death by regulation of Bax/Bcl-2 pathway. *Biogerontology* **2019**, *20*, 171–189. [CrossRef]

183. Zhang, Q.; Wu, Y.; Guan, Y.; Ling, F.; Li, Y.; Niu, Y. Epigallocatechin gallate prevents senescence by alleviating oxidative stress and inflammation in WI-38 human embryonic fibroblasts. *RSC Adv.* **2019**, *9*, 26787–26798. [CrossRef]

184. Dupont, C.; Armant, D.R.; Brenner, C.A. Epigenetics: Definition, mechanisms and clinical perspective. *Semin. Reprod. Med.* **2009**, *27*, 351–357. [CrossRef]

185. Fang, M.Z.; Wang, Y.; Ai, N.; Hou, Z.; Sun, Y.; Lu, H.; Welsh, W.; Yang, C.S. Tea polyphenol (−)-epigallocatechin-3-gallate inhibits DNA methyltransferase and reactivates methylation-silenced genes in cancer cell lines. *Cancer Res.* **2003**, *63*, 7563–7570.

186. Lee, W.J.; Shim, J.-Y.; Zhu, B.T. Mechanisms for the Inhibition of DNA Methyltransferases by Tea Catechins and Bioflavonoids. *Mol. Pharmacol.* **2005**, *68*, 1018–1030. [CrossRef]

187. Deb, G.; Shankar, E.; Thakur, V.S.; Ponsky, L.E.; Bodner, N.R.; Fu, P.; Gupta, S. Green tea-induced epigenetic reactivation of tissue inhibitor of matrix metalloproteinase-3 suppresses prostate cancer progression through histone-modifying enzymes. *Mol. Carcinog.* **2019**, *58*, 1194–1207. [CrossRef] [PubMed]

188. Nguyen, M.M.; Ahmann, F.R.; Nagle, R.B.; Hsu, C.-H.; Tangrea, J.A.; Parnes, H.L.; Sokoloff, M.H.; Gretzer, M.B.; Chow, H.-H.S. Randomized, Double-Blind, Placebo Controlled Trial of Polyphenon E in Prostate Cancer Patients before Radical Prostatectomy: Evaluation of Potential Chemopreventive Activities. *Cancer Prev. Res.* **2012**, *5*, 290–298. [CrossRef] [PubMed]

189. Mittal, A.; Piyathilake, C.; Hara, Y.; Katiyar, S.K. Exceptionally High Protection of Photocarcinogenesis by Topical Application of (−)-Epi gal locatechin-3-Gal late in Hydrophilic Cream in SKH-1 Hairless Mouse Model: Relationship to Inhibition of UVB-Induced Global DNA Hypomethylation. *Neoplasia* **2003**, *5*, 555–565. [CrossRef]

190. Nandakumar, V.; Vaid, M.; Katiyar, S.K. (−)-Epigallocatechin-3-gallate reactivates silenced tumor suppressor genes, Cip1/p21 and p16INK4a, by reducing DNA methylation and increasing histones acetylation in human skin cancer cells. *Carcinogenesis* **2011**, *32*, 537–544. [CrossRef] [PubMed]

191. Wong, C.P.; Nguyen, L.P.; Noh, S.K.; Bray, T.M.; Bruno, R.S.; Ho, E. Induction of regulatory T cells by green tea polyphenol EGCG. *Immunol. Lett.* **2011**, *139*, 7–13. [CrossRef] [PubMed]

192. Wu, D.-S.; Shen, J.-Z.; Yu, A.-F.; Fu, H.-Y.; Zhou, H.-R.; Shen, S.-F. Epigallocatechin-3-gallate and trichostatin A synergistically inhibit human lymphoma cell proliferation through epigenetic modification of p16INK4a. *Oncol. Rep.* **2013**, *30*, 2969–2975. [CrossRef]

193. Mirza, S.; Sharma, G.; Parshad, R.; Gupta, S.D.; Pandya, P.; Ralhan, R. Expression of DNA Methyltransferases in Breast Cancer Patients and to Analyze the Effect of Natural Compounds on DNA Methyltransferases and Associated Proteins. *J. Breast Cancer* **2013**, *16*, 23–31. [CrossRef]

194. Tyagi, T.; Treas, J.N.; Mahalingaiah, P.K.S.; Singh, K.P. Potentiation of growth inhibition and epigenetic modulation by combination of green tea polyphenol and 5-aza-2′-deoxycytidine in human breast cancer cells. *Breast Cancer Res. Treat.* **2015**, *149*, 655–668. [CrossRef]

195. Jin, H.; Chen, J.X.; Wang, H.; Lu, G.; Liu, A.; Li, G.; Tu, S.; Lin, Y.; Yang, C.S. NNK-induced DNA methyltransferase 1 in lung tumorigenesis in A/J mice and inhibitory effects of (−)-epigallocatechin-3-gallate. *Nutr. Cancer* **2015**, *67*, 167–176. [CrossRef]

196. Zhou, X.-Q.; Xu, X.-N.; Li, L.; Ma, J.-J.; Zhen, E.-M.; Han, C.-B. Epigallocatechin-3-gallate inhibits the invasion of salivary adenoid cystic carcinoma cells by reversing the hypermethylation status of the RECK gene. *Mol. Med. Rep.* **2015**, *12*, 6031–6036. [CrossRef]

197. Khalil, H.; Tazi, M.; Caution, K.; Ahmed, A.; Kanneganti, A.; Assani, K.; Kopp, B.; Marsh, C.; Dakhlallah, D.; Amer, A.O. Aging is associated with hypermethylation of autophagy genes in macrophages. *Epigenetics* **2016**, *11*, 381–388. [CrossRef] [PubMed]

198. Caution, K.; Pan, A.; Krause, K.; Badr, A.; Hamilton, K.; Vaidya, A.; Gosu, H.; Daily, K.; Estfanous, S.; Gavrilin, M.A.; et al. Methylomic correlates of autophagy activity in cystic fibrosis. *J. Cyst. Fibros.* **2019**, *18*, 491–500. [CrossRef] [PubMed]

199. Zhong, J.; Xu, C.; Reece, E.A.; Yang, P. The green tea polyphenol EGCG alleviates maternal diabetes-induced neural tube defects by inhibiting DNA hypermethylation. *Am. J. Obstet. Gynecol.* **2016**, *215*, 368. [CrossRef] [PubMed]

200. Remely, M.; Ferk, F.; Sterneder, S.; Setayesh, T.; Roth, S.; Kepcija, T.; Noorizadeh, R.; Rebhan, I.; Greunz, M.; Beckmann, J.; et al. EGCG Prevents High Fat Diet-Induced Changes in Gut Microbiota, Decreases of DNA Strand Breaks, and Changes in Expression and DNA Methylation ofDnmt1andMLH1in C57BL/6J Male Mice. *Oxidative Med. Cell. Longev.* **2017**, *2017*, 1–17. [CrossRef]

201. Khan, M.A.; Hussain, A.; Sundaram, M.K.; Alalami, U.; Gunasekera, D.; Ramesh, L.; Hamza, A.; Quraishi, U. (−)-Epigallocatechin-3-gallate reverses the expression of various tumor-suppressor genes by inhibiting DNA methyltransferases and histone deacetylases in human cervical cancer cells. *Oncol. Rep.* **2015**, *33*, 1976–1984. [CrossRef]

202. Chen, L.-L.; Han, W.-F.; Geng, Y.; Su, J.-S. A genome-wide study of DNA methylation modified by epigallocatechin-3-gallate in the CAL-27 cell line. *Mol. Med. Rep.* **2015**, *12*, 5886–5890. [CrossRef]

203. Bartel, D.P. MicroRNAs: Genomics, biogenesis, mechanism, and function. *Cell* **2004**, *116*, 281–297. [CrossRef]

204. Siddiqui, I.A.; Asim, M.; Hafeez, B.B.; Adhami, V.M.; Tarapore, R.S.; Mukhtar, H. Green tea polyphenol EGCG blunts androgen receptor function in prostate cancer. *FASEB J. Off. Publ. Fed. Am. Soc. Exp. Biol.* **2011**, *25*, 1198–1207. [CrossRef]

205. Wang, H.; Bian, S.; Yang, C.S. Green tea polyphenol EGCG suppresses lung cancer cell growth through upregulating miR-210 expression caused by stabilizing HIF-1α. *Carcinogenesis* **2011**, *32*, 1881–1889. [CrossRef]

206. Zhou, H.; Chen, J.X.; Yang, C.S.; Yang, M.Q.; Deng, Y.; Wang, H. Gene regulation mediated by microRNAs in response to green tea polyphenol EGCG in mouse lung cancer. *BMC Genomics* **2014**, *15*, S3. [CrossRef]

207. Baselga-Escudero, L.; Blade, C.; Ribas-Latre, A.; Casanova, E.; Suarez, M.; Torres, J.L.; Salvado, M.J.; Arola, L.; Arola-Arnal, A. Resveratrol and EGCG bind directly and distinctively to miR-33a and miR-122 and modulate divergently their levels in hepatic cells. *Nucleic Acids Res.* **2014**, *42*, 882–892. [CrossRef]

208. Zhou, D.-H.; Wang, X.; Feng, Q. EGCG Enhances the Efficacy of Cisplatin by Downregulating hsa-miR-98-5p in NSCLC A549 Cells. *Nutr. Cancer* **2014**, *66*, 636–644. [CrossRef] [PubMed]

209. Li, B.-B.; Huang, G.-L.; Li, H.-H.; Kong, X.; He, Z.-W. Epigallocatechin-3-gallate Modulates MicroRNA Expression Profiles in Human Nasopharyngeal Carcinoma CNE2 Cells. *Chin. Med. J.* **2017**, *130*, 93–99. [CrossRef] [PubMed]

210. Chen, Y.; Huang, L.; Wang, L.; Chen, L.; Ren, W.; Zhou, W. Differential expression of microRNAs contributed to the health efficacy of EGCG inin vitrosubarachnoid hemorrhage model. *Food Funct.* **2017**, *8*, 4675–4683. [CrossRef] [PubMed]

211. Zhu, Y.; Huang, Y.; Liu, M.; Yan, Q.; Zhao, W.; Yang, P.; Gao, Q.; Wei, J.; Zhao, W.; Ma, L. Epigallocatechin gallate inhibits cell growth and regulates miRNA expression in cervical carcinoma cell lines infected with different high-risk human papillomavirus subtypes. *Exp. Ther. Med.* **2019**, *17*, 1742–1748. [CrossRef] [PubMed]

212. Zhu, K.; Wang, W. Green tea polyphenol EGCG suppresses osteosarcoma cell growth through upregulating miR-1. *Tumor Biol.* **2016**, *37*, 4373–4382. [CrossRef]

213. Zhang, S.; Al-Maghout, T.; Bissinger, R.; Zeng, N.; Pelzl, L.; Salker, M.S.; Cheng, A.; Singh, Y.; Lang, F. Epigallocatechin-3-gallate (EGCG) up-regulates miR-15b expression thus attenuating store operated calcium entry (SOCE) into murine CD4(+) T cells and human leukaemic T cell lymphoblasts. *Oncotarget* **2017**, *8*, 89500–89514. [CrossRef]

214. Allegri, L.; Rosignolo, F.; Mio, C.; Filetti, S.; Baldan, F.; Damante, G. Effects of nutraceuticals on anaplastic thyroid cancer cells. *J. Cancer Res. Clin. Oncol.* **2018**, *144*, 285–294. [CrossRef]

215. Gordon, M.; Yan, F.; Zhong, X.; Mazumder, P.; Xu-Monette, Z.; Zou, D.; Young, K.; Ramos, K.; Li, Y.J.M.c. Regulation of p53-targeting microRNAs by polycyclic aromatic hydrocarbons: Implications in the etiology of multiple myeloma. *Mol. Carcinog.* **2015**, *54*, 1060–1069. [CrossRef]

216. Appari, M.; Babu, K.R.; Kaczorowski, A.; Gross, W.; Herr, I. Sulforaphane, quercetin and catechins complement each other in elimination of advanced pancreatic cancer by miR-let-7 induction and K-ras inhibition. *Int. J. Oncol.* **2014**, *45*, 1391–1400. [CrossRef]

217. Neuhaus, T.; Pabst, S.; Stier, S.; Weber, A.-A.; Schrör, K.; Sachinidis, A.; Vetter, H.; Ko, Y.D. Inhibition of the vascular-endothelial growth factor-induced intracellular signaling and mitogenesis of human endothelial cells by epigallocatechin-3 gallate. *Eur. J. Pharmacol.* **2004**, *483*, 223–227. [CrossRef] [PubMed]

218. Fassina, G.; Morini, M.; Minghelli, S.; Benelli, R.; Venè, R.; Noonan, D.M.; Albini, A. Mechanisms of Inhibition of Tumor Angiogenesis and Vascular Tumor Growth by Epigallocatechin-3-Gallate. *Clin. Cancer Res.* **2004**, *10*, 4865–4873. [CrossRef] [PubMed]

219. Jankun, J.; Selman, S.H.; Swiercz, R.; Skrzypczak-Jankun, E. Why drinking green tea could prevent cancer. *Nature* **1997**, *387*, 561. [CrossRef] [PubMed]

220. Franko, A.; Camargo, D.C.R.; Böddrich, A.; Garg, D.; Camargo, A.R.; Rathkolb, B.; Janik, D.; Aichler, M.; Feuchtinger, A.; Neff, F.; et al. Epigallocatechin gallate (EGCG) reduces the intensity of pancreatic amyloid fibrils in human islet amyloid polypeptide (hIAPP) transgenic mice. *Sci. Rep.* **2018**, *8*, 1116. [CrossRef]

221. Bonanomi, M.; Natalello, A.; Visentin, C.; Pastori, V.; Penco, A.; Cornelli, G.; Colombo, G.; Malabarba, M.G.; Doglia, S.M.; Relini, A.; et al. Epigallocatechin-3-gallate and tetracycline differently affect ataxin-3 fibrillogenesis and reduce toxicity in spinocerebellar ataxia type 3 model. *Hum. Mol. Genet.* **2014**, *23*, 6542–6552. [CrossRef]

222. Wei, J.C.-C.; Huang, H.-C.; Chen, W.-J.; Huang, C.-N.; Peng, C.-H.; Lin, C.-L. Epigallocatechin gallate attenuates amyloid β-induced inflammation and neurotoxicity in EOC 13.31 microglia. *Eur. J. Pharmacol.* **2016**, *770*, 16–24.

223. Li, X.; Chen, Y.; Shen, J.Z.; Pan, Q.; Yang, W.; Yan, H.; Liu, H.; Ai, W.; Liao, W.; Guo, S.; et al. Epigallocatechin Gallate Inhibits Hepatic Glucose Production in Primary Hepatocytes via Downregulating PKA Signaling Pathways and Transcriptional Factor FoxO1. *J. Agric. Food Chem.* **2019**, *67*, 3651–3661. [CrossRef]

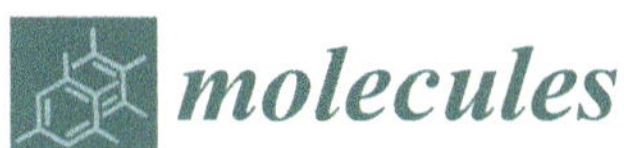 *molecules*

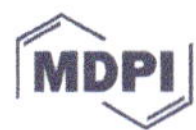

Review

Antidepressant Potential of Cinnamic Acids: Mechanisms of Action and Perspectives in Drug Development

Lúcio Ricardo Leite Diniz [1], Marilia Trindade de Santana Souza [1], Joice Nascimento Barboza [2], Reinaldo Nóbrega de Almeida [3] and Damião Pergentino de Sousa [2,*]

[1] Departament of Pharmacy, Federal University of Sergipe, São Cristóvão SE 49100-000, Brazil; luciodiniz@yahoo.com.br (L.R.L.D.); biomari@hotmail.com (M.T.d.S.S.)
[2] Departament of Pharmaceutical Sciences, Federal University of Paraíba, João Pessoa PB 58051-970, Brazil; joicenascimentobarboza@gmail.com
[3] Department of Physiology and Pathology, Federal University of Paraíba, João Pessoa PB 58051-970, Brazil; reinaldoan@uol.com.br
* Correspondence: damiao_desousa@yahoo.com.br; Tel.: +55-833-216-7347

Academic Editor: Raffaele Pezzani
Received: 15 November 2019; Accepted: 28 November 2019; Published: 6 December 2019

Abstract: Depression is a health problem that compromises the quality of life of the world's population. It has different levels of severity and a symptomatic profile that affects social life and performance in work activities, as well as a high number of deaths in certain age groups. In the search for new therapeutic options for the treatment of this behavioral disorder, the present review describes studies on antidepressant activity of cinnamic acids, which are natural products found in medicinal plants and foods. The description of the animal models used and the mechanisms of action of these compounds are discussed.

Keywords: natural products; phenylpropanoids; phenolic acids; plants; depression; behavioral disorders; forced swim test; tail suspension test

1. Introduction

Depression is a widespread chronic psychiatric disease, characterized by low mood, lack of energy, sadness, insomnia, and high morbidity, that affects more than 300 million people worldwide [1,2]. This illness can affect anyone, regardless of age, sex, social status, education, nationality or ethnic origin [3,4]. It is the leading cause of disability and is directly associated with a remarkable number of suicides cases around the world [5,6].

Despite the physiopathological mechanism of depression remaining not widely elucidated and unclear, numerous studies have shown a multifactorial origin, involving genetics, environmental, psychological, and social factors, as well as dysfunction in multiple brain areas such as the hippocampus, prefrontal cortex, nucleus accumbens, and amygdale [7–10]. Recent findings of the presence of inflammatory process and oxidative stress in the pathophysiology of depression provide new pathways and treatment targets for improvement of pharmacological approach in depression [11]. Recently, Réus et al. (2019) have reported a microglial activation with formation of intracellular multiprotein complexes, the inflammasomes, which in turn activate interleukin-1β (IL-1β) that leads to a significant increase in the production and expression of tumor necrosis factor-α (TNF-α), IL-1β, reactive species of oxygen (ROS), and nitric oxide (NO) [12]. This finding is in accordance with a previous study performed by Oglodek (2017), in which it was identified that major depressive disorders, associated or not to posttraumatic stress disorder, present changes in the cytokines and increased oxidative stress [13].

Although efforts to increase knowledge and skills for healthcare providers have been made, depression remains both underdiagnosed and undertreated [14]. Actually, the therapeutics tools used in the treatment of depression have not produced satisfactory outcomes as necessary novel strategies to improve treatment outcomes [15,16]. Figure 1 summarizes the main mechanisms of action of antidepressant drugs.

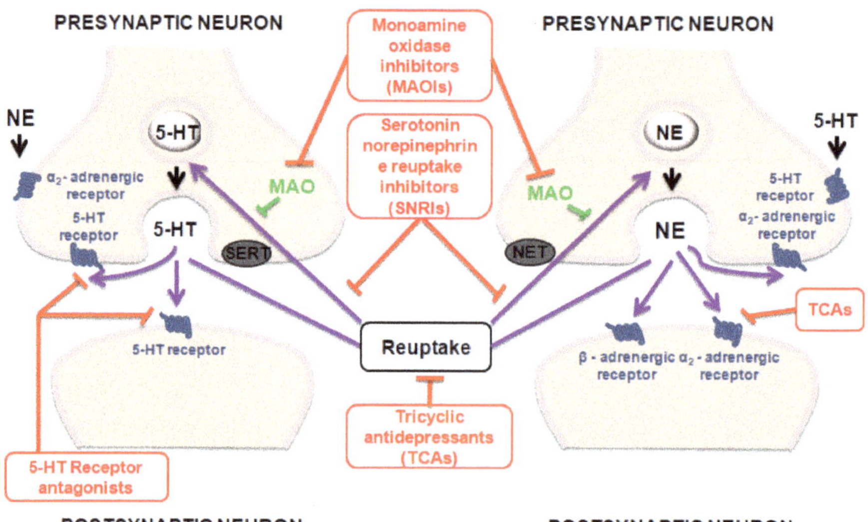

Figure 1. Mechanisms of action of antidepressant drugs.

Natural products have been important sources of new drugs against various pathologies. Reports of antidepressant activity on these compounds indicate that they may be an alternative treatment option for depression [17]. Cinnamic acids are a group of aromatic carboxylic acids with carbonic skeleton C_6–C_3 (Figure 2) found in a variety of plants and foods, for which the biosynthetic route can generate several secondary metabolites such as coumarins, lignans, isoflavonoids, flavonoids, and others natural products [18].Cinnamic acids and their derivatives have attracted the attention of researchers due to their wide distribution in nature, low toxicity, structural diversity, and pharmacological actions [19], as anti-inflammatory [20], antioxidant [21], antitumor [22], hypoglycemic [23], antidepressant [24], and cytoprotective actions of neuroinflammation in neurodegenerative diseases [25]. Considering the importance of cinnamic acids as bioactive substances and their presence in various foods and medicinal plants, this review discusses the antidepressant action mechanisms of these compounds, demonstrating their therapeutic potential for depressive disorders.

Figure 2. Chemical structure of cinnamic acid.

2. Materials and Methods

The present study was carried out based on the literature review of cinnamic acids with antidepressant activity. The survey, conducted in the Pubmed database, for studies published from January 2002 to October 2019, used the following keywords: Cinnamic acid, coumaric acid, para-coumaric acid, meta-coumaric acid, ortho-coumaric acid, ferulic acid, caffeic acid, sinapic acid, trimethoxycinnamic acid, methylenedioxycinnamic acid, methoxycinnamic acid, dimethoxycinnamic acid, antidepressant, and depression. The scientific publications were selected from studies published in English language.

3. Antidepressant Activity of Cinnamic Acids

Based on increasing evidence of the contributions of neuronal pro-inflammatory mediators and oxidative stress in the pathogenesis and development of depression, new therapeutic tools have been experimentally tested in order to improve the current treatment of depressive disorders. In this context, hydroxylated and/or methoxylated aromatic acids have shown promising results as neuroprotective agents [25]. Among these acids, there are phenolic acids, which are divided into hydroxybenzoic acids and hydroxycinnamic acids, based on C_6–C_1 and C_6–C_3 skeletons, respectively [26]. According to the literature, phenolic acids have potentially antioxidant properties due to the presence of a phenolic ring that promotes the electron donation and hydrogen atom transfer to free radicals, acting as free-radical scavengers, reducing agents, and quenchers of single oxygen formation [27,28]. It has been reported that phenolic compounds produce a significant reduction of pro-inflammatory cytokines, including TNF-α and IL-1β, and stimulate a concomitant increase of anti-inflammatory cytokines as interleukin-8 (IL-8) in different in vitro and in vivo models of inflammation [29–32]. Here, the antidepressant effect of cinnamic acids was investigated, specifically the trimethoxycinnamic acids, p-coumaric acid, caffeic acid, and ferulic acid on animal models and their relevance to the treatment of depression. The last three compounds are classified as phenolic acids.

Fifteen studies were found on cinnamic acids in experimental models of depression; the chemical structures of these acids are shown in Figure 3. Basically, the experimental model used in almost all studies for assessing antidepressant-like activity of cinnamic acids were the forced swim test (FST) and the tail suspension test (TST). Both tests are validated animal models fundamental for understanding the pathogenesis and treatment of mood and anxiety disorders, such as depression. The FST is based on the immersion of rodents in a beaker of water without a possible escape—a compound qualifies as a potential antidepressant if it reverts or delays the initial attempts to escape (active behavior) and promotes a progressive increase in the frequency and duration of episodes of immobile floating (passive behavior). The TST is based on the fact that animals subjected to the short-term, inescapable stress of being suspended by their tail, will develop an immobile posture [33,34]. Other important tests used to evaluate the effect of cinnamic acids on anxiety behaviors were the elevated plus maze (EPM) test, sucrose preference test, and open field test (OFT). In the EPM, the measure for anxiety is calculated by percentage of the total number of arm entries and the period of time spent on the open arms. Open-arm entries indicate security and low anxiety, while closed-arm entries, a sign of need for security. Decreased sucrose preference indicates the loss of the ability to feel pleasure (anhedonia), a common symptom of depression [34,35]. The OFT measures locomotor activity, including ambulation, exploration, latency, escape attempts, exploration, and the aversions of rodents to novel, brightly lit, open environments. In the OFT, reduced locomotor activity suggests anxiety-like behaviors associated with depression [34].

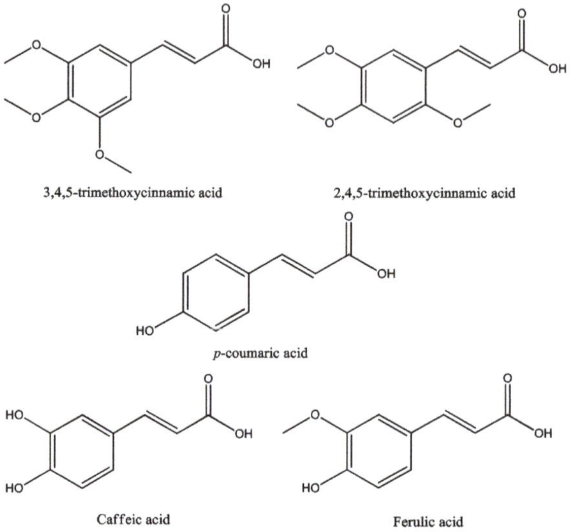

Figure 3. Chemical structures of antidepressant cinnamic acids.

In the literature, two studies have reported the effects of trimethoxycinnamic acid (TMCA) on depressive behaviors, showing divergences in results. In Nakazawa et al. (2003), 2,4,5-trimethoxycinnamic acid failed to alter the duration of immobility in FST for Male ddY mice intraperitoneally treated with TMCA, at a dose ranging from 25–200 mg/kg. Differently, Leem and Oh (2015) have shown that Male C57BL/6J mice, orally treated with 3,4,5-trimethoxycinnamicacid (50 mg/kg) for 15 days, showed reduced immobility in the FST and higher time and frequency of visits in the open arms than the control group in the EPM. The data suggest an antidepressant effect of 3,4,5-trimethoxycinnamic acid, which the authors have attributed to increased expression of the ΔFosB protein on the nucleus accumbens observed in TMCA-treated animals. There were differences in some methodological aspects between the two investigative approaches. Thus, it is difficult to conclude about the presence or absence of antidepressant effect of TMCA based on only two experimental studies that used different routes of administration, species of mice, and experimental protocols. In addition, antidepressant activity may be related to the position of the methoxyl group in the aromatic ring, since animals treated with 3,4,5-trimethoxycinnamic acid had antidepressant effects, which did not occur in those treated with 2,4,5-trimethoxycinnamic acid [36,37].

Some studies performed by Takeda and his group have shown that male ICR mice subjected to intraperitoneal treatment with caffeic acid, at a dose of 4 mg/kg, exhibit decreased immobility time in the FST, as well as a reduction in the duration of freezing of mice in the conditioned fear stress test. According to authors, the caffeic acid's ability to reduce depressive behavior might be attributed to, at least in part, an indirect modulation of the α1A-adrenoceptor and α1-adrenoceptor system and regulation of brain-derived neurotrophic factor (BDNF) expression in the frontal cortex caused by caffeic acid [38–40]. These data corroborate a study by Dzitoyeva and colleagues in which caffeic acid demonstrated antidepressant activity, attenuating BDNF mRNA decrease, by forced swimming test, using wild type mice and a 5-lipoxygenase (5-LOX) deficient group—previous studies have shown that caffeic acid inhibits 5-LOX. However, in this study it was observed that attenuation occurred only in wild rats, indicating that this acid can be used as a tool to study the regulation of the 5-LOX pathway of BDNF expression [41]. Therefore, antidepressant activity of caffeic acid may be related to its ability to regulate inflammation, as observed in the study by Huang et al. (2018), in which this acid inhibited dose-dependent increase in inflammatory and inducing cytokines affecting 5-HT, DA, and

NE metabolism, such as tyrosine (Tyr), 3-methoxy-4-hydroxyphenylglycol (MHPG), Tryptophan (Trp), and 5-hydroxyindoleacetic acid (5-HIAA), improving the behavior of depressed rats [42].

The antidepressant activity of ferulic acid is the most investigated among hydroxycinnamic acids [32,43]. According to Zeni and colleagues, ferulic acid exhibits major effects on free radical and inflammatory messengers and has the ability to counteract the reduction in reward-seeking behavior that tends to occur with depression. Animals also exhibit decreased immobility time in the FST and TST, using ferulic acid oral treatment ranging from 0.001–80 mg/kg/day. Moreover, several studies show that ferulic acid has no effect on locomotor activity in the OFT, indicating its specificity, while others show a reversal of decreased locomotor activity, suggesting ferulic acid's ability to reduce anxiety-like behaviors associated with depression. The antidepressant effect of ferulic acid has been attributed to diverse mechanisms, including modulation of serotonergic system by signaling pathway of protein kinase A (PKA), Ca^{2+}/calmodulin-dependent protein kinase II (CaMKII), protein kinase C (PKC), mitogen-activated protein kinases/extracellular signal-regulated kinases (MAPK/ERK), and phosphoinositide 3-kinases (PI3K) [44,45].

Ferulic acid acts as some of the antidepressant drugs from the pharmaceutical market, as shown by the study by Chen et al. (2015), in which there is an increase on the concentrations of monoamines serotonin and norepinephrine in the hippocampus and frontal cortex through the inhibition of monoamine oxidase A (MAO-A) activity in male ICR mice treated with ferulic acid [46]. However, unlike commercially available selective serotonin reuptake inhibitor (SSRI) drugs, which may cause bowel movement inhibition, ferulic acid exhibited both antidepressant and prokinetic activity. The Zhang et al. study performed the TST on rats, noting a reduction in immobility time, and increased locomotor activity, associated with an increase in gastric emptying speed [47].

In addition, it was noted that oral administration of ferulic acid at a dose of 5 mg/kg in male ICR mice for 7 days decreased TST immobility due to up regulation of gene expression associated with cell survival and proliferation, energy metabolism, and synthesis of dopamine in the limbic system of the brain of mice [48].

Lenziet al. (2015) have related ferulic acid's antioxidant activity and its effects on the central nervous system, evidenced by increasing superoxide dismutase (SOD), catalase (CAT) activities, and low thiobarbituric acid reactive substances (TBARS) levels found in hippocampus of ferulic acid-treated male swiss mice [49]. Furthermore, Li et al. attributed the ferulic acid's ability to reduce depressive-like behaviors, suggested by reducing immobility time in the FST and TST, observed in ferulic acid-treated male ICR mice to anti-inflammatory mechanisms [50]. In addition, a study of Liu et al. (2017) reported that ferulic acid increased the levels of BDNF and synaptic proteins (synapsin I and PSD-95) in the prefrontal cortex and hippocampus, as well as inhibited microglia activation, pro-inflammatory cytokines expression, nuclear factor kappa B (NF-κB) signaling, and decreased PYD domains-containing protein 3 NLRP3 [51].

A similar study by Zheng and colleagues demonstrated the relationship between the antidepressant effect and the anti-inflammatory activity of ferulic acid in prenatally-stressed offspring rats. In this work, it was noted that the administration of ferulic acid decreased the time of immobility and total number of crossing, rearing, grooming, and increased sucrose intake in the animals. Furthermore, it was able to reduce the concentration of inflammatory cytokines such as IL-6, IL-1, and TNF-α, and increase IL-10. As such, it was concluded that the antidepressant activity of ferulic acid occurs in part due to its anti-inflammatory activity and regulation on hypothalamic-pituitary-adrenal (HPA) axis [52].

In the study of Lee et al., it was observed that the antidepressant effects of *p*-coumaric acid may be related to its anti-inflammatory activity, as has also been shown in studies with caffeic acid. In this study, *p*-coumaric acid reduced lipopolysaccharide-induced tumor necrosis factor-α (LPS)-induced despair-related behavioral symptoms in the FST, TST, and sucrose splash test (SST), preventing the increase of inflammatory cytokines such as cyclooxygenase-2 and lipopolysaccharide-induced tumor necrosis factor-α (LPS), as well as inhibiting BDNF reduction [53].

Medicinal plants used to treat behavioral disorders that contain these psychoactive acids may have antidepressant action such as *Eugenia catharinensis* D. Legrand. Ethyl acetate extract of this species had antioxidant and antidepressant-like action in mice treated with corticosterone. Analysis of the extract using HPLC-ESI-MS/MS demonstrated the presence of several phenolic compounds, mainly phenolic acids, such as *p*-coumaric acid, ferulic acid, and caffeic acid. The authors suggest that chemical constituents are the active principles of antidepressant action [54]. Antidepressant action also was demonstrated for butanol fraction of *Olax subscorpioidea* Oliv. and was involved in the monoaminergic mechanism. Analysis of the chemical composition by HPLC indicated caffeic acid as one of the active ingredients of the plant [55]. In another study, ethyl acetate fraction from *Tabernaemontana catharinensis* A. DC. leaves showed antidepressant activity in animal models. Analysis of the chemical composition of this fraction proposes that the pharmacological action may be dependent on the presence of *p*-coumaric acid in the plant [56]. Therefore, the collection of studies discussed in this review (Table 1) show the pharmacological effect of cinnamic acids against the name Table 1 was added in text.

Depressive disorders. Figure 4 summarizes the main effects of cinnamic acids as antidepressants.

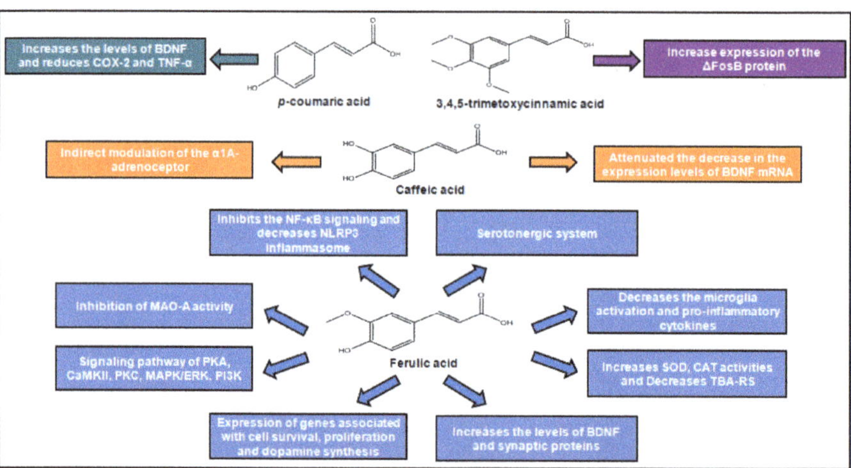

Figure 4. Antidepressant action of cinnamic acids.

Table 1. Cinnamic acids studied in experimental depression.

Compound	Animal Species	Dose and via of Administration	Behavioral Test	Observed Effects	Mechanism of Action	Reference
2,4,5-Trimethoxy-cinnamic acid (TMCA)	Male ddY mice	25, 50, 100 and 200 mg/kg, i.p.	FST	The treatment failed to alter the duration of immobility	-	[36]
3,4,5-Trimethoxy-cinnamic acid (TMCA)	Male C57BL/6J mice	25 and 50 mg/kg, p.o.	EPM; FST	The dose 50 mg/kg of treatment increased time and frequency of visits in the open arms of the EPM and showed reduced immobility in the FST	Increase expression of the ΔFosB protein on the nucleus accumbens	[37]
Caffeic acid	Male ICR mice	1, 2 and 4 mg/kg, i.p.	FST; spontaneous motor activity	The dose 4.0 mg/kg reduced the duration of immobility of mice	-	[38]
Caffeic acid	Male ICR mice and ddY mice	4 mg/kg,i.p.	Conditioned fear stress test	Reduced the duration of immobility of mice in the forced swimming test and reduced the duration of freezing of mice in the conditioned fear stress test	Indirect modulation of the α1A-adrenoceptor and α1-adrenoceptor system	[39]
Caffeic acid	Male ICR mice	4 mg/kg,i.p.	FST	Reduced the duration of immobility of mice in the forced swimming test	Attenuated the decrease in the expression levels of BDNF mRNA in the frontal cortex of mice following forced swimming	[40]
Caffeic acid	Male 5-LOX deficient mice and wild type	4 mg/kg,i.p.	FST	The pre-treatment was able to attenuate this decrease in the wild-type group	Caffeic acid can be used as a tool to study 5-lipoxygenase (5-LOX) pathway regulation of brain-derived neurotrophic factor (BDNF) expression	[41]
Caffeic acid	Male Sprague-Dawley rats	50, 75 and 100 mg/kg, i.p	OFT; FST	Inhibited the decrease of NE and the increase of Trp and MHPG in a dose-dependent manner	The inhibition of AA-COX-2/5-LOX pathways can improve the behaviors of depression rats	[42]
Ferulic acid	Male Sprague–Dawley rats	25 and 50 mg/kg, p.o.	FST; OFT	The dose 50 mg/kg reduced the duration of immobility of mice	Involvement of serotonergic system	[47]
Ferulic acid	Male Swiss mice	0.001, 0.01, 0.1, 1 and 10 mg/kg, p.o.	FST; TST; OFT	The doses 0.01, 0.1, 1 and 10 mg/kg reduced the duration of immobility of mice	Involvement of serotonergic system	[44]
Ferulic acid	Male Swiss mice	0.01 mg/kg, p.o.	TST; OFT	The dose 0.01 mg/kg reduced the duration of immobility of mice	Involvement signaling pathway of PKA, CaMKII, PKC, MAPK/ERK and PI3K	[44]
Ferulic acid	Male ICR mice	10, 20, 40 and 80 mg/kg, p.o.	FST; TST	The doses 40 and 80 mg/kg showed reduced immobility in the tests	The increase on the concentrations of monoamines 5-HT and norepinephrine in the hippocampus and frontal cortex through inhibition monoamine oxidase A (MAO-A) activity	[46]
Ferulic acid	Male Swiss mice	0.01, 0.1, 1 and 10 mg/kg/day, p.o.	FST; TST; OFT	The dose 1.0 mg/kg reduced the duration of immobility of mice	Increases SOD, CAT activities and decreases TBA-RS levels in hippocampus	[49]

Table 1. *Cont.*

Compound	Animal Species	Dose and via of Administration	Behavioral Test	Observed Effects	Mechanism of Action	Reference
Ferulic acid	Male ICR mice	3, 10, 30 and 90 mg/kg, p.o.	TST; FST; Locomotor activity	All doses reduced the duration of immobility of mice	-	[50]
Ferulic acid	Male ICR mice	20 and 40 mg/kg, p.o.	FST	The dose 40 mg/kg reduced the duration of immobility of mice	Increased the levels of BDNF and synaptic proteins (synapsin I and PSD-95) in both the prefrontal cortex and hippocampus.	[51]
Ferulic acid	Male ICR mice	20, 40 or 80 mg/kg, p.o.	SST; TST	All doses reduced the duration of immobility of mice	Inhibition of the microglia activation, pro-inflammatory cytokines expression, NF-κB signaling and decreased NLRP3 inflammasome	[51]
Ferulic acid	Male Swiss mice	1 mg/kg, p.o.	TST; OFT; SST	The dose 1.0 mg/kg reduced the duration of immobility of mice	-	[45]
Ferulic acid	Male ICR mice	5 mg/kg, p.o	TST	The dose 5 mg/kg reduced the duration of immobility of mice	Upregulates the expression of several genes associated with cell survival and proliferation, energy metabolism, and dopamine synthesis in mice limbic system of brain	[48]
Ferulic acid	Male Sprague-Dawley rats prenatally	12.5, 25, and 50 mg/kg, i.g.	SST, FST, OFT	Increased sucrose intake, and decreased immobility time and total number of crossings, rearing and grooming	Decreased concentration of inflammatory cytokines such as IL-6, IL-1 and TNF-α and increases IL-10	[52]
p-Coumaric acid	Male Sprague-Dawley rats	10 and 30 mg/kg p.o	FST; TST; SST	Improved LPS-induced despair-related behavioral symptoms	Prevented the increase of inflammatory cytokines in the hippocampus and the reduction of BDNF	[53]

4. Conclusions

Despite the few studies with cinnamic acids in animal depression models, the results indicate their potential applicability as candidates for antidepressant drugs. The studies discussed show that the antidepressant action of these natural products occurs via important neurotransmitters such as serotonin, as well as via the participation of inflammation-related metabolites such as AA-COX-2/5-LOX and BDNF. In some reports, there is a similarity in the mechanism of action with commercial antidepressant drugs. This data confirms the therapeutic potential of these compounds against behavioral disorders, such as depression. The availability of these compounds via commercial companies or laboratory synthesis, and the low cost of some acids, such as ferulic acid, make them interesting prototypes to advance the development of new antidepressant agents.

Author Contributions: Investigation, Methodology and Writing—Original Draft Preparation, L.R.L.D., M.T.d.S.S., J.N.B.; Formal Analysis, R.N.d.A.; Writing—Review and Editing, Supervision, D.P.d.S.

Funding: This research received no external funding.

Acknowledgments: This research was supported by the Conselho Nacional de Desenvolvimento Científico e Tecnológico (CNPq) and Coordenação de Aperfeiçoamento de Pessoal de Nível Superior (CAPES).

Conflicts of Interest: The authors declare no conflict of interest

Abbreviations

5-HIAA	5-Hydroxyindoleacetic acid
5-HT	Serotonin
5-LOX	5-Lipoxygenase
BDNF	Brain-derived neurotrophic factor
CaMKII	Ca^{2+}/calmodulin-dependent protein kinase II
CAT	Catalase
COX-2	Cyclooxygenase-2
EPM	Elevated plus maze test
FST	Forced swim test
IL-1β	Interleukin-1β
IL-8	Interleukin-8
LPS	Lipopolysaccharide
MAO	Monoamine oxidase
MAO-A	Monoamine oxidase A
MAPK/ERK	Mitogen-activated protein kinases/extracellular signal-regulated kinases
MHPG	3-Methoxy-4-hydroxyphenylglycol
NF-κB	Nuclear factor kappa B
NE	Norepinephrine
NET	Norepinephrine transporter
NO	Nitric oxide
OFT	Open field test
PI3K	Phosphoinositide 3-kinases
PKA	Protein kinase A
PKC	Protein kinase C
ROS	Reactive species of oxygen
SERT	Serotonin transporter
SNRI	Serotonin norepinephrine reuptake inhibitors
SOD	Superoxide dismutase
SSRI	Selective serotonin reuptake inhibitor
SST	Sucrose splash test

TBARS	Thiobarbituric acid reactive substances
TCA	Tricyclic antidepressants
TYR	Tyrosine
TMCA	2,4,5-Trimethoxycinnamic acid
TNF-α	Tumor necrosis factor-α
TRP	Tryptophan
TST	Tail suspension test

References

1. Peres, M.F.P.; Mercante, J.P.P.; Tobo, P.R.; Kamei, H.; Bigal, M.E. Anxiety and depression symptoms and migraine: A symptom-based approach research. *J. Headache Pain* **2017**, *18*, 37. [CrossRef] [PubMed]
2. Smith, K. Mental health: A world of depression. *Nature* **2014**, *515*, 181. [CrossRef] [PubMed]
3. Bravender, T. Mental Disorders and Learning Disabilities in Children and Adolescents: Depression in Adolescents. *FP Essent.* **2018**, *475*, 30. [PubMed]
4. Wang, S.; Blazer, D.G. Depression and cognition in the elderly. *Annu Rev. Clin. Psychol.* **2015**, *11*, 331. [CrossRef]
5. Gournellis, R.; Tournikioti, K.; Touloumi, G.; Thomadakis, C.; Michalopoulou, P.G.; Michopoulos, I.; Christodoulou, C.; Papadopoulou, A.; Douzenis, A. Psychotic (delusional) depression and completed suicide: A systematic review and meta-analysis. *Ann. Gen. Psychiatry* **2018**, *17*, 39. [CrossRef]
6. Hawton, K.; Casanas, I.C.C.; Haw, C.; Saunders, K. Risk factors for suicide in individuals with depression: A systematic review. *J. Affect. Disord.* **2013**, *147*, 17. [CrossRef]
7. Krishnan, V.; Nestler, E.J. The molecular neurobiology of depression. *Nature* **2008**, *455*, 894. [CrossRef]
8. Peng, G.J.; Tian, J.S.; Gao, X.X.; Zhou, Y.Z.; Qin, X.M. Research on the Pathological Mechanism and Drug Treatment Mechanism of Depression. *Curr. Neuropharmacol.* **2015**, *13*, 514. [CrossRef]
9. Ruiz, N.A.L.; Del Angel, D.S.; Olguin, H.J.; Silva, M.L. Neuroprogression: The hidden mechanism of depression. *Neuropsychiatr. Dis. Treat.* **2018**, *14*, 2837. [CrossRef]
10. Uchida, S.; Yamagata, H.; Seki, T.; Watanabe, Y. Epigenetic mechanisms of major depression: Targeting neuronal plasticity. *Psychiatry Clin. Neurosci* **2018**, *72*, 212. [CrossRef]
11. Liu, C.H.; Zhang, G.Z.; Li, B.; Li, M.; Woelfer, M.; Walter, M.; Wang, L. Role of inflammation in depression relapse. *J. Neuroinflammation* **2019**, *16*, 90. [CrossRef] [PubMed]
12. Reus, G.Z.; Silva, R.H.; de Moura, A.B.; Presa, J.F.; Abelaira, H.M.; Abatti, M.; Vieira, A.; Pescador, B.; Michels, M.; Ignacio, Z.M.; et al. Early Maternal Deprivation Induces Microglial Activation, Alters Glial Fibrillary Acidic Protein Immunoreactivity and Indoleamine 2,3-Dioxygenase during the Development of Offspring Rats. *Mol. Neurobiol.* **2019**, *56*, 1096. [CrossRef] [PubMed]
13. Oglodek, E.A. Changes in the concentrations of inflammatory and oxidative status biomediators (MIP-1 alpha, PMN elastase, MDA, and IL-12) in depressed patients with and without posttraumatic stress disorder. *Pharmacol Rep.* **2018**, *70*, 110. [CrossRef] [PubMed]
14. Stanners, M.N.; Barton, C.A.; Shakib, S.; Winefield, H.R. Depression diagnosis and treatment amongst multimorbid patients: A thematic analysis. *BMC Fam. Pract.* **2014**, *15*, 124. [CrossRef] [PubMed]
15. Blackburn, T.P. Depressive disorders: Treatment failures and poor prognosis over the last 50 years. *Pharmacol. Res. Perspect.* **2019**, *7*, e00472. [CrossRef] [PubMed]
16. Hollon, S.D.; Cohen, Z.D.; Singla, D.R.; Andrews, P.W. Recent Developments in the Treatment of Depression. *Behav. Ther.* **2019**, *50*, 257. [CrossRef]
17. López-Rubalcava, C.; Estrada-Camarena, E. Mexican medicinal plants with anxiolytic or antidepressant activity: Focus on preclinical research. *J. Ethnopharmacol.* **2016**, *20*, 377–391.
18. Guzman, J.D.; Mortazavi, P.N.; Munshi, T.; Evangelopoulos, D.; Mchugh, T.D.; Gibbons, S.; Malkinson, J.; Bhakta, S. 2-Hydroxy-substituted cinnamic acids and acetanilides are selective growth inhibitors of Mycobacterium tuberculosis. *MedChemComm* **2014**, *5*, 47–50. [CrossRef]
19. Tian, Y.; Liu, W.; Lu, Y.; Wang, Y.; Chen, X.; Bai, S.; Zhao, Y.; He, T.; Lao, F.; Shang, Y.; et al. Naturally Occurring Cinnamic Acid Sugar Ester Derivatives. *Molecules* **2016**, *21*, 1402. [CrossRef]
20. de Cássia, D.S.E.S.; Andrade, L.N.; Dos Reis, B.D.O.R.; de Sousa, D.P. A review on anti-inflammatory activity of phenylpropanoids found in essential oils. *Molecules* **2014**, *19*, 1459–1480. [CrossRef]

21. Sova, M. Antioxidant and antimicrobial activities of cinnamic acid derivatives. *Mini Rev. Med. Chem.* **2012**, *12*, 749–767. [CrossRef] [PubMed]
22. Anantharaju, P.G.; Gowda, P.C.; Vimalambike, M.G.; Madhunapantula, S.V. An overview on the role of dietary phenolics for the treatment of cancers. *Nutr. J.* **2016**, *15*, 99. [CrossRef] [PubMed]
23. Alam, M.A.; Subhan, N.; Hossain, H.; Hossain, M.; Reza, H.M.; Rahman, M.M.; Ullah, M.O. Hydroxycinnamic acid derivatives: A potential class of natural compounds for the management of lipid metabolism and obesity. *Nutr. Metab.* **2016**, *13*, 27. [CrossRef] [PubMed]
24. Liu, P.; Hu, Y.; Guo, D.H.; Wang, D.X.; Tu, H.H.; Ma, L.; Xie, T.T.; Kong, L.Y. Potential antidepressant properties of Radix polygalae (Yuan Zhi). *Phytomedicine* **2010**, *17*, 794–799. [CrossRef]
25. Szwajgier, D.; Borowiec, K.; Pustelniak, K. The Neuroprotective Effects of Phenolic Acids: Molecular Mechanism of Action. *Nutrients* **2017**, *9*, 477. [CrossRef]
26. Magoulas, G.E.; Papaioannou, D. Bioinspired syntheses of dimeric hydroxycinnamic acids (lignans) and hybrids, using phenol oxidative coupling as key reaction, and medicinal significance thereof. *Molecules* **2014**, *19*, 19769. [CrossRef]
27. Bialecka-Florjanczyk, E.; Fabiszewska, A.; Zieniuk, B. Phenolic Acids Derivatives-Biotechnological Methods of Synthesis and Bioactivity. *Curr. Pharm. Biotechnol.* **2018**, *19*, 1098. [CrossRef]
28. Wu, S.; Zhang, Y.; Ren, F.; Qin, Y.; Liu, J.; Liu, J.; Wang, Q.; Zhang, H. Structure-affinity relationship of the interaction between phenolic acids and their derivatives and beta-lactoglobulin and effect on antioxidant activity. *Food Chem.* **2018**, *245*, 613. [CrossRef]
29. Dludla, P.V.; Nkambule, B.B.; Jack, B.; Mkandla, Z.; Mutize, T.; Silvestri, S.; Orlando, P.; Tiano, L.; Louw, J.; Mazibuko-Mbeje, S.E. Inflammation and Oxidative Stress in an Obese State and the Protective Effects of Gallic Acid. *Nutrients* **2019**, *11*, 23. [CrossRef]
30. Oliviero, F.; Scanu, A.; Zamudio-Cuevas, Y.; Punzi, L.; Spinella, P. Anti-inflammatory effects of polyphenols in arthritis. *J. Sci. Food Agric.* **2018**, *98*, 1653. [CrossRef]
31. Gaspar, A.; Garrido, E.M.; Esteves, M.; Quezada, E.; Milhazes, N.; Garrido, J.; Borges, F. New insights into the antioxidant activity of hydroxycinnamic acids: Synthesis and physicochemical characterization of novel halogenated derivatives. *Eur. J. Med. Chem.* **2009**, *44*, 2092. [CrossRef] [PubMed]
32. Razzaghi-Asl, N.; Garrido, J.; Khazraei, H.; Borges, F.; Firuzi, O. Antioxidant properties of hydroxycinnamic acids: A review of structure- activity relationships. *Curr. Med. Chem.* **2013**, *20*, 4436. [CrossRef] [PubMed]
33. Castagne, V.; Moser, P.; Roux, S.; Porsolt, R.D. Rodent models of depression: Forced swim and tail suspension behavioral despair tests in rats and mice. *Curr. Protoc. Neurosci.* **2011**, *55*, 8–10. [CrossRef] [PubMed]
34. Yan, H.C.; Cao, X.; Das, M.; Zhu, X.H.; Gao, T.M. Behavioral animal models of depression. *Neurosci. Bull.* **2010**, *26*, 327. [CrossRef]
35. Abelaira, H.M.; Reus, G.Z.; Quevedo, J. Animal models as tools to study the pathophysiology of depression. *Braz. J. Psychiatry* **2013**, *35*, S112–S120. [CrossRef]
36. Nakazawa, T.; Yasuda, T.; Ueda, J.; Ohsawa, K. Antidepressant-like effects of apigenin and 2, 4, 5-trimethoxycinnamic acid from Perilla frutescens in the forced swimming test. *Biol. Pharm. Bull.* **2003**, *26*, 474–480. [CrossRef]
37. Leem, Y.H.; Oh, S. 3, 4, 5-Trimethoxycinnamin acid ameliorates restraint stress-induced anxiety and depression. *Neurosci. Lett.* **2015**, *585*, 54–59. [CrossRef]
38. Takeda, H.; Tsuji, M.; Inazu, M.; Egashira, T.; Matsumiya, T. Rosmarinic acid and caffeic acid produce antidepressive-like effect in the forced swimming test in mice. *Eur. J. Pharmacol.* **2002**, *449*, 261–267. [CrossRef]
39. Takeda, H.; Tsuji, M.; Miyamoto, J.; Masuya, J.; Iimori, M.; Matsumiya, T. Caffeic acid produces antidepressive-and/or anxiolytic-like effects through indirect modulation of the α1A-adrenoceptor system in mice. *Neuroreport* **2003**, *14*, 1067–1070. [CrossRef]
40. Takeda, H.; Tsuji, M.; Yamada, T.; Masuya, J.; Matsushita, K.; Tahara, M.; Matsumiya, T.; Limore, M.; Matsumiya, T. Caffeic acid attenuates the decrease in cortical BDNF mRNA expression induced by exposure to forced swimming stress in mice. *Eur. J. Pharmacol.* **2006**, *534*, 115–121. [CrossRef]
41. Dzitoyeva, S.; Imbesi, M.; Uz, T.; Dimitrijevic, N.; Manev, H.; Manev, R. Caffeic acid attenuates the decrease of cortical BDNF transcript IV mRNA induced by swim stress in wild-type but not in 5-lipoxygenase-deficient mice. *J. Neural Transm. Suppl.* **2008**, *115*, 823–827. [CrossRef] [PubMed]

42. Huang, D.; Zhang, L.; Yang, J.Q.; Luo, Y.; Cui, T.; Du, T.T.; Jiang, X.H. Evaluation on monoamine neurotransmitters changes in depression rats given with sertraline, meloxicam or/and caffeic acid. *Genes Dis.* **2019**, *6*, 167–175. [CrossRef] [PubMed]

43. Zdunska, K.; Dana, A.; Kolodziejczak, A.; Rotsztejn, H. Antioxidant Properties of Ferulic Acid and Its Possible Application. *Skin Pharmacol. Physiol.* **2018**, *31*, 332. [CrossRef] [PubMed]

44. Zeni, A.L.B.; Zomkowski, A.D.E.; Maraschin, M.; Rodrigues, A.L.S.; Tasca, C.I. Ferulic acid exerts antidepressant-like effect in the tail suspension test in mice: Evidence for the involvement of the serotonergic system. *Eur. J. Pharmacol.* **2012**, *679*, 68–74. [CrossRef]

45. Zeni, A.L.B.; Camargo, A.; Dalmagro, A.P. Ferulic acid reverses depression-like behavior and oxidative stress induced by chronic corticosterone treatment in mice. *Steroids* **2017**, *125*, 131–136. [CrossRef]

46. Chen, J.; Lin, D.; Zhang, C.; Li, G.; Zhang, N.; Ruan, L.; Yan, K.; Li, J.; Yu, X.; Xie, X.; et al. Antidepressant-like effects of ferulic acid: Involvement of serotonergic and norepinergic systems. *Metab. Brain Dis.* **2015**, *30*, 129–136. [CrossRef]

47. Zhang, Y.J.; Huang, X.; Wang, Y.; Xie, Y.; Qiu, X.J.; Ren, P.; Gao, L.C.; Zhou, H.H.; Zhange, H.Y.; Qiao, M.Q. Ferulic acid-induced anti-depression and prokinetics similar to Chaihu–Shugan–San via polypharmacology. *Brain Res. Bull.* **2011**, *86*, 222–228. [CrossRef]

48. Sasaki, K.; Iwata, N.; Ferdousi, F.; Isoda, H. Antidepressant-Like Effect of Ferulic Acid via Promotion of Energy Metabolism Activity. *Mol. Nutr. Food Res.* **2019**, *63*, 1900327. [CrossRef]

49. Lenzi, J.; Rodrigues, A.F.; de Sousa Rós, A.; de Castro, B.B.; de Lima, D.D.; Dal Magro, D.D.; Zeni, A.L.B. Ferulic acid chronic treatment exerts antidepressant-like effect: Role of antioxidant defense system. *Metab. Brain Dis.* **2015**, *30*, 1453–1463. [CrossRef]

50. Li, G.; Ruan, L.; Chen, R.; Wang, R.; Xie, X.; Zhang, M.; Chen, L.; Yan, Q.; Reed, M.; Chen, J.; et al. Synergistic antidepressant-like effect of ferulic acid in combination with piperine: Involvement of monoaminergic system. *Metab. Brain Dis.* **2015**, *30*, 1505–1514. [CrossRef]

51. Liu, Y.M.; Hu, C.Y.; Shen, J.D.; Wu, S.H.; Li, Y.C.; Yi, L.T. Elevation of synaptic protein is associated with the antidepressant-like effects of ferulic acid in a chronic model of depression. *Physiol. Behav.* **2017**, *169*, 184–188. [CrossRef] [PubMed]

52. Zheng, X.; Cheng, Y.; Chen, Y.; Yue, Y.; Li, Y.; Xia, S.; Li, Y.; Deng, H.; Zang, J.; Cao, Y. Ferulic Acid Improves Depressive-Like Behavior in Prenatally-Stressed Offspring Rats via Anti-Inflammatory Activity and HPA Axis. *Int. J. Mol. Sci.* **2019**, *20*, 493. [CrossRef] [PubMed]

53. Lee, S.; Kim, H.B.; Hwang, E.S.; Kim, E.S.; Kim, S.S.; Jeon, T.D.; Song, M.; Li, J.S.; Chung, M.C.; Maeng, S.; et al. Antidepressant-like effects of *p*-coumaric acid on LPS-induced depressive and inflammatory changes in rats. *Exp. Neurobiol.* **2018**, *27*, 189–199. [CrossRef] [PubMed]

54. Barauna, S.C.; Delwing-Dal, M.D.; Brueckheimer, M.B.; Maia, T.P.; Sala, G.A.B.N.; Döhler, A.W.; Harger, M.C.; de Melo, D.F.M.; de Gasper, A.L.; Alberton, M.D.; et al. Antioxidant and antidepressant-like effects of *Eugenia catharinensis* D. Legrand in an animal model of depression induced by corticosterone. *Metab. Brain Dis.* **2018**, *33*, 1985–1994. [CrossRef] [PubMed]

55. Adeoluwa, A.O.; Aderibigbe, O.A.; Agboola, I.O.; Olonode, T.E.; Ben-Azu, B. Butanol Fraction of *Olax subscorpioidea* Produces Antidepressant Effect: Evidence for the Involvement of Monoaminergic Neurotransmission. *Drug Res. (Stuttg).* **2019**, *69*, 53–60. [CrossRef]

56. Pauleti, N.N.; Mello, J.; Siebert, D.A.; Micke, G.A.; de Albuquerque, C.A.C.; Alberton, M.; Barauna, S.C. Characterisation of phenolic compounds of the ethyl acetate fraction from *Tabernaemontana catharinensis* and its potential antidepressant-like effect. *Nat. Prod. Res.* **2018**, *32*, 1987–1990. [CrossRef]

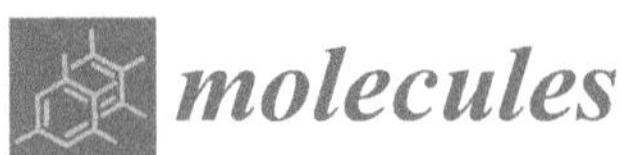 *molecules*

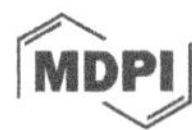

Article

Mahonia aquifolium Extracts Promote Doxorubicin Effects against Lung Adenocarcinoma Cells In Vitro

Ana Damjanović [1], Branka Kolundžija [1], Ivana Z. Matić [1], Ana Krivokuća [1], Gordana Zdunić [2], Katarina Šavikin [2], Radmila Janković [1], Jelena Antić Stanković [3,*] and Tatjana P. Stanojković [1]

[1] Department for Experimental Oncology, Institute of Oncology and Radiology of Serbia, 11 000 Belgrade, Serbia; zaanu011@gmail.com (A.D.); branka.kolundzija@gmail.com (B.K.); ivanamatic2103@gmail.com (I.Z.M.); krivokuca.ana@gmail.com (A.K.); jankovicr@ncrc.ac.rs (R.J.); stanojkovict@ncrc.ac.rs (T.P.S.)

[2] Department for Pharmaceutical Investigations and Development, Institute for Medicinal Plant Research, Dr. Josif Pančić, 11 070 Belgrade, Serbia; gzdunic@mocbilja.rs (G.Z.); katarina.savikin@gmail.com (K.Š.)

[3] Department for Microbiology and Immunology, Faculty of Pharmacy, University of Belgrade, 11 221 Belgrade, Serbia

* Correspondence: jelena.stankovic@pharmacy.bg.ac.rs; Tel.: +381113951224; Fax: +381113951840

Academic Editors: Raffaele Pezzani and Sara Vitalini

Received: 1 September 2020; Accepted: 26 October 2020; Published: 10 November 2020

Abstract: *Mahonia aquifolium* and its secondary metabolites have been shown to have anticancer potential. We performed MTT, scratch, and colony formation assays; analyzed cell cycle phase distribution and doxorubicin uptake and retention with flow cytometry; and detected alterations in the expression of genes involved in the formation of cell–cell interactions and migration using quantitative real-time PCR following treatment of lung adenocarcinoma cells with doxorubicin, *M. aquifolium* extracts, or their combination. MTT assay results suggested strong synergistic effects of the combined treatments, and their application led to an increase in cell numbers in the subG1 phase of the cell cycle. Both extracts were shown to prolong doxorubicin retention time in cancer cells, while the application of doxorubicin/extract combination led to a decrease in *MMP9* expression. Furthermore, cells treated with doxorubicin/extract combinations were shown to have lower migratory and colony formation potentials than untreated cells or cells treated with doxorubicin alone. The obtained results suggest that nontoxic *M. aquifolium* extracts can enhance the activity of doxorubicin, thus potentially allowing the application of lower doxorubicin doses in vivo, which may decrease its toxic effects in normal tissues.

Keywords: doxorubicin; *Mahonia aquifolium*; matrix metalloproteinases; cytotoxicity; human lung adenocarcinoma

1. Introduction

Doxorubicin (DOX) is a first-line anticancer agent that is highly effective against a wide spectrum of malignancies, including breast, lung, gastric, ovarian, and thyroid ones, as well as lymphoma, myeloma, sarcoma, and some forms of pediatric neoplasms. Despite good clinical effectiveness, DOX induces cumulative, dose-dependent toxicity and adverse effects, such as cardiotoxicity, and affects the brain, kidney, and liver [1]. Currently, both cancer treatments and in vivo studies are usually based on combined therapies that include various antineoplastic agents, possibly resulting in drug–drug interactions and even an increase in toxicity [2]. Studies investigating the management of DOX-induced toxicity have focused on the administration of antioxidant and/or antiapoptotic compounds in combination with DOX, the development of effective delivery systems, and the synthesis of DOX analogs [1]. One potential approach to the minimization of adverse effects is reducing the therapeutic dose of DOX by combining its application with that of other anticancer and/or organ-protective agents [3]. However, although some of these strategies fail to decrease DOX toxicity, recent investigations have demonstrated that certain phytocompounds in combination with DOX can ultimately be more successful [4,5].

The genus *Mahonia* includes approximately 60 species, which are widely distributed throughout Asia, North America, and Europe. Species belonging to the genus *Mahonia*, including the *Mahonia aquifolium* plant, have been shown to have antibacterial, antifungal, anti-inflammatory, and antioxidant effects and have been used in traditional Chinese and North American medicine [6]. Some research has shown that several representatives of this genus, such as *Mahonia oiwakensis* and *Mahonia bealei*, which are native to China, demonstrate antiproliferative activity against human cancer cells as well [7,8]. Berberine and similar alkaloids represent a major class of secondary metabolites of the *Mahonia* genus with a wide spectrum of different properties. These alkaloids have been reported to significantly inhibit growth of cancer cells and exhibit other anticancer effects [9–12]. Although *M. aquifolium* has been used in traditional medicine solely for treatment of inflammatory skin disorders [13], its chemical composition, as well as previously obtained results demonstrating the activity of different plants belonging to this genus, suggest that this plant possesses anticancer properties as well, as we have previously confirmed and reported [14].

Previous studies have demonstrated that the phytocompound berberine in combination with DOX can effectively limit the toxicity and adverse effects of DOX [4] and that *M. aquifolium*, whose main constituents are berberine and protoberberine alkaloids, has anticancer properties [14,15]. Therefore, we investigated the anticancer efficacy of the combination of DOX and water or ethanol extracts of *M. aquifolium* (MAW and MAE, respectively) in vitro.

The objective of our study was to elucidate the effects of DOX and MAW or MAE combinations on proliferation, migratory potential, and invasiveness of malignant cells. Furthermore, we examined the influence of these extracts on cellular uptake and retention of DOX. In order to understand the mechanisms underlying the effects of these extracts on migration and invasiveness, we analyzed gene expression changes of matrix metalloproteinases 2 and 9 (*MMP2* and *MMP9*), occludin (*OCLN*), catenin beta-1 (*CTNNB1*), and excision repair cross-complementation group 1 (*ERCC1*) in the treated human malignant cells.

2. Results

2.1. Cytotoxic Activity In Vitro

2.1.1. Cytotoxic Activity of Extracts and DOX

MAW and MAE showed moderate cytotoxic activities against A549 cells. After 72 h of treatment with extracts, MAW IC_{50} value was shown to be 56.36 ± 0.30 µg/mL, while MAE IC_{50} was 51.97 ± 3.27 µg/mL. The IC_{50} of DOX was 0.44 ± 0.02 µg/mL.

2.1.2. Cytotoxic Activity of DOX in Combination with Extracts

The combined extracts and DOX effects were evaluated using an isobolographic analysis method. After incubating cells with subtoxic concentrations of extracts in combination with DOX, there was an increase in cytotoxicity compared to the controls (Table 1). The CI values ranged from 0.14 to 0.38 for DOX/MAW and from 0.12 to 0.4 for DOX/MAE treatment, suggesting strong synergism (Table 2).

Table 1. Concentrations of doxorubicin alone or in combination with extracts that induced 50% decrease in cell survival after 72 h of treatment.

	IC_{50} (μg/mL)
	A549
DOX	0.4457 ± 0.0154
DOX + 5 μg/mL MAW	0.0234 ± 0.0022
DOX + 10 μg/mL MAW	0.0141 ± 0.0046
DOX + 20 μg/mL MAW	0.0067 ± 0.0018
DOX + 5 μg/mL MAE	0.0113 ± 0.0006
DOX + 10 μg/mL MAE	0.0103 ± 0.0016
DOX + 20 μg/mL MAE	0.0036 ± 0.0012

IC_{50} values are presented as the mean $\pm$ standard deviation (SD) from three independent experiments; DOX: doxorubicin; MAW: water extract of *M. aquifolium*; MAE: ethanol extract of *M. aquifolium*.

Table 2. Isobolographic analysis.

	CI
Treatment	A549
DOX + 5 μg/mL MAW	0.14
DOX + 10 μg/mL MAW	0.21
DOX + 20 μg/mL MAW	0.38
DOX + 5 μg/mL MAE	0.12
DOX + 10 μg/mL MAE	0.22
DOX + 20 μg/mL MAE	0.40

CI: combination index.

2.2. Cell Cycle Analysis

A549 cells treated with subtoxic concentrations of both MAE and MAW extracts for 24 h showed a slight increase in the percentage of cells in the G2/M phase of the cell cycle, but the changes induced by this treatment did not significantly differ from those in the controls. However, treatment of cells with IC_{20} and IC_{50} DOX led to a significant increase in the percentage of cells in the G2/M phase (Figure 1A), while cells treated with combination of DOX (IC_{20} or IC_{50}) and MAW or MAE (20 μg/mL) were shown to accumulate in the G1 phase compared to those treated with DOX alone (Figure 1B). Samples treated with combinations of DOX (IC_{20} or IC_{50}) and extracts showed an increase in the subG1 phase as well, compared to samples treated with DOX alone, and this increase in the number of subG1 cells was shown to be statistically significant for cells treated with combination of DOX and MAE (Figure 1B).

2.3. Cellular Uptake and DOX Retention

No significant changes in DOX uptake were observed following treatment with extracts (Table 3). However, the effects of extract treatment on DOX retention were more pronounced. Cells treated with extracts after DOX treatment retained considerably more DOX (up to 22% more) than cells treated with DOX and medium only (Table 3).

Table 3. Effects of *M. aquifolium* water and ethanol extracts on the uptake and retention of doxorubicin in A549 cells.

Treatment	Uptake	Retention
DOX IC_{50}	100	100
DOX IC_{50} + MAW (40 μg/mL)	92.34 ± 6.64	112.97 ± 0.25
DOX IC_{50} + MAE (40 μg/mL)	96.58 ± 2.77	122.23 ± 1.60

The results are presented as the mean $\pm$ standard deviation (SD) from three independent experiments.

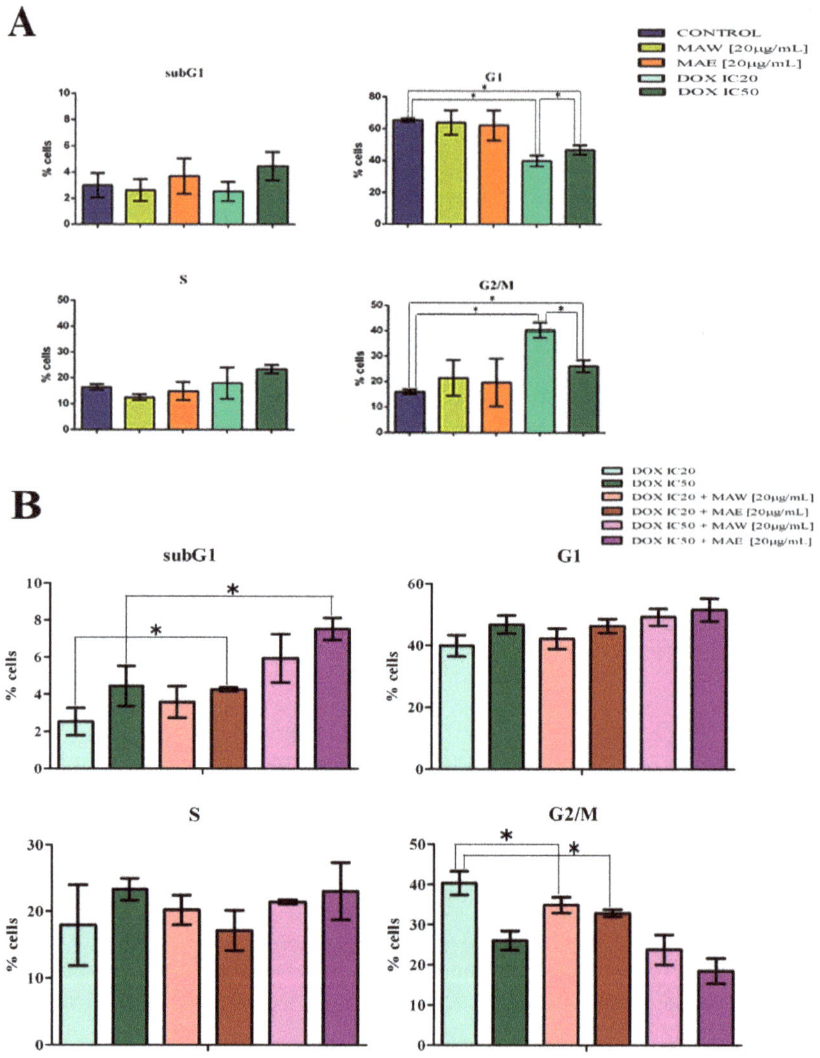

Figure 1. Changes in the cell cycle phase distribution of A549 cells after 24 h of treatment induced by (**A**) MAW (20 µg/mL), MAE (20 µg/mL), DOX IC20, or DOX IC50 compared to the control and (**B**) combination DOX/extract treatment compared to DOX treatment alone.

2.4. Cell Migration

Both extracts demonstrated an improved ability to reduce cell migration compared to the control or DOX (Figure 2). After 48 h, this decrease was shown to be statistically significant in both extract-treated samples. Cells treated with DOX alone did not show any significant variation, while the migratory ability of cells treated with DOX and MAE or MAW was shown to be considerably lower after 48 h (Figure 2B).

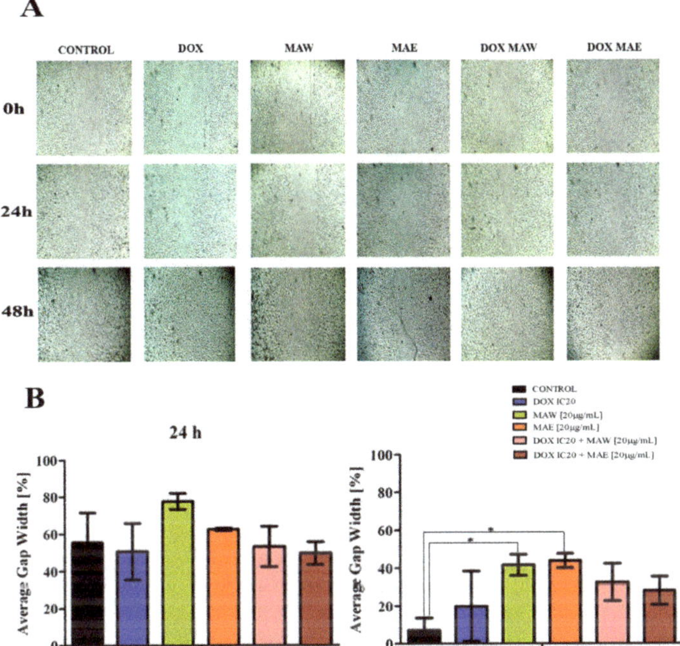

Figure 2. Effects of *M. aquifolium* extracts and DOX on migration of A549 cells. The cells were treated with DOX IC20, MAW (20 µg/mL), MAE (20 µg/mL), or their combinations. (**A**) Representative images of one of three independent experiments. (**B**) Quantitative analysis of results presented in (A).

2.5. Colony Formation

As shown in Figure 3, DOX considerably affected the ability of cells to form colonies even when applied in subtoxic concentrations, unlike MAW and MAE extracts, which caused only a slight decrease in the colony-forming ability. However, combinations of DOX and MAE/MAW extracts were shown to lead to an even more pronounced decrease in the colony-forming ability of the treated cells compared to DOX treatment alone.

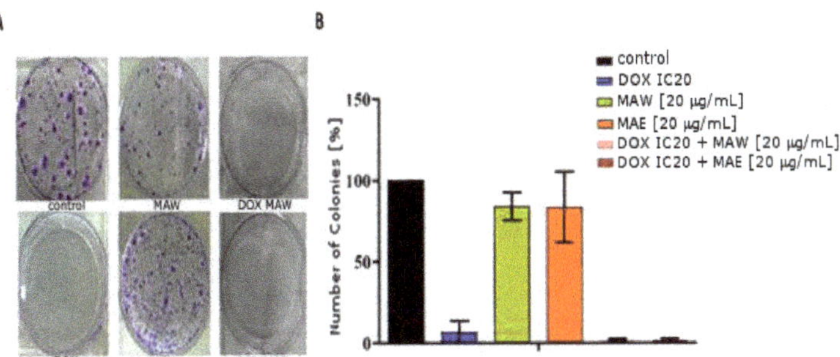

Figure 3. Effects of *M. aquifolium* extracts and DOX on A549 colony forming ability. (**A**) Representative images of colonies stained with Coomassie Brilliant Blue following treatment with DOX IC20, MAW (20 µg/mL), MAE (20 µg/mL), or their combinations. Experiments were performed at least three times. (**B**) Quantitative analysis of results presented in (A).

2.6. Gene Expression Analyses

We investigated the gene expression involved in the formation of cell junctions, in cell migration, and in DNA repair, as well as whether this gene expression is associated with the metastatic potential of cells (*MMP2*, *MMP9*, *OCLN*, *CTNNB1*, and *ERCC1*). Gene expression levels in the treated A549 cells were compared with those measured in the untreated, control cells grown only in the nutrient medium (Figure 4).

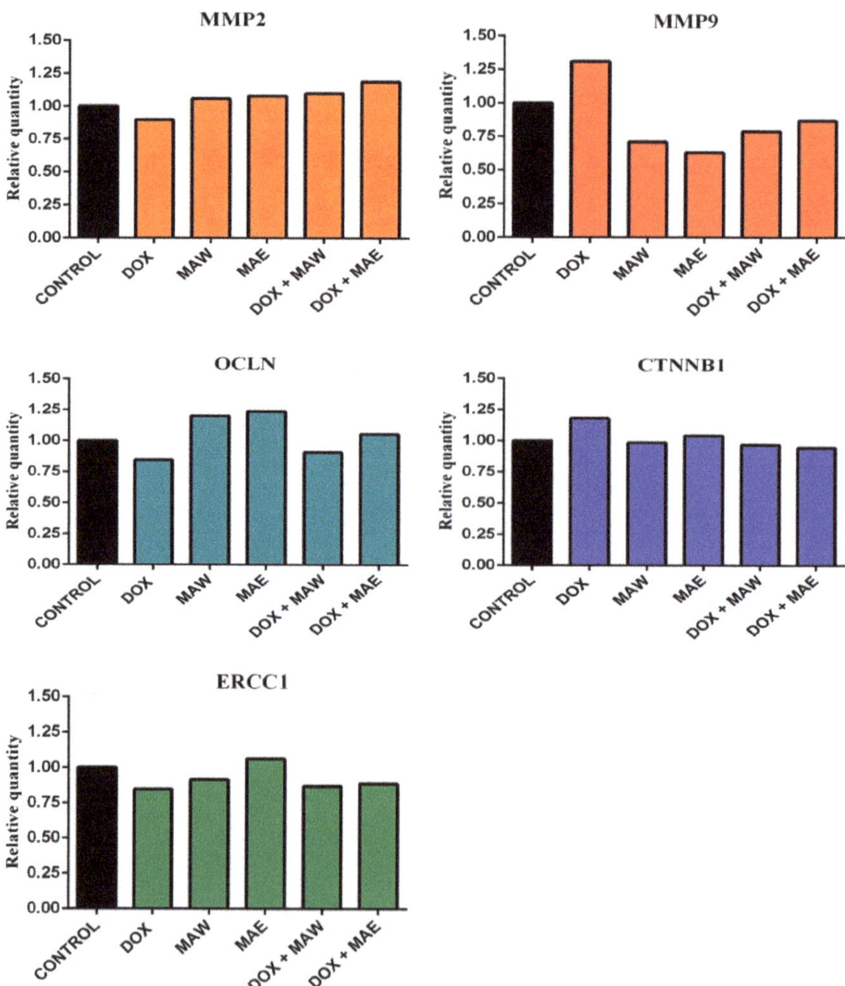

Figure 4. Effects of DOX IC20, MAE (20 µg/mL), MAW (20 µg/mL), or their combinations on gene expression.

DOX treatment was shown to decrease *MMP2* expression, while both the applied extracts and DOX/extract combinations slightly increased the expression of this gene (Figure 4). In contrast to this, *MMP9* expression was considerably lower after treatment with combination of the cytostatic and the investigated plant extracts (Figure 4), but it increased after treatment with DOX alone, in contrast to the control. Furthermore, DOX treatment was shown to inhibit the expression of *OCLN* and induce

CTNNB1 expression. Both the investigated extracts alone and the DOX/MAE combination treatment induced expression of *OCLN* (Figure 4) as opposed to the control cells, while its expression in cells treated with the DOX/MAW combination was higher than in cells treated with DOX alone. There were no alterations in *CTNNB1* expression after treatment with the DOX/MAW combination, while its expression was shown to be slightly lower after treatment of cells with the DOX/MAE combination than in the untreated cells (Figure 4).

Cells treated with MAE alone showed a slight increase in *ERCC1* expression levels, while inhibition of this gene expression was observed in samples treated with DOX, in those treated with MAW, as well as in those treated with the DOX/plant extract combination (Figure 4).

3. Discussion

Despite decades of good results in the clinical application of DOX in cancer therapy, this drug induces cumulative, dose-dependent adverse effects. Our previous studies have demonstrated that ethanol and water extracts obtained from *M. aquifolium* show good anticancer potential and that berberine and berberine-type alkaloids can be detected in both extracts [14]. Higher content of berberine was detected in MAE extract (2.44%) compared to MAW extract (1.34%) (LC-MC analyses).

Furthermore, after identifying cytotoxic metabolites from *M. aquifolium* using ^{1}H NMR-based metabolomic approach, we concluded that alkaloids with the highest cytotoxicity in our extracts are berberine, palmatine, and the bisbenzylisoquinoline alkaloid berbamine [15]. It has previously been reported that berberine and similar alkaloids can inhibit the growth of cancer cells [9], effectively limiting the toxicity of DOX [4].

Our initial screenings demonstrated that, of the tested cell lines, A549 cells were the least sensitive to the cytotoxic activity of MAE and MAW [14]. Nonsmall cell lung cancer patients often show resistance to therapy [16], and several mechanisms underlying the development of multidrug resistance in lung cancer have been identified, such as overexpression of drug efflux proteins and ATP-binding cassette (ABC) transporters [17]. Many studies have confirmed the presence of ABC transporters, breast cancer-resistant protein (BCRP), and lung resistance-related protein (LRP) in A549 cells, which have been shown to be related to anticancer drug resistance [18–20]; therefore, we selected the A549 cell line for all further experiments. The results obtained here demonstrate that the IC_{50} concentration of DOX can be multiply reduced (19 to 123 times) when DOX is combined with *M. aquifolium* extracts, suggesting that the same antiproliferative effects can be achieved using much lower concentrations of this drug. Furthermore, DOX and the plant extracts showed strong synergistic effects, clearly demonstrating that the individual anticancer activities of both constituents were preserved. It has been reported that cardiomyophaty, the most important adverse effect of DOX, primarily depends on the applied dose [21]. Doses below 450 mg/m^2 reduce the frequency of on-treatment events, but the cumulative effects lead to the development of late-onset adverse events [22,23]. Based on this, we hereby propose that coadministration of DOX with an additional agent with a synergistic effect may decrease the toxicity of this treatment without affecting the anticancer activity of DOX. Our previous studies have shown that *M. aquifolium* extracts are several times less cytotoxic to normal, healthy cells than to cancer cells in vitro [14], indicating good selectivity and potential for their use in anticancer therapy.

We conducted the experiments on A549 cells, which are the most invasive but also the least sensitive to DOX, which is part of medical therapy in the treatment of lung cancer. Previous research has shown that both berberine and berbamine can inhibit the growth of lung cancer cells in in vivo systems [24,25], and based on these results, we can conclude that the active principles of our extracts have potential to reach this target in the body.

A549 cell cycle analysis has demonstrated that DOX induces a strong G2/M transition block [26] as well as a considerable increase in the percentage of cells in the subG1 phase in contrast to that in the control sample, indicating that treated cells cannot pass through mitosis, which ultimately leads to apoptosis [27,28]. We demonstrated that the percentage of cells in the subG1 phase was similar when cells were treated with IC_{50} DOX alone or with plant extracts and IC_{20} DOX combined, confirming that the extracts allowed maintenance of the anticancer activity of DOX even when applying lower drug doses. Furthermore, we observed an increase in the number of cells in the G1 phase following treatment of cells with DOX/plant extract combinations in contrast to the number of cells in the G1 phase treated with DOX alone. As one of the goals of drug discovery efforts today is identifying the agents that target cell cycle checkpoints responsible for the control of progression through the cell cycle [29], we believe that the results obtained may be very important. Cell percentage increase in the G1 and subG1 phases observed in samples treated with DOX/plant extract combinations may suggest that this G1 block is irreversible and that treatment induces apoptosis, which leads to an increase in the number of cells in the subG1 phase. This significantly higher percentage in samples treated with the DOX/MAE combination than in the control sample, as well as the existing DOX-induced G2/M arrest observed after the treatment of cells with both MAE/MAW and DOX combinations, additionally confirms their synergistic effects.

Although extracts did not affect DOX uptake, we have demonstrated that they induce the retention of DOX up to 20% more than in untreated samples. Increasing drug dose to overcome drug resistance in cancer therapy is not feasible due to numerous potential side effects [30], and alternative approaches include improving accumulation, prolonging retention of drugs in cancer cells [31], and reducing drug exposure time [32]. The inhibition of drug efflux transporters p-glycoprotein (Pgp) and BCRP restores the intracellular levels of drug in DOX-resistant osteosarcoma cells and leads to the retention of DOX [33]. Our research suggests that the investigated extracts inhibit one or more of these proteins and induce the retention of DOX. Furthermore, this may be a mechanism underlying the activation of apoptosis and increase in the subG1 phase cell numbers after the DOX/extract treatment [33]. Our further studies should clarify the mechanisms of DOX retention.

The inhibitors of matrix metalloproteinases are considered potential novel agents able to inhibit tumor growth and metastases, but they were shown to be unsuccessful in several clinical trials, which may result from the dual role of matrix metalloproteinases during cancer cell invasion and metastases [34]. These enzymes can degrade extracellular matrix as well as promote cancer cell invasion, migration, and neovascularization [35], but, on the other hand, they are able to reduce cancer growth and vascularization by inducing the generation of angiogenesis inhibitors (angiostatin and tumstatin) [35–38]. Scientists [39] concluded that MMP-2 and MMP-9 drive metastatic pathways, migration, viability, and secretion of angiogenic factors in two cell lines representing the metastatic and nonmetastatic forms of retinoblastoma cells. The observed inhibition of MMP9 expression in cells treated with the extracts was maintained even after combining these extracts with DOX. Chen et al. [34] showed that the increase in plasma levels of MMP9 promotes tumorigenicity in vivo, and these tumors are smaller and less vascularized compared with those grown in mice with lower MMP9 levels, which is explained by MMP9-induced angiostatin synthesis. MMP9 inhibitors lead to a decrease in the number of tumor colonies, but tumors in vivo are larger and more vascularized, which may provide a rationale for the coadministration of MMP inhibitors and antiangiogenic agents [34]. Our previous study [14] showed good antiangiogenic potential of *M. aquifolium* extracts, especially MAE, and this effect may indicate that these agents are suitable for overcoming the aforementioned issue of tumor vascularization and growth at lower MMP9 levels, while lower MMP9 expression in cells treated with extracts may reduce the metastatic potential of cancer cells. However, further experiments with a broader range of extract doses must be carried out to establish the proapoptotic activity of M. *aquifolium*.

Berberine, the main plant alkaloid of the genus *Mahonia* and the constituent of both *M. aquifolium* extracts involved [14], exhibits antimetastatic potential as well by blocking Wnt/β-catenin signaling pathway [40–42]. Furthermore, berberine can activate ZO-1 (Zonula Occludance-1), which participates in the formation of cell-tight junctions and indirectly reduces cell mobility [43]. We have investigated the influence of DOX, extracts, and their combinations on the expression of genes that participate in cell adherence and tight junction formation. *CTNNB1* encodes β-catenin, while *OCLN* encodes the occludin protein, one of the main components of tight junctions. Taken together, the results obtained here suggest that a decrease in *MMP9* and an increase in *OCLN* expression levels following treatment with a combination of DOX and the investigated extracts may lead to inhibition of cell migration and reduction of the metastatic potential of the treated cells. We have also examined the effects of plant extracts on cell migration, showing that both extracts, alone or in combination with DOX, inhibit cell migration, unlike DOX alone. Colony formation analysis results support our observations that the investigated plant extracts work together with DOX, enhancing its anticancer effects.

4. Materials and Methods

4.1. Plant Extracts/LC-MC Analyses

The stem bark of cultivated *Mahonia aquifolium* (Pursh) Nutt. was collected in the National Garden park in Pančevo, Serbia, in October 2014. The voucher specimen is deposited at the herbarium of the Institute for Medicinal Plants Research "Dr Josif Pančić ", Belgrade (No. 046/14).

Both dry extracts were obtained from air-dried and finely powdered stem bark of cultivated *M. aquifolium*. MAE was extracted with 70% EtOH at room temperature for 24 h (1:5, *w/v*), while MAW was prepared by ultrasound-assisted extraction with water (1:10, *w/v*) for 30 min. Dry extracts were analyzed by the LC/MS method on Agilent 1200 Series, Agilent Technologies, with a DAD detector on the column Zorbax Eclipse XDB-C18 (RRHT, 50 × 4.6 mm i.d.; 1.8 μm) in combination with 6210 time-of-flight LC/MS system (Agilent Technologies) [14].

4.2. Reagents

High-capacity cDNA reverse transcription kit was obtained from Thermo Fisher Scientific (Waltham, MA, USA). All other reagents were purchased from Sigma-Aldrich (St. Louis, MO, USA), unless otherwise specified.

4.3. Cell Lines

Human lung adenocarcinoma (A549) cells (ATCC, Manassas, VA, USA) were maintained in RPMI-1640 medium at 37 °C in humidified atmosphere with 5% CO_2 [44].

4.4. MTT Assay

Stock solutions of MAW, MAE, and DOX were dissolved in dimethyl sulfoxide (DMSO) at the concentration of 50 mg/mL (extracts) or 1 mM (DOX). Cells were seeded into 96-well microtiter plates at a density of 5000 cells/well. After 24 h, they were treated with five different extract concentrations (12.5, 25, 50, 100, and 200 μg/mL) or DOX (0.31, 0.62, 1.25, 2.5, and 5 μM). To determine the combined effect of DOX and extracts, cells were treated with various concentrations of DOX in the presence of subtoxic concentrations of MAW or MAE (5, 10, or 20 μg/mL). The control cells were grown in culture medium only. After an additional 72 h of incubation, cell survival was determined by MTT test, as described elsewhere [44–46]. The absorbance was measured at 570 nm using Multiskan EX reader (Thermo Labsystems Beverly, MA, USA). The experiments were performed in triplicate, and the data are presented as mean ± standard deviation (SD) of the results obtained in three independent experiments.

Combination index (CI) was used to determine the degree of interaction between DOX and *M. aquifolium*, and its formula is the sum of the ratio of the dose of each drug in the compound to the dose when used alone when the combination and compound produce 50% efficacy [47].

The CI values represent the mean of three experiments with the following values: CI 1.3: antagonism; CI 1.1–1.3: moderate antagonism; CI 0.9–1.1: additive effect; CI 0.8–0.9: slight synergism; CI 0.6–0.8: moderate synergism; CI 0.4–0.6: synergism; and CI 0.2–0.4: strong synergism [48,49].

4.5. Cell Cycle Analysis

A549 cells were seeded into six-well plates (2×10^5 cells/well). After 24 h, the cells were treated with concentrations corresponding to IC_{20} or IC_{50} values of DOX with 20 μg/mL of extracts or with combination of IC_{20} or IC_{50} DOX with 20 μg/mL of extracts. The cells were incubated, collected, and fixed. Afterward, the cells were washed, treated with RNase A, stained with propidium iodide, and analyzed using FACSCalibur flow cytometer (BD Biosciences Franklin Lakes, NJ, USA) and CELLQuest software (BD Biosciences) [44]. The obtained results are presented as mean ± SD of the results obtained in three independent experiments.

4.6. Cellular Uptake and Retention of Doxorubicin

A549 cells were seeded in six-well plates (2×10^5 cells/well). For DOX uptake experiments, the cells were treated with IC_{50} DOX alone or in combination with 40 μg/mL of extracts. After 24 h, the cells were washed with the medium and analyzed using FACSCalibur. For DOX retention, the cells were treated with IC_{50} of DOX for 24 h, and afterward, the samples were washed and treated with 40 μg/mL of extracts or with the nutrient medium only. After 24 h, the treated cells were washed again and analyzed. Fluorescence intensity measured in cells treated with DOX alone was used as a mark of 100% DOX retention/uptake. All data are presented as mean ± SD obtained in three independent experiments.

4.7. Scratch Assay

A549 cells were seeded in 24-well plates (7×10^4 cells/well), where they formed confluent monolayers after 24 h. The monolayers were scraped with a 200 μL pipette tip, and straight, cell-free gaps in the middle of cell monolayers were created. The cells were subsequently washed with nutrient medium and treated with IC_{20} concentration of DOX in the presence or absence of the subtoxic extract concentration (20 μg/mL) or with 20 μg/mL extracts only. The control cells were maintained in nutrient medium only. Images were obtained immediately after making the scratches and after 24 and 48 h of incubation. Three independent experiments were performed. Three representative points were selected in each image; the widths of the gap were measured and averaged. The average gap width at 0 h was considered 100%, and other average gap widths (%) were calculated relative to this value.

4.8. Colony Formation Assay

A549 cells (5×10^4 cells/well) were seeded into six-well plates and incubated for 24 h. Subsequently, they were treated with 0.11 μg/mL (IC_{20}) of DOX alone, subtoxic concentrations of MAE or MAW (20 μg/mL), or their combination. After an additional 24 h of treatment, the medium was removed from the wells, cells were harvested by trypsinization and replated at different densities, and they were left to grow for 1 week. Afterward, the colonies were stained, and the total number of colonies per well was counted. The experiments were performed in triplicate and repeated three times. For each treatment, the obtained number of colonies/well was divided by the cell-seeding density, and these results were averaged.

4.9. Gene Expression Analyses

A549 cells were seeded in 75 cm^2 cell culture flasks (3×10^6 cells/flasks) and grown for 24 h. Afterward, the cells were treated with subtoxic IC_{20} concentrations of DOX, 20 μg/mL extracts, or combination of IC_{20} DOX and 20 μg/mL extracts for 24 h. The control cells were grown in the culture medium. Following incubation, cells were collected by trypsinization, washed using PBS, and the collected cell pellet was stored at −80 °C until further experiments.

Total RNA was extracted from cells using TRI Reagent BD kit in line with the manufacturer's recommendations. RNA bands were visualized on a UV transilluminator, and RNA concentration was determined spectrophotometrically (BioSpec Nano, Shimadzu, Kyoto, Japan). Primary cDNA was prepared with RT-PCR using random primers, and 2 μg of total RNA was used as a template for MultiScribe reverse transcriptase in a high-capacity cDNA reverse transcription kit in line with the manufacturer's instructions.

4.10. Real-Time PCR Amplification

All target transcripts were detected using quantitative real-time PCR (qPCR) and TaqMan assays. TaqMan gene expression assays (*OCLN*: Hs00170162_m1, *CTNNB1*: Hs00355049_m1, *MMP2*: Hs01548727_m1, *MMP9*: Hs00234579_m1, and *ERCC1*: Hs01012158_m1) contained 20× mix of unlabeled PCR primers and TaqMan (Minor groove blinder (MGB)) probes (FAM dye-labeled). Glyceraldehyde-3-phosphate dehydrogenase (*GAPDH*) levels obtained using TaqMan control reagents (Hs02758991_g1) were used as an endogenous control. PCR reactions were performed using an ABI Prism 7500 sequence detection system (Applied Biosystems) under previously described conditions [50].

4.11. Statistical Analysis

One-way ANOVA with Tukey's multiple comparison test was used for multiple data comparisons and p value < 0.05 was considered statistically significant.

5. Conclusions

Taken together, our results show that *M. aquifolium* extracts and their active principles should be investigated further, either on their own or in combination with other anticancer drugs similar to DOX. It remains to be determined whether changes in MMP9 expression and DOX retention underlie these effects and which alkaloids are responsible for the anticancer activities against A549 cells. In addition, the synergistic effects of extracts with DOX in other systems remain to be confirmed.

Author Contributions: Conceptualization, A.D., B.K. and T.P.S.; methodology, A.D., B.K., I.Z.M. and A.K., investigation, A.D., B.K. and J.A.S.; resources, G.Z. and K.Š.; data curation, A.D.; writing—original draft preparation, A.D. and B.K.; writing—review and editing, R.J., K.Š. and J.A.S.; supervision, T.P.S. and J.A.S.; project administration, T.P.S. and R.J.; funding acquisition, T.P.S., R.J. and J.A.S. All authors have read and agreed to the published version of the manuscript.

Funding: This work was supported by the Ministry of Education, Science, and Technological Development of the Republic of Serbia (Grant No.451-03-68/2020-14/200026 and Grant No. 451-03-68/2020-14/200043).

References

1. Carvalho, C.; Santos, R.X.; Cardoso, S.; Correia, S.; Oliveira, P.J.; Santos, M.S.; Moreira, P.I. Doxorubicin: The Good, the Bad and the Ugly Effect. *Curr. Med. Chem.* **2009**, *16*, 3267–3285. [CrossRef] [PubMed]
2. Thorn, C.F.; Oshiro, C.; Marsh, S.; Hernandez-Boussard, T.; McLeod, H.; Klein, T.E.; Altman, R.B. Doxorubicin pathways: Pharmacodynamics and adverse effects. *Pharm. Genom.* **2011**, *21*, 440–446. [CrossRef] [PubMed]
3. Bamodu, O.A.; Huang, W.C.; Tzeng, D.T.; Wu, A.; Wang, L.S.; Yeh, C.T.; Chao., T.Y. Ovatodiolide sensitizes aggressive breast cancer cells to doxorubicin, eliminates their cancer stem cell-like phenotype, and reduces doxorubicin-associated toxicity. *Cancer Lett.* **2015**, *364*, 125–134. [CrossRef] [PubMed]
4. Zhao, X.; Zhang, J.; Tong, N.; Liao, X..; Wang, E.; Li, Z.; Luo, Y.; Zuo, H. Berberine attenuates doxorubicin-induced cardiotoxicity in mice. *J. Int. Med. Res.* **2011**, *39*, 1720–1775. [CrossRef] [PubMed]
5. Osman, A.M.; Bayoumi, H.M.; Al-Harthi, S.E.; Damanhouri, Z.A.; Elshal, M.F. Modulation of doxorubicin cytotoxicity by resveratrol in a human breast cancer cell line. *Cancer Cell Int.* **2012**, *12*, 47. [CrossRef] [PubMed]
6. He, J.M.; Mu, Q. The medicinal uses of the genus Mahonia in traditional Chinese medicine: An ethnopharmacological, phytochemical and pharmacological review. *J. Ethnopharmacol.* **2015**, *175*, 668–683. [CrossRef] [PubMed]
7. Wong, B.S.; Hsiao, Y.C.; Lin, T.W.; Chen, K.S.; Chen, P.N.; Kuo, W.H.; Hsieh, Y.S. The in vitro and in vivo apoptotic effects of *Mahonia oiwakensis* on human lung cancer cells. *Chem. Biol. Interact.* **2009**, *180*, 165–174. [CrossRef]

8. Hu, W.; Yu, L.; Wang, M.H. Antioxidant and antiproliferative properties of water extract from *Mahonia bealei* (Fort.) *Carr. leaves. Food Chem. Toxicol.* **2011**, *49*. [CrossRef]

9. Kumar, A.; Ekavali, K.; Chopra, M.; Mukherjee, R.; Pottabathini, M.; Dhull, D.K. Current knowledge and pharmacological profile of berberine: An update. *Eur. J. Pharmacol.* **2015**, *761*, 288–297. [CrossRef]

10. Zhao, T.F.; Wang, X.K.; Rimando, A.M.; Che, C.T. Folkloric medicinal plants: *Tinospora sagittata* var. *cravaniana* and *Mahonia bealei. Planta Med.* **1991**, *57*, 505–510. [CrossRef]

11. Cernáková, M.; Kost'álová, D.; Kettmann, V.; Plodová, M.; Tóth, J.; Drímal, J. Potential antimutagenic activity of berberine, a constituent of Mahonia aquifolium. *BMC Complementary Altern. Med.* **2002**, *2*, 2. [CrossRef] [PubMed]

12. Racková, L.; Májeková, M.; Kost'álová, D.; Stefek, M. Antiradical and antioxidant activities of alkaloids isolated from Mahonia aquifolium. Structural aspects. *Bioorganic Med Chem.* **2004**, *12*, 4709–4715. [CrossRef] [PubMed]

13. Kost'álová, D.; Kardosová, A.; Hajnická, V. Effect of *Mahonia aquifolium* stem bark crude extract and one of its polysaccharide components on production of IL-8. *Fitoterapia* **2001**, *72*, 802–806. [CrossRef]

14. Damjanović, A.; Zdunić, G.; Šavikin, K.; Mandić, B.; Jadranin, M.; Matić, I.Z.; Stanojković, T.P. Evaluation of the anti-cancer potential of Mahonia aquifolium extracts via apoptosis and anti-angiogenesis. *Bangladesh J. Pharmacol.* **2016**, *11*, 741–774. [CrossRef]

15. Gođevac, D.; Damjanović, A.; Stanojković, T.P.; Anđelković, B.; Zdunić, G. Identification of cytotoxic metabolites from *Mahonia aquifolium* using1H NMR-based metabolomics approach. *J. Pharm. Biomed. Anal.* **2017**, *150*, 9–14. [CrossRef] [PubMed]

16. Ihde, D.C.; Minna, J.D. Non-small cell lung cancer. Part II: Treatment. *Curr. Probl. Cancer* **1991**, *15*, 105–154. [CrossRef]

17. Borst, P.; Evers, R.; Kool, M.; Wijnholds, J. A family of drug transporters: The multidrug resistance-associated proteins. *J. Natl. Cancer Inst.* **2000**, *92*, 1295–1302. [CrossRef]

18. Salomon, J.J.; Ehrhardt, C. Nanoparticles attenuate P-glycoprotein/MDR1function in A549 human alveolar epithelial cells. *Eur. J. Pharm. Biopharm.* **2011**, *77*, 392–397. [CrossRef]

19. Lee, E.; Lim, S.J. The association of increased lung resistance protein expression with acquired etoposide resistance in human H460 lung cancer cell lines. *Arch. Pharmacal Res.* **2006**, *29*, 1018–1023. [CrossRef]

20. Meschini, S.; Marra, M.; Calcabrini, A.; Monti, E.; Gariboldi, M.; Dolfini, E.; Arancia, G. Role of the lung resistance-related protein (LRP) in the drug sensitivity of cultured tumor cells. *Toxicol. Vitr.* **2002**, *16*, 389–398. [CrossRef]

21. Chatterjee, K.; Zhang, J.; Honbo, N.; Karliner, J.S. Doxorubicin cardiomyopathy. *Cardiology* **2009**, *115*, 155–162. [CrossRef]

22. De Angelis, A.; Urbanek, K.; Cappetta, D.; Piegari, E.; Ciuffreda, L.P.; Rivellino, A.; Esposito, G.; Rossi, F.; Berrino, L. Doxorubicin cardiotoxicity and target cells: A broader perspective. *Cardio-Oncol.* **2016**, *2*, 1. [CrossRef]

23. Lipshultz, S.E.; Lipsitz, S.R.; Sallan, S.E.; Dalton, V.M.; Mone, S.M.; Gelber, R.D.; Colan, S.D. Chronic progressive cardiac dysfunction years after doxorubicin therapy for childhood acute lymphoblastic leukemia. *J. Clin. Oncol.* **2005**, *23*, 2629–2636. [CrossRef] [PubMed]

24. Xu, J.; Long, Y.; Ni, L. Anticancer effect of berberine based on experimental animal models of various cancers: A systematic review and meta-analysis. *BMC Cancer* **2019**, *19*, 589. [CrossRef] [PubMed]

25. Hou, Z.B.; Lu, K.J.; Wu, X.L.; Chen, C.; Huang, X.E.; Yin, H.T. In vitro and in vivo antitumor evaluation of berbamine for lung cancer treatment. *Asian Pac. J. Cancer Prev.* **2014**, *15*, 1767–1769. [CrossRef] [PubMed]

26. Miwa, S.; Yano, S.; Kimura, H.; Yamamoto, M.; Toneri, M.; Matsumoto, Y.; Uehara, F.; Hiroshima, Y.; Murakami, T.; Hayashi, K.; et al. Cell-cycle fate-monitoring distinguishes individual chemosensitive and chemoresistant cancer cells in drug-treated heterogeneous populations demonstrated by real-time FUCCI imaging. *Cell Cycle (Georget. Tex.)* **2014**, *14*, 621–629. [CrossRef]

27. Wlodkowic, D.; Telford, W.; Skommer, J.; Darzynkiewicz, Z. Apoptosis and beyond: Cytometry in studies of programmed cell death. *Methods Cell Biol.* **2011**, *103*, 55–98.

28. Vermes, I.; Haanen, C. Reutelingsperger. Flow cytometry of apoptotic cell death. *J. Immunol. Methods* **2000**, *243*, 167–190. [CrossRef]

29. DiPaola, R.S. To arrest or not to G(2)-M Cell-cycle arrest: Commentary re: A. K. Tyagi et al., Silibinin strongly synergizes human prostate carcinoma DU145 cells to doxorubicin-induced growth inhibition, G(2)-M arrest, and apoptosis. *Clin. Cancer Res.* **2002**, *8*, 3311–3314.

30. Tipton, J.M. Side effects of cancer chemotherapy. In *Handbook of Cancer Chemotherapy*; Skeel, R.T., Ed.; Lippincott Williams & Wilkins: Philadelphia, PA, USA, 2003; pp. 561–580.

31. Wong, H.L.; Bendayan, R.; Rauth, A.M.; Xue, H.Y.; Babakhanian, K.; Wu, X.Y. A mechanistic study of enhanced doxorubicin uptake and retention in multidrug resistant breast cancer cells using a polymer-lipid hybrid nanoparticle system. *J. Pharmacol. Exp. Ther.* **2006**, *317*, 1372–1381. [CrossRef]

32. Millenbaugh, N.J.; Wientjes, M.G.; Au, J.L. A pharmacodynamic analysis method to determine the relative importance of drug concentration and treatment time on effect. *Cancer Chemother. Pharmacol.* **2000**, *45*, 265–272. [PubMed]

33. Gonçalves, C.; Martins-Neves, S.R.; Paiva-Oliveira, D.; Oliveira, V.E.; Fontes-Ribeiro, C.; Gomes, C.M. Sensitizing osteosarcoma stem cells to doxorubicin-induced apoptosis through retention of doxorubicin and modulation of apoptotic-related proteins. *Life Sci.* **2015**, *130*, 47–56. [CrossRef] [PubMed]

34. Chen, X.; Su, Y.; Fingleton, B.; Acuff, H.; Matrisian, L.M.; Zent, R.; Pozzi, A. Increased plasma MMP9 in integrin alpha1-null mice enhances lung metastasis of colon carcinoma cells. *Int. J. Cancer* **2005**, *116*, 52–61. [CrossRef]

35. Hiraoka, N.; Allen, E.; Apel, I.J.; Gyetko, M.R.; Weiss, S.J. Matrix metalloproteinases regulate neovascularization by acting as pericellular Fibrinolysins. *Cell* **1998**, *95*, 365–377. [CrossRef]

36. Cornelius, L.A.; Nehring, L.C.; Harding, E.; Bolanowski, M.; Welgus, H.G.; Kobayashi, D.K.; Shapiro, S.D. Matrix metalloproteinases generate angiostatin: Effects on neovascularization. *J. Immunol.* **1998**, *161*, 6845–6852.

37. Sang, Q.X. Complex role of matrix metalloproteinases in angiogenesis. *Cell Res.* **1998**, *8*, 171–177. [CrossRef]

38. Hamano, Y.M.; Zeisberg, Y.H.; Sugimoto, H.J.C.; Lively, J.C.Y.; Maeshima, Y.C.; Yang, C.; Kalluri, R. Physiological levels of tumstatin, a fragment of collagen IV alpha3 chain, are generated by MMP-9 proteolysis and suppress angiogenesis via alphaV beta3 integrin. *Cancer Cell* **2003**, *3*, 589–601. [CrossRef]

39. Webb, A.H.; Gao, B.T.; Goldsmith, Z.K.; Morales-Tirado, V.M. Inhibition of MMP-2 and MMP-9 decreases cellular migration, and angiogenesis in in vitro models of retinoblastoma. *BMC Cancer* **2017**, *17*, 434. [CrossRef]

40. Park, K.S.; Kim, J.B.; Bae, J.; Park, S.Y.; Jee, H.G.; Lee, K.E.; Youn, Y.K. Berberine inhibited the growth of thyroid cancer cell lines 8505C and TPC1. *Yonsei Med. J.* **2012**, *53*, 346–351. [CrossRef]

41. Albring, K.F.; Weidemüller, J.; Mittag, S.; Weiske, J.F.; Geroni, M.C.; Lombardi, P.; Huber, O. Berberine acts as a natural inhibitor of Wnt/β-catenin signaling–identification of more active 13-arylalkyl derivatives. *Biofactors* **2013**, *39*, 652–662. [CrossRef] [PubMed]

42. Kaboli, J.; Rahmat, P.; Ismail, A.; Ling, K.H. Targets and mechanisms of berberine, a natural drug with potential to treat cancer with special focus on breast cancer. *Eur. J. Pharmacol.* **2014**, *740*, 584–595. [CrossRef] [PubMed]

43. Liu, J.; He, C.; Zhou, K.; Wang, J.; Kang, J.X. Coptis extracts enhance the anticancer effect of estrogen receptor antagonists on human breast cancer cells. *Biochem. Biophys. Res. Commun.* **2009**, *378*, 174–178. [CrossRef] [PubMed]

44. Matić, I.Z.; Aljančić, I.; Žižak, Ž.; Vajs, V.; Jadranin, M.; Milosavljević, S.; Juranić, Z.D. In vitro antitumor actions of extracts from endemic plant *Helichrysum zivojinii*. *Bmc Complementary Altern. Med.* **2013**, *13*, 36. [CrossRef] [PubMed]

45. Mosmann, T. Rapid colorimetric assay for cellular growth and survival: Application to proliferation and cytotoxicity assays. *J. Immunol. Methods* **1983**, *65*, 55–63. [CrossRef]

46. Ohno, M.; Abe, T. Rapid colorimetric assay for the quantification of leukemia inhibitory factor (LIF) and interleukin-6 (IL-6). *J. Immunol. Methods* **1991**, *145*, 199–203. [CrossRef]

47. Huang, R.Y.; Pei, L.; Liu, Q. Isobologram Analysis: A Comprehensive Review of Methodology and Current Research. *Front. Pharmacol.* **2019**, *10*, 1222. [CrossRef]

48. Forner, A.; Llovet, J.M.; Bruix, J. Hepatocellular carcinoma. *Lancet* **2012**, *379*, 1245–1255. [CrossRef]

49. Khan, M.A.; Singh, M.; Khan, M.S.; Najmi, A.K.; Ahmad, S. Caspase mediated synergistic effect of Boswellia serrata extract in combination with doxorubicin against human hepatocellularcarcinoma. *Biomed. Res. Int.* **2014**, *2014*, 294143. [CrossRef]

50. Zec, M.; Srdic-Rajic, T.; Krivokuca, A.; Jankovic, R.; Todorovic, T.; Andelkovic, K.; Radulovic, S. Novel selenosemicarbazone metal complexes exert anti-tumor effect via alternative, caspase- independent necroptotic cell death. *Med. Chem.* **2014**, *10*, 759–771. [CrossRef]

Sample Availability: Samples of the compounds are available from the authors.

Publisher's Note: MDPI stays neutral with regard to jurisdictional claims in published maps and institutional affiliations.

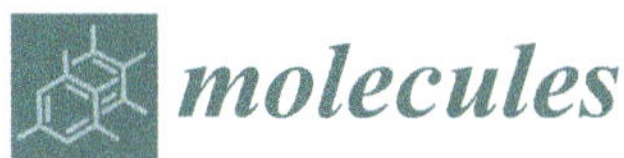 *molecules*

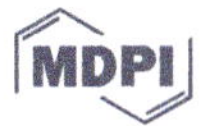

Article

Active Compound of *Pharbitis* Semen (*Pharbitis nil* Seeds) Suppressed KRAS-Driven Colorectal Cancer and Restored Muscle Cell Function during Cancer Progression

Jisu Song [1,2], Heejung Seo [1,3], Mi-Ryung Kim [1], Sang-Jae Lee [1], Sooncheol Ahn [2,*] and Minjung Song [1,4,*]

[1]   Department of Food Biotechnology, School of Medical and Life Science, Silla University, Busan 46958, Korea; jisu632@naver.com (J.S.); ssk4623@naver.com (H.S.); haha7kmr@silla.ac.kr (M.-R.K.); sans76@silla.ac.kr (S.-J.L.)
[2]   Department of Medical Science, School of Medicine, Pusan National University, Yangsan 50612, Korea
[3]   Department of Cogno-Mechatronics Engineering, College of Nanoscience & Nanotechnology, Pusan National University, Busan 46241, Korea
[4]   WT-MRC Institute of Metabolic Science, University of Cambridge, Cambridge CB20QQ, UK
*   Correspondence: ahnsc@pusan.ac.kr (S.A.); ms2700@medschl.cam.ac.uk (M.S.)

Academic Editor: Raffaele Pezzani
Received: 21 May 2020; Accepted: 18 June 2020; Published: 22 June 2020

Abstract: Kirsten rat sarcoma viral oncogene homolog (KRAS)-driven colorectal cancer (CRC) is notorious to target with drugs and has shown ineffective treatment response. The seeds of *Pharbitis nil*, also known as morning glory, have been used as traditional medicine in East Asia. We focused on whether *Pharbitis nil* seeds have a suppressive effect on mutated KRAS-driven CRC as well as reserving muscle cell functions during CRC progression. Seeds of *Pharbitis nil* (*Pharbitis* semen) were separated by chromatography and the active compound of *Pharbitis* semen (PN) was purified by HPLC. The compound PN efficiently suppressed the proliferation of mutated KRAS-driven CRC cells and their clonogenic potentials in a concentration-dependent manner. It also induced apoptosis of SW480 human colon cancer cells and cell cycle arrest at the G2/M phase. The CRC related pathways, including RAS/ERK and AKT/mTOR, were assessed and PN reduced the phosphorylation of AKT and mTOR. Furthermore, PN preserved muscle cell proliferation and myotube formation in cancer conditioned media. In summary, PN significantly suppressed mutated KRAS-driven cell growth and reserved muscle cell function. Based on the current study, PN could be considered as a promising starting point for the development of a nature-derived drug against KRAS-mutated CRC progression.

Keywords: *Pharbitis nil*; colorectal cancer; KRAS; muscle function

---

1. Introduction

Colorectal cancer (CRC) is the third most diagnosed cancer worldwide. Recent statistics showed CRC caused 832,000 deaths and nearly 1.6 million new cases were diagnosed [1]. Among the various CRCs, Kirsten rat sarcoma viral oncogene homolog (KRAS) genetic mutation driven-CRC are known to be difficult to target, and prone to drug-induced side effects [2,3]. Mutated KRAS proteins cause persistent activation of GTP, which endlessly send signals to the RAS/extracellular signal–regulated kinases (RAS/ERK) or protein kinase B/mammalian target of rapamycin (AKT/mTOR) cell regulation pathways [2]. ERK or mTOR proteins activate transcription factors involved in cell death, cell cycle progression, and transcription [2,4]. To inhibit RAS activation, antibody therapy was developed to target EGFR, such as Cetuximab, but various drug-resistance issues were documented [5–7]. Therefore, novel medicinal substances with effective anti-cancer properties are needed and plant-derived foods or medicinal plants can offer potential means.

Several natural products have exhibited anti-CRC activity. For example, Danshen (*Salvia miltiorrhiza*) improved the survival rate of patients with colorectal cancer [8]. Triterpenoids from *Rhus chinensis* Mill [9], protopine from *Nandina domestica* [10], Paris saponin VII from *Trillium tschonoskii* [11] and protein hydrolysates from Fenugreek (*Trigonella foenum graecum*) [12] suppressed the proliferation and induced apoptosis of CRC cells. Additionally, rosemary (*Rosmarinus officinalis*) inhibited CRC growth by inducing necrosis [13]. However, limited studies have examined the effects of natural extracts targeting mutated KRAS-driven CRC and none of these studies tested the efficacy of these extracts on muscle function. In our previous study, *Cordyceps militaris* germinated soybeans suppressed mutated KRAS-driven CRC via the RAS/ERK pathway [14]. *Phellinus linteus* grown on germinated brown rice increased the sensitivity of Cetuximab to inhibit KRAS-CRC progression both in vitro and in vivo [15]. Although the two natural compounds have anti-CRC activities, more medicinal substances are needed to target the notorious and drug-resistant nature of mutated KRAS-driven CRC.

Morning glory (*Pharbitis nil*) is a well-known ornamental plant, and its seeds have been used in traditional medicine to treat various cancers and inflammatory diseases in Korea, China, and Japan [16]. Recent studies have demonstrated its suppressive effects on breast cancer [17], lung cancer [18] and gastric cancer cells [19]. In addition, the seed of *Pharbitis nil* is the main constitute of the approved drug, DA-9701 (Motilitone) [20]. DA-9701 is a botanical drug for treating functional dyspepsia and composed of the seed of *Pharbitis nil* and *Corydalis* tuber. Therefore, we anticipated its safety on human and can be adapted for therapies in a relatively short timeframe if proven its efficiency. In view of its anticancer effects, we considered the active compound of *Pharbitis* semen (PN) may inhibit the proliferation and progression of mutated KRAS-driven CRC without inducing serious side effects.

In addition to the suppressive effect of PN on CRCs, we evaluated the effect of compound PN on muscle cell function. During the course of CRC, cachexia, a complex syndrome showing severe muscle weight loss, is often accompanied with CRC progression and worsened treatment therapies [21–23]. Therefore, treating cachexia becomes an important combinational therapy in the treatment of CRCs. We mimicked cancer-associated environment with conditioned media and evaluated the effect of PN on muscle cells.

In the present study, the anticancer activity of PN was investigated by examining its anti-proliferation and clonogenic features in five different CRC cell models. Cell cycle and apoptotic analyses were performed, and the changes in RAS/ERK and AKT/mTOR pathways were investigated. Finally, we assessed the effect of the compound PN on muscle cell proliferation and function.

2. Results and Discussion

2.1. PN Suppressed Colorectal Cancer Cell Progress

To investigate the anti-proliferative effects of PN on mutated KRAS-driven CRC, KRAS mutated SW480 and HCT116 cells as well as KRAS-wild type (WT) HT29 and WiDr were evaluated. Cells were treated with PN at 0, 0.1, 0.5, 1, 2, or 4 µg/mL and incubated for 48 or 72 h in triplicate. Cetuximab which has been used to treat mutated KRAS-driven CRCs was used as a control. Figure 1A summarized the proliferation profiles. PN inhibited cell growth in a concentration dependent manner in mutated KRAS-driven cell lines at 48 and 72 h. At 72 h, SW480 viability was decreased to 41.6 ± 1.0% when treated with PN at 2 µg/mL and to 26.0 ± 4.5% when treated with 4 µg/mL PN. When compared to control drug of Cetuximab, PN showed higher suppressive effect from 2 µg/mL concentration. Data also indicated that KRAS mutated cell lines responded more sensitively on PN treatment compared to KRAS wild type cells of HT-29 and WiDr. In KRAS wild type cells, PN treatment did not show statistical decrease on proliferation at 48 h. The IC_{50} values of KRAS mutated cells at 72 h are 1.74 and 2.78 µg/mL on SW480 and HCT116 cells, whereas they are 4.14 and 4.46 µg/mL on KRAS WT cells of HT29 and

WiDr cells. IC_{50} values of KRAS mutated cells are relatively low compared to other natural extract such as pogostone (HCT116: 18.7 ± 1.93 µg/mL) [24].

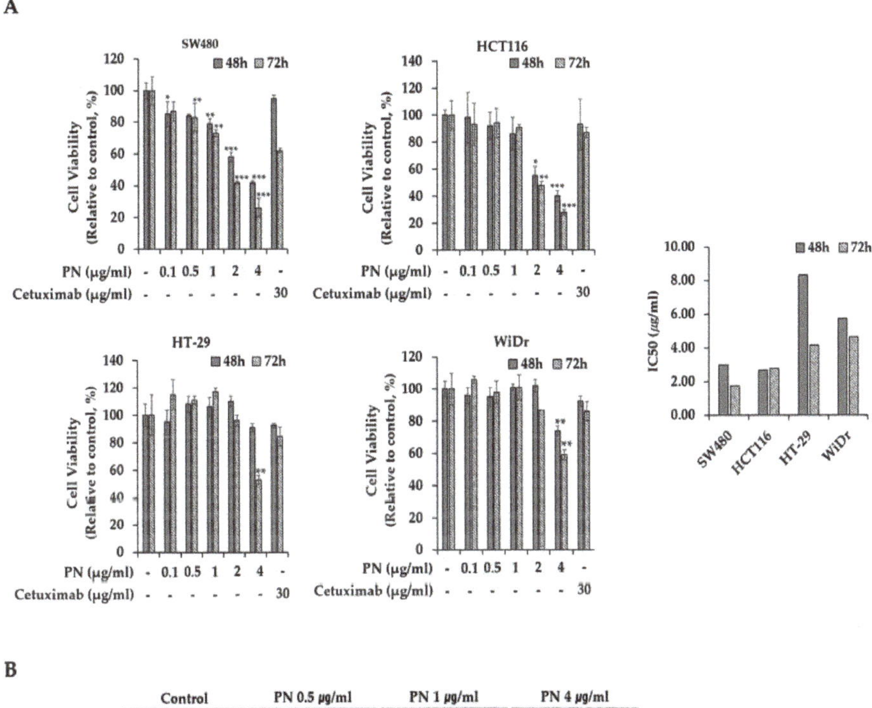

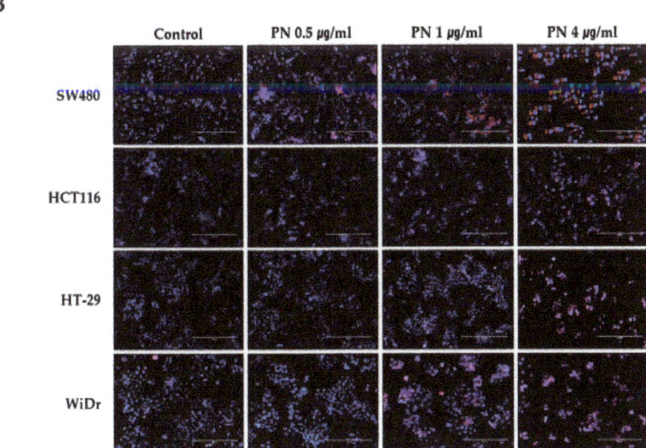

Figure 1. (**A**) PN suppressive effect on KRAS-mutated colorectal cancer cells of SW480 (KRAS[G12V]) and HCT116 (KRAS[G13D]), and KRAS-wild types CRCs of HCT116 and WiDr. Cells were treated for 48 and 72 h under PN treatment (0, 0.1, 0.5, 1, 2 and 4 µg/mL) and Cetuximab (30 µg/mL). IC_{50} values are calculated. Results are presented as means ± S.D. of three independent experiments. * $p < 0.05$, ** $p < 0.01$, *** $p < 0.001$. (**B**) Representative colorectal cancer cell images under PN treatment (0, 0.5, 1 and 4 µg/mL). Blue represents the DAPI-stained cell nuclei, and the propidium iodide-stained dead cells are red. Scale bar = 500 µm. DAPI, 4′,6-diamidino-2-phenylindole; PI, propidium iodide.

Cells were stained with DAPI and PI for live and dead cell detection. Cell nuclei were stained with DAPI (blue) which represent all cells, and dead cells were stained with PI (red). Most cells in control group were stained with DAPI and little PI staining after 48 h of cultivation indicating most cells are alive (Figure 1B). In contrast, cells treated with PN began to appear dead PI stained cells from 0.5 μg/mL.

By assessing clonogenic potentials, we evaluated if PN inhibited tumorogeneity. As shown in Figure 2, PN dose-dependently suppressed colony formation by the KRAS mutated cell lines SW480, and HCT116. For example, PN treatment at 1 μg/mL suppressed SW480 cell colony formation to 26%. Surprisingly, almost no colony formation was observed by KRAS mutated CRCs treated with 4 μg/mL of PN. In contrast, HT29 and WiDr colonies are still visible even at the highest concentration. These findings show that PN sensitively suppress proliferation rate and tumor forming abilities in the long-term aspects of mutated KRAS-driven CRC cells. Further mechanistic and molecular studies were performed with SW480 cells at PN concentrations ranging from 0.1 to 4 μg/mL.

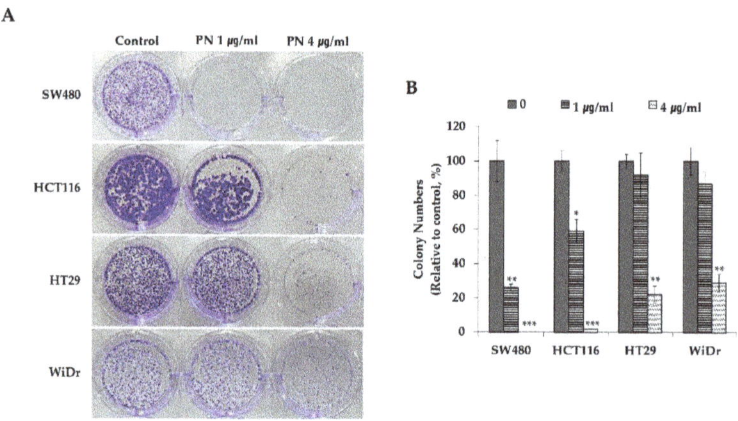

Figure 2. (**A**) Clonogenic potential after the PN treatment (0, 1 and 4 μg/mL) on KRAS-mutated colorectal cell lines of SW480 (KRAS^{G12V}) and HCT116 (KRAS^{G13D}) and KRAS-WT cells of HT29 and WiDr. (**B**) Relative colony numbers upon the PN treatment were calculated compared to the control. Results are presented as means ± S.D. of three independent experiments. * $p < 0.05$, ** $p < 0.01$, *** $p < 0.001$.

Seeds of *Pharbitis nil* contains several bioactive compounds such as polysaccharides [16], pharbitin (resin glycosides) [25], anthocyanins, diterpenoids [26], triterpene saponins [27], pharbilignan C [17], neolignane, and monoterpene glycosides [28]. Pharbilignan C has been reported to induce human breast cancer cell apoptosis via the mitochondria-medicated intrinsic pathway [17], and lignans exhibited anti-inflammatory and anti-cancer activities [29]. Thus, the observed suppressive effects of PN on CRC cell-lines may have been due to the presence of these functional compounds.

2.2. PN Induced Apoptosis and Cell Cycle Arrest in the G2/M Phase

To investigate the mechanism of cell death in mutated KRAS-driven human colorectal cell lines induced by PN, we analyzed apoptosis and cell cycles. For detecting apoptotic cells, Annexin V-FITC and PI staining was used. Annexin V binds specifically to a phosphatidylserine residue that is externalized by cells undergoing apoptosis. As seen in Figure 3, PN substantially increased the percentage of apoptotic cells in a concentration-dependent manner. Early (Annexin V FITC$^+$/PI$^-$) and late (Annexin V FITC$^+$/PI$^+$) apoptosis counts were increased up to 28.6 ± 1.4 % and 40.2 ± 2.7 % at 2 or

4 µg/mL PN treatment for 48 h, respectively. These observations suggest PN inhibits CRC proliferation by inducing apoptosis.

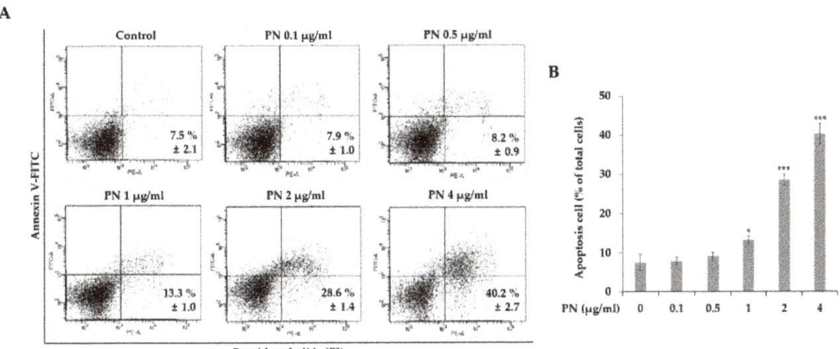

Figure 3. (**A**) Flow cytometric apoptosis images PN treatment using Annexin V-FITC/PI staining. SW480 cells were stained with Annexin V-FITC/PI upon PN treatment (0, 0.1, 0.5, 1, 2, and 4 µg/mL). (**B**) The percentage of apoptotic cells upon the PN treatment were compared. Asterisks (*) indicate statistical differences compared to untreated control (n = 3). * $p < 0.05$, ** $p < 0.01$, *** $p < 0.001$; Student's *t* test. Statistical differences among the experimental groups were confirmed via one-way ANOVA test. FITC, fluorescein isothiocyanate; PI, propidium iodide.

Cell cycle is progressed into four phases: gap1 (G1), DNA synthesis (S), gap2 (G2) and mitosis (M). Arresting cancer cells at a certain stage are often viewed as therapeutic targets [30]. The cell cycle after exposing SW480 cells at concentrations of 0.5–4 µg/mL of PN was investigated. As seen in Figure 4A, cell cycle analysis showed PN concentration-dependently induced accumulation in the G2/M phase and a concomitant reduction in the G0/G1 phase. For example, the proportions of cells in the G2/M phase after treatment with 1 or 4 µg/mL of PN were 28.5 ± 0.3% and 41.2 ± 6.7%, respectively, which demonstrated PN inhibited cell growth by arresting cells in the G2/M phase. Then, we investigated expression levels of the cdc2 and cyclin B1, which are proteins for cell cycle progression from G2/M to G0/G1. Indeed, western blot images revealed that PN concentration-dependently reduced the levels of both proteins (Figure 4B).

PN was found to arrest cells in the G2/M phase to reduce the number of cells in the G0/G1 phase (Figure 4), therefore less cells enter into mitosis. This is interesting in that most of the cell cycle arrests caused by natural extracts reported to date have occurred in the G0/G1 or G2/M stages. [21,31,32]. For example, pogostone induced G0/G1 arrest in a KRAS mutated HCT116 cell-line [24].

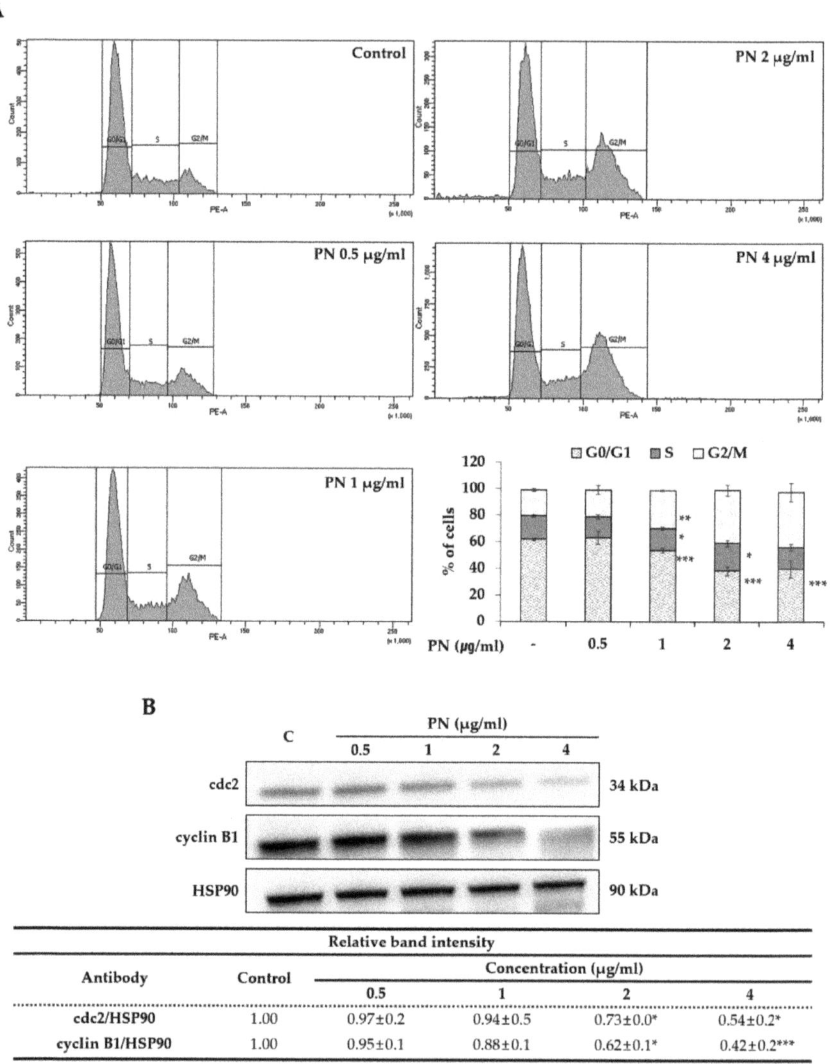

Figure 4. (**A**) Cell cycle analysis upon PN treatment (0, 0.5, 1, 2, and 4 µg/mL). Images represent the SW480 cell response under PN treatment. Percentages in each cell cycle phase (G0/G1, S, G2/M) are calculated and G2/M phase are increased as concentration dependent manner. Asterisks indicates statistical differences compared to untreated control through Student's *t*-test (* $p < 0.05$, ** $p < 0.01$, *** $p < 0.001$). (**B**) Expression of G2/M phase related proteins of cdc2 and cyclin B1 upon PN treatment. HSP90 was used as a loading control and the protein intensity was analyzed in triplicate. The ratios of cdc2/HSP90 and cyclin B1/HSP90 were calculated and analyzed by Student *t*-test * $p < 0.05$, ** $p < 0.01$, *** $p < 0.001$.

2.3. Inhibition of the AKT/mTOR Pathway Enhanced PN-Induced Cell Death

Mutated KRAS-driven CRC signals are through the ERK/MEK or AKT/mTOR pathways [3,4]. During mutated KRAS-driven CRC progression, mutant RAS constitutively activates ERK/MEK or AKT/mTOR phosphorylation, and as a result promotes cancer cell proliferation. To determine whether

SW480 growth inhibition by PN is regulated by RAS/ERK or AKT/mTOR pathways, cells are treated with PN for 48 h and protein levels of KRAS, p-ERK, p-AKT, and p-mTOR were assessed by western blot. As shown in Figure 5, PN significantly and concentration-dependently suppressed p-AKT and p-mTOR phosphorylation. For example, the expression of p-AKT was reduced to 0.31 in PN 4 μg/mL treated cells as compared with 1.0 in the non-treated control. The level of KRAS and ERK phosphorylation was similar in all groups as observed in Figure 5. These results demonstrated that PN suppressed CRC progression predominantly via the AKT/mTOR pathway. The AKT/mTOR and ERK/MEK pathways are known to be major regulatory signaling pathways that relate to CRC cell proliferation, metabolism, and survival [2,4,33]. Our observations suggest that the antitumor effect of PN is caused by reductions in the phosphorylations of AKT and mTOR.

A

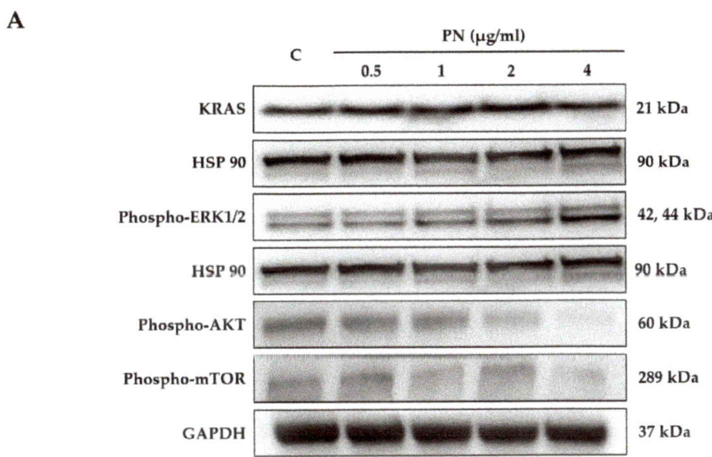

B

Antibody	Control	Relative band intensity Concentration (μg/ml)			
		0.5	1	2	4
KRAS / HSP90	1.00	1.26±0.1	1.44±0.5	1.4±0.2	1.15±0.0
Phospho-ERK1/2 / HSP90	1.00	1.00±0.0	1.12±0.5	0.95±0.6	1.31±0.5
Phospho-AKT / GAPDH	1.00	0.86±0.3	0.84±0.2**	0.56±0.0***	0.31±0.0***
Phospho-mTOR / GAPDH	1.00	0.89±0.4	0.77±0.3**	0.57±0.2*	0.57±0.2**

Figure 5. (**A**) Representative western blot images of KRAS, HSP90, phospho-p42/44 MAPK (phospho-ERK1/2), phospho-AKT, phospho-mTOR protein expression in SW480 cells treated with the compound PN (0, 0.5, 1, 2 and 4 μg/mL). (**B**) The ratios of KRAS/HSP90, phospho-ERK1/2/HSP90, and phospho-AKT/GAPDH, phospho-mTOR/GAPDH were calculated and compared to the control. (N = 3; mean SEM, * $p < 0.05$, ** $p < 0.01$, *** $p < 0.001$; Student's *t* test).

2.4. PN Restores Muscle Cell Function during Cancer Progression

During cancer progression, skeletal muscles are weakened which causes progressive functional impairment, called cachexia [21–23]. Accordingly, it is important aspects that agents targeting cancers do not adversely affect muscle cells. Thus, we examined the proliferation and function of muscle cells of myoblast, treated with different concentrations of PN (0, 0.1, 0.5, 1, 2, or 4 μg/mL) for 48 or 72 h. In Figure 6A, PN did not inhibit cell proliferation up to 2 μg/mL concentrations. After 72 h of treatment with 2 or 4 μg/mL of PN, cell viabilities remained at 97% and 61% of non-treated control levels. Next, we examined if PN affected muscle functions of myotube formation by inducing myogenic differentiation. Phenotypes were detected by myosin heavy chain (MyHC) immunostaining and fusion indices were calculated. Surprisingly, PN treatment did not inhibit myogenic differentiation as determined by MyHC staining and fusion indices (Figure 6B,C). In fact, fusion indices even improved at all PN treated groups. Our data suggest that PN has a beneficial effect on muscle cell function.

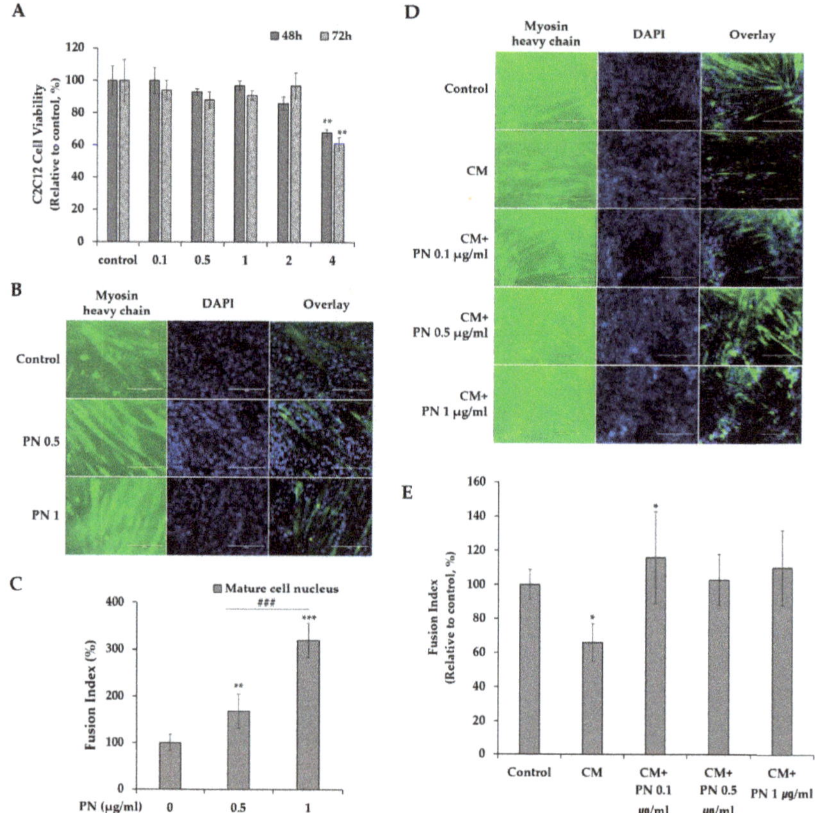

Figure 6. (**A**) C2C12 cells were treated with different PN concentrations (0, 0.1, 0.5, 1, 2 and 4 µg/mL) for 48 and 72 h. Results are presented as means ± S.D. of 3 independent experiments, * $p < 0.05$, ** $p < 0.01$, *** $p < 0.001$. (**B**) Immunofluorescence microscopy for the expression of the myogenic markers Myosin heavy Chain (MyHC) and DAPI. Myogenesis was induced in differentiation media and treated for 5 days with different PN concentration (0, 0.5 and 1 µg/mL). (**C**) Fusion indexes were calculated as the % of the nuclei inside myotubes compared to the total number of nuclei. (N= 3 independent experiments; mean SEM, * $p < 0.05$, ** $p < 0.01$, *** $p < 0.001$; Student's *t* test). Between experimental groups, statistical difference was found via one-way ANOVA (### $p < 0.001$). (**D**) Representative images of myotube formation on cancer conditioned media upon PN treatment (0, 0.1, 0.5 and 1 µg /mL). Myotube was detected with MyHC (green) immunostaining and nuclear counterstained DAPI (blue). Scale bar = 200 µm. (**E**) Fusion index were calculated as the % of the nuclei inside myotubes compared to the total number of nuclei. (Data were from three independent experiments; mean SEM, * $p < 0.05$; Student's *t* test).

Because PN did not impair and rather supported C2C12 myogenic differentiation into myotube formation, we further investigated if PN could attenuate conditioned media (CM)-mediated muscle function impairment. In Figure 6D,E, reduced myotube numbers and MyHC expression were observed on PN-untreated control, which indicated cancer environment significantly impaired muscle cell function. However, PN-treatment rescued C2C12 muscle cell dysfunctions. In detail, increased myotube formation and MyHC expression compared to the SW480 control CM were observed (Figure 6D,E).

During cancer progression, cancer-associated cachexia is common [21], and one of the problems posed by anti-cancer drugs is that they impair normal cell proliferation and function. Therefore, the maintenance of muscle cell proliferation and myogenic differentiation are important aspects at the cancer therapeutic development. Interestingly, we found PN did not impair muscle cell proliferation, but actually restored muscle cell function.

3. Materials and Methods

3.1. Preparation of PN from the Seeds of Pharbitis nil

PN was prepared as previously reported [34]. In brief, dried seeds of *Pharbitis nil* (1 kg) were ground. Then, ground *Pharbitis nil* was immersed in methanol (MeOH) at room temperature for 48 h and extracted. The MeOH extract was filtered with 5 μm filter paper and concentrated using a rotary evaporator (Tokyo Rikakikai, Tokyo, Japan). To purify compound PN, the MeOH extract (5 g) was dissolved in 50% MeOH and chromatographed on a Diaion HP-20 column by the gradient MEOH (50%, 80%, 100%, each fraction 500 mL). The 100% MeOH fraction (800 mg) was further chromatographed on reversed-phase C-18 and Sephadex LH-20 column using 100% MeOH as mobile phase, simultaneously. The 250 mg of purified compound PN was confirmed by high performance liquid chromatography (HPLC) in our previous study.

3.2. Cell Culture and Treatment

The human CRC cell-lines, SW480, HCT116, HT29 and WiDR were purchased from the American Type Culture Collection (Rockville, MD, USA). G12V KRAS mutated SW480 ($KRAS^{G12V}$), G13D KRAS mutated HCT116 ($KRAS^{G13D}$), KRAS wild types of HT29 and WiDR were cultured in RPMI-1640 supplemented with 10% fetal bovine serum (FBS; Invitrogen), and 1% penicillin-streptomycin (P/S; Sigma, St. Louis, MO, USA). C2C12 cells were purchased from ATCC and cultured in DMEM (Dulbecco's modified Eagle's medium) containing 10% FBS and 1% P/S in a 5% CO_2 atmosphere at 37 °C.

3.3. Cell Proliferation by MTS Assay

An MTS (3-(4,5-dimethylthiazol-2-yl)-5-(3-carboxymethoxyphenyl)-2-(4-sulfophenyl)-2H-tetrazolium) assay (Promega, Fitchburg, WA, USA) was used to determine the anti-proliferative effect of PN on CRC cell lines and its toxic effect on C2C12 muscle cells. For each cell line tested, 2×10^4 cells per well were seeded onto 96-well plates and allowed to attach. Cells were treated with PN at 0.1, 0.5, 1, 2, or 4 μg/mL and incubated for 48 and 72 h. Cetuximab of 30 μg/mL was added as a control. MTS solution (20 μL) was then added and cells were incubated at 37 °C for 1 h. Absorbance were measured at 490 nm (Model 550, Bio-Rad, Hercules, CA, USA). The experiments were performed in triplicate. IC_{50} values (concentrations that inhibited cell growth by 50%) were compared.

3.4. DAPI/PI Staining

Cells were treated with PN for 48 h, fixed with 4% paraformaldehyde (Sigma), washed with PBS, and stained with DAPI (4′,6-diamidino-2-phenylindole, Sigma) to detect cell nuclei and with PI (propidium iodide, Sigma) to detect dead cells in the dark. Stained cells were then observed under a fluorescence microscope (EVOS®, Thermo Scientific, Waltham, MA, USA).

3.5. Clonogenic Assay

Human CRC cell lines were seeded at 1×10^3 cell/well onto six-well plates. After cells had completely attached, they were treated with 1 or 4 μg/mL of PN, and 10 days later, fixed with

4% paraformaldehyde for 10 min, dried, and stained with 0.05% crystal violet (Sigma) for 15 min. The experiments were performed in triplicate.

3.6. Cell Apoptosis Analysis

Human CRC cells were treated with PN at 0.1, 0.5, 1, 2, or 4 µg/mL for 48 h, harvested, stained with Annexin V-FITC and PI for 15 min in the dark, according to the manufacturer's instructions (BD Biosciences, San Jose, CA, USA). Apoptotic cells were analyzed by flow cytometry (FC 500, Beckman Coulter, Indianapolis, IN, USA). The experiments were performed in triplicate.

3.7. Cell Cycle Analysis

Cell cycles were analyzed by flow cytometry in triplicate. Cells were seeded, treated with PN at 0.5, 1, 2, or 4 µg/mL for 24 h, detached, fixed in ice-cold 70% ethanol, and stained with PI solution containing RNase for 10 min in the dark. Cell cycle distributions were analyzed by flow cytometry (FC 500).

3.8. Western Blotting

Western blot analysis was performed in triplicate as previously described [14]. Cells were treated with compound PN (0.5–4 µg/mL) for 48 h and detached with trypsin-EDTA. Proteins were isolated with RIPA buffer containing protease inhibitors (Sigma) and quantified using a bicinchoninic acid (BCA) assay (Thermo Scientific). Proteins were separated in precast SDS-PAGE gels (10%, Invitrogen) and transferred to membranes using the iBlot system (Thermo Scientific). Membranes were blocked with 5% skimmed milk in Tris buffered saline (TBS) and incubated with the following primary antibodies overnight at 4 °C; cdc2, cyclin B1, HSP90, phospho-mTOR, GAPDH, KRAS, phospho-ERK1/2, and phospho-AKT. Membranes were then washed and incubated with HRP-conjugated goat anti-rabbit or anti-mouse antibodies (Pierce, Rockford, IL, USA). Densitometric analysis was performed using ImageJ software (NIH, Bethesda, MD, USA) and ratios of proteins versus the loading control were calculated.

3.9. Myogenic Differentiation

C2C12 myoblasts were seeded onto six-well plates (4×10^4 cells/well) in triplicate and cultured for 2 days in DMEM. Myogenesis was induced by culturing cells in differentiation medium (DMEM, 2% Horse serum, 1% P/S) containing PN at 0.5, 1 µg/mL for 5 days [35]. Differentiated muscle cells were immunostained for fast myosin heavy chain (f-MyHC, a marker of terminal myogenic differentiation), fixed with 4% paraformaldehyde, blocked with 5% goat serum, and incubated at room temperature with myosin 4 monoclonal antibody (MF20)-Alexa Fluor 488 (Thermo Scientific) overnight at 4 °C. The nuclei were visualized by staining with DAPI (Sigma) for 10 min. Total cell nuclei and nuclei within f-MyHC-positive myofibers in at least 15 fields of three replicate platings were counted by using ImageJ. Myotube fusion indices were calculated by expressing the number of cells expressing f-MyHC (green) as a percentage of total nuclei (DAPI, blue) [35,36].

3.10. Preparation of SW480-Conditioned Media

To prepare conditioned media, SW480 cells were cultured on the 100 mm cell culture dish with the concentration of 5×10^4 cells/seeding. After 24 h, cells were washed with 1× PBS and changed to serum-free DMEM. Upon one day of incubation, media were collected and supernatant parts were filtered through 0.2 µm syringe filter for conditioned media (CM).

3.11. C2C12 Myogenic Differentiation in Cancer Conditioned Media

To investigate the effect of PN on C2C12 myogenic differentiation under during cancer progression, conditioned media (CM) were applied as follows. First of all, C2C12 myoblasts were seeded onto six-well plates (4×10^4 cells/well) and cultured for 2 days in regular DMEM. After cells are attached, the mixture of CM and differentiation media (2% horse serum in DMEM) with the ratio of 1:3 were added and PN with the concentrations of 0.1, 0.5 and 1 µg/mL were treated.

3.12. Statistical Analysis

Results were reported as means ± standard errors of means (SEM) of experiments performed in triplicate. Comparisons among experimental groups were performed by one-way ANOVA using SPSS ver. 12.0 (SPSS, IBM, USA). *p*-values of <0.05 were deemed significant.

4. Conclusions

The results of the present study showed two beneficial effect of PN on KRAS-mutated CRC. Firstly, it significantly suppressed KRAS-mutated CRC progression. Cell proliferation and clonogenic potential were decreased at relatively low concentrations via apoptosis and G2/M phase arrest. The mechanism responsible for the effects of PN may be associated with the AKT/mTOR signaling pathway. Secondly, PN rescued muscle cells dysfunction under cancer progression. Collectively, our results provide support for the incorporation of PN into therapeutic regimens targeting mutated KRAS-driven CRC. For future research, the toxicity and efficacy of PN needs to be performed in animal studies.

Author Contributions: J.S. carried out most of the experiments and contributed data interpretation; H.S. contributed to the experimental design and performed clonogenic potential and Western blot experiments; M.-R.K. contributed to data interpretation; S.-J.L. contributed to the conception; S.A. prepared compound PN and contributed to the conception; M.S. contributed to the conception and design of the entire study and wrote the manuscript. All authors have read and agreed to the published version of the manuscript.

Funding: This research was funded by Brain Korea 21 (NRF-2016R1A1A1A05921948) and by Basic Research of the NRF (NRF-2020R1F1A1076624). The APC was funded by NRF-2020R1F1A1076624.

Acknowledgments: The authors thank to KyungA Rhu and Heebang Cho on analyzing cell images.

Conflicts of Interest: The authors have nothing to declare.

References

1. Siegel, R.L.; Miller, K.D.; Jemal, A. Cancer statistics, 2018. *CA* **2018**, *68*, 7–30. [CrossRef] [PubMed]
2. McCormick, F. KRAS as a Therapeutic Target. *Clin. Cancer Res.* **2015**, *21*, 1797–1801. [CrossRef]
3. Misale, S.; Yaeger, R.; Hobor, S.; Scala, E.; Janakiraman, M.; Liska, D.; Valtorta, E.; Schiavo, R.; Buscarino, M.; Siravergna, G.; et al. P2.08 Emergence of Kras Mutations and Acquired Resistance to Anti Egfr Therapy in Colorectal Cancer. *Ann. Oncol.* **2012**, *23*, v24. [CrossRef]
4. Lee, S.K.; Hwang, J.H.; Choi, K.Y. Interaction of the Wnt/beta-catenin and RAS-ERK pathways involving co-stabilization of both beta-catenin and RAS plays important roles in the colorectal tumorigenesis. *Adv. Biol. Regul.* **2018**, *68*, 46–54. [CrossRef] [PubMed]
5. Van Cutsem, E.; Köhne, C.-H.; Hitre, E.; Zaluski, J.; Chien, C.-R.C.; Makhson, A.; D'Haens, G.; Pinter, T.; Lim, R.; Bodoky, G.; et al. Cetuximab and Chemotherapy as Initial Treatment for Metastatic Colorectal Cancer. *N. Engl. J. Med.* **2009**, *360*, 1408–1417. [CrossRef] [PubMed]
6. Bardelli, A.; Siena, S. Molecular Mechanisms of Resistance to Cetuximab and Panitumumab in Colorectal Cancer. *J. Clin. Oncol.* **2010**, *28*, 1254–1261. [CrossRef] [PubMed]
7. Lièvre, A.; Bachet, J.-B.; Le Corre, D.; Boige, V.; Landi, B.; Emile, J.-F.; Côté, J.-F.; Tomasic, G.; Penna, C.; Ducreux, M.; et al. KRAS Mutation Status Is Predictive of Response to Cetuximab Therapy in Colorectal Cancer. *Cancer Res.* **2006**, *66*, 3992–3995. [CrossRef]
8. Lin, Y.-Y.; Lee, I.-Y.; Huang, W.-S.; Lin, Y.-S.; Kuan, F.-C.; Shu, L.-H.; Cheng, Y.-C.; Yang, Y.; Wu, C.-Y. Danshen improves survival of patients with colon cancer and dihydroisotanshinone I inhibit the proliferation of colon cancer cells via apoptosis and skp2 signaling pathway. *J. Ethnopharmacol.* **2017**, *209*, 305–316. [CrossRef]
9. Wang, G.; Wang, Y.-Z.; Yu, Y.; Wang, J.-J. Inhibitory ASIC2-mediated calcineurin/NFAT against colorectal cancer by triterpenoids extracted from Rhus chinensis Mill. *J. Ethnopharmacol.* **2019**, *235*, 255–267. [CrossRef]
10. Son, Y.; An, Y.; Jung, J.; Shin, S.; Park, I.; Gwak, J.; Ju, B.G.; Chung, Y.; Na, M.; Oh, S. Protopine isolated from Nandina domestica induces apoptosis and autophagy in colon cancer cells by stabilizing p53. *Phytotherapy Res.* **2019**, *33*, 1689–1696. [CrossRef]

11. Zhou, H.; Sun, Y.; Zheng, H.; Fan, L.; Mei, Q.; Tang, Y.; Duan, X.; Li, Y. Paris saponin VII extracted from trillium tschonoskii suppresses proliferation and induces apoptosis of human colorectal cancer cells. *J. Ethnopharmacol.* **2019**, *239*, 111903. [CrossRef]

12. Allaoui, A.; Gascón, S.; Benomar, S.; Quero, J.; De La Osada, J.; Nasri, M.; Yoldi, M.J.R.; Boualga, A. Protein Hydrolysates from Fenugreek (Trigonella foenum graecum) as Nutraceutical Molecules in Colon Cancer Treatment. *Nutrients* **2019**, *11*, 724. [CrossRef] [PubMed]

13. Pérez-Sánchez, A.; Barrajón-Catalán, E.; Ruiz-Torres, V.; Agulló-Chazarra, L.; Herranz-López, M.; Valdés, A.; Cifuentes, A.; Micol, V. Rosemary (Rosmarinus officinalis) extract causes ROS-induced necrotic cell death and inhibits tumor growth in vivo. *Sci. Rep.* **2019**, *9*, 808. [CrossRef]

14. Seo, H.; Song, J.; Kim, M.; Han, D.-W.; Park, H.-J.; Song, M. Cordyceps militaris Grown on Germinated Soybean Suppresses KRAS-Driven Colorectal Cancer by Inhibiting the RAS/ERK Pathway. *Nutrients* **2018**, *11*, 20. [CrossRef] [PubMed]

15. Park, H.-J.; Park, J.-B.; Lee, S.-J.; Song, M. Phellinus linteus Grown on Germinated Brown Rice Increases Cetuximab Sensitivity of KRAS-Mutated Colon Cancer. *Int. J. Mol. Sci.* **2017**, *18*, 1746. [CrossRef]

16. Wang, Q.; Sun, Y.; Yang, B.; Wang, Z.; Liu, Y.; Cao, Q.; Sun, X.; Kuang, H.-X. Optimization of polysaccharides extraction from seeds of Pharbitis nil and its anti-oxidant activity. *Carbohydr. Polym.* **2014**, *102*, 460–466. [CrossRef]

17. Park, Y.J.; Choi, C.-I.; Chung, H.; Kim, K.H. Pharbilignan C induces apoptosis through a mitochondria-mediated intrinsic pathway in human breast cancer cells. *Bioorganic Med. Chem. Lett.* **2016**, *26*, 4645–4649. [CrossRef] [PubMed]

18. Jung, H.J.; Kang, J.-H.; Choi, S.; Son, Y.K.; Lee, K.R.; Seong, J.K.; Kim, S.Y.; Oh, S.H. Pharbitis Nil (PN) induces apoptosis and autophagy in lung cancer cells and autophagy inhibition enhances PN-induced apoptosis. *J. Ethnopharmacol.* **2017**, *208*, 253–263. [CrossRef]

19. Ko, S.-G.; Koh, S.-H.; Jun, C.-Y.; Nam, C.-G.; Bae, H.; Shin, M.-K. Induction of Apoptosis by Saussurea lappa and Pharbitis nil on AGS Gastric Cancer Cells. *Boil. Pharm. Bull.* **2004**, *27*, 1604–1610. [CrossRef]

20. Lee, T.H.; Jung, I.C.; Kim, N.H.; Choi, S.; Lee, K.R.; Son, M.; Jin, M. Gastroprokinetic effects of DA-9701, a new prokinetic agent formulated with Pharbitis Semen and Corydalis Tuber. *Phytomedicine* **2008**, *15*, 836–843. [CrossRef]

21. Bruggeman, A.R.; Kamal, A.H.; Leblanc, T.W.; Ma, J.D.; E Baracos, V.; Roeland, E. Cancer Cachexia: Beyond Weight Loss. *J. Oncol. Pract.* **2016**, *12*, 1163–1171. [CrossRef] [PubMed]

22. De Castro, G.S.; Simoes, E.; Lima, J.D.; Ortiz-Silva, M.; Festuccia, W.T.; Tokeshi, F.; Alcântara, P.S.; Otoch, J.P.; Coletti, D.; Seelaender, M.C.L. Human Cachexia Induces Changes in Mitochondria, Autophagy and Apoptosis in the Skeletal Muscle. *Cancers* **2019**, *11*, 1264. [CrossRef]

23. Villars, F.O.; Pietra, C.; Giuliano, C.; Lutz, T.A.; Riediger, T. Oral Treatment with the Ghrelin Receptor Agonist HM01 Attenuates Cachexia in Mice Bearing Colon-26 (C26) Tumors. *Int. J. Mol. Sci.* **2017**, *18*, 986. [CrossRef] [PubMed]

24. Cao, Z.-X.; Yang, Y.-T.; Yu, S.; Li, Y.-Z.; Wang, W.-W.; Huang, J.; Xie, X.-F.; Xiong, L.; Lei, S.; Peng, C. Pogostone induces autophagy and apoptosis involving PI3K/Akt/mTOR axis in human colorectal carcinoma HCT116 cells. *J. Ethnopharmacol.* **2017**, *202*, 20–27. [CrossRef] [PubMed]

25. Ono, M.; Takigawa, A.; Mineno, T.; Yoshimitsu, H.; Nohara, T.; Ikeda, T.; Fukuda-Teramachi, E.; Noda, N.; Miyahara, K. Acylated Glycosides of Hydroxy Fatty Acid Methyl Esters Generated from the Crude Resin Glycoside (Pharbitin) of Seeds ofPharbitis nilby Treatment with Indium(III) Chloride in Methanol. *J. Nat. Prod.* **2010**, *73*, 1846–1852. [CrossRef] [PubMed]

26. Kim, K.H.; Choi, S.U.; Lee, K.R. Diterpene Glycosides from the Seeds ofPharbitis nil. *J. Nat. Prod.* **2009**, *72*, 1121–1127. [CrossRef]

27. Jung, D.Y.; Ha, H.; Lee, H.Y.; Kim, C.; Lee, J.-H.; Bae, K.; Kim, J.S.; Kang, S.S. Triterpenoid saponins from the seeds of Pharbitis nil. *Chem. Pharm. Bull.* **2008**, *56*, 203–206. [CrossRef]

28. Lee, S.; Moon, E.; Kim, K.H. Neolignan and monoterpene glycoside from the seeds of Pharbitis nil. *Phytochem. Lett.* **2017**, *20*, 98–101. [CrossRef]

29. Kim, K.H.; Woo, K.W.; Moon, E.; Choi, S.U.; Kim, S.Y.; Choi, S.Z.; Son, M.W.; Lee, K.R. Identification of Antitumor Lignans from the Seeds of Morning Glory (Pharbitis nil). *J. Agric. Food Chem.* **2014**, *62*, 7746–7752. [CrossRef]

30. Evan, G.I.; Vousden, K.H. Proliferation, cell cycle and apoptosis in cancer. *Nature* **2001**, *411*, 342–348. [CrossRef]

31. Mollah, M.L.; Park, D.K.; Park, H.J. Cordyceps militaris Grown on Germinated Soybean Induces G2/M Cell Cycle Arrest through Downregulation of Cyclin B1 and Cdc25c in Human Colon Cancer HT-29 Cells. *Evid Based Complement Altern. Med.* **2012**, *2012*, 249217. [CrossRef] [PubMed]

32. Zhang, Z.; Wang, C.Z.; Du, G.J.; Qi, L.W.; Calway, T.; He, T.C.; Du, W.; Yuan, C.S. Genistein induces G2/M cell cycle arrest and apoptosis via ATM/p53-dependent pathway in human colon cancer cells. *Int. J. Oncol.* **2013**, *43*, 289–296. [CrossRef] [PubMed]

33. Ponnurangam, S.; Standing, D.; Rangarajan, P.; Subramaniam, D. Tandutinib inhibits the Akt/mTOR signaling pathway to inhibit colon cancer growth. *Mol. Cancer Ther.* **2013**, *12*, 598–609. [CrossRef] [PubMed]

34. Choi, H.D.; Yu, S.N.; Park, S.-G.; Kim, Y.W.; Nam, H.W.; An, H.H.; Kim, S.H.; Kim, K.-Y.; Ahn, S.C. Biological Activities of Pharbitis nil and Partial Purification of Anticancer Agent from Its Extract. *J. Life Sci.* **2017**, *27*, 225–232. [CrossRef]

35. Nie, Y.; Chen, H.; Guo, C.; Yuan, Z.; Zhou, X.; Zhang, Y.; Zhang, X.; Mo, D.; Chen, Y. Palmdelphin promotes myoblast differentiation and muscle regeneration. *Sci. Rep.* **2017**, *7*, 41608. [CrossRef] [PubMed]

36. Pavlidou, T.; Rosina, M.; Fuoco, C.; Gerini, G.; Gargioli, C.; Castagnoli, L.; Cesareni, G. Regulation of myoblast differentiation by metabolic perturbations induced by metformin. *PLoS ONE* **2017**, *12*, e0182475. [CrossRef] [PubMed]

Sample Availability: Samples of the compound PN are not available from the authors.

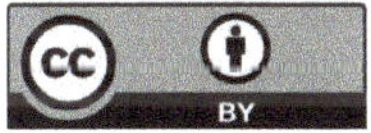

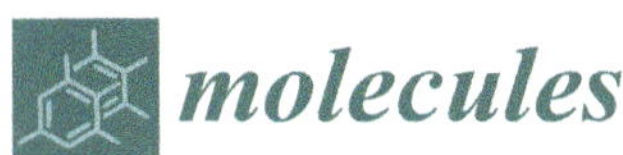 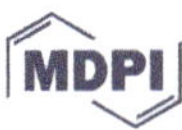

Article

Multifloroside Suppressing Proliferation and Colony Formation, Inducing S Cell Cycle Arrest, ROS Production, and Increasing MMP in Human Epidermoid Carcinoma Cell Lines A431

Xin Zhang [1,2,†], Yamei Li [1,2,†], Zhengping Feng [1,2], Yaling Zhang [1,2,*], Ye Gong [1,2], Huanhuan Song [1,2], Xiaoli Ding [1,2] and Yaping Yan [1,2,*]

[1] National Engineering Laboratory for Resource Development of Endangered Crude Drugs in Northwest of China; College of Life Science, Shaanxi Normal University, Xi'an 710062, China; zhang1xin@126.com (X.Z.); yummylee@snnu.edu.cn (Y.L.); fengzhengping@snnu.edu.cn (Z.F.); gongye@snnu.edu.cn (Y.G.); 15667085859@163.com (H.S.); dingding@snnu.edu.cn (X.D.)

[2] Key Laboratory of the Ministry of Education for Medicinal Resources and Natural Pharmaceutical Chemistry, College of Life Science, Shaanxi Normal University, Xi'an 710062, China

* Correspondence: zy114l@snnu.edu.cn (Y.Z.); yaping.yan@snnu.edu.cn (Y.Y.); Tel./Fax: +86-029-8531-0623 (Y.Y.)

† These authors contributed equally to this article.

Academic Editors: Raffaele Pezzani and Sara Vitalini

Received: 23 November 2019; Accepted: 16 December 2019; Published: 18 December 2019

Abstract: Multifloroside (**4**), together with 10-hydroxyoleoside 11-methyl ester (**1**), 10-hydroxyoleoside dimethyl ester (**2**), and 10-hydroxyligustroside (**3**), are all secoiridoids, which are naturally occurring compounds that possess a wide range of biological and pharmacological activities. However, the anti-cancer activity of **1–4** has not been evaluated yet. The objective of this work was to study the anti-cancer activities of **1–4** in the human epidermoid carcinoma cell lines A431 and the human non-small cell lung cancer (NSCLC) cell lines A549. The results indicate that **1–4** differ in potency in their ability to inhibit the proliferation of human A431 and A549 cells, and multifloroside (**4**) display the highest inhibitory activity against A431 cells. The structure-activity relationships suggest that the *o*-hydroxy-*p*-hydroxy-phenylethyl group may contribute to the anti-cancer activity against A431 cells. Multifloroside treatment can also inhibit cell colony formation, arrest the cell cycle in the S-phase, increase the levels of reactive-oxygen-species (ROS), and mitochondrial membrane potential (MMP), but it did not significantly induce cell apoptosis at low concentrations. The findings indicated that multifloroside (**4**) has the tendency to show selective anti-cancer effects in A431 cells, along with suppressing the colony formation, inducing S cell cycle arrest, ROS production, and increasing MMP.

Keywords: anti-cancer activities; multifloroside; 10-oxyderivatives of oleoside secoiridoids; structure-activity relationship; flow cytometry

---

1. Introduction

Cancer is currently the second leading cause of death globally [1–3]. While great strides have been made in the treatment of cancer in recent decades, we still face many open challenges to existing cancer therapies, such as adaptive resistance [4]. Throughout the development of human society, the importance of natural products [4–9] and their derivatives [10–12] in cancer treatment or prevention is supported by abundant evidence from cancer research [3,13,14], and give hopes to cancer patients.

The *Oleaceae* is a botanical family of woody dicotyledonous plants that are important in daily lives of many people due to their broad economic, food, and medicinal values. As previously reported, a total of 232 secoiridoids (glycosides, aglycones, derivatives, and dimers) have been isolated from species in the *Oleaceae*. Multifloroside (**4**), together with 10-hydroxyoleoside 11-methyl ester (**1**), 10-hydroxyoleoside dimethyl ester (**2**), and 10-hydroxyligustroside (**3**), are 10-oxyderivatives of oleoside secoiridoid (Figure 1), and have been isolated from many *Oleaceae* plants, such as *Osmanthus asiaticus Nakai* [15], *Jasminum lanceolarium* Roxb [16,17], *Jasminum multiflorum* extract [18], and *Jasminum elongatum* (Bergius) Willd [19] (Figure 1). These four 10-oxyderivatives of oleoside secoiridoids (**1–4**) are similar in structure, with a hydroxyl substituent at 10 position, one of substituents, such as hydroxyl, methyl, *p*-hydroxy-phenylethyl, or *o*-hydroxy-*p*-hydroxy-phenylethyl, at 7 position, and one of substituents, such as methyl or *o*-hydroxy-*p*-hydroxy-phenylethyl, at 11 position.

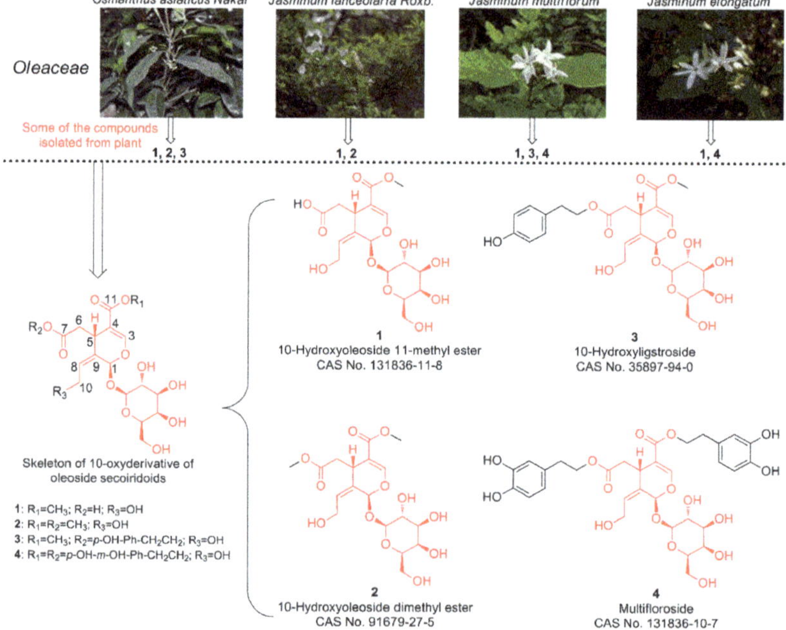

Figure 1. Chemical structures of four 10-oxyderivative of oleoside secoiridoids (**1–4**) isolated from plants in the Oleaceae family. The images of the *Oleaceae* plants were downloaded from the Chinese Field Herbarium website (http://www.cfh.ac.cn/default.html).

No previous anti-cancer studies on **1–4** have been reported. Therefore, the study was basically aimed at helping us understand in vitro anti-cancer effect of **1–4** against the human epidermoid carcinoma cell lines A431 and the non-small cell lung cancer (NSCLC) cell lines A549. The structure-activity relationships (SAR) and their effect on cell colony formation, apoptosis, cell-cycle distribution, intracellular reactive-oxygen-species (ROS) generation, and the mitochondrial membrane potential (MMP) were also demonstrated in the present study.

2. Results

2.1. Anti-Proliferative Activity of **1–4** In Vitro

The 3-(4,5-dimethylthiazol-2-yl)-2,5-diphenyltetrazolium bromide (MTT) assay [20,21] was used to evaluated the anti-proliferative activities of **1–4** against the human epidermoid carcinoma cell lines A431 and human NSCLC cell lines A549. Cells were cultured with indicated concentrations (250, 200, 100, and 25 µM) of **1–4** or the reference compound gefitinib (an epidermal growth factor receptor inhibitor) for 72 h, and living cells were detected by MTT assay. The results are shown in

Figure 2. When against A549 cells, compared with the control cells, significant growth inhibitor effect could be observed when cells were treated with 200 µM of **1**, 200, 100, and 50 µM of **3**, 250 µM of **4**, and 250, 200, 100, and 50 µM of gefitinib (Figure 2A). When against A431 cells, compared with the control cells, significant growth inhibitor effect could be observed when cells were treated by 250 µM of **1**, 200 µM of **2**, and 250, 200, 100, and 50 µM of **4** and gefitinib (Figure 2B). The results are further shown in Figure 2C and D, when A549 cells were treated with 250 µM of **4** (multifloroside) or 25 µM of gefitinib, cell viabilities decreased markedly to 30.30% and 70.85% compared with the control group, respectively ($p < 0.001$), when A431 cells were treated with 250, 200, 100, 50, and 25 µM of **4** (multifloroside) or 25 µM of gefitinib, cell viabilities decreased markedly to 7.21%, 12.44%, 70.29%, 75.87%, 84.62%, and 34.02% compared with the control group, respectively ($p < 0.001$), and the inhibitory effect was concentration-dependent. The above results suggest that **1–4** possess different anti-proliferative activities against A549 and A431 cells, and **4** (multifloroside) is the most potent agent against A431 cells.

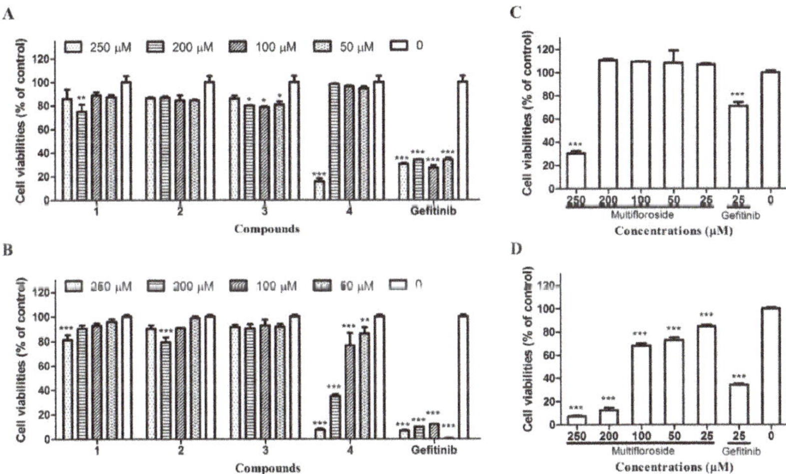

Figure 2. Anti-proliferative activity of compounds in two human cancer cell lines (A549 and A431) as determined by the MTT assay. (**A**) **1–4** against A549 cells, (**B**) **1–4** against A431 cells, (**C**) Multifloroside (**4**) against A549 cells, (**D**) Multifloroside (**4**) against A431 cells. All results are shown as the mean ± SEM ($n = 3$). * $p < 0.05$, ** $p < 0.01$, and *** $p < 0.001$ indicate significant differences compared with the control.

2.2. The Structure-Activity Relationships (SAR)

The structure-activity relationships were analyzed basing on the MTT results, and we found that, in the core structure of 10-oxyderivatives of oleoside secoiridoids, **1–4** all had a hydroxyl substituent at the 10 position and only differed at the 7 and 11 positions. **1** had a hydroxyl group at the 7 position and a methyl group at the 11 position, **2** had methyl groups at the 7 and 11 positions, and **3** had a *p*-hydroxy-phenylethyl group at the 7 position and a methyl group at the 11 position, while **4** (multifloroside) had an *o*-hydroxy-*p*-hydroxy-phenylethyl group at both the 7 and 11 positions (Figure 1), which indicated that the *o*-hydroxy-*p*-hydroxy-phenylethyl group may contribute to the anti-proliferative activity of multifloroside against A431 cells.

2.3. Multifloroside Inhibits Tumor Cell Colony Formation

Encouraged by the above results, we further investigated the bioactivity of multifloroside. First, the inhibitory effect of multifloroside on the proliferative ability of A431 cells was determined via colony formation assay. Herein, A431 cells were seeded into a 6-well cell culture plate at a density of 400 cells/well and treated with multifloroside at several concentrations (200, 100, 50, and 25 µM), gefitinib (25 µM) or 0.5% DMSO for 12 days, and then stained with crystal violet. As shown in Figure 3, multifloroside resulted in a significant suppression of cell colony formation. When the cells were incubated with multifloroside (200 and 100 µM) or gefitinib (25 µM), colony formation were completely suppressed. In addition, the cells incubated with multifloroside (50 and 25 µM) formed fewer and smaller colonies in a concentration-dependent manner compared to the control group. There were 337 viable colonies when A431 cells were treated with 0.5% DMSO, but only 183 and 76 colonies were observed when the cells were exposed to multifloroside at concentrations of 50 and 25 µM, respectively. Therefore, the plating efficiency (PE) showed a significant decrease compared to the control ($p < 0.001$). The PEs were 84%, 46%, and 24% for the control, and the 25 µM and 50 µM multifloroside treatments, respectively, and were 0 for the other groups. These results demonstrate that multifloroside inhibits the growth of A431 cells and that the inhibitory effect of multifloroside persists for a significant period of time.

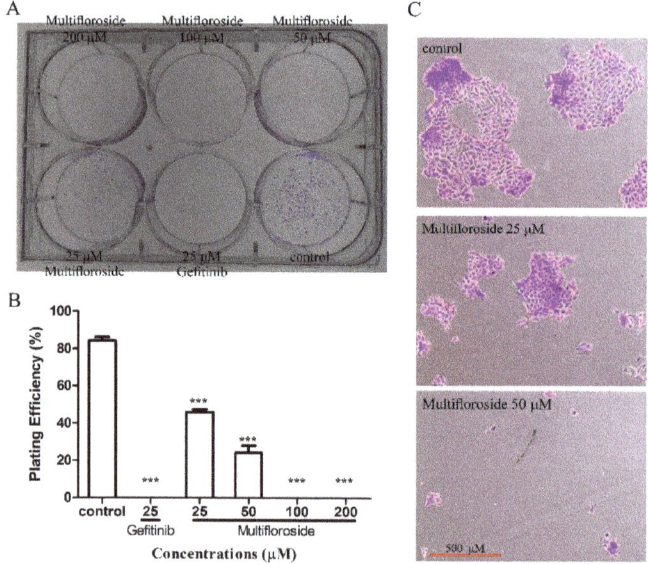

Figure 3. Colony formation of A431 cells inhibited by multifloroside. (**A**) A431 cells were incubated with the indicated concentrations of multifloroside or gefitinib and fixed with 4% paraformaldehyde and stained with 0.2% crystal violet 12 days after cell treatment. (**B**) Bar chart showing the decrease in the number of colonies after incubation with multifloroside. (**C**) Micrographs showing differences between the cell colonies. Images were taken of stained single colonies observed under a microscope. A single colony was defined to be an aggregate of >50 cells. Data are shown as mean ± SEM ($n = 3$), *** $p < 0.001$ indicates a significant difference compared with the control.

2.4. Effect of Multifloroside on Cell Apoptosis in A431 Cells

After treatment with multifloroside for 48 h, apoptosis of A431 cells was measured by flow cytometry using annexin V-FITC and PI labeling. As shown in Figure 4, 96.30% of A431 cells were in their normal state in the untreated control groups. When cells were treated with multifloroside (200 µM) or gefitinib (25 µM), the numbers of early apoptotic cells were significantly higher than in the control groups ($p < 0.001$). However, there were no significant differences in the numbers of early apoptotic cells when cells exposed to lower concentrations of multifloroside (25, 50 and 100 µM). In addition, there were no significant differences in the numbers of late apoptotic cells and necrotic cells when cells were treated with multifloroside at 25, 50, 100, and 200 µM and gefitinib at 25 µM. These results indicate not only that early apoptosis of A431 cells was not significantly influenced by treatment with low concentrations of multifloroside but also that late apoptosis was not significantly affected by multifloroside at the tested concentrations (25–200 μM).

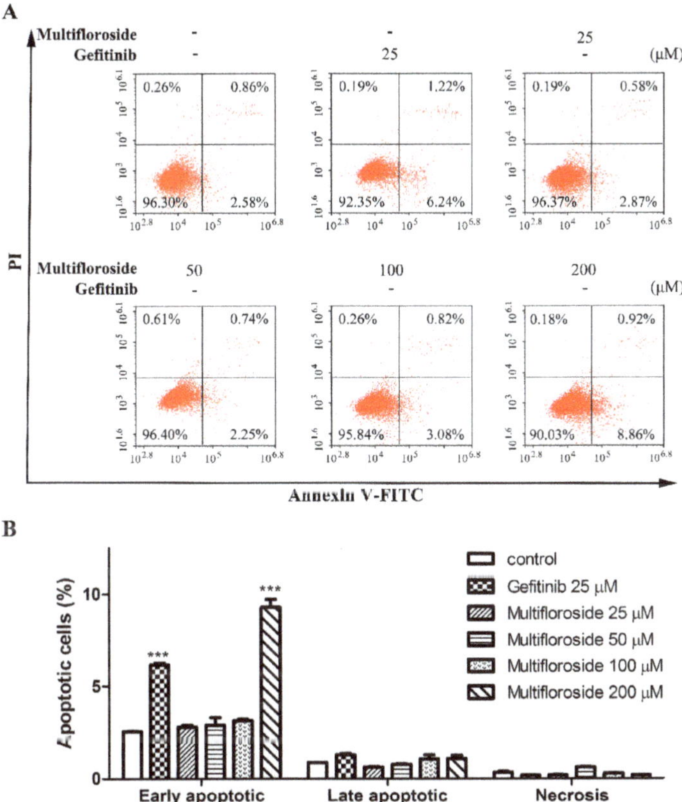

Figure 4. Effect of multifloroside on cell apoptosis in A431 cells. (**A**) Representative histograms of apoptosis in the cells treated with multifloroside for 48 h, (**B**) Percentages of apoptotic cells in each group from (**A**). All values are expressed as mean ± SEM (n = 3). *** p < 0.001 indicates a significant differences compared with the control at the same group.

2.5. S-Phase Cell Cycle Arrest Induced by Multifloroside

In order to study the relationship between the anti-proliferative activity of multifloroside and cell cycle arrest, A431 cells were treated with multifloroside or gefitinib for 48 h, after which the cells were stained with PI and examined using flow cytometry. As shown in Figure 5, when cells were treated with multifloroside at four different concentrations (25, 50, 100 and 200 μM), the number of A431 cells in S phase were significantly increased (p < 0.001), from 28.55% to 31.78%, 49.29%, and 55.30%, respectively, accompanied by a decrease in the number of cells in G0/G1 and G2/M. In the gefitinib (25 μM) treated cells, the percentage of cells in G0/G1, S, and G2/M were 77.54%, 16.17%, and 6.29%, respectively. These results indicate, unlike gefitinib which arrests the A431 cells in the G0/G1-phase, multifloroside can arrest the cell cycle of A431 cells in the S-phase and showed concentration-dependent activity.

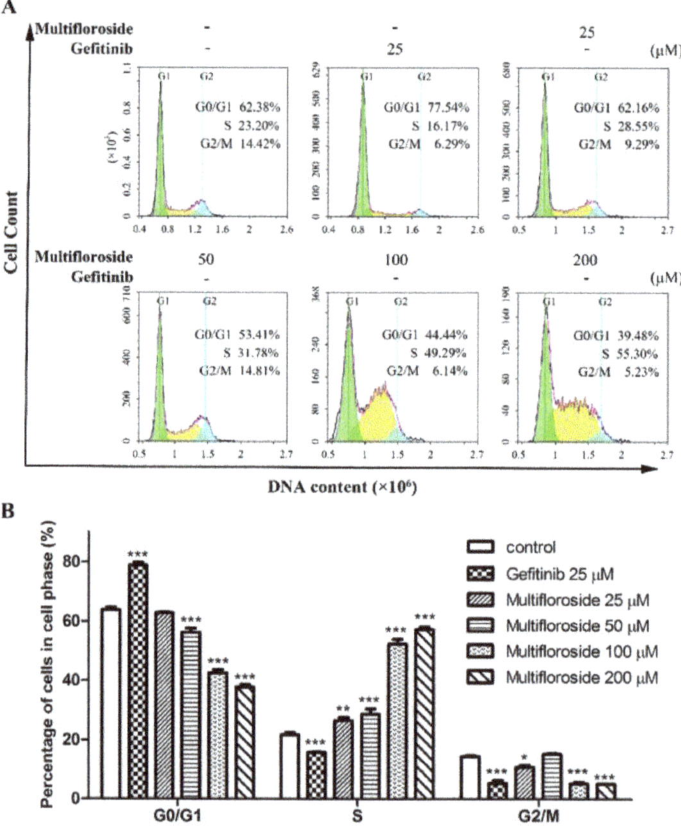

Figure 5. Effect of multifloroside on the cell cycle phase distribution in A431 cells. (**A**) Representative histograms of DNA content in the cells treated with multifloroside for 48 h, and (**B**) percentages of cell populations in the G0/G1, S and G2/M phases from (**A**). All values are expressed as mean ± SEM (n = 3). * $p < 0.05$, ** $p < 0.01$, and *** $p < 0.001$ indicate significant differences compared with the control at the same phase.

2.6. Intracellular ROS Production Induced by Multifloroside

Intracellular ROS generation was evaluated via MitoSox red reagent staining and flow cytometry analysis. As shown in Figure 6, treatment with gefitinib (25 μM) significantly increased the fluorescence intensity ($p < 0.001$), and treatment with multifloroside at high concentrations (50 and 100 μM) also significantly increased the fluorescence intensity ($p < 0.001$) in a dose-dependent manner. Treatment with multifloroside at a low concentration (25 μM) also increased the fluorescence intensity, but the difference was not statistically significant ($p > 0.05$). These results indicate that ROS production can be induced by multifloroside at the tested concentrations.

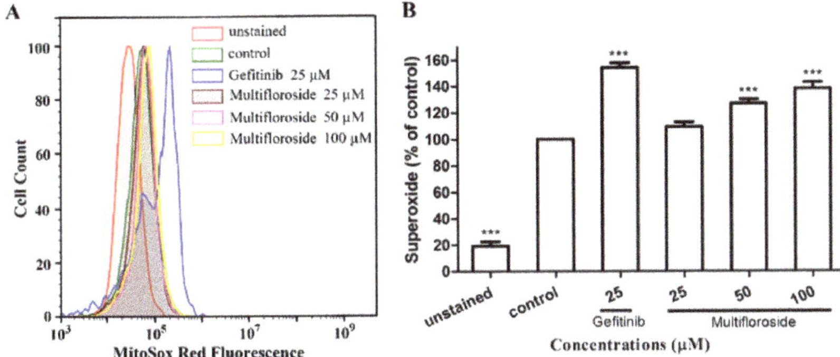

Figure 6. Effect of multifloroside on ROS production. A431 cells were treated with different concentrations of multifloroside for 48 h, then MitoSox red reagent (5 µM) was loaded and the cells were analyzed by flow cytometry for the quantification of multifloroside-induced oxidative stress in A431 cells. The fluorescence intensity of MitoSox Red reagent in cells was obtained by FACS (**A**) and the data was analyzed using GraphPad Prism 5 (**B**). The values are presented as mean ± SEM ($n = 3$). *** $p < 0.001$ indicates a significant differences compared with the control.

2.7. Effect of Multifloroside on the MMP

MMP of A431 cells stained with JC-10 was assayed by flow cytometry. As shown in Figure 7, the JC-10 fluorescence ratio (% of J-aggregates with Red Fluorescence divided by the % of J-monomers with Green Fluorescence) decreased but was not significantly different ($p > 0.05$) when cells were treated with gefitinib (25 µM), while the ratios increased when cells were treated with multifloroside (25, 50, and 100 µM). Moreover, the differences in the JC-10 fluorescence ratios were not significant when cells were treated with multifloroside at 25 and 100 µM, and they were significant when cells were treated with 50 µM multifloroside ($p < 0.01$). The above results indicate the MMP did not decrease, but rather increased, with multifloroside treatment

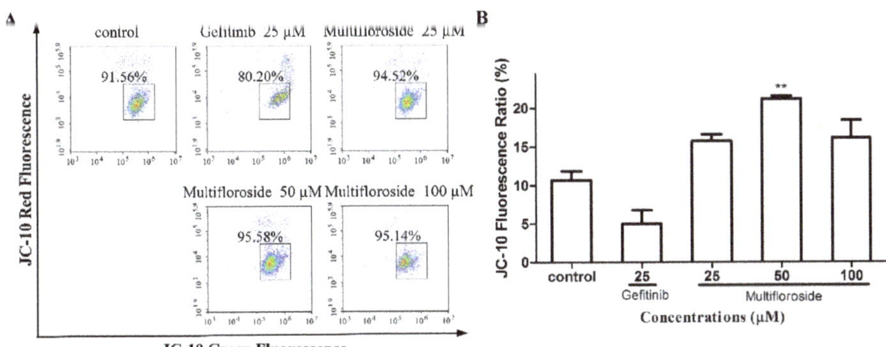

Figure 7. Effect of multifloroside on the MMP of A431 cells. A431 cells were treated with different concentrations of multifloroside for 48 h and analyzed by flow cytometry after JC-10 staining. The fluorescent intensity of JC-10 in cells was obtained by FACS (**A**) and the data was analyzed by GraphPad Prism 5 (**B**). The percentage of cells with JC-10 red fluorescence is indicated. JC-10 fluorescence ratio (%) equals the red/green fluorescence intensity ratio. The values are presented as mean ± SEM ($n = 3$). ** $p < 0.01$ indicates a significant differences compared with the control.

3. Discussion

Cancer incidence and mortality are rising rapidly worldwide. Throughout the development of human society, nature has catered to the basic needs of humans, not the least of which is the provision of medicines for the treatment of a wide spectrum of diseases [22,23]. There is growing evidence that specific bioactive compounds present in plants used as spices, fruits, vegetables, and nuts can be effective against some cancers. Secoiridoids, isolated from *Oleaceae* family, which are now widely used in the fields of food and medicine, have been extensively investigated in recent years and have been shown to possess a variety of pharmacological effects [24–29], such as anti-diabetic [30,31], anti-oxidant [32,33], anti-inflammatory [34–36], immunosuppressive [37], neuroprotective [36,38,39], and anti-cancer [1,40–42]. Multifloroside (**4**), together with 10-hydroxyoleoside 11-methyl ester (**1**), 10-hydroxyoleoside dimethyl ester (**2**), and 10-hydroxyligustroside (**3**), are all 10-oxyderivatives of oleoside secoiridoids.

1–3, together with other eight secoiridoid glycosides, were isolated from the bark of *Osmanthus asiaticus Nakai in 1993* [15]; **2** was isolated from *Jasminum lanceolarium* Roxb in 1997 and 2007 [16,17]; **1** was also isolated from *Jasminum lanceolarium* Roxb in 2007 [16]; **1**, **3**, and **4** were isolated from the water soluble fraction of *Jasminum multiflorum* extract [18]; **1** and **4**, with the other 11 types of iridoid glycosides and 15 other compounds, were identified by UPLC-MS in extracts of *Jasminum elongatum* (Bergius) Willd in 2016 [19]. However, by now, only **1** and **4** have been found to possess coronary dilating and cardiotropic activities [18]. Therefore, we aimed to investigate the in vitro anti-cancer activities of **1–4** in this study. Cancer is characterized by uncontrolled cell growth, invasiveness, and formation of metastasis, and the cells of most of malignant tumors are proliferate intensively [14]. Thus, we first evaluated the anti-proliferative activities of **1–4** against A431 human epidermoid carcinoma cells and A549 human NSCLC cells. The results showed that **1–4** possess different anti-proliferative activities against A549 and A431 cells, and that **4** (multifloroside) had the most potent inhibitory activity against A431 cells (Figure 2). As reported, it appears that the best way to prevent cancer is through rational dietary habits and behaviors, and consumption of sufficient amounts of antioxidants and bioactive plant-derived compounds that demonstrate protective effects against carcinogenesis in pre-clinical and clinical studies [43], **4** (multifloroside) and its derivatives may be the way to prevent epidermoid carcinoma cancer. The SAR were analyzed, and we found that the *o*-hydroxy-*p*-hydroxy-phenylethyl group may contribute to the anti-proliferative activity of multifloroside against A431 cells. In a future study, it may be advantageous to study other oleoside secoiridoids with *o*-hydroxy-*p*-hydroxy-phenylethyl substituents in order to identify the most potent compounds in the *Oleaceae* that can protect against the epidermoid carcinomas.

Second, a colony formation assay was performed to detect the inhibitory effect of multifloroside on the proliferative ability of A431 cells. The assay is now widely used to examine the effect of agents with potential clinical applications [44], and it shows the ability of a cancer cell to produce a viable colony after drug treatment; thus, the results obtained may help to predict the efficacy of agents in vivo [45]. Similarly to other reported plant anti-cancer molecules and their derivatives, such as panaxatriol [46], cycloartenol [47], and oridonin derivatives [48], the number and the size of tumor cell colonies were significantly decreased when A431 cell were treated by 200, 100, 50, and 25 μM multifloroside (Figure 3). These results all illustrate that multifloroside can significantly inhibit the growth of A431 cells, which is consistent with the results of MTT assay.

As reported, most of malignant tumors whose cells proliferate intensively, represent very dynamic structures that create numerous mutations resulting in new tumor cell lines with different genotypes and phenotypes within the tumor mass. In such malignancies, a highly variable sensitivity to therapeutics can be observed, and some of cell lines develop resistance to the treatment [14,49]. Therefore, the biological effects of combining various plant molecules (phytochemicals) with proven cytotoxic effects administered together with conventional therapy to target a markedly wider range of signaling pathways in cancer cells should be superior compared to single compound in cancer treatment and thus may delay the development of drug resistance in cancer [43]. So, further urgent research is needed for the identification of new molecules (including plant-derived compounds) with well-validated anticancer properties within combinational clinical approach in oncology. Further studies were then done to elucidate the mechanism of action of multifloroside on A431 cells. In general, drug-induced apoptosis is one major mechanism of action for the treatment of cancer, and various signaling pathways are involved in the process [50]. However, the apoptotic assay suggested multifloroside at high concentration (200 µM) induced cell apoptosis but that at lower concentrations (100, 50, and 25 µM) could not (Figure 4). Cell cycle regulating is a key method in controlling tumor propagation [50]. As reported, most antitumor compounds inhibit cell proliferation by inducing cell cycle arrest [48]. Cell-cycle analyses indicated the cell-cycle distribution was significantly changed, and was also different from that resulting from gefitinib, where the cells were arrested in the G0/G1-phase, multifloroside-treated cells were arrested cells in the S-phase (Figure 5). Mitochondria are the main source of cellular ROS, which have a double-edged sword role in cytotoxicity in cancer cells [51,52]. Herein, ROS levels were significantly increased after cells were treated with multifloroside at 50 and 100 µM for 48 h (Figure 6). Similarly, the MMP was increased when cells were treated with multifloroside at the tested concentrations compared with the control group (Figure 7). JC-10 forms "J-aggregates" displaying red fluorescence in healthy cells, in contrast, as the membrane potential decreases, JC-10 monomers are generated, resulting in a shift to green fluorescence [52]. These results all suggest that multifloroside may exert its anti-cancer effect through cell-cycle arrest and an increase in the ROS and MMP in A431 cells. The above gives a well-validated anticancer properties for multifloroside and suggests multifloroside may be the potential one in applying to anti-epidermoid carcinoma cancer.

4. Methods

4.1. Chemicals and Other Reagents

10-hydroxyoleoside 11-methyl ester (**1**, $C_{17}H_{24}O_{12}$, CAS No. 131836-11-8, MW 420.37, purity 98%), 10-hydroxyoleoside dimethyl ester (**2**, $C_{18}H_{26}O_{12}$, CAS No. 91679-27-5, MW 434.39, purity 98%), 10 hydroxyligustroside (**3**, $C_{25}H_{32}O_{13}$, CAS No. 35897-94-0, MW 540.51, purity 97%) and multifloroside (**4**, $C_{32}H_{38}O_{16}$, CAS No. 131836-10-7, MW 678.64, purity 98%) (Figure 1) were purchased from BioBioPha Co., Ltd. (Kunming, China). MTT was from Merck Millipore. The Annexin V-FITC/PI double staining apoptosis assay kit and Cell Cycle Detection Kit were from KeyGEN Bio Tech (Nanjing, China). MitoSox Red mitochondrial superoxide indicator was obtained from Thermo Fisher (Shanghai, China). The JC-10 Mitochondrial Membrane Potential Assay Kit was from Mybiotech, (Xi'an, China). Dulbecco's Modified Eagle's Medium (DMEM) and fetal bovine serum (FBS) were purchased from Gibco (Carlsbad, California, USA). Trypsin, penicillin, streptomycin and L-glutamate were purchased from MP Biomedicals, LLC (Santa Ana, CA, USA). All other chemicals used in this work were analytical grade and were purchased from local commercial suppliers and used without further purification unless otherwise noted.

4.2. Chemicals and Other Reagents

Human epidermoid carcinoma cell lines A431 and human NSCLC cell lines A549 were purchased from the Cell Bank of the Chinese Academy of Sciences (Shanghai, China). Cells were maintained in 60 mm cell culture dishes and cultured using DMEM supplemented with 10% FBS, 100 units/mL penicillin, 100 µg/mL streptomycin, and 2 mM L-glutamate at 37 °C in a 5% CO_2 atmosphere with 95% humidity.

4.3. MTT Assay for In Vitro Anti-Proliferative Activity

The effect of compounds on cell proliferation was determined using the MTT assay, which is one of the most versatile and popular assays to assess the rate of cell proliferation caused by drugs and cytotoxic agents [53]. The assays were performed as previously described [52,54,55].

4.4. Colony Formation Assay

Cell colony formation assay was performed according to the reference methods [45,48]. Firstly, cells were digested, harvested, and suspended using DMEM medium, and 400 cells/well were seeded into 6-well cell culture plates and incubated with multifloroside (25-200 μM) or gefitinib (25 μM) for 12 days, until the cells in the control dishes had formed visible colonies. Then the colonies were washed three times with PBS and fixed with 4% paraformaldehyde for 20 min. All cells were stained with 0.2% crystal violet for 20 min. The stained colonies were counted and compared with the control samples. The medium was changed every three days.

4.5. Cell Apoptosis Analysis

Following treatment with different concentrations of multifloroside for 48 h, the apoptosis of A431 cells was measured using the Annexin V-FITC/PI apoptosis detection kit according to the manufacturer's instructions. Apoptosis of the treated cells was then detected by flow cytometry (ACEA NovoCyte™, ACEA Biosciences, San Diego, CA, USA).

4.6. Cell Cycle Analysis

Following treatment with different concentrations of multifloroside for 48 h, the distribution of cell cycle was measured using the cell cycle detection kit according to the manufacturer's instructions. The cell cycle of the treated cells was then detected by flow cytometry to quantify the amount of DNA in each cell (ACEA NovoCyte™, ACEA Biosciences, San Diego, CA, USA).

4.7. Detection of Intracellular ROS

Intracellular ROS production was examined using MitoSox Red mitochondrial superoxide indicator according to the manufacturer's protocol and following our previously described method [52]. In brief, 24 h after plating the cells, the culture medium was replaced with fresh medium containing various concentrations of multifloroside (25-100 μM) or gefitinib (25 μM). After incubation for 48 h, cells were trypsinized, washed, and stained with MitoSox. Next, cells were washed, centrifuged to remove the supernatant, and resuspended in HBSS. Finally, ROS production in the cells was immediately monitored by flow cytometry (ACEA NovoCyte™, ACEA Biosciences, San Diego, CA, USA).

4.8. Mitochondrial Membrane Potential (MMP) Assay

MMP was analyzed using the JC-10 Mitochondrial Membrane Potential Assay Kit according to the manufacturer's instructions and following our previously described protocol [52]. In brief, 24 h after plating the cells, the culture medium was replaced with fresh medium containing various concentrations of multifloroside (25-100 μM) or gefitinib (25 μM). After incubation for 48 h, cells were trypsinized, washed, and stained with JC-10 dye. Next, cells were washed, centrifuged to remove the supernatant, and resuspended in PBS. Finally, the red/green fluorescence was detected by flow cytometry (ACEA NovoCyte™, ACEA Biosciences, San Diego, CA, USA).

4.9. Statistical Analysis

All measurements were made in triplicate, and all data are expressed as means ± SEM of three independent experiments. The significant differences from the respective control for each experimental group were examined by one-way analysis of variance (ANOVA) using GraphPad Prism 5 software. A value of $p < 0.05$ was considered to be statistically significant, and values of $p < 0.01$ or $p < 0.001$ indicated extremely significant differences.

5. Conclusions

In summary, multifloroside (**4**), together with other three 10-oxyderivatives of oleoside secoiridoids (**1–3**), were evaluated for their anti-cancer activities in *vitro*. These four compounds differ in their inhibition potency against human cancer cell lines A431 and A549, and interestingly, only multifloroside exhibited the most potent inhibitory activity against A431 cells. Further studies on multifloroside suggest that it can inhibit cell colony formation, arrest the cell cycle in the S-phase, and increase the level of ROS and MMP but cannot exert significant changes in cell apoptosis. These findings can help us understand the structure-activity relationships behind the tumor-inhibitory effect of **1–4** against the two tumor cell lines and have important implications for the potential use of multifloroside in the treatment of human epidermoid carcinoma. In a subsequent study, we will identify and design novel derivatives of multifloroside, investigate their activities in vitro and in vivo, and provide additional information on the ability of these compounds to protect against epidermoid carcinoma cancer.

Author Contributions: Y.Z. and Y.Y. designed the experiments. X.Z. and Y.L. conducted the experiments. X.Z., Z.F. and Y.Z. drafted the manuscript. Z.F., Y.G. and H.S. helped to conduct some experiments. X.D. conducted some of the data analysis and assisted in figures making. Y.Y. contributed to the discussion section and revised the manuscript. All authors have read and agreed to the published version of the manuscript.

Funding: This work was supported by grants from the National Natural Science Foundation of China (81571596, 81601044 and 81771279), the Fundamental Research Funds for the Central Universities (GK201906010, GK201701009 and GK201603110), and the Postdoctoral Science Foundation of Shaanxi Normal University.

Conflicts of Interest: The authors declare no conflict of interests.

References

1. Celano, M.; Maggisano, V.; Lepore, S.M.; Russo, D.; Bulotta, S. Secoiridoids of olive and derivatives as potential coadjuvant drugs in cancer: A critical analysis of experimental studies. *Pharmacol. Res.* **2019**, *142*, 77–86. [CrossRef] [PubMed]

2. Zhang, Q.Y.; Wang, F.X.; Jia, K.K.; Kong, L.D. Natural Product Interventions for Chemotherapy and Radiotherapy-Induced Side Effects. *Front. Pharmacol.* **2018**, *9*, 1253. [CrossRef] [PubMed]

3. Das, B.; Satyalakshmi, G. Natural products based anticancer agents. *Mini-Rev. Org. Chem.* **2012**, *9*, 169–177. [CrossRef]

4. Chamberlin, S.R.; Blucher, A.; Wu, G.; Shinto, L.; Choonoo, G.; Kulesz-Martin, M.; McWeeney, S. Natural Product Target Network Reveals Potential for Cancer Combination Therapies. *Front. Pharmacol.* **2019**, *10*, 557. [CrossRef] [PubMed]

5. Yuan, T.; Ling, F.; Wang, Y.; Teng, Y. A natural product atalantraflavone inhibits non-small cell lung cancer progression via destabilizing Twist1. *Fitoterapia* **2019**, *137*, 104275. [CrossRef]

6. Xu, X.; Peng, W.; Liu, C.; Li, S.; Lei, J.; Wang, Z.; Kong, L.; Han, C. Flavone-based natural product agents as new lysine-specific demethylase 1 inhibitors exhibiting cytotoxicity against breast cancer cells in vitro. *Bioorg. Med. Chem.* **2019**, *27*, 370–374. [CrossRef]

7. Huang, P.; Sun, L.Y.; Zhang, Y.Q. A Hopeful Natural Product, Pristimerin, Induces Apoptosis, Cell Cycle Arrest, and Autophagy in Esophageal Cancer Cells. *Anal. Cell Pathol. (Amst)* **2019**, *2019*, 6127169. [CrossRef]

8. Guzman, E.A.; Pitts, T.P.; Diaz, M.C.; Wright, A.E. The marine natural product Scalarin inhibits the receptor for advanced glycation end products (RAGE) and autophagy in the PANC-1 and MIA PaCa-2 pancreatic cancer cell lines. *Investig. New Drugs* **2019**, *37*, 262–270. [CrossRef]

9. Rakariyatham, K.; Yang, X.; Gao, Z.; Song, M.; Han, Y.; Chen, X.; Xiao, H. Synergistic chemopreventive effect of allyl isothiocyanate and sulforaphane on non-small cell lung carcinoma cells. *Food Funct.* **2019**, *10*, 893–902. [CrossRef]

10. Liang, J.W.; Wang, M.Y.; Wang, S.; Li, X.Y.; Meng, F.H. Fragment-Based Structural Optimization of a Natural Product Itampolin A as a p38alpha Inhibitor for Lung Cancer. *Mar. Drugs* **2019**, *17*, 53. [CrossRef]

11. Cowan, J.; Shadab, M.; Nadkarni, D.H.; Kc, K.; Velu, S.E.; Yusuf, N. A Novel Marine Natural Product Derived Pyrroloiminoquinone with Potent Activity against Skin Cancer Cells. *Mar. Drugs* **2019**, *17*, 443. [CrossRef] [PubMed]

12. Okayama, M.; Kitabatake, S.; Sato, M.; Fujimori, K.; Ichikawa, D.; Matsushita, M.; Suto, Y.; Iwasaki, G.; Yamada, T.; Kiuchi, F.; et al. A novel derivative (GTN024) from a natural product, komaroviquinone, induced the apoptosis of high-risk myeloma cells via reactive oxygen production and ER stress. *Biochem. Biophys. Res. Commun.* **2018**, *505*, 787–793. [CrossRef] [PubMed]

13. Park, M.N.; Song, H.S.; Kim, M.; Lee, M.J.; Cho, W.; Lee, H.J.; Hwang, C.H.; Kim, S.; Hwang, Y.; Kang, B.; et al. Review of Natural Product-Derived Compounds as Potent Antiglioblastoma Drugs. *Biomed. Res. Int.* **2017**, *2017*, 8139848. [CrossRef] [PubMed]

14. Liskova, A.; Kubatka, P.; Samec, M.; Zubor, P.; Mlyncek, M.; Bielik, T.; Samuel, S.M.; Zulli, A.; Kwon, T.K.; Busselberg, D. Dietary Phytochemicals Targeting Cancer Stem Cells. *Molecules* **2019**, *24*, 899. [CrossRef]

15. Sugiyama, M.; Machida, K.; Matsuda, N.; Kikuchi, M. A secoiridoid glycoside from Osmanthus asiaticus. *Phytochemistry* **1993**, *34*, 1169–1170. [CrossRef]

16. Sun, J. Studies on the Chemical Constituents of Jasminum lanceolarium and Lobelia sessilifolia, Dissertation Institute of Medicinal Plant Development. Ph.D. Thesis, Peking Union Medical College & Chinese Academy of Medical Sciences, Beijing, China, 2007.

17. Shen, Y.-C.; Lin, S.-L.; Chein, C.-C. Three secoiridoid glucosides from Jasminum lanceolarium. *Phytochemistry* **1997**, *44*, 891–895. [CrossRef]

18. Shen, Y.C.; Lin, C.Y.; Chen, C.H. Secoiridoid glycosides from Jasminum multiflorum. *Phytochemistry* **1990**, *29*, 2905–2912. [CrossRef]

19. Wang, F.; Han, L.; Song, Y. UPLC/Q-TOF-MS based rapid analysis and identification of chemical composition of Jasminum elongatum (Bergius) Willd. *Guangdong Yaoxueyuan Xuebao* **2016**, *32*, 55–60.

20. Kong, L.Y.; Xue, M.; Zhang, Q.C.; Su, C.F. In vivo and in vitro effects of microRNA-27a on proliferation, migration and invasion of breast cancer cells through targeting of SFRP1 gene via Wnt/beta-catenin signaling pathway. *Oncotarget* **2017**, *8*, 15507–15519. [CrossRef]

21. Zhang, Y.; Chen, L.; Xu, H.; Li, X.; Zhao, L.; Wang, W.; Li, B.; Zhang, X. 6,7-Dimorpholinoalkoxy quinazoline derivatives as potent EGFR inhibitors with enhanced antiproliferative activities against tumor cells. *Eur. J. Med. Chem.* **2018**, *147*, 77–89. [CrossRef]

22. Cragg, G.M.; Grothaus, P.G.; Newman, D.J. Impact of natural products on developing new anti-cancer agents. *Chem. Rev.* **2009**, *109*, 3012–3043. [CrossRef] [PubMed]

23. Nepali, K.; Sharma, S.; Ojha, R.; Dhar, K.L. Vasicine and structurally related quinazolines. *Med. Chem. Res.* **2012**, *22*, 1–15. [CrossRef]

24. Huang, Y.L.; Oppong, M.B.; Guo, Y.; Wang, L.Z.; Fang, S.M.; Deng, Y.R.; Gao, X.M. The Oleaceae family: A source of secoiridoids with multiple biological activities. *Fitoterapia* **2019**, *136*, 104155. [CrossRef] [PubMed]

25. Ghisalberti, E.L. Biological and pharmacological activity of naturally occurring iridoids and secoiridoids. *Phytomedicine* **1998**, *5*, 147–163. [CrossRef]

26. Pérez, J.A.; Hernández, J.M.; Trujillo, J.M.; López, H. Iridoids and secoiridoids from Oleaceae. *Stud. Nat. Prod. Chem.* **2005**, *32*, 303–363.

27. Dinda, B.; Debnath, S.; Harigaya, Y. Naturally occurring secoiridoids and bioactivity of naturally occurring iridoids and secoiridoids. A review, part 2. *Chem. Pharm. Bull.* **2017**, *55*, 689–728. [CrossRef]

28. Dinda, B.; Chowdhury, D.R.; Mohanta, B.C. Naturally occurring iridoids, secoiridoids and their bioactivity. An updated review, part 3. *Chem. Pharm. Bull.* **2009**, *57*, 765–796. [CrossRef]

29. Dinda, B.; Debnath, S.; Banik, R. Naturally occurring iridoids and secoiridoids. An updated review, part 4. *Chem. Pharm. Bull.* **2011**, *59*, 803–833. [CrossRef]

30. Liu, Q.; Kim, S.H.; Kim, S.B.; Jo, Y.H.; Kim, E.S.; Hwang, B.Y.; Oh, K.; Lee, M.K. Anti-obesity effect of (8-E)-nuzhenide, a secoiridoid from Ligustrum lucidum, in high-fat diet-induced obese mice. *Nat. Prod. Commun.* **2014**, *9*, 1399–1401. [CrossRef]

31. Vaidya, H.B.; Ahmed, A.A.; Goyal, R.K.; Cheema, S.K. Glycogen phosphorylase-a is a common target for anti-diabetic effect of iridoid and secoiridoid glycosides. *J. Pharm. Pharm. Sci.* **2013**, *16*, 530–540. [CrossRef]

32. Varga, E.; Barabas, C.; Toth, A.; Boldizsar, I.; Noszal, B.; Toth, G. Phenolic composition, antioxidant and antinociceptive activities of Syringa vulgaris L. bark and leaf extracts. *Nat. Prod. Res.* **2019**, *33*, 1664–1669. [CrossRef] [PubMed]

33. Giardinieri, A.; Schicchi, R.; Geraci, A.; Rosselli, S.; Maggi, F.; Fiorini, D.; Ricciutelli, M.; Loizzo, M.R.; Bruno, M.; Pacetti, D. Fixed oil from seeds of narrow-leaved ash (F. angustifolia subsp. angustifolia): Chemical profile, antioxidant and antiproliferative activities. *Food Res. Int.* **2019**, *119*, 369–377. [CrossRef] [PubMed]

34. Jin, C.; Jin, M.; Li, R.; Diao, S.; Sun, J.; Ma, Y.J.; Zhou, W.; Li, G. Isolation of a new natural kingiside aglucone derivative and other anti-inflammatory constituents from Syringa reticulate. *Nat. Prod. Res.* **2018**. [CrossRef] [PubMed]

35. Silvan, J.M.; Pinto-Bustillos, M.A.; Vasquez-Ponce, P.; Prodanov, M.; Martinez-Rodriguez, A.J. Olive mill wastewater as a potential source of antibacterial and anti-inflammatory compounds against the food-borne pathogen Campylobacter. *Innovative Food Sci. Emerging Technol.* **2019**, *51*, 177–185. [CrossRef]

36. Suh, W.S.; Kwon, O.K.; Lee, T.H.; Subedi, L.; Kim, S.Y.; Lee, K.R. Secoiridoid glycosides from the twigs of Ligustrum obtusifolium possess anti-inflammatory and neuroprotective effects. *Chem. Pharm. Bull.* **2018**, *66*, 78–83. [CrossRef] [PubMed]

37. Ngo, Q.-M.T.; Lee, H.-S.; Nguyen, V.T.; Woo, M.H.; Kim, J.A.; Min, B.S. Chemical constituents from the fruits of Ligustrum japonicum and their inhibitory effects on T cell activation. *Phytochemistry* **2017**, *141*, 147–155. [CrossRef]

38. Dinda, B.; Dinda, M.; Kulsi, G.; Chakraborty, A.; Dinda, S. Therapeutic potentials of plant iridoids in Alzheimer's and Parkinson's diseases: A review. *Eur. J. Med. Chem.* **2019**, *169*, 185–199. [CrossRef] [PubMed]

39. Park, K.J.; Suh, W.S.; Subedi, L.; Kim, S.Y.; Choi, S.U.; Lee, K.R. Secoiridoid Glucosides from the Twigs of Syringa oblata var. dilatata and Their Neuroprotective and Cytotoxic Activities. *Chem. Pharm. Bull.* **2017**, *65*, 359–364. [CrossRef] [PubMed]

40. Wei, W.; Hao, E.-W.; Zhang, M.; Pan, X.-L.; Qin, J.-F.; Xie, J.-L.; Deng, J.-G.; Wei, W.; Hao, E.-W.; Zhang, M.; et al. Chemical constituents from Jasminum pentaneurum Hand.-Mazz and their cytotoxicity against human cancer cell lines. *Nat. Prod. Res.* **2019**. [CrossRef]

41. Essafi Rhouma, H.; Trabelsi, N.; Chimento, A.; Benincasa, C.; Tamaalli, A.; Perri, E.; Zarrouk, M.; Pezzi, V. Olea europaea L. Flowers as a new promising anticancer natural product: phenolic composition, antiproliferative activity and apoptosis induction. *Nat. Prod. Res.* **2019**. [CrossRef]

42. Fabiani, R. Anti-cancer properties of olive oil secoiridoid phenols: A systematic review of in vivo studies. *Food Funct.* **2016**, *7*, 4145–4159. [CrossRef] [PubMed]

43. Kapinova, A.; Stefanicka, P.; Kubatka, P.; Zubor, P.; Uramova, S.; Kello, M.; Mojzis, J.; Blahutova, D.; Qaradakhi, T.; Zulli, A.; et al. Are plant-based functional foods better choice against cancer than single phytochemicals? A critical review of current breast cancer research. *Biomed. Pharmacother.* **2017**, *96*, 1465–1477. [CrossRef] [PubMed]

44. Munshi, A.; Hobbs, M.; Meyn, R.E. Clonogenic cell survival assay. *Methods Mol. Med.* **2005**, *110*, 21–28. [PubMed]

45. Nieddu, V.; Pinna, G.; Marchesi, I.; Sanna, L.; Asproni, B.; Pinna, G.A.; Bagella, L.; Murineddu, G. Synthesis and Antineoplastic Evaluation of Novel Unsymmetrical 1,3,4-Oxadiazoles. *J. Med. Chem.* **2016**, *59*, 10451–10469. [CrossRef]

46. Yu, R.; Zhang, Y.; Xu, Z.; Wang, J.; Chen, B.; Jin, H. Potential antitumor effects of panaxatriol against DU-15 human prostate cancer cells is mediated via mitochondrial mediated apoptosis, inhibition of cell migration and sub-G1 cell cycle arrest. *J. BUON* **2018**, *23*, 200–204.

47. Niu, H.; Li, X.; Yang, A.; Jin, Z.; Wang, X.; Wang, Q.; Yu, C.; Wei, Z.; Dou, C. Cycloartenol exerts anti-proliferative effects on Glioma U87 cells via induction of cell cycle arrest and p38 MAPK-mediated apoptosis. *J. BUON* **2018**, *23*, 1840–1845.

48. Xu, S.; Yao, H.; Luo, S.; Zhang, Y.-K.; Yang, D.-H.; Li, D.; Wang, G.; Hu, M.; Qiu, Y.; Wu, X.; et al. A Novel Potent Anticancer Compound Optimized from a Natural Oridonin Scaffold Induces Apoptosis and Cell Cycle Arrest through the Mitochondrial Pathway. *J. Med. Chem.* **2017**, *60*, 1449–1468. [CrossRef]

49. Abotaleb, M.; Kubatka, P.; Caprnda, M.; Varghese, E.; Zolakova, B.; Zubor, P.; Opatrilova, R.; Kruzliak, P.; Stefanicka, P.; Busselberg, D. Chemotherapeutic agents for the treatment of metastatic breast cancer: An update. *Biomed. Pharmacother.* **2018**, *101*, 458–477. [CrossRef]

50. Lou, C.; Xu, X.; Chen, Y.; Zhao, H.; Alisol, A. Suppresses Proliferation, Migration, and Invasion in Human Breast Cancer MDA-MB-231 Cells. *Molecules* **2019**, *24*, 3651. [CrossRef]

51. Ye, Y.; Zhang, T.; Yuan, H.; Li, D.; Lou, H.; Fan, P. Mitochondria-Targeted Lupane Triterpenoid Derivatives and Their Selective Apoptosis-Inducing Anticancer Mechanisms. *J. Med. Chem.* **2017**, *60*, 6353–6363. [CrossRef]

52. Zhang, Y.; Hou, Q.; Li, X.; Zhu, J.; Wang, W.; Li, B.; Zhao, L.; Xia, H. Enrichment of novel quinazoline derivatives with high antitumor activity in mitochondria tracked by its self-fluorescence. *Eur. J. Med. Chem.* **2019**, *178*, 417–432. [CrossRef] [PubMed]

53. Wu, Q.; Kroon, P.A.; Shao, H.; Needs, P.W.; Yang, X. Differential Effects of Quercetin and Two of Its Derivatives, Isorhamnetin and Isorhamnetin-3-glucuronide, in Inhibiting the Proliferation of Human Breast-Cancer MCF-7 Cells. *J. Agric. Food. Chem.* **2018**, *66*, 7181–7189. [CrossRef] [PubMed]

54. Zhang, Y.; Zhang, Y.; Liu, J.; Chen, L.; Zhao, L.; Li, B.; Wang, W. Synthesis and in vitro biological evaluation of novel quinazoline derivatives. *Bioorg. Med. Chem. Lett.* **2017**, *27*, 1584–1587. [CrossRef] [PubMed]

55. Chen, L.; Zhang, Y.; Liu, J.; Wang, W.; Li, X.; Zhao, L.; Wang, W.; Li, B. Novel 4-arylaminoquinazoline derivatives with (E)-propen-1-yl moiety as potent EGFR inhibitors with enhanced antiproliferative activities against tumor cells. *Eur. J. Med. Chem.* **2017**, *138*, 689–697. [CrossRef] [PubMed]

Sample Availability: Not available.

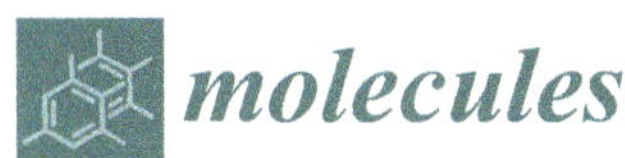 *molecules*

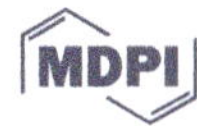

Article

Phenolic Compounds in Extracts of *Hibiscus acetosella* (Cranberry Hibiscus) and Their Antioxidant and Antibacterial Properties

Jae Il Lyu [1], Jaihyunk Ryu [1], Chang Hyun Jin [1], Dong-Gun Kim [1,2], Jung Min Kim [1,3], Kyoung-Sun Seo [4], Jin-Baek Kim [1], Sang Hoon Kim [1], Joon-Woo Ahn [1], Si-Yong Kang [5] and Soon-Jae Kwon [1,*]

[1] Advanced Radiation Technology Institute, Korea Atomic Energy Research Institute, Jeongup 56212, Korea; jaeil@kaeri.re.kr (J.I.L.); jhryu@kaeri.re.kr (J.R.); chjin@kaeri.re.kr (C.H.J.); dgkim@kaeri.re.kr (D.-G.K.); jmkim0803@kaeri.re.kr (J.M.K.); jbkim74@kaeri.re.kr (J.-B.K.); shkim80@kaeri.re.kr (S.H.K.); joon@kaeri.re.kr (J.-W.A.)
[2] Department of Life-Resources, Graduate School, Sunchon National University, Suncheon 57922, Korea
[3] Division of Plant Biotechnology, College of Agriculture and Life Science, Chonnam National University, Gwangju 61186, Korea
[4] Jangheung Research Institute for Mushroom Industry, Jangheung 59338, Korea; astragali@daum.net
[5] Department of Horticulture, College of Industrial Sciences, Kongju National University, Yesan, Chungnam Province 32439, Korea; sykang@kongju.ac.kr
* Correspondence: soonjaekwon@kaeri.re.kr; Tel.: +82-63-570-3312

Academic Editor: Raffaele Pezzani
Received: 14 August 2020; Accepted: 11 September 2020; Published: 12 September 2020

Abstract: Hibiscus species are rich in phenolic compounds and have been traditionally used for improving human health through their bioactive activities. The present study investigated the phenolic compounds of leaf extracts from 18 different *H. acetosella* accessions and evaluated their biofunctional properties, focusing on antioxidant and antibacterial activity. The most abundant phenolic compound in *H. acetosella* was caffeic acid, with levels ranging from 14.95 to 42.93 mg/100 g. The antioxidant activity measured by the ABTS assay allowed the accessions to be classified into two groups: a high activity group with red leaf varieties (74.71–84.02%) and a relatively low activity group with green leaf varieties (57.47–65.94%). The antioxidant activity was significantly correlated with TAC (0.933), Dp3-Sam (0.932), Dp3-Glu (0.924), and Cy3-Sam (0.913) contents ($p < 0.001$). The *H. acetosella* phenolic extracts exhibited antibacterial activity against two bacteria, with zones of inhibition between 12.00 and 13.67 mm (*Staphylococcus aureus*), and 10.67 and 13.33 mm (*Pseudomonas aeruginosa*). All accessions exhibited a basal antibacterial activity level (12 mm) against the Gram-positive *S. aureus*, with PI500758 and PI500764 exhibiting increased antibacterial activity (13.67 mm), but they exhibited a more dynamic antibacterial activity level against the Gram-negative *P. aeruginosa*.

Keywords: *Hibiscus acetosella*; phenolic compound; antioxidant; antibacterial; UPLC

1. Introduction

Hibiscus acetosella, a member of the Malvaceae family, is an amphidiploid plant native to Africa and is usually consumed as a green vegetable. In the traditional medicine of western and central Africa, decoction drinks have been prepared from extracts of the leaves and shoots because of their anti-anemic and antipyretic properties [1]. The presence of a wide variety of biochemical compounds, such as polyphenols, flavonoids, and anthocyanins have been reported in Hibiscus species [2,3]. Two examples, *H. cannabinus* and *H. sabdariffa*, have been studied most regarding the relationship between their biochemical compounds in the plant leaves and their biofunctional activity [4–7], while *H. acetosella* has been much less studied.

Phenolic compounds found in Hibiscus plants consist of phenolic acids such as hibiscus, protocatechuic, gallic, chlorogenic and caffeic acids, and the organic acid, citric acid. Flavonoids such as kaempferitrin, gallocatechin, quercetin, and luteolin are also present in these plants. Anthocyanins, detected mostly in flowers with calyces and some of the red-colored leaves, include cyanidin-3-glucoside, delphinidin-3-galactoside, delphinidin-3-glucoside, cyanidin-3-sambubioside, and delphinidin-3-sambubioside [8–10]. These compounds possess antioxidant properties shown by their effective scavenging activity on reactive oxygen species (ROS) and free radicals. Generally, to investigate the antioxidant activity of Hibiscus plants based on phenolic compound levels, the 2,2′-azino-bis (3-ethylbenzthiazoline-6-sulfonic acid) (ABTS) hydroxyl radical scavenging assay and 2,2-diphenyl-1-picryl-hydrazyl-hydrate (DPPH) free radical assay have been widely used [4,7,11]. Kapepula et al. [12] investigated the ability of *H. cannabinus*, *H. sabdariffa*, and *H. acetosella* to scavenge free radicals and reported IC_{50} values ranging from 43 to 186 µg/mL from ABTS and DPPH assays, although the three species differed in the composition of their phenolic compounds.

In terms of pharmacological effects, Hibiscus plants have also attracted interest because of their biological activities, which include antibacterial, anti-inflammatory, antigenotoxic, hepatoprotective, and antimutagenic activities [13–16]. In particular, the antibacterial activity of *H. sabdariffa* has been well-studied as well as other biological activities of extracts of its leaves and flowers [4,17,18], while *H. acetosella* has been reported as having anti-inflammatory [12] and antimutagenic activity [16], but no antibacterial activity.

The present study therefore aimed to determine the composition of phenolic compounds in the extracts of leaves from 18 *H. acetosella* accessions using UPLC analysis and to assess their bioactive properties, antioxidant and antibacterial activities, using the ABTS assay and agar-well diffusion test, respectively. The relationship between phenolic extracts and their biofunctional properties will also be evaluated using statistical analysis.

2. Results and Discussion

2.1. Phenolic Composition of H. acetosella Leaf Extracts

First, before measuring the content of phenolic compounds, the color characteristics of the *H. acetosella* leaves were investigated (Figure 1). The leaf color is usually green, but three accessions appeared red (PI500777, PI500801, and PI500805). The petiole colors could be divided into four types: 7 accessions were green, 5 accessions green-red, 2 accessions light-red, and 4 accessions red (Table 1). The phenolic compounds of the *H. acetosella* accessions were detected by UV-spectrophotometry and UPLC (Table 2). The total phenolic content (TPC) and total flavonoid content (TFC) levels ranged from 193.14 to 434.67, and 199.10 to 262.19 mg/100 g, respectively, with the highest level in PI500707. A previous study on *H. acetosella*, investigating a different variety using a different extraction method, reported TPC and TFC levels of 1730 and 775 mg/100 g, respectively, values more than three times those found in the present study [19]. Phenolic compounds play an important role in the adaptation of plants to the environment, and their content is determined by the origin, harvesting time, and cultivation conditions [3,20]. Previous data has shown that the TPC and TFC contents can vary by approximately three times according to the region where the plants are collected [21,22]. In the present study, the major polyphenols in *H. acetosella* were identified as caffeic acid (CA) and chlorogenic acid (CGA), while gallocatechin (GC) and gallic acid (GAL) were present in relatively small amounts (Table 2). In particular, CA is present in three Hibiscus plants, *H. cannabinus*, *H. sabdariffa*, and *H. acetosella*, with the highest amounts in *H. acetosella* [12]. CGA is also a major phenolic compound in *H. sabdariffa* aqueous extract [23]. The PI500707 accession also exhibited significantly higher levels of polyphenols such as GC (1.57 mg/100 g), GAL (1.97 mg/100 g), CGA (41.56 mg/100 g), and CA (42.93 mg/100 g) in the collected accessions. As expected, the TAC level was associated with the coloration of the leaf, as well as with the anthocyanins content. In green leaves, the TAC content was less than 1 mg/100 g, but in three accessions with red leaves, the contents ranged from 17.25 to 19.98 mg/100 g (Table 2). Three anthocyanins, delphinidin-3-sambubioside (Dp3-Sam), delphinidin-3-glucoside (Dp3-Glu), and cyanidin-3-sambubioside (Cy3-Sam), were only detected in red leaves but also seen in UPLC 3D profiling (Figure S1). Similar findings have also been reported in a previous study of phenolic compounds in Hibiscus plants [4,6,24].

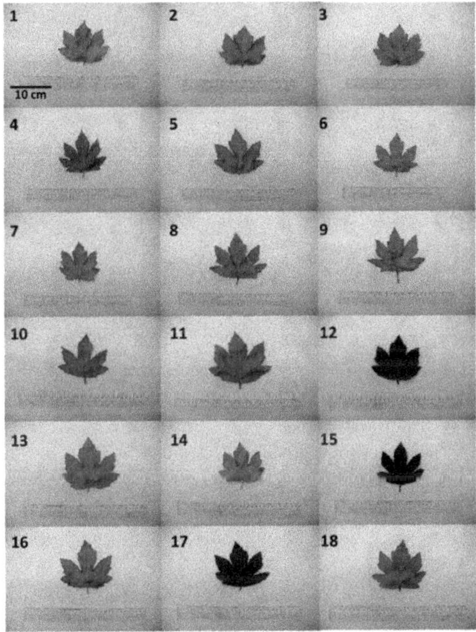

Figure 1. Leaf color of the 18 different *H. acetosella* accessions used in this study.

Table 1. Leaf and petiole color of the 18 different *H. acetosella* accessions used in this study.

Number	ID	Leaf Color	Petiole Color
1	PI 500707	Green	Green-red
2	PI 500730	Green	Green-red
3	PI 500744	Green	Green-red
4	PI 500749	Green	Green
5	PI 500755	Green	Green
6	PI 500756	Green	Green
7	PI 500758	Green	Green
8	PI 500761	Green	Red
9	PI 500764	Green	Light-red
10	PI 500765	Green	Light-red
11	PI 500766	Green	Green-red
12	PI 500777	Red	Red
13	PI 500778	Green	Green
14	PI 500794	Green	Green
15	PI 500801	Red	Red
16	PI 500804	Green	Green
17	PI 500805	Red	Red
18	PI 591552	Green	Green-red

Table 2. Contents of phenolic compounds in leaf extracts from 18 different *H. acetosella* accessions (mean value ± S.D., n = 3).

Accessions	TPC	TFC	TAC	GC	GAL	CGA	CA	Dp3-Sam	Dp3-Glu	Cy3-Sam
PI 500707	434.67 ± 16.0 [a*]	262.19 ± 11.6 [a]	0.47 ± 0.11 [a]	1.57 ± 0.07 [a]	1.97 ± 0.8 [b]	41.56 ± 5.74 [a]	42.93 ± 7.11 [a]	Nd [(1)]	nd	nd
PI 500730	297.52 ± 27.8 [d]	229.69 ± 9.7 [b]	0.44 ± 0.10 [a]	0.95 ± 0.04 [f]	0.67 ± 0.2 [a]	13.2 ± 3.18 [de]	27.72 ± 0.49 [de]	nd	nd	nd
PI 500744	291.62 ± 23.8 [de]	227.57 ± 7.0 [bc]	0.35 ± 0.08 [a]	0.96 ± 0.05 [f]	0.86 ± 0.38 [a]	8.66 ± 1.02 [f]	30.5 ± 0.57 [cd]	nd	nd	nd
PI 500749	283.58 ± 12.0 [de]	222.03 ± 6.5 [bc]	0.3 ± 0.06 [a]	0.68 ± 0.04 [h]	0.52 ± 0.12 [a]	5.28 ± 0.59 [fg]	35.83 ± 0.24 [bc]	nd	nd	nd
PI 500755	282.72 ± 25.0 [de]	210.71 ± 8.9 [cd]	0.12 ± 0.03 [a]	0.74 ± 0.03 [gh]	0.91 ± 0.42 [a]	18.45 ± 3.13 [cd]	24.49 ± 0.09 [ef]	nd	nd	nd
PI 500756	302.04 ± 23.1 [d]	217.42 ± 7.2 [bc]	0.13 ± 0.04 [a]	0.77 ± 0.04 [gh]	0.87 ± 0.4 [a]	16 ± 3.07 [d]	31.35 ± 0.24 [cd]	nd	nd	nd
PI 500758	288.29 ± 29.6 [de]	210.27 ± 8.7 [cd]	0.15 ± 0.05 [a]	0.83 ± 0.05 [fg]	0.98 ± 0.44 [a]	21.25 ± 3.21 [cd]	35.03 ± 7.74 [bc]	nd	nd	nd
PI 500761	248.2 ± 21.9 [ef]	219.24 ± 10.3 [bc]	0.59 ± 0.15 [a]	1.07 ± 0.07 [de]	0.63 ± 0.14 [a]	5.4 ± 1.19 [fg]	22.79 ± 0.14 [ef]	nd	nd	nd
PI 500764	230.94 ± 7.3 [g]	199.1 ± 9.7 [f]	0.42 ± 0.08 [a]	0.73 ± 0.03 [gh]	0.59 ± 0.13 [a]	9.66 ± 2.38 [ef]	24.93 ± 1.09 [ef]	nd	nd	nd
PI 500765	378.5 ± 13.6 [b]	224.32 ± 8.3 [bc]	0.43 ± 0.08 [a]	0.8 ± 0.05 [gh]	1.05 ± 0.52 [a]	35.25 ± 1.08 [b]	32.23 ± 0.32 [cd]	nd	nd	nd
PI 500766	249.77 ± 27.6 [ef]	203.53 ± 14.2 [d]	0.32 ± 0.10 [a]	1.14 ± 0.10 [cd]	0.94 ± 0.48 [a]	17.35 ± 1.49 [cd]	14.95 ± 1.83 [f]	nd	nd	nd
PI 500777	409.81 ± 37.6 [ab]	254.03 ± 4.9 [a]	19.98 ± 4.5 [b]	1.15 ± 0.07 [cd]	1.13 ± 0.61 [a]	18.37 ± 1.62 [cd]	38.28 ± 2.46 [ab]	9.37	0.65	2.00
PI 500778	276.25 ± 30.0 [de]	211.46 ± 7.8 [cd]	0.1 ± 0.03 [a]	0.78 ± 0.02 [gh]	0.85 ± 0.37 [a]	16.53 ± 3.01 [d]	35.59 ± 7.81 [bc]	nd	nd	nd
PI 500794	289.39 ± 15.1 [de]	207.26 ± 9.3 [d]	0.17 ± 0.04 [a]	0.69 ± 0.02 [h]	0.87 ± 0.39 [a]	21.7 ± 3.02 [c]	26.58 ± 0.44 [de]	nd	nd	nd
PI 500801	309.72 ± 15.6 [d]	227.99 ± 6.8 [bc]	17.25 ± 3.7 [b]	1.29 ± 0.13 [b]	0.95 ± 0.51 [a]	5.7 ± 0.25 [fg]	32.01 ± 0.56 [cd]	8.20	0.42	1.88
PI 500804	235.17 ± 19.5 [g]	204.19 ± 9.3 [d]	0.16 ± 0.05 [a]	0.95 ± 0.09 [f]	0.82 ± 0.36 [a]	10.2 ± 2.63 [ef]	21.87 ± 0.07 [ef]	nd	nd	nd
PI 500805	360.67 ± 20.6 [c]	227.65 ± 9.7 [bc]	18.3 ± 4.0 [b]	1.26 ± 0.13 [bc]	1.11 ± 0.59 [a]	20.49 ± 1.69 [cd]	31.67 ± 0.46 [bc]	9.02	0.46	1.68
PI 591552	193.14 ± 14.0 [h]	199.74 ± 12.6 [df]	0.42 ± 0.12 [a]	1.01 ± 0.10 [ef]	0.73 ± 0.36 [a]	3.02 ± 0.42 [h]	16.64 ± 0.61 [e]	nd	nd	nd

Phenolic compounds (mg/100 g): total phenolic contents (TPC), total flavonoid contents (TFC), total anthocyanin contents (TAC), gallocatechin (GC), gallic acid (GAL), chlorogenic acid (CGA), caffeic acid (CA); anthocyanins (mg CGE/g): delphinidin-3-sambubioside (Dp3-Sam), delphinidin-3-glucoside (Dp3-Glu), cyanidin-3-sambubioside (Cy3-Sam). * The letters adjacent to mean value indicate the result of Duncan's multiple range test at the 5% probability level (n = 3); [(1)] not detectable.

2.2. Effects of Phenolic Extracts on the Radical Cation Scavenging Activity

To compare the antioxidant properties of the 18 *H. acetosella* accessions, the radical cation scavenging activity of their phenolic extracts (10 times diluted) was determined using the ABTS assay (Table 3). The ABTS assay mainly depends on hydrogen peroxide in the presence of ABTS to produce the radical cation and has been previously used for measuring the total antioxidant activity in a wide variety of plants rich in polyphenols [25]. The antioxidant activity varied from the highest value of 84.02% (PI500805) to the lowest value of 57.47% (PI500756) in the *H. acetosella* extracts, with that of the control ascorbic acid (500 µM) at 99.83%. These values of antioxidant activity were higher than those previously reported for *H. acetosella* [26]. The activity of the phenolic compounds from the ABTS assay increased with the contents of the related anthocyanins, TAC, Dp3-Sam, Dp3-Glu, and Cy3-Sam (Table 3). For example, PI500801 (74.71%), PI500777 (82.34%) and PI500805 (84.02%) exhibited the highest antioxidant activity, as well as abundant TAC and anthocyanins contents. In contrast, 15 *H. acetosella* accessions with no detectable anthocyanins contents, showed a slightly decreased antioxidant activity from 57.47% (PI500756) to 65.94% (PI500707). The antioxidant effect of the extracts was probably caused by flavonoids and anthocyanins, especially anthocyanins, which have been reported to exhibit excellent antioxidant activity in Hibiscus plants [27,28]. Interestingly, Maciel et al. [29] have purified anthocyanins such as Dp3-Sam, Dp3-Glu, Cy3-Sam, and cyanidin-3-glucoside (Cy3-Glu) from a crude extract of the *H. sabdariffa* calyx, which exhibited a higher antioxidant activity from the DPPH assay than that of the crude extract. The present study attempted to make use of the DPPH radical activity assay, but an unknown precipitate was produced in the reaction mixture, which affected the measurements in the extracts from some of the accessions. This might have been caused by the reaction of unknown compounds with the organic solvent (Table S1). Nonetheless, all accessions, except for the four aberrant accessions, tended to exhibit a higher antioxidant activity measured by the DPPH assay than that measured by the ABTS activity assay. The antioxidant and bioactive properties of anthocyanins have also been linked to health benefits such as anti-cancer, anti-inflammatory, and anti-diabetic activities [30–34]. Consequently, these results are consistent with previous studies, indicating that anthocyanin compounds were the main contributors to the antioxidant activity of *H. acetosella*.

Table 3. Antioxidant and antibacterial activities of 18 different *H. acetosella* accessions.

ID	Antioxidant Activity	Antibacterial Activities (mm) [2]	
	ABTS (%)	*S. aureus*	*P. aeruginosa*
Control [1]	99.83 ± 0.18	12.80 ± 0.34	13.10 ± 0.42
PI 500707	65.94 ± 0.18 [h]	12.00 ± 1.00 [a]	11.33 ± 0.58 [ab]
PI 500730	59.36 ± 0.13 [bc]	12.33 ± 0.58 [ab]	13.00 ± 0.00 [de]
PI 500744	64.47 ± 0.18 [fg]	13.33 ± 0.58 [bc]	12.33 ± 0.58 [cd]
PI 500749	62.25 ± 0.22 [de]	12.00 ± 0.00 [a]	12.00 ± 0.00 [bc]
PI 500755	59.44 ± 0.99 [bc]	12.00 ± 0.00 [a]	12.00 ± 0.00 [bc]
PI 500756	57.47 ± 0.15 [a]	13.00 ± 0.00 [abc]	12.00 ± 0.00 [bc]
PI 500758	62.46 ± 0.15 [de]	13.67 ± 0.58 [c]	11.33 ± 0.58 [ab]
PI 500761	65.10 ± 0.15 [gh]	13.33 ± 0.58 [bc]	13.33 ± 0.58 [e]
PI 500764	61.91 ± 0.23 [d]	13.67 ± 0.58 [c]	12.00 ± 0.00 [bc]
PI 500765	64.05 ± 0.36 [f]	12.67 ± 0.58 [abc]	12.00 ± 0.00 [bc]
PI 500766	60.11 ± 0.51 [c]	12.00 ± 0.00 [a]	11.67 ± 0.58 [bc]
PI 500777	82.34 ± 0.23 [j]	12.67 ± 0.58 [abc]	11.33 ± 0.58 [ab]
PI 500778	61.75 ± 0.40 [d]	12.33 ± 0.58 [ab]	12.00 ± 0.00 [bc]
PI 500794	63.00 ± 0.38 [e]	12.67 ± 0.58 [abc]	11.67 ± 0.58 [bc]
PI 500801	74.71 ± 0.07 [i]	12.67 ± 0.58 [abc]	11.67 ± 0.58 [bc]
PI 500804	58.56 ± 0.08 [b]	13.33 ± 0.58 [bc]	12.00 ± 0.00 [bc]
PI 500805	84.02 ± 0.15 [k]	13.33 ± 0.58 [bc]	11.33 ± 0.58 [ab]
PI 591552	65.61 ± 0.08 [h]	12.67 ± 0.58 [abc]	10.67 ± 0.58 [a]

[1] Control used were: ascorbic acid (500 µM) in antioxidant assay and gentamicin (5 µg) (antibacterial assay).
[2] Inhibition zone of *H. acetosella* leaf extract against *Staphylococcus aureus* (Gram-positive) and *Pseudomonas aeruginosa* (Gram-negative). The results are shown as the mean ± standard error of three replicates. Mean with the same letter are not significantly different at the 5% probability level (Duncan's multiple range test). nd; not detectable.

2.3. Inhibitory Effects of Phenolic Extracts against Gram-Positive and Gram-Negative Bacteria

The inhibitory effects of the phenolic extracts of *H. acetosella* leaves on the Gram-positive (*Staphylococcus aureus* ATCC 6538) and Gram-negative (*Pseudomonas aeruginosa* ATCC 9027) bacteria are shown in Table 3. Distilled water, used as the negative control, exhibited no inhibitory effect against the two bacteria (Figure S2), but gentamicin (5 µg), used as the positive control, exhibited inhibition zones against the two bacteria of 12.80 ± 0.34 mm (*S. aureus*) and 13.10 ± 0.42 mm (*P. aeruginosa*). The phenolic extracts of the 18 *H. acetosella* accessions showed antibacterial activity against two bacteria, the zones of inhibition ranging from 12.00 to 13.67 mm (*S. aureus*) and from 10.67 to 13.33 mm (*P. aeruginosa*). For the *S. aureus* bacteria, all accessions exhibited a basal antibacterial activity level (12 mm), with PI500758 and PI500764 exhibiting an increased level of antibacterial activity (13.67 mm), but the Gram-negative (*P. aeruginosa*) bacteria exhibited a wider range of levels of antibacterial activity (Table 3). These antibacterial activities were exhibited similar levels against both Gram-positive and Gram-negative bacteria in *H. sabdariffa* [4,31,35]. The present study first confirmed the presence of antibacterial activity against two bacteria among the phenolic extracts of the 18 different *H. acetosella* accessions as a basis for optimization in future research using a formal antibacterial measuring method.

2.4. Relationship between Phenolic Extracts and Biofunctional Properties

The Pearson correlation coefficient and hierarchical clustering were used to assess the relationship between the contents of phenolic compounds in the extracts and the biofunctional properties (antioxidant and antibacterial activities) in the 18 *H. acetosella* accessions (Table 4, Figure 2). The antioxidant activity (ABST) was significantly correlated with TAC (0.933), Dp3-Sam (0.932), Dp3-Glu (0.924), and Cy3-Sam (0.913) contents ($p < 0.001$). The TPC, TFC, and GC contents also exhibited significant correlation coefficients ranging between 0.526 and 0.567 ($p < 0.05$). Consequently, the antioxidant activity in *H. acetosella* was strongly correlated with its contents of phenolic compounds, with the related anthocyanin contents also being involved in the antioxidant activity. In contrast, the antibacterial activity against Gram-positive bacteria was not significantly correlated with the content of phenolic compounds but antibacterial activity against Gram-negative bacteria was negatively correlated with the GAL content (-0.433, $p < 0.05$). However, the content of GAL is too low in *H. acetosella* to produce an antibacterial response. Overall, the antibacterial activity varied between the accessions, suggesting the involvement of other specific phenolic compounds present in their extracts. Borrás-Linares et al. [4] have also reported that the antimicrobial assay revealed no significant or a negative correlation between phenolic contents and antibacterial activity in *H. sabdariffa*, suggesting a similar response. Hierarchical clustering classified the accessions and measurements according to their chemical and biofunctional similarities. The accessions divided into two clusters: the first cluster contained high contents of anthocyanins and the second cluster according to the status of the phenolic compounds and biofunctional properties. The measurements were classified into three clusters: cluster I contained antibacterial activities, cluster II contained phenolic compounds without anthocyanins, and cluster III contained antioxidant activity with anthocyanins (Figure 2). These results, as mentioned earlier, indicated that the antioxidant activity was strongly associated with the levels of anthocyanins such as TAC, Dp3-Sam, Dp3-Glu, and Cy3-Sam.

Table 4. Correlation coefficients between the contents of phenclic compcunds and antioxidant/bacterial activities.

	TPC	TFC	TAC	GC	GAL	CGA	CA	Dp3-Sam	Dp3-Glu	Cy3-Sam	ABST	S. aureus	P. aeruginosa
TPC	1.000	0.887 ***	0.475 *	0.478 *	0.770 ***	0.730 ***	0.787 ***	0.471 *	0.499 *	0.462 *	0.528 *	−0.233	−0.175
TFC		1.000	0.470 *	0.636 **	0.685 **	0.475 *	0.747 ***	0.458 *	0.498 *	0.463 *	0.526 *	−0.265	−0.024
TAC			1.000	0.508 *	0.223	−0.040	0.307	1.000 ***	0.989 ***	0.997 ***	0.933 ***	0.101	−0.317
GC				1.000	0.693 **	0.258	0.199	0.501 *	0.475 *	0.501 *	0.567 *	−0.117	−0.250
GAL					1.000	0.8_1 ***	0.532 **	0.223	0.228	0.216	0.317	−0.254	−0.433 *
CGA						1.000	0.491 *	−0.037	−0.021	−0.058	0.063	−0.255	−0.245
CA							1.000	0.306	0.328	0.309	0.349	−0.095	−0.115
Dp3-Sam								1.000	0.986 ***	0.996 ***	0.932 ***	0.106	−0.323
Dp3-Glu									1.000	0.986 ***	0.924 ***	0.084	−0.325
Cy3-Sam										1.000	0.913 ***	0.086	−0.315
ABST											1.000	0.145	−0.380 *
S. aureus												1.000	0.090
P. aeruginosa													1.000

Significant levels are indicated as; * (0.05 > p > 0.01), ** (0.01 > p > 0.001), *** (0.001 > p).

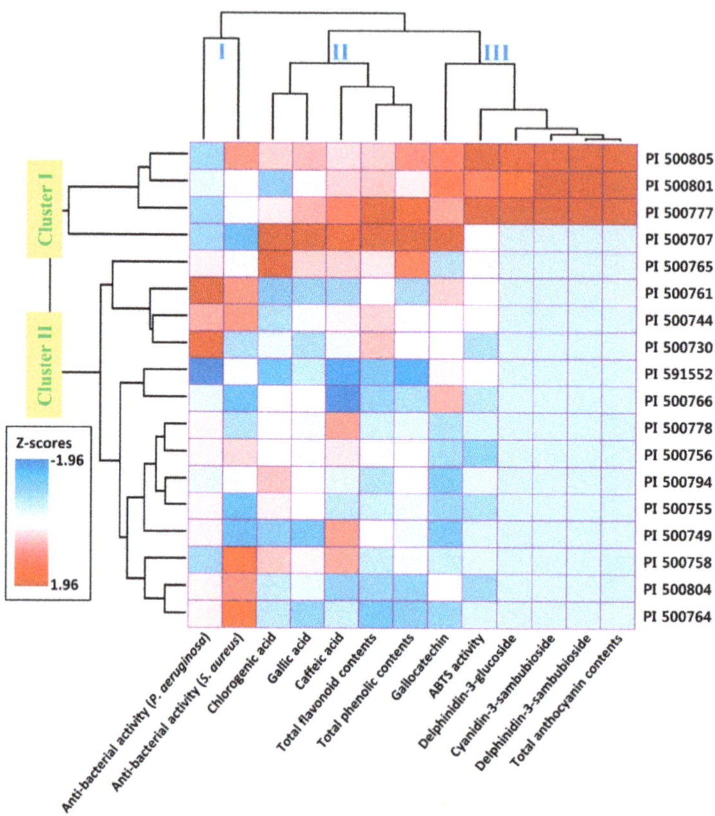

Figure 2. Hierarchical cluster analysis of the 18 different *H. acetosella* accessions according to their phenolic compound contents and biofunctional properties.

3. Materials and Methods

3.1. Plant Materials

The 18 accessions studied (Table 1, Figure 1) were collected from the USDA and originated in Zambia. The leaves of the genotypes were harvested in August for each accession for the analysis of the functional compounds. The leaves were picked by hand from plants grown in three separate plots on the same plantation. The seeds were planted 20 cm apart in rows 60 cm apart in plots (3 × 4.2 m). Fertilizer (N:P:K 4:2:2 *w/w/w*) was applied at 550 kg/ha shortly after seeding. The experiment was conducted at the Korea Atomic Energy Research Institute (35°30′33.9″ N, 126°50′02.3″ E, Jeongeup, Korea). The plants' cultivation conditions between May and August 2017 were as follows: mean temperature 17.8–24.4 °C, relative humidity 66.0–80.9%, mean sunlight 10.4–7.0 h. All of these climate data were accessed through the Korea Meteorological Administration web portal (http://weather.go.kr/).

3.2. Phenolic Compounds Extraction

All samples were ground to achieve a particle sizeable to pass through a 500-mesh sieve. The ground samples (1 g) were extracted in 5 mL of distilled water for 16 h then filtered through a 0.45-μm membrane filter. The antioxidant and antibacterial activities were measured using these aqueous extracts.

3.3. Total Phenolic Content

The total phenolic content (TPC) was determined by the Folin–Ciocalteu colorimetric method [7]. A small quantity (0.2 mL) of each extract and 1.5 mL of Folin–Ciocalteu reagent (20% *v/v*) were mixed thoroughly. Four mL of Na_2CO_3 (7%) were added, then made up to 10 mL with water. The mixture was kept in the dark at room temperature for 90 min. The absorbance was then measured at 760 nm using a UV-spectrophotometer (UV-1800, Shimadzu, Kyoto, Japan). TPC was calculated using a calibration curve of gallic acid.

3.4. Total Flavonoid Content

The total flavonoid content (TFC) of the *H. acetosella* extracts was determined as described by Ryu et al. [7]. Each extract sample (0.2 mL) was added to 4 mL double-distilled water and 0.3 mL of 5% $NaNO_2$ in a flask. The samples were left for 5 min, then 0.3 mL of 10% $AlCl_3$ was added. After 6 min, 2 mL NaOH were added then made up to 10 mL with double-distilled water. The absorbance was then measured at 510 nm. TFC was calculated using a calibration curve of quercetin equivalents.

3.5. Total Anthocyanin Content

The total anthocyanin contents (TAC) of the *H. acetosella* extracts were determined as described by Sutharut et al. [36]. The pH differential method, consisting of a KCl buffer (0.025 M, pH 1.0) and a CH_3COONa buffer (0.4 M, pH 4.5), was used to determine the total anthocyanin content of the methanol extract prepared from each sample. A 1-mL aliquot of the extract was mixed with 4 mL of each of the buffers then incubated at 28 °C for 15 min so that the solution could equilibrate. The absorbance was measured at 510 nm and 700 nm using deionized water as a blank. The final result was converted to milligrams of cyanidin-3-glucoside equivalents (CGE) per gram dry weight (mg CGE/g dry weight).

3.6. UPLC Analysis

The phenolic compounds were analyzed using a ultra-high performance liquid chromatography (UPLC) system (CBM-20A, Shimadzu) with two gradient pump systems (LC-30AD, Shimadzu), a UV-detector (SPD-M30A, Shimadzu), an auto sample injector (SIL-30AC, Shimadzu), and a column oven (CTO-30A, Shimadzu). Separation was achieved on an XR-ODS column (3.0 × 100 mm, 1.8 μm, Shimadzu) using a linear gradient elution program with a mobile phase containing solvent A (0.1%, *v/v*, trifluoroacetic acid in distilled deionized water) and solvent B (0.1%, *v/v*, trifluoroacetic acid in acetonitrile). The phenolic compounds were separated using the following gradient: 0–5 min, 10–15% B; 5–10 min, 15–20% B; 10–15 min, 20–30% B; 15–25 min, 30–50% B; 25–30 min, 50–75% B; 30–35 min, 75–100% B; 35–40 min, 100–5% B; and 40–45 min, 5–0% B. The phenolic compounds and anthocyanins were detected at 280 nm and 520 nm, respectively. The chlorogenic acid (CGA), caffeic acid (CA), delphinidin-3-sambubioside (Dp3-Sam), delphinidin-3-glucoside (Dp3-Glu), cyanidin-3-sambubioside (Cy3-Sam), all obtained from Sigma-Aldrich Co. (St. Louis, MO, USA) were identified based on the retention times of commercial standards (UV spectrum). Gallocatechin (GC) and gallic acid (GAL) were identified as described in a previous study [16] and by their UV-visible spectral characteristics.

3.7. ABTS Radical Cation Scavenging Activity

Each extract sample was diluted 10-fold with water, then the ABTS value was evaluated as described by Re et al. [25]. In brief, ABTS was measured using pre-formed radical monocations. The mixtures, along with 7.4 mM ABTS solution and 2.6 mM potassium persulfate, were incubated at room temperature in the dark for 24 h. The ABTS solution was diluted with phosphate-buffered saline (pH 7.4) to achieve an absorbance of 0.7 ± 0.02 at 734 nm. Each sample (10 μL) was then reacted with 190 μL of the ABTS solution. The absorbance at 734 nm was measured 6 min after the reaction using the Benchmark Plus ELISA reader (Bio-Rad, Hercules, CA, USA).

3.8. Antibacterial Activity Assays

The antibacterial activities of the extracts were tested against two pathogenic species, a Gram-positive bacterium (*Staphylococcus aureus* ATCC 6538) and a Gram-negative bacterium (*Pseudomonas aeruginosa* ATCC 9027), using the agar-well diffusion method [4] with some modification. The two bacterial cultures were grown in Difco Nutrient Agar (BD Difco, Franklin Lakes, NJ, USA) for 24 h at 32 °C then diluted with sterile distilled water to obtain an inoculum concentration of 10^6 cfu/mL before the suspensions were spread on the nutrient agar medium. Aliquots of each phenolic extract (70 µL) were added to an 8-mm diameter paper disc placed on the plates then incubated at 32 °C for 24 h. The positive and negative controls used gentamicin (5 µg) (Merck, Kenilworth, NJ, USA) and sterile distilled water, respectively. The antibacterial activity was determined as the diameter of the inhibition zones (mm) around the discs from each extract.

3.9. Statistical Analysis

The chemical analysis and biofunctional assay data were assessed using multiple variance analysis (ANOVA) with Duncan's multiple range *post-hoc* test in the SPSS version 20 statistical software package (IBM Corp., Armonk, NY, USA). Differences between mean values were considered to be significant at $p < 0.05$. The hierarchical clustering analysis was performed using the complete linkage method based on the phenolic compound contents and biofunctional data from the 18 different *H. acetosella* accessions. The phenolic compounds were visualized as z-values on a heatmap.

4. Conclusions

In this study, the composition of phenolic compounds in the leaf extracts of 18 different *H. acetosella* accessions was determined and how it contributed to their antioxidant and antibacterial activities. The antioxidant activity was significantly associated with the level of anthocyanins in the phenolic extracts. This study is the first to report the antibacterial activity of *H. acetosella* against both Gram-positive and Gram-negative bacteria. These results could be useful for exploring the potential of medicinal crops as a valuable resource for discovering new pharmaceutical drugs.

Supplementary Materials: The Supplementary Materials are available online. Figure S1: Ultra-high performance liquid chromatography (UPLC) 3D profiles of the 18 *H. acetosella* accessions. The numbers in the boxes correspond to the numbers in column 1 of Table 1. Figure S2: Agar-well diffusion test demonstrating inhibition zones against *S. aureus* and *P. aeruginosa* bacteria. All test were performed three replicates. Table S1: DPPH radical activity of 18 different *H. acetosella accessions.*

Author Contributions: Conceptualization, J.I.L. and J.R.; formal analysis, J.I.L., J.R., K.-S.S., and C.H.J.; investigation, D.-G.K., J.M.K., and S.H.K.; writing—original draft preparation, J.I.L., J.R. and C.H.J.; writing—review and editing, J.I.L. and S.-J.K.; supervision, J.-B.K.; project administration, S.-Y.K.; funding acquisition, J.-W.A. All authors have read and agreed to the published version of the manuscript.

Funding: This work was supported by the research program of Korea Atomic Energy Research Institute, Republic of Korea and the Radiation Technology R&D Program (NRF-2017M2A2A6A05018538) through the National Research Foundation of Korea, funded by the Ministry of Science and ICT.

Acknowledgments: We thank Philip Creed, from Edanz Group (https://en-author-services.edanzgroup.com/) for editing a draft of this manuscript.

Conflicts of Interest: The authors declare no conflict of interest.

References

1. Ssegawa, P.; Kasenene, J.M. Medicinal plant diversity and uses in the Sango bay area, Southern Uganda. *J. Ethnopharmacol.* **2007**, *113*, 521–540. [CrossRef] [PubMed]
2. Pascoal, A.; Quirantes-Piné, R.; Fernando, A.L.; Alexopoulou, E.; Segura-Carretero, A. Phenolic composition and antioxidant activity of kenaf leaves. *Ind. Crops Prod.* **2015**, *78*, 116–123. [CrossRef]

3. Wang, J.; Cao, X.; Ferchaud, V.; Qi, Y.; Jiang, H.; Tang, F.; Yue, Y.; Chin, K.L. Variations in chemical fingerprints and major flavonoid contents from the leaves of thirty-one accessions of *Hibiscus sabdariffa* L. *Biomed. Chromatogr.* **2016**, *30*, 880–887. [CrossRef] [PubMed]

4. Borrás-Linares, I.; Fernández-Arroyo, S.; Arráez-Roman, D.; Palmeros-Suárez, P.; Del Val-Díaz, R.; Andrade-Gonzáles, I.; Fernández-Gutiérrez, A.; Gómez-Leyva, J.; Segura-Carretero, A. Characterization of phenolic compounds, anthocyanidin, antioxidant and antimicrobial activity of 25 varieties of Mexican Roselle (*Hibiscus sabdariffa*). *Ind. Crops Prod.* **2015**, *69*, 385–394. [CrossRef]

5. Formagio, A.; Ramos, D.; Vieira, M.; Ramalho, S.; Silva, M.; Zárate, N.; Foglio, M.; Carvalho, J. Phenolic compounds of Hibiscus sabdariffa and influence of organic residues on its antioxidant and antitumoral properties. *Braz. J. Biol.* **2015**, *75*, 69–76. [CrossRef] [PubMed]

6. Ifie, I.; Marshall, L.J.; Ho, P.; Williamson, G. *Hibiscus sabdariffa* (Roselle) extracts and wine: Phytochemical profile, physicochemical properties, and carbohydrase inhibition. *J. Agric. Food Chem.* **2016**, *64*, 4921–4931. [CrossRef]

7. Ryu, J.; Kwon, S.-J.; Ahn, J.-W.; Jo, Y.D.; Kim, S.H.; Jeong, S.W.; Lee, M.K.; Kim, J.-B.; Kang, S.-Y. Phytochemicals and antioxidant activity in the kenaf plant (*Hibiscus cannabinus* L.). *J. Plant Biotechnol.* **2017**, *44*, 191–202. [CrossRef]

8. Ryu, J.; Kwon, S.-J.; Kim, D.-G.; Lee, M.-K.; Kim, J.M.; Jo, Y.D.; Kim, S.H.; Jeong, S.W.; Kang, K.-Y.; Kim, S.W.; et al. Morphological characteristics, chemical and genetic diversity of kenaf (*Hibiscus cannabinus* L.) genotypes. *J. Plant Biotechnol.* **2017**, *44*, 416–430. [CrossRef]

9. Wang, J.; Cao, X.; Jiang, H.; Qi, Y.; Chin, K.L.; Yue, Y. Antioxidant activity of leaf extracts from different Hibiscus sabdariffa accessions and simultaneous determination five major antioxidant compounds by LC-Q-TOF-MS. *Molecules* **2014**, *19*, 21226–21238. [CrossRef]

10. Zhen, J.; Villani, T.S.; Guo, Y.; Qi, Y.; Chin, K.; Pan, M.-H.; Ho, C.-T.; Simon, J.E.; Wu, Q. Phytochemistry, antioxidant capacity, total phenolic content and anti-inflammatory activity of *Hibiscus sabdariffa* leaves. *Food Chem.* **2016**, *190*, 673–680. [CrossRef]

11. Thungmungmee, S.; Wisidsri, N.; Khobjai, W. *Antioxidant Activities of Chaba Maple (Hibiscus acetosella) Flower Extract*; Applied Mechanics and Materials; Trans Tech Publications: Freienbach, Switzerland, 2019; pp. 34–39.

12. Kapepula, P.M.; Kabamba Ngombe, N.; Tshisekedi Tshibangu, P.; Tsumbu, C.; Franck, T.; Mouithys-Mickalad, A.; Mumba, D.; Tshala-Katumbay, D.; Serteyn, D.; Tits, M. Comparison of metabolic profiles and bioactivities of the leaves of three edible Congolese Hibiscus species. *Nat. Prod. Res.* **2017**, *31*, 2885–2892. [CrossRef] [PubMed]

13. Chen, C.C.; Chou, F.P.; Ho, Y.C.; Lin, W.L.; Wang, C.P.; Kao, E.S.; Huang, A.C.; Wang, C.J. Inhibitory effects of Hibiscus sabdariffa L extract on low-density lipoprotein oxidation and anti-hyperlipidemia in fructose-fed and cholesterol-fed rats. *J. Sci. Food Agric.* **2004**, *84*, 1989–1996. [CrossRef]

14. Farombi, E.O.; Fakoya, A. Free radical scavenging and antigenotoxic activities of natural phenolic compounds in dried flowers of *Hibiscus sabdariffa* L. *Mol. Nutr. Food Res.* **2005**, *49*, 1120–1128. [CrossRef] [PubMed]

15. Lin, H.H.; Huang, H.P.; Huang, C.C.; Chen, J.H.; Wang, C.J. Hibiscus polyphenol-rich extract induces apoptosis in human gastric carcinoma cells via p53 phosphorylation and p38 MAPK/FasL cascade pathway. In *Molecular Carcinogenesis*; University of Texas MD Anderson Cancer Center: Houston, TX, USA, 2005; Volume 43, pp. 86–99.

16. Vilela, T.C.; Leffa, D.D.; Damiani, A.P.; Damazio, D.D.C.; Manenti, A.V.; Carvalho, T.J.G.; Ramlov, F.; Amaral, P.A.; Andrade, V.M. *Hibiscus acetosella* extract protects against alkylating agent-induced DNA damage in mice. *An. Acad. Bras. Ciênc.* **2018**, *90*, 3165–3174. [CrossRef] [PubMed]

17. Abdallah, E.M. Antibacterial efficiency of the Sudanese Roselle (*Hibiscus sabdariffa* L.), a famous beverage from Sudanese folk medicine. *J. Intercult. Ethnopharmacol.* **2016**, *5*, 186. [CrossRef] [PubMed]

18. Jung, E.; Kim, Y.; Joo, N. Physicochemical properties and antimicrobial activity of Roselle (*Hibiscus sabdariffa* L.). *J. Sci. Food Agric.* **2013**, *93*, 3769–3776. [CrossRef]

19. Tsumbu, C.N.; Deby-Dupont, G.; Tits, M.; Angenot, L.; Frederich, M.; Kohnen, S.; Mouithys-Mickalad, A.; Serteyn, D.; Franck, T. Polyphenol content and modulatory activities of some tropical dietary plant extracts on the oxidant activities of neutrophils and myeloperoxidase. *Int. J. Mol. Sci.* **2012**, *13*, 628–650. [CrossRef]

20. Ryu, J.; Kwon, S.-J.; Jo, Y.D.; Jin, C.H.; Nam, B.M.; Lee, S.Y.; Jeong, S.W.; Im, S.B.; Oh, S.C.; Cho, L. Comparison of phytochemicals and antioxidant activity in blackberry (*Rubus fruticosus* L.) fruits of mutant lines at the different harvest time. *Plant Breed. Biotechnol.* **2016**, *4*, 242–251. [CrossRef]

21. Babich, O.; Prosekov, A.; Zaushintsena, A.; Sukhikh, A.; Dyshlyuk, L.; Ivanova, S. Identification and quantification of phenolic compounds of Western Siberia Astragalus danicus in different regions. *Heliyon* **2019**, *5*, e02245. [CrossRef]

22. Jiang, B.; Zhang, Z.-W. Comparison on phenolic compounds and antioxidant properties of cabernet sauvignon and merlot wines from four wine grape-growing regions in China. *Molecules* **2012**, *17*, 8804–8821. [CrossRef]

23. De Leonardis, A.; Pizzella, L.; Macciola, V. Evaluation of chlorogenic acid and its metabolites as potential antioxidants for fish oils. *Eur. J. Lipid Sci. Technol.* **2008**, *110*, 941–948. [CrossRef]

24. Lyu, J.I.; Kim, J.M.; Kim, D.-G.; Kim, J.-B.; Kim, S.H.; Ahn, J.-W.; Kang, S.-Y.; Ryu, J.; Kwon, S.-J. Phenolic compound content of leaf extracts from different Roselle (*Hibiscus sabdariffa*) accessions. *Plant Breed. Biotechnol.* **2020**, *8*, 1–10. [CrossRef]

25. Re, R.; Pellegrini, N.; Proteggente, A.; Pannala, A.; Yang, M.; Rice-Evans, C. Antioxidant activity applying an improved ABTS radical cation decolorization assay. *Free Radic. Biol. Med.* **1999**, *26*, 1231–1237. [CrossRef]

26. Thisakorn, D.; Suradwadee, T.; Warachate, K.; Nakuntwalai, W.; Surachai, T. Antioxidant and free radical scavenging activity of *Hibiscus acetosella* leaves extracts. *Int. J. Appl. Pharm.* **2019**, *11*. [CrossRef]

27. Owoade, A.; Lowe, G.; Khalid, R. The in vitro antioxidant properties of Hibiscus anthocyanins rich extract (HAE). *Nat. Sci.* **2015**, *13*, 22–29.

28. Wu, H.-Y.; Yang, K.-M.; Chiang, P.-Y. Roselle anthocyanins: Antioxidant properties and stability to heat and pH. *Molecules* **2018**, *23*, 1357. [CrossRef]

29. Maciel, L.G.; do Carmo, M.A.V.; Azevedo, L.; Daguer, H.; Molognoni, L.; de Almeida, M.M.; Granato, D.; Rosso, N.D. *Hibiscus sabdariffa* anthocyanins-rich extract: Chemical stability, In Vitro antioxidant and antiproliferative activities. *Food Chem. Toxicol.* **2018**, *113*, 187–197. [CrossRef]

30. Da-Costa-Rocha, I.; Bonnlaender, B.; Sievers, H.; Pischel, I.; Heinrich, M. *Hibiscus sabdariffa* L.—A phytochemical and pharmacological review. *Food Chem.* **2014**, *165*, 424–443. [CrossRef]

31. Lim, H.-W.; Seo, K.-H.; Chon, J.-W.; Song, K.-Y. Antimicrobial activity of *Hibiscus sabdariffa* L. (Roselle) powder against food-borne pathogens present in dairy products: Preliminary study. *J. Dairy Sci. Biotechnol.* **2020**, *38*, 37–44. [CrossRef]

32. Olvera-García, V.; Castaño-Tostado, E.; Rezendiz-Lopez, R.; Reynoso-Camacho, R.; González de Mejía, E.; Elizondo, G.; Loarca-Piña, G. *Hibiscus sabdariffa* L. extracts inhibit the mutagenicity in microsuspension assay and the proliferation of HeLa cells. *J. Food Sci.* **2008**, *73*, T75–T81. [CrossRef]

33. Yang, M.-Y.; Peng, C.-H.; Chan, K.-C.; Yang, Y.-S.; Huang, C.-N.; Wang, C.-J. The hypolipidemic effect of Hibiscus sabdariffa polyphenols via inhibiting lipogenesis and promoting hepatic lipid clearance. *J. Agric. Food Chem.* **2010**, *58*, 850–859. [CrossRef] [PubMed]

34. Tsuda, T.; Horio, F.; Uchida, K.; Aoki, H.; Osawa, T. Dietary cyanidin 3-O-β-D-glucoside-rich purple corn color prevents obesity and ameliorates hyperglycemia in mice. *J. Nutr.* **2003**, *133*, 2125–2130. [CrossRef] [PubMed]

35. Zarkani, A.A. Antimicrobial activity of *Hibiscus sabdariffa* and *Sesbania grandiflora* extracts against some G–ve and G+ ve strains. *Banat. J. Biotechnol.* **2016**, *7*, 17–23. [CrossRef]

36. Sutharut, J.; Sudarat, J. Total anthocyanin content and antioxidant activity of germinated colored rice. *Int. Food Res. J.* **2012**, *19*, 215–221.

Sample Availability: Samples of the compounds are not available from the authors.

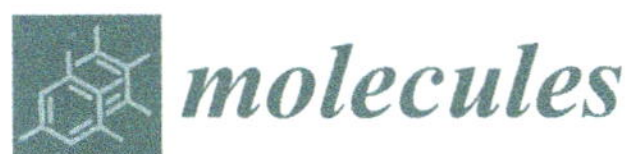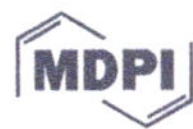

Article

The Impact of Maltodextrin and Inulin on the Protection of Natural Antioxidants in Powders Made of Saskatoon Berry Fruit, Juice, and Pomace as Functional Food Ingredients

Sabina Lachowicz [1,*], Anna Michalska-Ciechanowska [2] and Jan Oszmiański [2]

[1] Department of Fermentation and Cereals Technology, Faculty of Biotechnology and Food Science, Wrocław University of Environmental and Life Sciences, 51–630 Wrocław, Poland
[2] Department of Fruit, Vegetable and Plant Nutraceutical Technology, Faculty of Biotechnology and Food Science, Wrocław University of Environmental and Life Sciences, 51–630 Wrocław, Poland; anna.michalska@upwr.edu.pl (A.M.-C.); jan.oszmianski@upwr.edu.pl (J.O.)
* Correspondence: sabina.lachowicz@upwr.edu.pl

Academic Editors: Raffaele Pezzani and Sara Vitalini
Received: 10 March 2020; Accepted: 10 April 2020; Published: 15 April 2020

Abstract: The objective of this study was to examine the effect of inulin and maltodextrin applied during vacuum drying of Saskatoon berry fruit, juice, and pomace on the retention of bioactive compounds and antioxidant capacity (radical scavenging capacity (ABTS), ferric reducing antioxidant potential (FRAP)) of powders obtained. Ultra-high performance liquid chromatography (UPLC-PDA-ESI-MS/MS) was used to identify major groups of polyphenolic compounds, such as: flavan-3-ols (35% of all polyphenols for fruit powder, 33% for juice powder, and 39% for pomace powders of all polyphenols), anthocyanins (26% for fruit powder, 5% for juice powder, and 34% for pomace), phenolic acids (33% for fruit powder, 55% for juice powder, and 20% for pomace powder), and flavanols (6% for fruit powder, 6% for juice powder, and 7% for pomace powder). In general, the content of polyphenols was more dependent on the content than on the type of carrier used for drying, regardless of the matrix tested. The average sum of polyphenols and the antioxidant activity (for ABTS and FRAP assay) of the powders with 30% of carrier addition were 5054.2 mg/100 g dry matter (d.m.) as well as 5.3 and 3.6 mmol Trolox/100 g d.m. in the ABTS and FRAP tests, respectively. The increase in carrier concentration by 20% caused a decrease of 1.5-fold in the content of polyphenols and a 1.6-fold and 1.5-fold in the antioxidant potential, regardless of the matrix tested. The principal component analysis (PCA) analysis indicated that the freeze-drying process led to the lowest degradation of the identified compounds, regardless of the matrix tested, with the exception of juice and pomace powders dried by vacuum drying at 60 °C. In this case, the release of (−)-epicatechin was observed, causing an increase in the flavanol contents. Thus, this work demonstrated the effect of processing and matrix composition on the preservation of antioxidant bioactives in Saskatoon berry powders. Properly designed high-quality Saskatoon berry powders with the mentioned carriers may be used as nutraceutical additives to fortify food products and to improve their functional properties.

Keywords: *Amelanchier alnifolia* Nutt.; carriers; powders; bioactive compounds; functional food

---

1. Introduction

Saskatoon berry (*Amelanchier alnifolia* Nutt.) belongs to the *Rosaceae* family and is commonly found in the North America [1,2], and also in Poland. In folk medicine, it was used to combat many ailments [3]. Its fruits contain polyphenolic compounds, like e.g., anthocyanins, phenolic acids (mainly hydroxycinnamic acids), polymers of procyanidins, (+)-catechins, (−)-epicatechins, and quercetin derivatives [3,4]. These compounds have a wide spectrum of biological functions and biochemical activities, e.g., anti-diabetic, anti-inflammatory, antioxidant, and anti-cancer properties [1,3,5,6].

In order to preserve of bioactive constituents from fruits during processing, the powdering process has recently been proposed as one of the possible ways to obtain products with natural health-promoting constituents. The processing of fruits, including thermal treatment, causes significant changes in the composition of processed products compared to the raw materials [7]. The transformation of fruit material into powdered is made easier when the addition of a carrier agent is applied. Such an approach may lead to stability improvement of natural bioactive compounds during further processing. This may allow entrapping polyphenolic compounds in the carrier shell or matrix so that the thermolabile active substance gains protection against degradation and their stability [8–10]. The most commonly used carriers include maltodextrin, gums, proteins, and starches [11,12]. Recently, carriers with functional properties have been used during food the powdering process. In this study, we used two carriers: maltodextrin—because it is the most commonly used carrier, and inulin—due to its proven prebiotic effects and pro-health potential. What is more, the addition of maltodextrin and inulin improve the drying yield [13,14].

The selection of carriers, their concentration, and drying technique are all important factors that affect the profile and concentration of antioxidant compounds. Although the impact of carriers and their concentration on the profile of bioactive compounds in fruit powders has been evaluated in some previous studies [15,16], there is lack of information on the impact of these factors on the phytochemicals of *Amelanchier alnifolia* Nutt. Thus, the objective of the present study was to investigate the influence of maltodextrin and inulin used as a carrier and of their concentration on the quantitative and qualitative composition of polyphenolic profile of *Amelanchier alnifolia* Nutt. fruit, juice, and pomace powders obtained by freeze-drying and vacuum-drying at 50 and 60 °C. Polyphenol profile was determined by ultra-high performance liquid chromatography (UPLC-PDA-ESI-MS/MS) and their antioxidant properties determined by radical scavenging capacity (ABTS), and ferric reducing antioxidant potential (FRAP).

2. Results and Discussion

2.1. Polyphenolic Content and Chemical Profile

In the present study, polyphenolic compounds were determined using UPLC-PDA-ESI-MS/MS in Saskatoon berry powders with carriers considering the type of the material subjected to drying (whole fruit, juice, pomace), the drying method, and the type of carrier and its concentration (Table 1 and Tables S1–S4). Detailed analyses allowed identifying 42 compounds classified to four main groups as anthocyanins, phenolic acids, flavonols, and flavan-3-ols. Their presence in powders obtained from Saskatoon berry fruits was also confirmed in earlier works [1,2,4,6,17,18].

The most abundant group belonging to polyphenolic compounds was represented in the analyzed powders by flavan-3-ols (monomers, oligomers, and polymeric procyanidins). These compounds were previously identified in fruits by Lachowicz et al. [6,17]. This group accounted for 35% of total polyphenolic compounds in fruit powder, for 33% in juice powder, and for 39% in pomace powder. Among the monomers and oligomers, the presence of 14 compounds was identified; they accounted for 36% of total flavan-3-ols in fruit powder, for 67% in juice powder, and for 20% in pomace powder. In addition, the presence of polymeric procyanidins was determined by phloroglucinolysis (they accounted for 64% of total flavan-3-ols in fruit powder, for 33% in juice powder, and for 80% in pomace powder) (Table S1). In this research two monomers (main ion at m/z 289), two dimers (main ion at m/z 577), five trimers (main ion at m/z 863), and five tetramers (main ion at m/z 1153) were identified based on MS data and available literature [1,17].

Anthocyanins were the second abundant group determined in the powders [1] and constituted 26% of total polyphenolic compounds in fruit powder, 5% in juice powder, and 34% in pomace powder. Furthermore, six cyanidins were identified including four glycosides of cyanidins (cyanidin-3-*O*-galactoside: *m/z* 449, -3-*O*-glucoside: *m/z* 499, -3-*O*-xyloside: *m/z* 419, -3-*O*-arabinoside: *m/z* 419) and two cyanidin aglycons (*m/z* 287). Among the 6 identified compounds, the major compound belonging to anthocyanins was cyanidin-3-*O*-galactoside (it accounted for 69.9% of all anthocyanins). This was confirmed in earlier reports [2].

Phenolic acids were the next group of polyphenols that accounted for 33% of total polyphenolic compounds in fruit powder, for 55% in juice powder, and for 20% in pomace powder. According to the MS spectra, standards, and literature, eight hydroxycinnamic acids were determined, including: three isomers of caffeoylquinic acid (*m/z* 353), two coumaroylquinic acids (*m/z* 353), and three isomers of caffeic acids (*m/z* 341), as well as one hydroxybenzoic acid identified as protocatechuic acid (*m/z* 153). The major phenolic acids were 5-*O*-caffeoylquinic acid (56% of all phenolic acids), and 4-*O*-caffeoylquinic acid (19%). The mass noted on the negative mode was *m/z* 353 with similar MS spectra to those reported in literature [1,2].

The last and the smallest group of phenolic compounds was constituted by flavonols [17]. This group accounted for 6% of total flavonols in fruit powder, for 6% in juice powder, and for 7% in pomace powder; and the major compound was quercetin-3-*O*-galactoside [1,2] which represented 46% of all flavonols. In this work, thirteen flavonols were identified including ten glycosides of kaempferol and quercetin (based on ion at *m/z* 285 and 301, respectively), two acetylated compounds (*m/z* 507), and one quercetin aglycon (*m/z* 301) [1,2].

The average total content of identified polyphenols was 6535 mg/100 g d.m. in pomace powders. Their content was lower by 38% and 70% in fruit and juice powders, respectively (Table 1 and Tables S1–S4). This is due to the accumulation location of these constituents in the outer layer of the fruit that remains in the pomace during pressing [19,20]. In addition, the highest antioxidant capacity was found in pomace powders and was 3.4-fold (ABTS assay) and 3-fold (FRAP assay) higher when compared to the fruit powders as well as 7-fold (ABTS assay) and 6-fold (FRAP assay) compared to juice powders (Table 2). These relationships were also confirmed during the drying of chokeberry [21] and cranberry fruits [22] and can be explained by distribution of phenols, because they are not equally distributed in the plant material [22]. Anthocyanins and flavonols are mostly presented in the peel of berry, also polymeric procyanidins, monomers, and oligomers of flavan-3-ols are essentially located in the peel, but some content of these compounds occur in the pulp thus in the juice [21,22]. In addition, conditions of juice processing, mash maceration, and the type of enzymatic preparation may significantly impact the content of polyphenols in the juice and pomace of product [21,22]. This fact is widely known in the literature, but there is little information on the impact of carriers and their quantity and drying methods on the individual matrix, especially of Saskatoon berry. What is more, according to literature [1–3,17,23,24], the Saskatoon berry fruits are an excellent source of polyphenolic compounds and antioxidant properties responsible for their proved anti-inflammatory, antidiabetic, and chemo-protective effects. They have more bioactive compounds than e.g., blueberry, blackberry, bilberry, raspberry, and strawberry [25,26]. However, little is known about the use of this raw material as a functional additive. Available data relate only to Saskatoon berry supplements and used the accumulation of plasma levels of anthocyanins [27]. *Amelanchier alnifolia* Nutt. (90 g) were administered immediately after every low antioxidant meal. The authors noted plasma concentrations of cyanidin-3-*O*-xyloside and cyanidin-3-*O*-galactoside were significantly increased following 3 consecutive supplements 4 h apart. Therefore, they recommend that anthocyanin supplements with every meal would higher their plasma concentrations [27]. Another work concerned the prevention of diabetes in obese mice by consuming Saskatoon berry [28]. Male mice were served a control diet, high fat and high sucrose diet, and high fat and high sucrose with 5% of Saskatoon berry powder (weight/weight) diet for 15 weeks. The results showed that Saskatoon berry powder suppressed high fat, high sucrose diet-induced hyperglycemia, hyperlipidemia, insulin resistance, and vascular inflammation [28]. Therefore, research was undertaken to obtain new functional additives (powders) from various Saskatoon berry matrices with the highest possible content of antioxidant compounds.

2.2. Influence Type of Carriers on Polyphenolic Compounds and Antioxidant Capacity in Dependence on the Matrix

The principal component analysis (PCA) was used to study the impact of the type of carriers on the protection of polyphenolic compounds and their antioxidant activity depending on the matrix tested (Figure 1). It showed that in the case of fruit powders, drying in the presence of inulin was associated with a higher concentration and protection of flavan-3-ols group and their individual compounds ((+)-catechin, B-type procyanidin: dimer, and tetramer, and A-type procyanidin dimer), 3 and 4-*O*-caffeoylquinic acids, di-caffeoylquinic acid, and cyanidin-3-*O*-arabinoside. While maltodextrin caused the higher retention and ensured protection of polymeric procyanidins, total phenolic acids and their derivatives, total flavonols and their derivatives, total anthocyanins and their derivatives, and total phenolic acids and their antioxidant activity (strong correlation with the ferric reducing antioxidant potential (FRAP)) and positive correlation with the radical scavenging capacity (ABTS)). Bakowska-Barczak and Kołodziejczyk [29] also reported that the use of maltodextrin resulted in the highest contents of anthocyanins and polyphenols in black currant powders. The higher retention of polyphenolic compounds was also noted in cactus pear with maltodextrin when compared to inulin [30]. In turn, PCA analysis showed that in the case of juice powders, inulin had a stronger impact on total flavonols and their main derivatives, (+)-catechin, (−)-epicatechin, B-type procyanidin dimer, polymeric procyanidins, cyanidin-3-*O*-arabinoside, and 3-*O*-caffeoylquinic acid; while, maltodextrin led to the higher retention of total phenolic acid, total anthocyanins, total flavan-3-ols. What is more, the ability to scavenge the ABTS radicals was higher in the case of the juice powders with maltodextrin addition, whereas higher FRAP values were noted for the powders prepared with inulin. The addition of maltodextrin into juice powders affected the release of free cyanidin and quercetin aglycons. Whereas, in black currant juice powder, the use of inulin resulted in a 9% higher anthocyanin retention compared to the use of maltodextrin [16]. Furthermore, the PCA analysis of pomace powders showed that the product with inulin had higher contents of total of polyphenolic compounds, A and B-type procyanidin dimer, polymeric procyanidin, and quercetin-3-*O*-robinobioside, and also a higher degree of polymerization. This product had higher antioxidant potency, while maltodextrin was responsible for the protection of total anthocyanins and their derivatives, total flavan-3-ols and their derivatives, total phenolic acids and their derivatives, and total flavonols and their derivatives. Thus, the type of carrier and its impact on antioxidant compounds depended mainly on the analyzed matrix. The high antioxidant power of the juice and pomace powders with inulin and also of the fruit powders with maltodextrin can be affected by polymerized compounds. This can also be confirmed by a strong correlation between the polymerized compounds and antioxidant activity i.e., $r = 0.997$ for FRAP and 0.430 for ABTS (for fruit powders), $r = 0.995$ and 0.998 for FRAP and ABTS assay (juice powders), and $r = 0.997$ and 0.998 for FRAP and ABTS assay (pomace powders). Therefore, the choice of a carrier will largely depend on the desired composition of bioactive compounds with antioxidant activity for the functional additive regardless of the Saskatoon berry matrix tested.

A

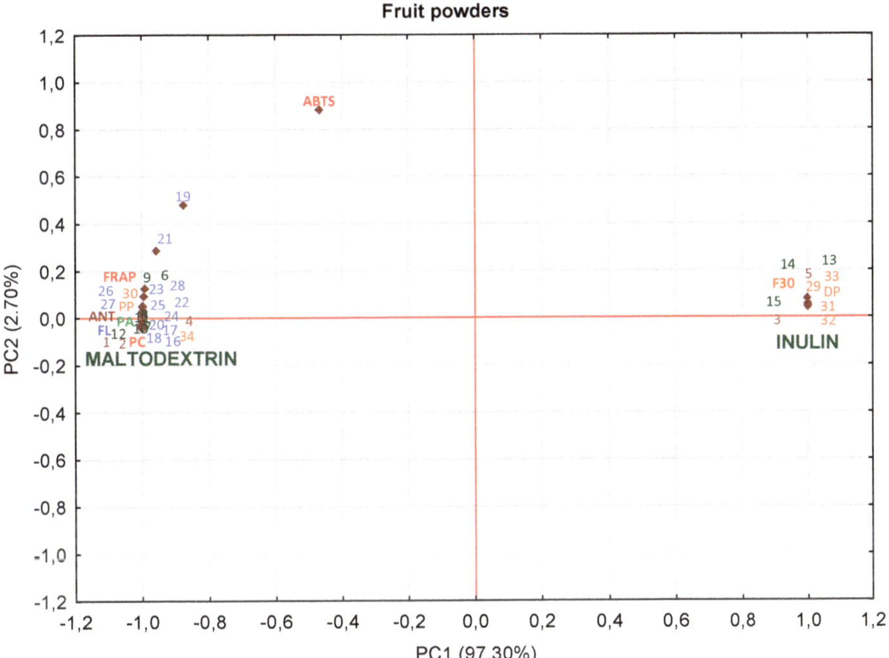

B

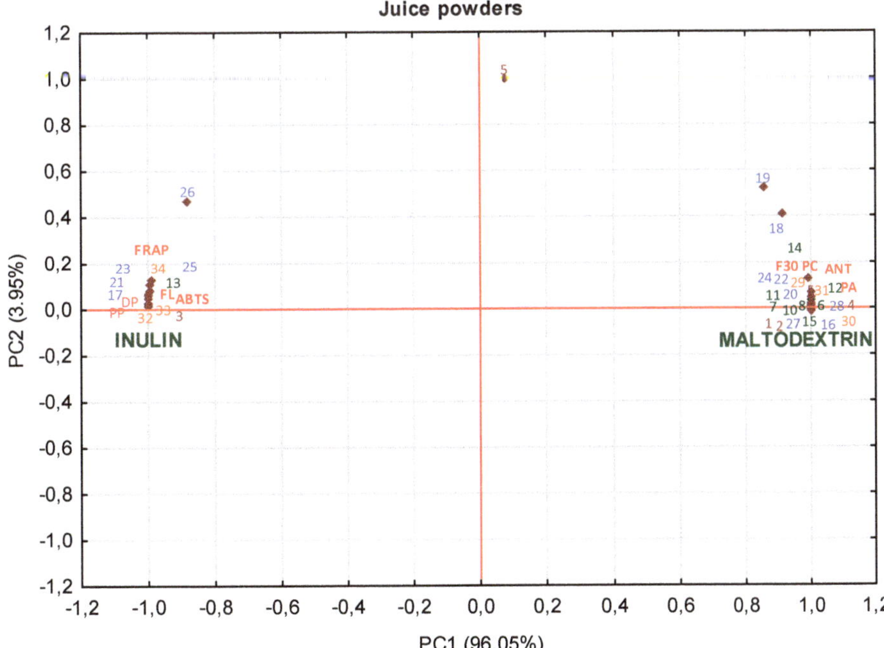

Figure 1. *Cont.*

C

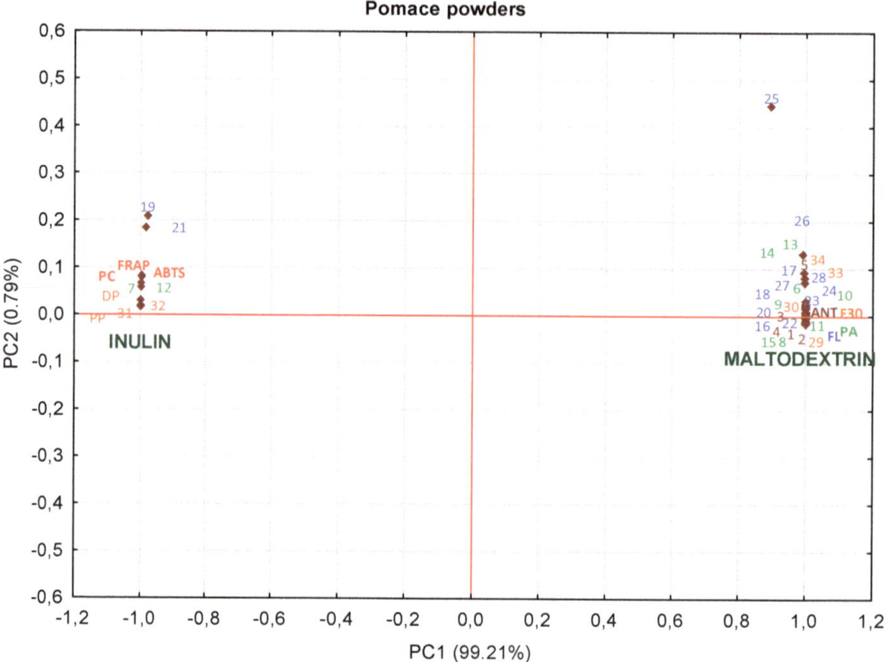

Figure 1. Principal component analysis (PCA) of the impact of type of carrier to phytochemical parameter in fruit (**A**), juice (**B**), pomace (**C**) powders. *Abbreviations:* ANT—sum of anthocyanins; FL—sum of flavonols; PA—sum of phenolic acid; PP—polymeric procyanidins; F3O—sum of flavan-3-ols (monomers and oligomers); DP—degree of polymerization; PC—sum of polyphenolic compounds; **1**—cyanidin-3-*O*-galactoside; **2**—cyanidin-3-*O*-glucoside; **3**—cyanidin-3-*O*-arabinoside; **4**—cyanidin-3-*O*-xyloside; **5**—cyanidin; **6**—protocatechuic acid; **7**—caffeic acid glucoside; **8**—caffeoylhexose; **9**—acid isomers; **10**—3-*O*-caffeoylquinic acid; **11**—5-*O*-caffeoylquinic acid; **12**—4-*O*-caffeoylquinic acid; **13**—3-*O*-*p*-coumaroylquinic acid; **14**—di-caffeoylquinic acid; **15**—di-caffeoylquinic acid; **16**—kaempferol-3-*O*-galactoside; **17**—quercetin-3-*O*-arabinobioside; **18**—kampferol-3-*O*-glucoside; **19**—quercetin; **20**—quercetin-3-*O*-rutinoside; **21**—quercetin-3-*O*-robinobioside; **22**—quercetin-3-*O*-galactoside; **23**—quercetin-3-*O*-glucoside; **24**—quercetin-3-*O*-arabinoside; **25**—quercetin-3-*O*-xyloside; **26**—quercetin-3-*O*-(6″-acetyl)glucoside; **27**—quercetin-3-*O*-(6″-acetyl)galactoside; **28**—quercetin-deoxyhexo-hexoside; **29**—sum of B-type procyanidin tetramer; **30**—sum of B-type procyanidin trimer; **31**—sum of B-type procyanidin dimer; **32**—A-type procyanidin dimer; **33**—(-)-epicatechin; **34**—(+)-catechin.

2.3. Impact of the Amount of Added Carriers' on Polyphenols Content and Antioxidant Capacity in Dependence on the Matrix

The concentration of carriers had a stronger impact on the retention of polyphenolic compounds than the type of carrier or drying method. A similar observation was made for black currant powders with the use of the mentioned-above carriers for drying [16]. In turn, addition of maltodextrin at the level of 15% was found to protect the bioactive compounds from thermal degradation [31]. The principal component analysis (PCA) was used to evaluate the influence of the concentration of carriers on the protection of antioxidant compounds depending on the matrix tested (Figure 2). PCA graph for powders with 30% of carriers showed by 20% and 37% higher content of total polyphenols, and by 29% and 47% higher antioxidant potential determined with ABTS and FRAP assays compared to the powders obtained with 40% and 50% of carriers, respectively, regardless of the matrix tested. Probably, the content of phenolics was affected by the dilution effect with the carrier; the higher the carrier concentration, the lower the content of bioactive compounds. A similar observation was made in the case of *Eugenia dysenterica* DC. powders pointing to a concentration of a carrier on the content of polyphenols. Samples obtained using 10% of carriers showed the highest content of polyphenols, while the powders with 30% of carrier presenting the lowest amount of phenols [32]. This can also be confirmed by a strong positive correlation between individual polyphenolic compounds (anthocyanins, phenolic acids, flavonols, flavan-3-ols) and antioxidant activity (ABTS assay) of $r = 0.979, 0.999, 0.998,$ 0.992 (for fruit powders), $r = 0.993, 0.974, 0.998, 0.999$ (juice powders), and $r = 0.958, 0.993, 0.994, 0.998$ (pomace powders). Depending on the matrix, the lowest loss of polyphenolic compounds was noted in juice powders and it was 17% and 21% with 40% and 50% of carriers compared to the powders with 30% of carriers. While in fruit and pomace powders losses were 11% and 18% higher. Greater degradation of flavan-3-ols (monomers and oligomer) and polymeric procyanidin was found in the fruit and pomace powders than in the juice powders; it reached ca. 24% and 30%. As for the anthocyanins, the greatest degradation was found in fruit powder (ca. 43% in product with 50% of carrier) > pomace powder (around 40%) > juice powders (38%). While, the smallest degradation of phenolic acids and flavonols was found in the pomace powders—around 15% and 26% and 12% and 28% in products with 40% and 50% of carriers, respectively, compared to the final product with 30% of carrier. Probably high stability can be due to presence of cell wall polysaccharide compounds e.g., pectins, whether lower water activity [21,22]. Additionally, it might be due to the better encapsulation process of these samples, which is confirmed by Daza et al. [32] who followed the highest retentions of bioactive compounds in cagaita powders with 20%–30% of carriers. However, the higher carrier concentration affected the protection of individual compounds, e.g., in the case of fruit powders—40% of carrier influenced higher protection of cyanidin-3-O-arabinose and a higher degree of polymerization, but 50% of carrier affected the B-type procyanidin tetramer. Whereas in the case of juice powders—40% of carrier caused high retention of quercetin-3-O-robinobioside, -3-O-arabinoside, -3-O-glucoside, and protocatechuic acid, but 50% of carrier caused a high degree of polymerization. Finally, in the case of pomace powders—40% of carrier caused a high degree of polarization just like in the fruit powders. Indicating that might have led to a release of the compounds from more polymerized structures. Similarly as with pulp and juice powders made from cagaita and plum, the concentration of carriers had a strong influence on the decrease of total polyphenolic compounds [32,33]. Thus, the higher carrier concentration led to a lower polyphenol content and lower antioxidant activity, indicating the strong effect of the initial composition of the matrix tested. Moreover, dried products with carriers showed a 1.6 and 1.9, and 1.5 times higher protection of the antioxidant capacity and phenolic compounds, than the products without carriers [17]. Which is also confirmed by other authors who confirmed that the use of carriers affects the protection of bioactive compounds [32,33]. Different interactions between the powders compounds and the carrier might also occur compared to the powders without a carrier [32].

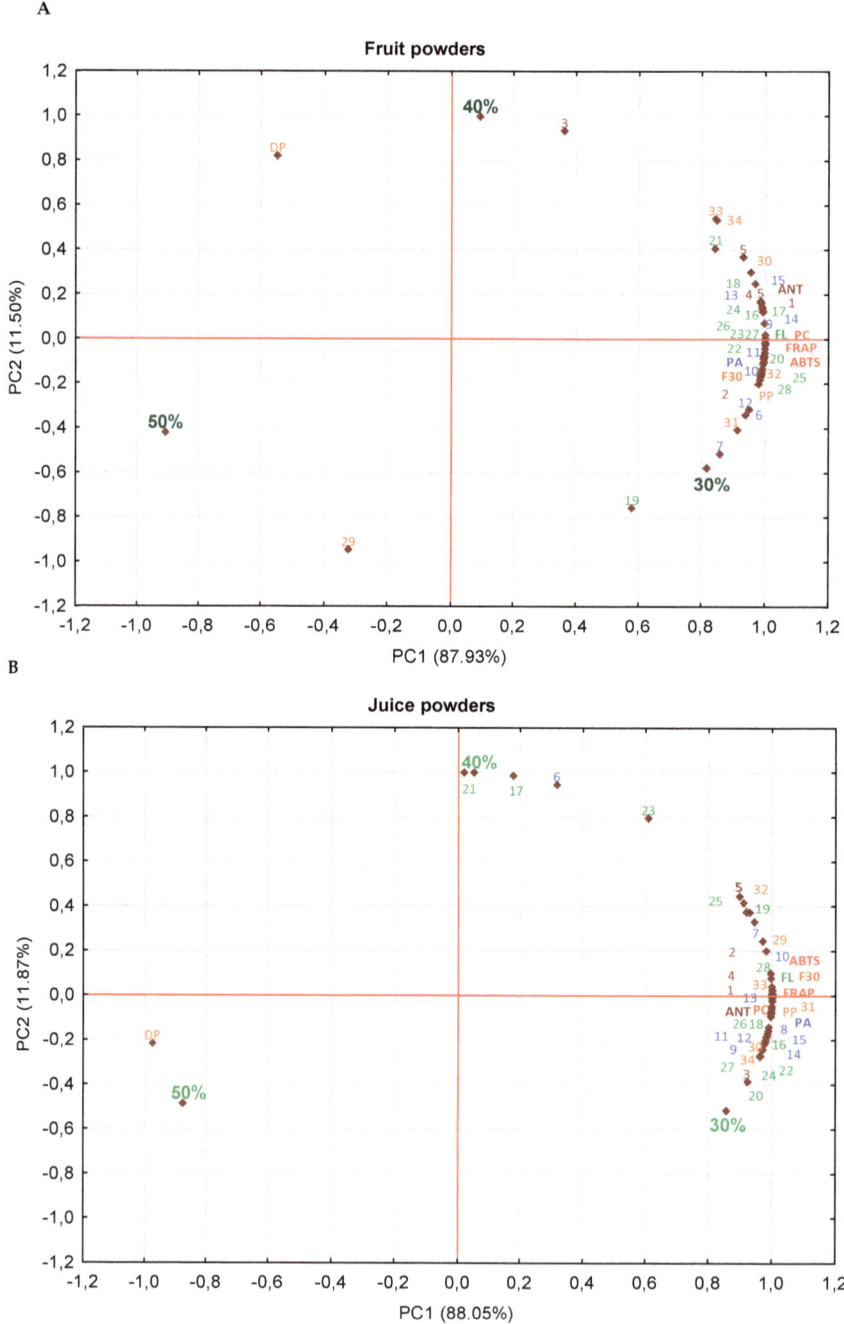

Figure 2. *Cont.*

C

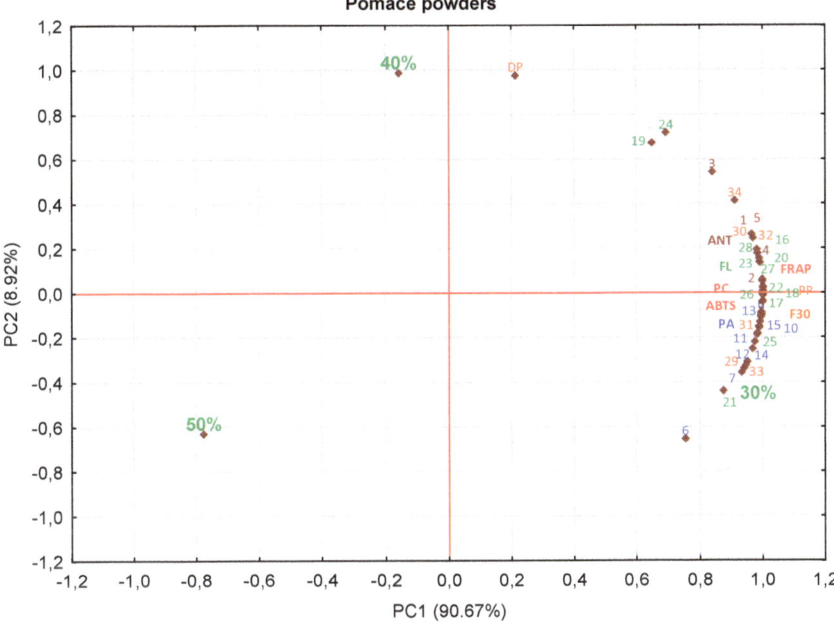

Figure 2. Principal component analysis (PCA) of the impact of carriers' concentration on phytochemicals in fruit (**A**), juice (**B**), pomace (**C**) powders. *Abbreviations:* 30%, 40%, 50%, concentration; ANT—sum of anthocyanins; FL—sum of flavonols; PA—sum of phenolic acid; PP—polymeric procyanidins; F3O—sum of flavan-3-ols (monomers and oligomers); DP—degree of polymerization; PC—sum of polyphenolic compounds; **1**—cyanidin-3-*O*-galactoside; **2**—cyanidin-3-*O*-glucoside; **3**—cyanidin-3-*O*-arabinoside; **4**—cyanidin-3-*O*-xyloside; **5**—cyanidin; **6**—protocatechuic acid; **7**—caffeic acid glucoside; **8**—caffeoylhexose; **9**—trihydroxycinnamoylquinic acid isomers; **10**—3-*O*-caffeoylquinic acid; **11**—5-*O*-caffeoylquinic acid; **12**—4-*O*-caffeoylquinic acid; **13**—3-*O*-*p*-coumaroylquinic acid; **14**—di-caffeoylquinic acid; **15**—di-caffeoylquinic acid; **16**—kaempferol-3-*O*-galactoside; **17**—quercetin-3-*O*-arabinobioside; **18**—kaempferol-3-*O*-glucoside; **19**—quercetin; **20**—quercetin-3-*O*-rutinoside; **21**—quercetin-3-*O*-robinobioside; **22**—quercetin-3-*O*-galactoside; **23**—quercetin-3-*O*-glucoside; **24**—quercetin-3-*O*-arabinoside; **25**—quercetin-3-*O*-xyloside; **26**—quercetin-3-*O*-(6″-acetyl)glucoside; **27**—quercetin-3-*O*-(6″-acetyl)galactoside; **28**—quercetin-deoxyhexo-hexoside; **29**—sum of B-type procyanidin tetramer; **30**—sum of B-type procyanidin trimer; **31**—sum of B-type procyanidin dimer; **32**—A-type procyanidin dimer; **33**—(-)-epicatechin; **34**—(+)-catechin.

2.4. Impact of the Type of Drying Method on Polyphenolic Compounds and Antioxidant Capacity in Dependence on the Matrix

The PCA analyses showed that the powders produced after the freeze-drying process had the highest content of almost all polyphenolic compounds and antioxidant activity, regardless of the matrix tested (Figure 3). Similar observations were made during drying *Averrhoa carambola* pomace. The freeze-drying with carriers was more effective in ensuring the retention of polyphenolic compounds when compared to spray drying [12]. Moreover, after freeze-drying *Averrhoa carambola* pomace, it was noted that the higher the drying process temperature, the lower the antioxidant activity, while opposite observation was made for the juice powder. The higher the vacuum drying temperature, the stronger the degradation of anthocyanins in juice powders made from black currant. However, vacuum drying at 50 °C affected high retained phenolic acids and flavonols [16]. The best effect of drying cranberry products was obtained after spray-drying and freeze-drying, while an increase in aglycon of quercetin after vacuum-drying at 60 °C was observed [31]. Therefore, it can be concluded that the antioxidant activity of the tested material was dependent on the content of polyphenolic compounds, which did not degrade under mild freeze-drying conditions.

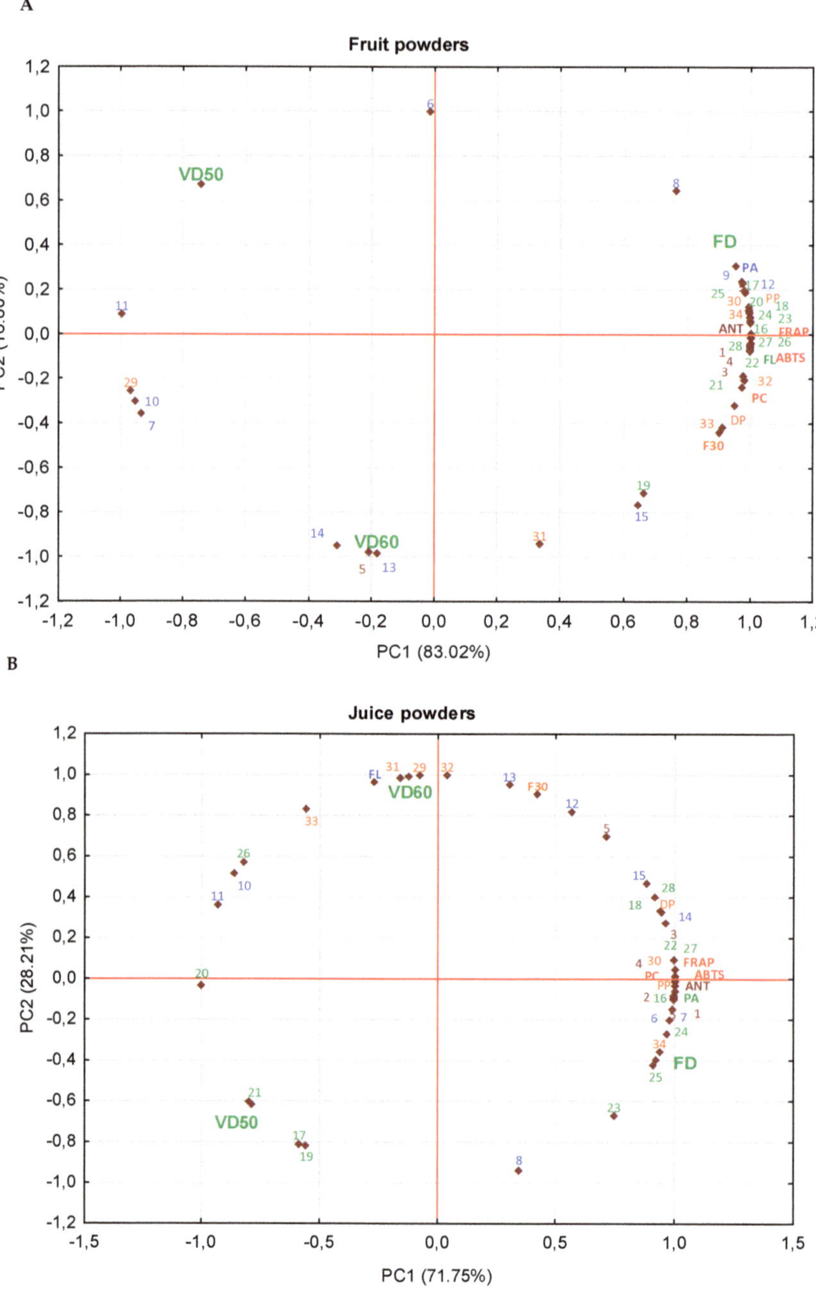

Figure 3. *Cont.*

C

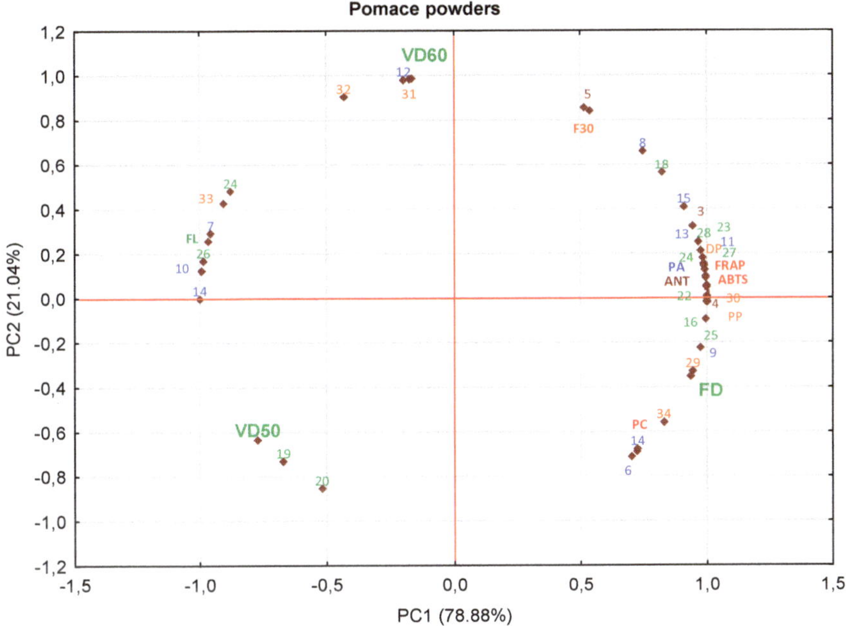

Figure 3. Principal component analysis (PCA) of the impact of drying method on phytochemicals in fruit (**A**), juice (**B**), pomace (**C**) powders. *Abbreviations:* FD, freeze-drying; VD/50, vacuum-drying in 50 °C; VD/60, vacuum-drying in 60 °C; ANT—sum of anthocyanins; FL—sum of flavonols; PA—sum of phenolic acid; PP—polymeric procyanidins; F3O—sum of flavan-3-ols (monomers and oligomers); DP—degree of polymerization; PC—sum of polyphenolic compounds, **1**—cyanidin-3-*O*-galactoside; **2**—cyanidin-3-*O*-glucoside; **3**—cyanidin-3-*O*-arabinoside; **4**—cyanidin-3-*O*-xyloside; **5**—cyanidin; **6**—protocatechuic acid; **7**—caffeic acid glucoside; **8**—caffeoylhexose; **9**—trihydroxycinnamoylquinic acid isomers; **10**—3-*O*-caffeoylquinic acid; **11**—5-*O*-caffeoylquinic acid; **12**—4-*O*-caffeoylquinic acid; **13**—3-*O*-*p*-coumaroylquinic acid; **14**—di-caffeoylquinic acid; **15**—di-caffeoylquinic acid; **16**—kaempferol-3-*O*-galactoside; **17**—quercetin-3-*O*-arabinobioside; **18**—kampferol-3-*O*-glucoside; **19**—quercetin; **20**—quercetin-3-*O*-xrutinoside; **21**—quercetin-3-*O*-robinobioside; **22**—quercetin-3-*O*-galactoside; **23**—quercetin-3-*O*-glucoside; **24**—quercetin-3-*O*-arabinoside; **25**—quercetin-3-*O*-xyloside; **26**—quercetin-3-*O*-(6''-acetyl)glucoside; **27**—quercetin-3-*O*-(6''-acetyl)galactoside; **28**—quercetin-deoxyhexo-hexoside; **29**—sum of B-type procyanidin tetramer; **30**—sum of B-type procyanidin trimer; **31**—sum of B-type procyanidin dimer; **32**—A-type procyanidin dimer; **33**—(-)-epicatechin; **34**—(+)-catechin.

Vacuum drying method affected the retention of individual compounds: for fruit powders, vacuum drying at 50 °C resulted in a higher retention of hydroxybenzoic acid (protocatechuic acid), and hydroxycinnamic acid (caffeic acid) in powders whereas drying at 60 °C had an impact on B-type procyanidin dimer, and tetramer, 4, 3-*O*-caffeoylquinic acids, di-caffeoylquinic acid, free cyanidin, and quercetin aglycon. In the case of juice powders, application of the temperature of 50 °C during vacuum drying resulted in a higher retention of quercetin-3-*O*-robinobioside, -3-*O*-arabinoside, and quercetin aglycon. Drying at 60 °C influenced a higher content of total flavonols and their derivatives, flavan-3-ols and their monomers and oligomers, and free cyanidin aglycon. However, in blackcurrant juice powders, the vacuum drying at 50 °C and 70 °C caused a higher retention of anthocyanins, and according to the authors, this could be due to the inactivation of polyphenol oxidase [16]. In the present study, the higher temperature contributed only to the release of free aglycon of anthocyanins. As far as the pomace powders are concerned, the vacuum drying at 50 °C had a strong impact on the content of free aglycon, and quercetin-3-*O*-rutinoside. The drying at 60 °C influenced the retention of monomers ((−)-epicatechin) and oligomers of flavan-3-ols, and total flavonols and their derivatives. On the other hand, among all compounds identified in flavan-3-ols group, (−)-epicatechin content in juice powders was 2.8 times higher after vacuum drying at 60 °C when compared to the freeze-drying. This suggests the temperature-depended release of this compound from polymerized structures. A similar observation was made for blackcurrant juice the vacuum drying of which at 90 °C resulted in 130 times higher (+)-catechin content compared to vacuum drying at 50 °C. The authors concluded that the controlled release of compounds from polymerized structures during drying may be helpful in obtaining the desired content of polyphenolic compounds in the powders [16]. In turn, a similar increase of flavonols aglycon content under the influence of high temperature as a result of the deglycosylation of flavonol glycosides was observed in cranberry products [31,34]. In addition, similarly to cranberry juice powders [31], the temperature influenced the retention of total flavonols in juice and pomace powders made from Saskatoon berry. This can also be confirmed by negative correlation between flavonols and antioxidant activity of $r = -0.265$ for ABTS assay, and $r = -0.253$ for FRAP assay (for juice powders), and $r = -0.925$ for ABTS assay, and $r = -0.890$ for FRAP assay (pomace powders). Moreover, the increased content of flavonols and their derivatives was also observed upon vacuum drying of juice and pomace powders made of black currant at 50 °C and 70 °C [16,35]; however, the authors observed that an increase of temperature above 80 °C and 90 °C decreased flavonols content. Among all of the compounds tested, anthocyanins were the most unstable constituents when the higher temperature of drying was applied. Their average amount after vacuum drying at 50 °C was 42% lower when compared to the freeze-drying. Moreover, the increase of the temperature during vacuum drying by 10 °C caused their 13% loss. Bakowska-Barczak and Kołodziejczyk [29] reported that the higher the temperature during drying black current powder, the stronger the degradation of anthocyanins. Cai and Corke [36] also noted that a higher drying temperature had a stronger effect on amaranthus betacyanins degradation. On the other hand, depending on the matrix tested, the smallest degradation of anthocyanins was noted in the pomace powder after freeze-drying and it was 1.4 and 1.7 times lower when compared to vacuum drying at 50 and 60 °C, respectively. While, degradation of anthocyanins in the fruit and juice powder after vacuum drying at 50 and 60 °C was 56% and 65%. Probably the highest retention of compounds from pomace can be due to lower water activity, and also with location of compounds because most of them are distributed in berry skin which does not lead to their complete degradation during heat conditions [21,22]. Thus, the research confirmed that mild conditions of freeze-drying ensured the protection of anthocyanins, and this was in line with the previous reports showing that the temperature strongly affected their degradation [37–39]. Moreover, the higher the drying temperature is, the greater the degradation of the polyphenolic compounds and their antioxidant activity. The temperature of 50 °C influenced the release of quercetin aglycon. Regardless of the matrix tested, the temperature of 60 °C used for vacuum drying resulted in greater retention of phenolic acid derivatives as well as flavan-3-ols monomers ((−)-epicatechin) and oligomers. It could be due to the partial inactivation of polyphenol oxidase, because Siddiq et al. [40] noted that PPO lost about partial inactivation during thermal treatment of blueberry at 55 and 65 °C [40]. Therefore, the selection of drying technique for the preparation of Saskatoon berry powders is highly important when the retention of bioactive compounds is concerned.

Table 1. The sum of anthocyanins, phenolic acids, flavan-3-ols, polymeric procyanidins, and total polyphenolic compounds [mg/100 g d.m.] in the fruit, juice, and pomace powders made form Saskatoon berry.

Drying Method	Type of Carriers	Con. [%]	Anthocyanins	Phenolic Acids	Flavonols	Flavavan-3-ols	Polymeric Procyanidins	Total of Polyphenolic Compounds
			FRUIT					
FD	Inulin	30	2457.6 ± 662.6 [1]	1572.4 ± 266.0	365.1 ± 57.5	597.7 ± 493.3	2537.6 ± 493.3	6625.0 ± 1177.7
		40	1887.7 ± 489.4	1175.5 ± 195.0	311.0 ± 46.6	557.5 ± 194.0	1313.9 ± 194.0	4423.7 ± 791.3
		50	1282.0 ± 335.9	932.5 ± 161.6	254.4 ± 35.9	510.6 ± 166.6	1149.0 ± 166.6	3399.4 ± 578.2
	Maltodextrin	30	2195.9 ± 608.3	1505.3 ± 259.5	408.5 ± 64.0	592.8 ± 447.0	2354.3 ± 447.0	6119.6 ± 1073.5
		40	1497.8 ± 382.9	1337.0 ± 230.6	329.4 ± 49.5	560.6 ± 236.3	1490.9 ± 236.3	4375.3 ± 724.0
		50	1111.8 ± 305.1	907.1 ± 147.8	231.0 ± 31.1	463.7 ± 134.6	975.0 ± 134.6	3025.0 ± 505.7
VD/50	Inulin	30	741.3 ± 243.9	1831.3 ± 306.8	342.7 ± 54.4	550.6 ± 381.0	2049.7 ± 381.0	4676.7 ± 959.1
		40	809.5 ± 262.6	1312.9 ± 232.1	271.1 ± 40.0	532.5 ± 261.9	1557.8 ± 261.9	3720.2 ± 687.4
		50	617.5 ± 208.6	980.3 ± 175.5	229.6 ± 31.3	437.7 ± 142.8	973.5 ± 142.8	2602.6 ± 460.4
	Maltodextrin	30	897.8 ± 303.4	1905.5 ± 326.2	359.7 ± 56.5	517.2 ± 269.2	1576.6 ± 269.2	4436.4 ± 841.3
		40	681.7 ± 217.8	1474.7 ± 263.5	270.7 ± 40.2	500.6 ± 177.8	1183.7 ± 177.8	3380.3 ± 645.4
		50	496.6 ± 165.4	963.4 ± 165.6	217.5 ± 29.9	440.5 ± 121.7	885.1 ± 121.7	2375.0 ± 440.6
VD/60	Inulin	30	874.5 ± 288.3	1743.3 ± 288.3	352.2 ± 56.6	575.9 ± 369.3	2029.3 ± 369.3	4703.8 ± 916.3
		40	665.9 ± 215.0	1280.0 ± 208.8	266.0 ± 39.3	497.6 ± 186.1	1218.0 ± 186.1	3203.2 ± 594.7
		50	555.8 ± 189.4	868.5 ± 144.8	222.0 ± 30.5	468.5 ± 210.7	1283.5 ± 210.7	2738.3 ± 540.5
	Maltodextrin	30	735.2 ± 242.1	1708.9 ± 281.9	352.6 ± 56.5	529.3 ± 200.9	1314.4 ± 200.9	3814.9 ± 742.4
		40	592.4 ± 192.4	1200.8 ± 190.7	262.6 ± 39.5	416.0 ± 114.0	835.0 ± 114.0	2667.7 ± 503.9
		50	493.7 ± 164.4	919.0 ± 146.4	226.8 ± 31.3	433.5 ± 84.6	699.4 ± 84.6	2143.5 ± 392.1
			POMACE					
FD	Inulin	30	3711.7 ± 928.2	1783.7 ± 286.1	740.3 ± 133.6	532.1 ± 753.6	3481.1 ± 753.6	7873.7 ± 1464.8
		40	3139.3 ± 790.5	1512.9 ± 241.2	636.5 ± 111.8	491.8 ± 626.2	2942.1 ± 626.2	6834.5 ± 1262.3
		50	2287.2 ± 576.1	1173.9 ± 178.0	652.0 ± 126.6	415.9 ± 539.1	2521.5 ± 539.1	7533.7 ± 1611.3
	Maltodextrin	30	3399.8 ± 859.5	1730.9 ± 285.0	820.1 ± 141.1	511.3 ± 495.5	2454.2 ± 495.5	7465.6 ± 1348.2
		40	2475.3 ± 622.3	1361.2 ± 220.8	654.6 ± 109.3	512.9 ± 608.6	2896.2 ± 608.6	6654.0 ± 1259.2
		50	2267.8 ± 570.9	1001.0 ± 154.0	481.8 ± 76.9	408.0 ± 647.5	2937.6 ± 647.5	6390.0 ± 1329.4
VD/50	Inulin	30	2374.5 ± 806.6	1560.8 ± 238.1	565.1 ± 94.6	465.2 ± 637.0	2956.9 ± 637.0	6336.2 ± 1211.3
		40	1723.9 ± 583.8	1302.5 ± 221.5	431.1 ± 69.8	431.3 ± 535.7	2524.8 ± 535.7	5470.4 ± 1040.6
		50	1573.3 ± 533.4	1201.1 ± 214.4	380.4 ± 58.9	412.3 ± 364.5	1835.5 ± 364.5	5669.8 ± 1089.7
	Maltodextrin	30	2574.3 ± 870.2	1582.5 ± 235.2	555.1 ± 90.8	522.1 ± 620.2	2951.2 ± 620.2	6785.3 ± 1247.4
		40	2160.8 ± 733.1	1388.8 ± 215.5	471.1 ± 73.5	471.1 ± 407.2	2066.5 ± 407.2	5093.3 ± 883.4
		50	1564.5 ± 530.7	1243.7 ± 208.2	369.5 = 56.0	427.4 ± 310.9	1642.3 ± 310.9	4647.2 ± 791.1

Table 1. *Cont.*

Drying Method	Type of Carriers	Con. [%]	Anthocyanins	Phenolic Acids	Flavonols	Flavavan-3-ols	Polymeric Procyanidins	Total of Polyphenolic Compounds
VD/60	Inulin	30	1705.3 ± 574.1	1293.1 ± 196.9	495.0 ± 78.3	533.5 ± 528.1	2604.6 ± 528.1	5639.4 ± 1076.5
		40	1663.4 ± 562.1	1138.9 ± 180.3	450.3 ± 68.4	545.7 ± 486.5	2452.5 ± 486.5	4529.9 ± 1013.9
		50	870.2 ± 284.1	1096.7 ± 170.4	321.6 ± 44.3	465.5 ± 421.3	2112.7 ± 421.3	5998.2 ± 1201.2
	Maltodextrin	30	2744.5 ± 924.5	1345.0 ± 190.2	597.1 ± 93.1	548.4 ± 560.0	2743.8 ± 560.0	6186.0 ± 1163.4
		40	2004.1 ± 680.3	1166.4 ± 176.7	475.2 ± 70.4	513.0 ± 449.6	2275.3 ± 449.6	4850.6 ± 932.4
		50	1338.5 ± 451.5	1048.4 ± 168.4	368.4 ± 53.7	456.5 ± 312.0	1674.1 ± 312.0	3008.6 ± 767.9
JUICE								
FD	Inulin	30	232.5 ± 60.4	1400.3 ± 215.1	187.2 ± 26.5	449.0 ± 94.9	770.2 ± 94.9	2330.2 ± 644.0
		40	157.7 ± 40.7	1077.5 ± 186.9	143.6 ± 17.1	406.5 ± 93.6	715.8 ± 93.6	2008.0 ± 490.3
		50	133.3 ± 30.7	867.8 ± 151.0	137.2 ± 14.4	324.2 ± 94.0	630.4 ± 94.0	1671.1 ± 403.8
	Maltodextrin	30	197.6 ± 49.8	1418.7 ± 223.1	188.8 ± 26.1	447.5 ± 69.0	622.4 ± 69.0	2206.2 ± 640.4
		40	158.5 ± 39.6	1162.6 ± 191.8	155.0 ± 18.9	407.4 ± 62.2	525.9 ± 62.2	1843.6 ± 520.9
		50	139.0 ± 34.2	875.4 ± 156.5	129.4 ± 13.3	373.7 ± 59.6	460.9 ± 59.6	1404.4 ± 407.3
VD/50	Inulin	30	136.1 ± 46.2	1249.8 ± 186.7	189.5 ± 27.2	428.0 ± 90.2	725.5 ± 90.2	2052.6 ± 595.7
		40	54.9 ± 19.3	1008.2 ± 166.1	157.0 ± 19.9	380.2 ± 85.7	668.0 ± 85.7	1788.4 ± 479.2
		50	50.1 ± 17.7	824.7 ± 136.3	138.7 ± 15.1	387.9 ± 85.2	653.5 ± 85.2	1582.1 ± 408.5
	Maltodextrin	30	92.3 ± 31.6	1263.1 ± 193.4	187.9 ± 27.0	433.2 ± 61.1	556.5 ± 61.1	1915.9 ± 582.3
		40	88.7 ± 29.7	1095.0 ± 176.2	164.1 ± 21.1	403.2 ± 60.0	503.4 ± 60.0	1659.1 ± 510.8
		50	69.4 ± 23.0	844.4 ± 139.9	137.9 ± 15.3	375.9 ± 57.5	443.8 ± 57.5	1325.9 ± 400.3
VD/60	Inulin	30	39.6 ± 12.1	1155.5 ± 158.7	195.8 ± 28.5	483.3 ± 94.1	782.4 ± 94.1	2000.8 ± 570.2
		40	22.4 ± 7.8	914.9 ± 146.5	142.7 ± 16.6	408.3 ± 88.2	684.5 ± 88.2	1710.7 ± 446.0
		50	34.4 ± 11.0	878.7 ± 125.9	170.2 ± 21.5	390.4 ± 89.3	680.6 ± 89.3	1661.0 ± 435.7
	Maltodextrin	30	94.6 ± 31.0	1271.5 ± 172.6	212.7 ± 32.2	456.9 ± 71.4	628.0 ± 71.4	1989.0 ± 593.4
		40	80.2 ± 26.0	1078.1 ± 159.3	176.0 ± 23.0	415.6 ± 64.3	529.1 ± 64.3	1630.2 ± 538.9
		50	57.3 ± 18.7	825.4 ± 125.9	137.9 ± 15.0	377.9 ± 62.8	458.2 ± 62.8	1298.6 ± 413.3

[1] Values are expressed as the mean ($n = 3$) ± standard deviation. ND, not detected; FD, freeze-drying; VD/50, vacuum-drying at 50 °C; VD/60, vacuum-drying at 60 °C.

Table 2. Antioxidant activity [mmol Trolox/100 g d.m.] of the fruit, juice, and pomace powders made from Saskatoon berry.

Drying Method	Type of Carriers	Con. [%]	Antioxidant Capacity [mmol Trolox/100 g d.m.]	
			ABTS	FRAP
		FRUIT		
FD	Inulin	30	5.2 ± 0.4 [1]	3.4 ± 0.1
		40	3.9 ± 0.1	2.5 ± 0.1
		50	3.8 ± 0.2	2.1 ± 0.2
	Maltodextrin	30	5.4 ± 0.1	4.0 ± 0.1
		40	4.4 ± 0.1	3.1 ± 0.3
		50	2.4 ± 0.1	1.9 ± 0.2
VD/50	Inulin	30	4.9 ± 0.1	3.0 ± 0.1
		40	4.2 ± 0.3	2.7 ± 0.1
		50	3.1 ± 0.1	2.0 ± 0.2
	Maltodextrin	30	4.9 ± 0.1	3.4 ± 0.1
		40	3.2 ± 0.1	2.2 ± 0.1
		50	1.9 ± 0.1	1.5 ± 0.1
VD/60	Inulin	30	5.8 ± 0.5	3.9 ± 0.1
		40	3.4 ± 0.1	2.4 ± 0.2
		50	2.7 ± 0.3	2.1 ± 0.2
	Maltodextrin	30	4.9 ± 0.6	3.3 ± 0.3
		40	2.9 ± 0.5	2.3 ± 0.2
		50	2.5 ± 0.1	1.5 ± 0.1
		POMACE		
FD	Inulin	30	10.0 ± 0.9	7.3 ± 0.1
		40	9.0 ± 0.2	6.7 ± 0.5
		50	7.9 ± 0.3	4.9 ± 0.2
	Maltodextrin	30	11.6 ± 0.5	7.9 ± 0.2
		40	9.7 ± 0.4	6.9 ± 0.1
		50	6.9 ± 0.2	5.3 ± 0.5
VD/50	Inulin	30	9.6 ± 0.4	6.0 ± 0.4
		40	7.7 ± 0.3	4.8 + 0.1
		50	5.7 ± 0.1	4.1 ± 0.5
	Maltodextrin	30	8.6 ± 0.1	5.4 ± 0.1
		40	7.7 ± 0.5	4.8 ± 0.2
		50	6.1 ± 0.3	3.8 ± 0.4
VD/60	Inulin	30	7.9 ± 0.2	4.8 ± 0.3
		40	6.3 ± 0.5	4.0 ± 0.1
		50	5.7 ± 0.5	3.7 ± 0.1
	Maltodextrin	30	7.7 ± 0.1	4.7 ± 0.6
		40	6.6 ± 0.2	4.0 ± 0.3
		50	5.3 ± 0.4	3.0 ± 0.1
		JUICE		
FD	Inulin	30	1.7 ± 0.1	1.2 ± 0.1
		40	1.1 ± 0.1	0.8 ± 0.1
		50	0.8 ± 0.1	0.6 ± 0.1
	Maltodextrin	30	1.5 ± 0.1	1.1 ± 0.1
		40	0.9 ± 0.2	0.8 ± 0.1
		50	0.7 ± 0.1	0.5 ± 0.1

Table 2. *Cont.*

Drying Method	Type of Carriers	Con. [%]	Antioxidant Capacity [mmol Trolox/100 g d.m.]	
			ABTS	**FRAP**
VD/50	Inulin	30	1.5 ± 0.1	1.2 ± 0.1
		40	1.2 ± 0.1	0.9 ± 0.1
		50	1.0 ± 0.1	0.7 ± 0.1
	Maltodextrin	30	1.4 ± 0.3	1.3 ± 0.1
		40	1.2 ± 0.1	0.8 ± 0.1
		50	0.7 ± 0.1	0.5 ± 0.1
VD/60	Inulin	30	1.6 ± 0.1	1.2 ± 0.1
		40	1.2 ± 0.1	0.7 ± 0.1
		50	0.9 ± 0.1	0.9 ± 0.1
	Maltodextrin	30	1.4 ± 0.2	1.1 ± 0.2
		40	1.1 ± 0.3	0.9 ± 0.1
		50	0.7 ± 0.2	0.5 ± 0.1

[1] Values are expressed as the mean (n = 3) ± standard deviation. ND, not detected; FD, freeze-drying; VD/50, vacuum-drying at 50 °C; VD/60, vacuum-drying at 60 °C.

3. Materials and Methods

3.1. Reagents

Acetonitrile, formic acid, methanol, ABTS (2,2′-azinobis(3-ethylbenzothiazoline-6-sulfonic acid), 6-hydroxy-2,5,7,8-tetramethylchroman-2-carboxylic acid (Trolox, Sigma-Aldrich, Steinheim, Germany), 2,4,6-tri(2-pyridyl)-s-triazine (TPTZ), acetic acid, and phloroglucinol were purchased from Sigma-Aldrich (Steinheim, Germany). (−)-Epicatechin, (+)-catechin, chlorogenic acid, di-caffeic quinic acid, procyanidin B2, procyanidin A2, *p*-coumaric acid, keampferol-3-*O*-galactoside, quercetin-3-*O*-galactoside, caffeic acid, cyanidin-3-*O*-galactoside, and cyanidin-3-*O*-glucoside standards were purchased from Extrasynthese (Lyon, France). Acetonitrile for ultra-phase liquid chromatography (UPLC; gradient grade) and ascorbic acid were from Merck (Darmstadt, Germany).

3.2. Material

The raw material used in the study included Saskatoon berries (*A. alnifolia* L.) *cv.* 'Smoky' that were purchased from the horticultural farm in Wojciechów near Lublin, Poland (51°14′08″N 22°14′41″E). This cultivar was chosen on the basis of the previous research (Lachowicz et al., 2019). The resulting fruit was ground in Thermomix (Wuppertal, Vorkwek, Germany) at 40 °C for 10 min. Then, the juice was extracted on a hydraulic press and centrifuged. Solutions with carrier concentrations of 30%, 40%, and 50% (*w/w*) were prepared. The carriers applied to produce powders were maltodextrin DE (20–40) and inulin (Beneo-Orafti, Belgium). The received fruit-carrier, juice-carrier, and pomace-carrier compositions were dried.

3.3. Methods

3.3.1. Drying Methods

Freeze-drying (FD, control) (ca. 100 g) was carried out in a freeze dryer (Christ Alpha 1–4 LSC; Osterode am Harz, Germany) for 24 h. The temperature within the drying chamber was −60 °C, while the heating plates had the temperature of 25 °C.

Vacuum drying (VD) was made in VACUCELL 111 ECO LINE vacuum dryer (MMM Medcenter Einrichtungen GmbH, Planegg, Germany) at 50 and 60 °C under pressure of 0.1 mbar for 24, and 16 h, respectively.

All drying experiment were performed in duplicate. The samples obtained were milled by laboratory mill (IKA A.11, Wilmington, NC, US), and vacuum sealed. The powders were kept in a freezer (−20 °C) until extracts' preparation.

3.3.2. Identification and Quantification of Polyphenols

Polyphenols were extracted from the fruit, juice, and pomace powders in triplicate ($n = 3$) according to Lachowicz et al. [17]. For polyphenolic compounds: wheat bread (1 g) were extracted with 10 mL of mixture containing UPLC-grade methanol (30 mL/100 mL), and acetic acid (1 mL/100 mL of reagent). The extraction was performed twice by incubation for 20 min under sonication (Sonic 6D, Polsonic, Warsaw, Poland) and with occasional shaking. Next, the slurry was centrifuged at 19,000× g for 10 min, and the supernatant was filtered through a hydrophilic PTFE 0.20 μm membrane (Millex Samplicity Filter, Merck, Darmstadt, Germany) and used for analysis.

Qualitative (LC-QTOF-MS) and quantitative (UPLC-PDA-FL) analysis of polyphenols (anthocyanins, flavan-3-ols, flavonols, and phenolic acids) was performed as previously described by Lachowicz et al. (2017). Separations of individual polyphenols were carried out using a UPLC BEH C$_{18}$ column (1.7 μm, 2.1 × 100 mm, Waters Corporation, Milford, MA, USA) at 30 °C. The samples (10 μL) were injected, and the elution was completed in 15 min with a sequence of linear gradients and isocratic flow rates of 0.45 mL/min. The mobile phase consisted of solvent A (2% formic acid; *v/v*) and solvent B (100% acetonitrile). The program began with isocratic elution with 99% solvent A (0–1 min), and then a linear gradient was used until 12 min, lowering solvent A to 0%; from 12.5 to 13.5 min, the gradient returned to the initial composition (99% A), and then it was held constant to re-equilibrate the column. Characterization of the single components was carried out via the retention time and the accurate molecular masses. Each compound was optimized to its estimated molecular mass [M − H]−/[M + H]+ in the negative and positive mode before and after fragmentation. The data obtained from UPLC-MS were subsequently entered into the MassLynx 4.0 ChromaLynx Application software (Waters Corporation, Milford, MA, USA). On the basis of these data, the software is able to scan different samples for the characterized substances. The runs were monitored at the wavelength of 360 nm for flavonol glycosides. The PDA spectra were measured over the wavelength range of 200–800 nm in steps of 2 nm. The retention times and spectra were compared to those of the pure standard. The calibration curves were run at 360 nm for the standard keampferol-3-O-galactoside, quercetin-3-O-galactoside, at 320 nm for the standard of chlorogenic, caffeic, di-caffeic quinic, and *p*-coumaric acids, at 520 nm for the standard cyanidin-3-O-galactoside and cyanidin-3-O-glucoside and at 280 nm for the standard (−) epicatechin, (+)-catechin, procyanidins B2 and A2, at concentrations ranging from 0.05–5 mg/mL (R^2 = 0.9999). The measurements were performed in triplicates. The results were expressed as mg per 100 g dry matter (d.m.).

3.3.3. Analysis of Proanthocyanidins by Phloroglucinolysis

Direct phloroglucinolysis of samples was performed as described by Lachowicz et al. [17]. Samples were weighed in an amount of 5 mg, then 0.8 mL of the methanolic solution of phloroglucinol (75 g/L) and ascorbic acid (15 g/L) were added. After addition of 0.4 mL of methanolic HCl (0.3 mol/L), the vials were incubated for 30 min at 50 °C with continuous vortexing in a thermo shaker (TS-100, BioSan, Riga, Latvia). The reaction was stopped by placing the vials in an ice bath with the addition of 0.6 mL of the sodium acetate 0.2 mol/L. Next the vials were centrifuged immediately at 20,000× g for 10 min at 4 °C. Samples were stored at 4 °C before reverse phase HPLC (RP-HPLC) analysis. All incubations were done in triplicate. Phloroglucinolysis products were separated on a Cadenza CD C18 (75 mm × 4.6 mm, 3 μm) column (Imtakt, Kyoto, Japan). The liquid chromatograph was a Waters (Milford, MA, USA) system equipped with diode array and scanning fluorescence detectors (Waters 474) and autosampler (Waters 717 plus). Solvent A (25 mL acetic acid and 975 mL water) and solvent B (acetonitrile) were used in the following gradients: initial, 5 mL/100 mL B; 0–15 min, to 10 mL/100 mL B linear; 15–25 min to 60 mL/100 mL B linear; followed by washing and reconditioning of the column. A flow rate of 1 mL/min and an oven temperature of 15 °C with the injection of the filtrate (20 μL) on the HPLC system. The fluorescence detection was recorded at excitation wavelength of 278 nm and emission wavelength of 360 nm. The calibration curves, which were based on peak area, were established using (+)-catechin, (−)-epicatechin, (+)-catechins, and (−)-epicatechin-phloroglucinol adduct standards. The average degree of polymerization was measured by calculating the molar ratio of all the flavan-3-ol units (phloroglucinol adducts + terminal units) to (−)-epicatechin and (+)-catechin, which correspond to terminal units. Quantification of the (+)-catechin, (−)-epicatechin, (+)-catechin, and (−)-epicatechin-phloroglucinol adducts was achieved by using the calibration curves of the corresponding standards (Extrasynthese). All data were obtained in triplicate. The results were expressed as mg per 100 g d.m.

3.3.4. Antioxidant Capacity

For antioxidant activity: the samples (1 g) were mixed with 10 mL of MeOH/water (80:20%, *v/v*) and with 1% of HCl, sonicated at 20 °C for 15 min and left for 24 h at 4 °C. Then the extract was again sonicated for 15 min, and centrifuged at 15,000g for 10 min. The ABTS and the FRAP assays were determined according to Re et al. [41] and Benzie and Strain [42], respectively, by Synergy H1 spectrophotometer (BioTek Instruments Inc., Winnoski, VT, USA). The antioxidant capacity was expressed as mmol of Trolox per 100 g d.m.

3.3.5. Statistical Analysis

Statistical analysis, one-way ANOVA and principal component analysis (PCA) were conducted using Statistica version 12.5 (StatSoft, Kraków, Poland). Significant differences ($p \leq 0.05$) between average values were evaluated by one-way ANOVA and HSD Tukey multiple range test.

4. Conclusions

The concentration of carriers had a stronger impact on the content of polyphenolic compounds and antioxidant capacity than the type of carrier or drying method. The choice of a carrier should be done in dependence of the matrix and of the desired composition of bioactive compounds and antioxidant activity. Therefore, maltodextrin can be recommended for powders obtained from the fruit and juice of Saskatoon berry, whereas inulin can be applied in order to produce pomace powders with better functional composition of bioactive compounds. In addition, PCA showed that the freeze-drying process led to the highest content of almost all polyphenolic compounds and their high antioxidant activity, regardless of the matrix tested.

Thus, in future research, properly prepared Saskatoon berry powders with the mentioned carriers will be used as functional additives to design functional food especially foodstuff for enhancing health benefit properties.

Supplementary Materials: The following are available online, Table S1. Identification and quantification of flavan-3-ols [mg/100 g d.m.] in fruit, juice, and pomace powders made form Saskatoon berry, Table S2. Identification and quantification of anthocyanins [mg/100 g d.m.] in the fruit, juice, and pomace powders made form Saskatoon berry, Table S3. Identification and quantification of phenolic acids [mg/100 g d.m.] in the fruit, juice, and pomace powders made form Saskatoon berry, Table S4. Identification and quantification of flavonols [mg/100 g d.m.] in the fruit, juice, and pomace powders made form Saskatoon berry.

Author Contributions: Conceptualization, S.L., A.M.-C.; methodology, S.L., A.M.-C., J.O.; writing—original draft preparation and editing, S.L., A.M.-C.; writing—review, S.L.; supervision, S.L.; project administration, S.L.; funding acquisition, S.L. All authors have read and agreed to the published version of the manuscript.

Funding: This research was supported by Wrocław University of Environmental and Life Sciences; grant name "Innovative scientist", grant number B030/0032/20".

Acknowledgments: The authors would like to thank BioGrim company for providing the raw material. The work was created in a leading research team 'Food&Health' (S.L.), and 'Plants4food' (A.M.-C.).

Conflicts of Interest: The authors declare no conflict of interest.

References

1. Lavola, A.; Karjalainen, R.; Julkunen-Tiitto, R. Bioactive Polyphenols in Leaves, Stems, and Berries of Saskatoon (*Amelanchier alnifolia* Nutt.) Cultivars. *J. Agric. Food Chem.* **2012**, *60*, 1020–1027. [CrossRef] [PubMed]
2. Bakowska-Barczak, A.M.; Kolodziejczyk, P. Evaluation of Saskatoon Berry (*Amelanchier alnifolia* Nutt.) Cultivars for their Polyphenol Content, Antioxidant Properties, and Storage Stability. *J. Agric. Food Chem.* **2008**, *56*, 9933–9940. [CrossRef] [PubMed]
3. Jurikova, T.; Balla, S.; Sochor, J.; Pohanka, M.; Mlcek, J.; Baron, M. Flavonoid Profile of Saskatoon Berries (*Amelanchier alnifolia* Nutt.) and Their Health Promoting Effects. *Molecules* **2013**, *18*, 12571–12586. [CrossRef] [PubMed]
4. Lachowicz, S.; Oszmiański, J.; Pluta, S. The composition of bioactive compounds and antioxidant activity of Saskatoon berry (*Amelanchier alnifolia* Nutt.) genotypes grown in central Poland. *Food Chem.* **2017**, *235*, 234–243. [CrossRef] [PubMed]
5. Rodríguez-Roque, M.J.; Rojas-Graü, M.A.; Elez-Martinez, P.; Martin-Belloso, O. Soymilk phenolic compounds, isoflavones and antioxidant activity as affected by in vitro gastrointestinal digestion. *Food Chem.* **2013**, *136*, 206–212.
6. Lachowicz, S.; Seliga, Ł.; Pluta, S. Distribution of phytochemicals and antioxidative potency in fruit peel, flesh, and seeds of Saskatoon berry. *Food Chem.* **2020**. [CrossRef]
7. Ioannou, I.; Hafsa, I.; Hamdi, S.; Charbonnel, C.; Ghoul, M. Review of the effects of food processing and formulation on flavonol and anthocyanin behaviour. *J. Food Eng.* **2012**, *111*, 208–217. [CrossRef]
8. Augustin, M.A.; Hemar, Y. Nano- and micro-structured assemblies for encapsulation of food ingredients. *Chem. Soc. Rev.* **2009**, *38*, 902–912. [CrossRef]
9. Fang, Z.; Bhandari, B. Effect of spray drying and storage on the stability of bayberry polyphenols. *Food Chem.* **2011**, *129*, 1139–1147. [CrossRef]
10. Kha, T.; Nguyen, M.H.; Roach, P. Effects of spray drying conditions on the physicochemical and antioxidant properties of the Gac (*Momordica cochinchinensis*) fruit aril powder. *J. Food Eng.* **2010**, *98*, 385–392. [CrossRef]
11. Wang, Y.; Lu, Z.; Lv, F.; Bie, X. Study on microencapsulation of curcumin pigments by spray drying. *Eur. Food Res. Technol.* **2009**, *229*, 391–396. [CrossRef]
12. Saikia, S.; Mahnot, N.K.; Mahanta, C.L. Optimisation of phenolic extraction from Averrhoa carambola pomace by response surface methodology and its microencapsulation by spray and freeze drying. *Food Chem.* **2015**, *171*, 144–152. [CrossRef] [PubMed]
13. Shoaib, M.; Shehzad, A.; Omar, M.; Rakha, A.; Raza, H.; Sharif, H.R.; Shakeel, A.; Ansari, A.; Niazi, S. Inulin: Properties, health benefits and food applications. *Carbohydr. Polym.* **2016**, *147*, 444–454. [CrossRef] [PubMed]
14. Silva, P.I.; Stringheta, P.C.; Teofilo, R.; Oliveira, I. Parameter optimization for spray-drying microencapsulation of jaboticaba (*Myrciaria jaboticaba*) peel extracts using simultaneous analysis of responses. *J. Food Eng.* **2013**, *117*, 538–544. [CrossRef]
15. Michalska-Ciechanowska, A.; Wojdyło, A.; Lech, K.; Łysiak, G.; Figiel, A. Physicochemical properties of whole fruit plum powders obtained using different drying technologies. *Food Chem.* **2016**, *207*, 223–232. [CrossRef]
16. Michalska-Ciechanowska, A.; Wojdyło, A.; Brzezowska, J.; Majerska, J.; Ciska, E. The Influence of Inulin on the Retention of Polyphenolic Compounds during the Drying of Blackcurrant Juice. *Molecules* **2019**, *22*, 4167. [CrossRef]
17. Lachowicz, S.; Michalska, A.; Lech, K.; Majerska, J.; Oszmiański, J.; Figiel, A. Comparison of the effect of four drying methods on polyphenols in saskatoon berry. *LWT* **2019**, *111*, 727–736. [CrossRef]
18. De Souza, D.R.; Willems, J.L.; Low, N.H. Phenolic composition and antioxidant activities of saskatoon berry fruit and pomace. *Food Chem.* **2019**, *290*, 168–177. [CrossRef]
19. Slimestad, R.; Torskangerpoll, K.; Nateland, H.S.; Johannessen, T.; Giske, N.H. Flavonoids from black chokeberries, Aronia melanocarpa. *J. Food Compos. Anal.* **2005**, *18*, 61–68. [CrossRef]
20. White, B.L.; Howard, L.R.; Prior, R.L. Proximate and Polyphenolic Characterization of Cranberry Pomace†. *J. Agric. Food Chem.* **2010**, *58*, 4030–4036. [CrossRef]
21. Oszmiański, J.; Lachowicz, S. Effect of the Production of Dried Fruits and Juice from Chokeberry (*Aronia melanocarpa* L.) on the Content and Antioxidative Activity of Bioactive Compounds. *Molecules* **2016**, *8*, 1098. [CrossRef]

22. Gouw, V.P.; Jung, J.; Zhao, Y. Functional properties, bioactive compounds, and in vitro gastrointestinal digestion study of dried fruit pomace powders as functional food ingredients. *LWT* **2017**, *80*, 136–144. [CrossRef]

23. Jurikova, T.; Sochor, J.; Rop, O.; Mlcek, J.; Balla, S.; Szekeres, L.; Žitný, R.; Zitka, O.; Adam, V.; Kizek, R. Evaluation of Polyphenolic Profile and Nutritional Value of Non-Traditional Fruit Species in the Czech Republic — A Comparative Study. *Molecules* **2012**, *17*, 8968–8981. [CrossRef] [PubMed]

24. Lachowicz, S.; Oszmiański, J.; Seliga, Ł.; Pluta, S. Phytochemical Composition and Antioxidant Capacity of Seven Saskatoon Berry (*Amelanchier alnifolia* Nutt.) Genotypes Grown in Poland. *Molecules* **2017**, *5*, 853. [CrossRef] [PubMed]

25. Mazza, G.; Cottrell, T. Carotenoids and cyanogenic glucosides in saskatoon berries (*Amelanchier alnifolia* Nutt.). *J. Food Compos. Anal.* **2008**, *21*, 249–254. [CrossRef]

26. Li, W.; Hydamaka, A.W.; Lowry, L.; Beta, T. Comparison of antioxidant capacity and phenolic compounds of berries, chokecherry and seabuckthorn. *Open Life Sci.* **2009**, *4*, 499–506. [CrossRef]

27. Fang, J.; Huang, J. Accumulation of plasma levels of anthocyanins following multiple saskatoon berry supplements. *Xenobiotica* **2019**, *50*, 454–457. [CrossRef]

28. Zhao, R.; Khafipour, E.; Sepehri, S.; Huang, F.; Beta, T.; Shen, G.X. Impact of Saskatoon berry powder on insulin resistance and relationship with intestinal microbiota in high fat-high sucrose diet-induced obese mice. *J. Nutr. Biochem.* **2019**, *69*, 130–138. [CrossRef]

29. Bakowska-Barczak, A.M.; Kolodziejczyk, P.P. Black currant polyphenols: Their storage stability and microencapsulation. *Ind. Crop. Prod.* **2011**, *34*, 1301–1309. [CrossRef]

30. Sáenz, C.; Tapia, S.; Chávez, J.; Robert, P. Microencapsulation by spray drying of bioactive compounds from cactus pear (*Opuntia ficus-indica*). *Food Chem.* **2009**, *114*, 616–622.

31. Michalska-Ciechanowska, A.; Wojdyło, A.; Honke, J.; Ciska, E.; Andlauer, W. Drying-induced physico-chemical changes in cranberry products. *Food Chem.* **2018**, *240*, 448–455. [CrossRef] [PubMed]

32. Daza, L.D.; Fujita, A.; Granato, D.; Favaro-Trindade, C.S.; Genovese, M.I. Functional properties of encapsulated Cagaita (*Eugenia dysenterica* DC.) fruit extract. *Food Biosci.* **2017**, *18*, 15–21. [CrossRef]

33. Michalska-Ciechanowska, A.; Wojdyło, A.; Łysiak, G.; Figiel, A. Chemical Composition and Antioxidant Properties of Powders Obtained from Different Plum Juice Formulations. *Int. J. Mol. Sci.* **2017**, *1*, 176. [CrossRef] [PubMed]

34. White, B.L.; Howard, L.R.; Prior, R.L. Impact of Different Stages of Juice Processing on the Anthocyanin, Flavonol, and Procyanidin Contents of Cranberries. *J. Agric. Food Chem.* **2011**, *59*, 4692–4698. [CrossRef] [PubMed]

35. Michalska-Ciechanowska, A.; Wojdyło, A.; Łysiak, G.; Lech, K.; Figiel, A. Functional relationships between phytochemicals and drying conditions during the processing of blackcurrant pomace into powders. *Adv. Powder Technol.* **2017**, *28*, 1340–1348. [CrossRef]

36. Cai, Y.; Corke, H. Production and Properties of Spray-dried Amaranthus Betacyanin Pigments. *J. Food Sci.* **2000**, *65*, 1248–1252. [CrossRef]

37. Patras, A.; Brunton, N.; O'Donnell, C.P.; Tiwari, B. Effect of thermal processing on anthocyanin stability in foods; mechanisms and kinetics of degradation. *Trends Food Sci. Technol.* **2010**, *21*, 3–11. [CrossRef]

38. Tiwari, U.; Cummins, E. Factors influencing levels of phytochemicals in selected fruit and vegetables during pre- and post-harvest food processing operations. *Food Res. Int.* **2013**, *50*, 497–506. [CrossRef]

39. Piga, A.; Del Caro, A.; Corda, G. From Plums to Prunes: Influence of Drying Parameters on Polyphenols and Antioxidant Activity. *J. Agric. Food Chem.* **2003**, *51*, 3675–3681. [CrossRef]

40. Siddiq, M.; Dolan, K. Characterization of polyphenol oxidase from blueberry (*Vaccinium corymbosum* L.). *Food Chem.* **2017**, *218*, 216–220. [CrossRef]

41. Re, R.; Pellegrini, N.; Proteggente, A.; Pannala, A.; Yang, M.; Rice-Evans, C. Antioxidant activity applying an improved ABTS radical cation decolorization assay. *Free. Radic. Boil. Med.* **1999**, *26*, 1231–1237. [CrossRef]

42. Benzie, I.; Strain, J. The Ferric Reducing Ability of Plasma (FRAP) as a Measure of "Antioxidant Power": The FRAP Assay. *Anal. Biochem.* **1996**, *239*, 70–76. [CrossRef] [PubMed]

Sample Availability: Samples of the compounds are available from the authors.

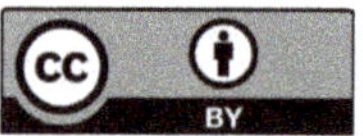

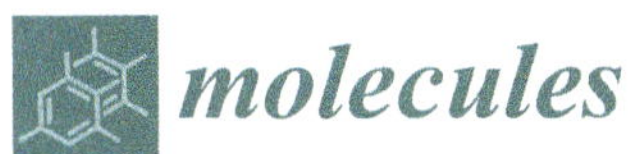 *molecules*

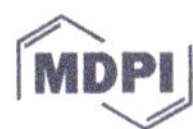

Article

Influence of the Phenological State of in the Antioxidant Potential and Chemical Composition of *Ageratina havanensis*. Effects on the P-Glycoprotein Function

Trina H. García [1], Claudia Quintino da Rocha [2], Livan Delgado-Roche [3], Idania Rodeiro [3],
Yaiser Ávila [4], Ivones Hernández [3], Cindel Cuellar [3], Miriam Teresa Paz Lopes [5], Wagner Vilegas [6],
Giulia Auriemma [7], Iraida Spengler [1,*] and Luca Rastrelli [7,*]

[1] Center for Natural Product Research, Faculty of Chemistry, University of Havana, Havana 10400, Cuba
[2] Department of Chemistry, Federal University of Maranhão, São Luis, Maranhão 65080-805, Brazil
[3] Department of Pharmacology, Institute of Marine Sciences (ICIMAR), Loma 14, Alturas del Vedado,
    Plaza de la Revolución, Havana 10400, Cuba
[4] Institute of Ecology and Systematics, Havana 10400, Cuba
[5] Laboratory of Antitumor Natural Substances, Department of Pharmacology, Institute of Biological Sciences,
    Federal University of Minas Gerais (UFMG), Belo Horizonte 31207-90, Brazil
[6] Experimental Campus of Sao Vicente, UNESP-Sao Paulo State University, Sao Vicente,
    Sao Paulo 11.330-900, Brazil
[7] Department of Pharmacy, University of Salerno, Via Giovanni Paolo II, 84084 Fisciano (SA), Italy
*   Correspondence: iraida@fq.uh.cu (I.S.); rastrelli@unisa.it (L.R.)

Academic Editors: Raffaele Pezzani and Carmen Formisano
Received: 31 March 2020; Accepted: 30 April 2020; Published: 2 May 2020

Abstract: *Ageratina havanensis* (Kunth) R. M. King & H. Robinson is a species of flowering shrub in the family Asteraceae, native to the Caribbean and Texas. The aim of this work was to compare the quantitative chemical composition of extracts obtained from *Ageratina havanensis* in its flowering and vegetative stages with the antioxidant potential and to determine the effects on P-glycoprotein (P-gp) function. The quantitative chemical composition of the extracts was determined quantifying their major flavonoids by UPLC-ESI-MS/MS and by PCA analysis. The effects of the extracts on P-gp activity was evaluated by Rhodamine 123 assay; antioxidant properties were determined by DPPH, FRAP and inhibition of lipid peroxidation methods. The obtained results show that major flavonoids were present in higher concentrations in vegetative stage than flowering stage. In particular, the extracts obtained in the flowering season showed a significantly higher ability to sequester free radicals compared to those of the vegetative season, meanwhile, the extracts obtained during the vegetative stage showed a significant inhibitory effect against brain lipid peroxidation and a strong reductive capacity. This study also showed the inhibitory effects of all ethanolic extracts on P-gp function in 4T1 cell line; these effects were unrelated to the phenological stage. This work shows, therefore, the first evidence on: the inhibition of P-gp function, the antioxidant effects and the content of major flavonoids of *Ageratina havanensis*. According to the obtained results, the species *Ageratina havanensis* (Kunth) R. M. King & H. Robinson could be a source of new potential inhibitors of drug efflux mediated by P-gp. A special focus on all these aspects must be taking into account for future studies.

Keywords: *Ageratina havanensis*; flavonoids; UPLC-ESI-MS/MS; P-glycoprotein; antioxidant potential

1. Introduction

Polyphenols, particularly flavonoids, have been widely studied for their bioactive properties and their strong antioxidant effects are well noted [1–3]. In addition, some plant antioxidant polyphenols exhibit anti-neoplastic activity by multiple pathways, including their potential to intensify the action of cytostatic drugs, through the attenuating the multidrug resistance (MDR) phenomenon [4]. The best recognized and the most frequent cause of the MDR involves an increased activity of ATP-binding cassette family transporters (ABC) [5]. A large number of compounds have been identified as MDR suppressors by interfering with the P-gp-mediated export of chemotherapeutic agents [6–9]. However, in many cases the high toxicity of these substances has limited their use [10]. Thus, natural antioxidants have been identified as novel potential candidates [11–16].

Different studies show that plants of the genus *Ageratina* contain a variety of flavonoids. Particularly, in our previous research studying the extracts obtained from the leaves of *Ageratina havanensis* (Kunth) R. M. King & H. Robinson, growing in Cuba, by chromatographic, spectroscopic and spectrometric methods, we identified a significant presence of flavonoids and their glucosides [17,18]. We also determined that the qualitative composition of the flavonoids in the plant is similar in two different phenological stages, that is flowering and vegetative state [18].

Taking into account the abundance of flavonoids in the extracts prepared from *Ageratina havanensis*, it is expected that these extracts have antioxidant properties [19–21]. As qualitative composition of flavonoids is similar in both phenological stages, it could be hypothesized that the biological activity in both stages is similar, too. Based on these considerations, in this paper we studied the *Ageratina havanensis* (Kunth) R. M. King & H. Robinson extracts to prove their ability to inhibit P-gp function under no cytotoxicity conditions, their antioxidant potential and the influence of their quantitative composition on the biological properties of the plant.

2. Results

2.1. P-gp Modulation by Extracts Obtained from Ageratina havanensis

The first step of this study was to investigate if the extracts obtained from *Ageratina havanensis* could inhibit P-gp activity under no cytotoxicity conditions. In order to mimic the chemo-resistance in humans, the cells chosen for this research were the well-characterized mouse mammary carcinoma 4T1 cells that express multi-resistance phenotype after exposure to different anticancer drugs mediated by P-gp.

Firstly, to determine the cytotoxic effects of the eleven extracts obtained from *Ageratina havanensis* on 4T1 cells, the MTT assay was employed. Table 1 reports the IC_{50} values calculated after exposure of the cells to the *Ageratina havanensis* extracts for 24 h. As shown, the treatments reduced cell viability showing only slight differences between the products. In all the cases, significant differences were observed in comparison with control cells for values above 250 µg/mL. Thus, a range of concentrations under IC_{50} values was selected for evaluating effects of the extracts on P-gp function.

Rho-123 is a fluorescent compound, which enters the cells passively and concentrates in mitochondria. As P-gp substrate, the intracellular loading of this probe is inversely proportional to P-gp activity. Intracellular fluorescence increased in a dose-dependent fashion in 4T1 cells exposed to Lf-EtOH until F-EtOH extract for 1 h, but important differences between the extracts were found. The percentage of the inhibitory effect on the activity of the transporter produced at the highest concentration tested (200 µg/mL) are showed in Table 1. As reported, all ethanolic extracts (Lf-EtOH, Lv-EtOH, Sf-EtOH and F-EtOH) showed promissory inhibitory effects. More in details, the inhibitory activity was above 50% for both Sf-EtOH and Sv-EtOH, the two extracts obtained from the stem bark, compared to controls. On the contrary, the F-EtOAc and F-*n*-BuOH extracts were not able to inhibit the function of the transporter under the same experimental conditions.

Table 1. Cytotoxicity and inhibitory effects on P-gp function of *Ageratina havanensis* (Kunth) R. M. King & H. Robinson extracts on breast cancer 4T1 cells.

Harvesting Stage	Plant Organs	Extracts	IC$_{50}$ (µg/mL)	Inhibition P-gp Function (%)
Flowering	Leaves	Lf-EtOH	381.6 ± 7.5	35
		Lf-EtOAc	252.5 ± 10.1	23
		Lf-*n*-BuOH	302.0 ± 8.0	19
		Lv-EtOH	392.8 ± 6.7	58
Vegetative stage		Lv-EtOAc	313.0 ± 12.1	45
		Lv-*n*-BuOH	496.5 ± 6.7	27
Flowering	Stems	Sf-EtOH	228.2 ± 8.7	84
Vegetative stage		Sv-EtOH	355.7 ± 7.6	65
Flowering	Flowers	F-EtOH	263.5 ± 8.2	85
		F-EtOAc	259.5 ± 10.6	-
		F-*n*-BuOH	315.5 ± 9.9	-

IC$_{50}$ is defined, as the concentration required achieving 50% inhibition over control cells, values are shown as mean ± SEM. %: represents the percentage of inhibition P-gp activity at the higher concentration tested (200 µg/mL) respect to control cells (untreated cells) after 1 h of exposure. Verapamil used as control positive was included, showing values of inhibition in the order of 300% to the activity exhibit by control cells. Values showed are from two independent experiments with three replicas.

2.2. Antioxidant Effects of Extracts Obtained from Ageratina havanensis

The screening of the antioxidant activity of the substances may require a combination of different methods to describe the background about the antioxidant properties of the samples. Here, the antioxidant potential of the *Ageratina havanensis* extracts was determined by using three in vitro methods, which previously have been used to predict the antioxidant capacity of several substances (DPPH free radical scavenging assay, FRAP assay and the determination of lipid peroxidation in brain rat homogenates) [22–24].

The model of scavenging the stable DPPH radical has been used method to evaluate the free radical scavenging ability of substances [23,24]. In this case, the antioxidant effect of the analyzed sample on DPPH radical scavenging may be due to their hydrogen donating ability and it reduce the stable violet DPPH radical to the yellow DPPH-H. Substances which are able to perform this reaction can be considered as antioxidants and therefore radical scavengers [25]. On the other hands, FRAP assay is based on the ability of antioxidant to reduce Fe^{3+} to Fe^{2+} in the presence of tripyridyltriazine (TPTZ), forming the intense blue Fe^{2+}–TPTZ complex with an absorption maximum at 593 nm; the absorbance increase is proportional to the antioxidant content [22]. As shown in Table 2, the radical scavenging activity of the eleven *Ageratina havanensis* extracts evaluated was significantly ($p < 0.05$) higher in the flowering compared to the vegetative season, meanwhile, the reductive capacity was significantly ($p < 0.05$) higher in vegetative state.

During the last years, lipid peroxidation has received renewed attention from the viewpoints of nutrition and medicine. Lipid peroxidation is implicated in the underlying mechanisms of several disorders and diseases such as cardiovascular diseases, cancer, neurodegenerative diseases, and even aging [26]. It is the accumulated result of reactive oxygen species and a chain reaction that causes the dysfunction of biological systems [27]. Furthermore, the extracts from the flowering season showed a significant ($p < 0.05$) inhibition of lipid peroxidation against brain phospholipid peroxidation compared with the extracts from the vegetative stage (Table 2).

Table 2. In vitro antioxidant capacity of *Ageratina havanensis* (Kunth) R. M. King & H. Robinson extracts.

Harvesting Stage	Plant Organs	Extracts	FRAP (μM of Ascorbic Acid Equivalents)	DPPH IC$_{50}$ (μg/mL)	Lipid Peroxidation Inhibition IC$_{50}$ (μg/mL)
Flowering	Leaves	Lf-EtOH	88.21 ± 3.77 [a]	22.65 ± 1.73 [a]	16.52 ± 2.19 [a]
		Lf-EtOAc	90.52 ± 3.61 [a]	39.27 ± 2.04 [a]	21.63 ± 1.78 [a]
		Lf-*n*-BuOH	63.51 ± 2.62 [a]	53.12 ± 0.92 [a]	38.91 ± 3.52 [a]
Vegetative stage		Lv-EtOH	279.42 ± 8.48 [b]	151.90 ± 3.71 [b]	41.66 ± 2.87 [b]
		Lv-EtOAc	234.70 ± 7.93 [b]	138.11 ± 2.67 [b]	46.23 ± 3.12 [b]
		Lv-*n*-BuOH	231.56 ± 10.14 [b]	84.24 ± 3.81 [b]	51.60 ± 2.04 [b]
Flowering	Stems	Sf-EtOH	88.43 ± 3.96 [a]	39.23 ± 1.92 [a]	37.21 ± 2.55 [a]
Vegetative stage		Sv-EtOH	197.21 ± 3.30 [b]	32.72 ± 7.23 [a]	48.32 ± 3.87 [b]
Flowering	Flowers	F-EtOH	169.91 ± 7.63 [a]	29.45 ± 1.99 [a]	21.35 ± 2.66 [a]
		F-EtOAc	167.21 ± 5.34 [a]	38.77 ± 2.64 [b]	32.34 ± 2.01 [b]
		F-*n*-BuOH	91.66 ± 3.21 [b]	54.13 ± 2.88 [c]	30.27 ± 3.81 [b]
Sakuranetin			319.38 ± 6.65	-	-
7-methoxyaromadendrin			238.45 ± 2.11	-	-
Ascorbic acid			-	21.97 ± 0.84	-
Trolox-C					10.64 ± 1.02

Values represent the mean ± SEM of the antioxidant activity of *A. havanensis* extracts. IC$_{50}$ values were calculated as the extract concentration required to scavenge 50% of DPPH$^{•}$, Ascorbic acid was employed as standard for DPPH$^{•}$ assay and Trolox-C for lipid peroxidation assay. Different letters in the same column represent statistical differences (ANOVA, Dunnet post-hoc test; $p < 0.05$). Comparisons were carried out between extracts according to the seasonal stage (leaves, stems or flowers) or according to the solvent (EtOH, EtOAc or *n*-BuOH). Three independent experiments were done and samples were analyzed by triplicate.

2.3. Quantification of Sakuranetin and 7-Methoxyromadendrin in the Extracts of Ageratina havanensis

The major flavonoids sakuranetin and 7-methoxyaromadendrin only differ for a hydroxyl group (Figure 1) and thus elute with very close retention times. Because of this, it was necessary to develop a rapid, sensitive and accurate method that would allow for their quantification in *Ageratina havanensis* extracts. UPLC-ESI-MS/MS system provides high separation capacity, high analytical speed and high analytical sensitivity. The addition of 0.1% formic acid to the mobile phase helped achieve satisfactory peak symmetry, good resolution, and significantly enhanced sensitivity. In this case, this method was useful for quantifying sakuranetin and 7-methoxyaromadendrin in the extracts of *Ageratina havanensis* collected in both seasons.

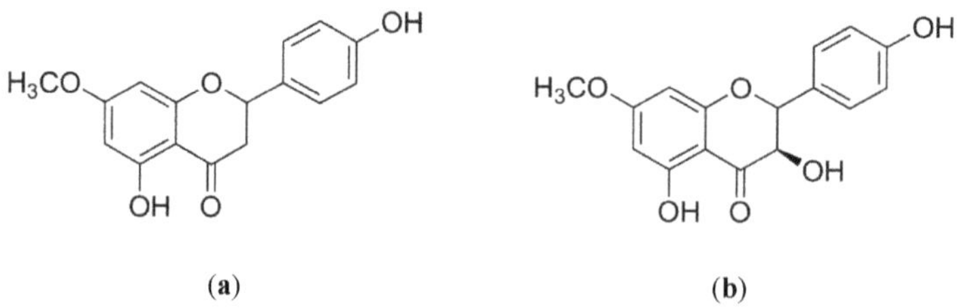

(a)   (b)

Figure 1. Chemical structures of: (**a**) sakuranetin; (**b**) 7-methoxyromadendrin.

2.3.1. Method Validation

Linearity, LDQ and LOQ

Calibration curves of the standard sakuranetin and 7-methoxyaromadendrin were established with negative UPLC-ESI-MS/MS on SRM mode. The validation data of the method showed good correlation coefficients, 0.9909 and 0.9928, respectively, in the mass concentration range of 1–50 ppm, Table S1.

Matrix Effect and Recovery

The recoveries after SPE were 93.2% and 97.4% for sakuranetin and 7-methoxyaromadendrin respectively, which means that 6.8 and 2.6% were lost in the solid phase extraction process. The ratios (A/B × 100)% were 88.3% for sakuranetin and 94.7% for 7-methoxyaromadendrin, so the presence of the matrix decreases the recovery of sakuranetin and 7-methoxyaromadendrin by 4.9% and 2.7% respectively. These results showed that all values were within acceptable ranges.

Precision and Accuracy of the System

In this method, injection errors, dilution, adduct formation etc. can occur. Therefore, precision and accuracy of the system were evaluated. The results suggest that both parameters were acceptable for the quantification method developed. In the case of precision, very similar % RSD were observed. The results of sakuranetin were less than 2.5% in the experiments intra-day and inter-day whereas for 7-methoxyaromadendrine were less than 3.5%. Accuracy showed results above 98% intra-day and inter-day in both standards for the concentrations tested, Table S2.

2.3.2. Concentration of Standards in the Extracts

The linear calibration curves were used for quantitative analyses of the standards in the extracts, Table 3. In general, the ethyl acetate extracts showed higher concentration of the analyzed patterns. The concentration of sakuranetin is approximately three times the concentration of 7-methoxyarycomadendrine. Extracts from the leaves of the vegetative season present a higher concentration of analyzed flavonoids than those from the flowering season.

Table 3. Concentration of sakuranetin and 7-methoxyaromadendrin in the extracts by UPLC/ESI/TQD/MS^n.

Harvesting Stage	Plant Organs	Extracts	Concentration (µg/mL)	
			Sakuranetin	7-Methoxyaromadendrin
Flowering	Leaves	Lf-EtOH	Below LOQ	1.27
		Lf-EtOAc	46.70	16.8
		Lf-*n*-BuOH	Below LOQ	Below LOQ
		Lv-EtOH	13.20	2.90
Vegetative stage		Lv-EtOAc	87.02	30.2
		Lv-*n*-BuOH	Below LOQ	Below LOQ
Flowering	Stems	Sf-EtOH	Below LOQ	Below LOQ
Vegetative stage		Sv-EtOH	Below LOQ	Below LOQ
Flowering	Flowers	F-EtOH	Below LOQ	Below LOQ
		F-EtOAc	29.90	6.30
		F-*n*-BuOH	Below LOQ	Below LOQ

2.3.3. Principal Component Analysis of Extracts

Principal component analysis (PCA) allowed comparing extracts of *Ageratina havanensis* according their chemical composition. The original variables were reduced to the two principal components PC1 (77.9%) and PC2 (5.6%) representing an 83.6% of the total data variance (Table S3). According to eigenvalues, peaks with *m/z* 447 gave principal contribution to PC1. Also, sakuranetin (*m/z* 285, [M − H]$^-$), 7-methoxyaromadendrin (*m/z* 301, [M − H]$^-$) and peaks with *m/z* 463 had great influence on the variability of the data in this component. From the extracts of *Ageratina havanensis*, were isolated and identified in previous studies three glycosides with *m/z* 447 and the same fragmentation ([286 + 162 − H]$^-$) in its MS^2 spectrum [17,18]. Because of that, it was concluded that the most influential variables in PC1 were the concentration of sakuranetin and 7-methoxy-aromadendrin. On the other hand, the glycosides (*m/z* 447 and *m/z* 463) were the variables that most influenced on PC2, Table S4.

Figure 2 shows that the ethyl acetate extract from the leaves collected in vegetative state (Lv-EtOAc) differs from the rest of the extracts with respect to PC1 followed by the ethyl acetate extract from the leaves collected in flowering state (Lf-EtOAc). The rest of the extracts showed similarity in PC1. According to this behavior, it was concluded that sakuranetin, 7-methoxyaromadendrin and the glycosides (the original variables that most influence CP1) were higher in the vegetative stage, mainly in the ethyl acetate extract of leaves. With respect to PC2, the *n*-butanol extract of the leaves collected in flowering state (Lf-*n*-BuOH) is different from the rest of the extracts. Sakuranetin and 7-methoxyaromadendrin in this case do not influence the total variability of the data but the glycosides have a significant influence. These results were expected since in the quantification, the concentration of both sakuranetin and 7-methoxyaromadendrin resulted higher in the extracts of ethyl acetate of the leaves, being greater in the vegetative state, whereas in the ethanolic and *n*-butanolic extracts, these flavonoids were below the limit of quantification.

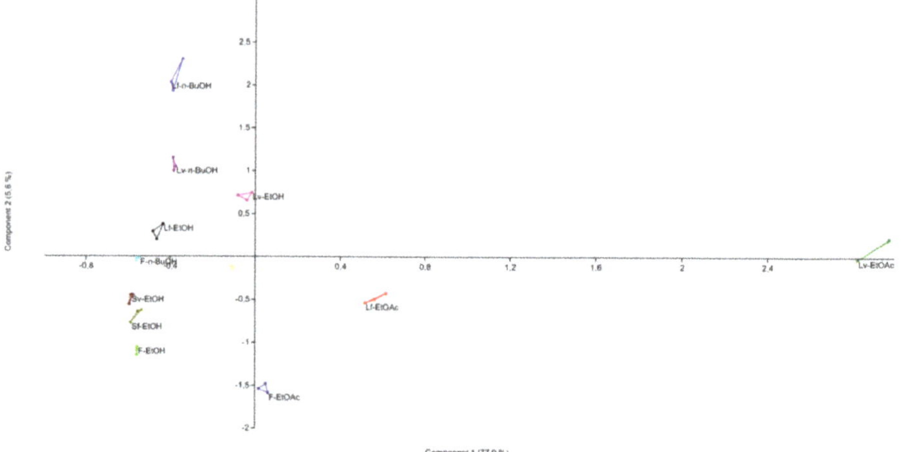

Figure 2. Scatter plot of PCA of the extracts on the first two principle components.

3. Discussion

Breast cancer is the most frequently diagnosed cancer and the leading cause of cancer-related death among women worldwide [28]. Despite the long list of drugs that have been used in the treatment of breast tumors, marked drug multi-resistance during treatment remains one of the main problems facing the clinic today when applying a therapy against breast cancer. Among various mechanisms of chemo-resistance, resistance due to the increased expression of P-gp is the best characterized and it is considered the most important in cancer therapy. The significance of the above mentioned is also supported by the fact that more than 50% of existing anticancer drugs are going to P-gp mediated efflux [29]. Since the results of clinical trials using P-gp inhibitors have not been very promising, the search for new modulators which selectively inhibit P-gp activity without significant negative side effects is currently under high interest and hopes are pinned on the application of some plant polyphenols [11].

P-gp may affect the pharmacokinetic parameters of drugs or other compounds, possibly leading to modifications of their bioavailability as well as of their distribution, metabolism, elimination and toxicity (ADMET) [30]. Together with several CYP450 isoenzymes, P-gp is involved in drug-drug, food-drug and, finally, herb-drug interactions [31]. Herbal medicines may interact with drugs at the intestine, liver, kidneys, and targets of action. Importantly, many of these drugs have very narrow therapeutic indices. Most of them are substrates for P-gp. The underlying mechanisms for most described herb-drug interactions are not entirely understood, and several pharmacokinetic and/or pharmacodynamic interferences are often implicated in these interactions. In particular, enzyme induction and inhibition may play an important role in the occurrence of some herb-drug interactions. Because herb-drug interactions can significantly affect circulating levels of drug and, hence, alter the clinical outcome, the identification of herb-drug interactions has important implications [32]. As present results suggest the species *Ageratina havanensis* (Kunth) R. M. King & H. Robinson could be a source of new potential inhibitors of drug efflux mediated by P-gp; focus on these aspects must be taking into account for future studies.

Today it is known that P-gp function and its regulation can be mediated via reactive oxidative species (ROS) [33–37]. Therefore, the transport of P-gp substrates may be altered by modulation of P-gp expression/activity under conditions of oxidative stress [38]. In this sense, natural antioxidants, such as polyphenols, could influence the function of this membrane transporter. It was reported that polyphenolic compounds, mainly flavonoids or their derivatives, can modulate the main ABC transporters responsible for cancer drug resistance, including P-gp [16,39–41].

The interest in health benefits of polyphenols has increased due to their powerful antioxidant and free radical scavenging activities observed in vitro [42]. Current evidence strongly supports a contribution of polyphenols, in particular flavonoids, to the prevention and therapy of cancer and other chronic diseases [1,43]. Literature data have shown that plant phenolic content and antioxidant activity depend on several factors, mainly environmental conditions [3]. Previous studies show that summer plants (reproductive stage) are richer in phenolic compounds than spring ones (vegetative stage), and consequently exhibit higher antioxidant activities [2,3]. Here, we evaluated the antioxidant potential of the *Ageratina havanensis* extracts by using three in vitro methods of well-established use to strongly predict the antioxidant capacity of several substances [22–24]. But surprisingly, the results of the performed studies showed the opposite, the concentration of flavonoids is higher in the vegetative state. In fact, we observed that *Ageratina havanensis* extracts possess higher reductive capacity in the vegetative period. This finding might be related to the content of sakuranetin and 7-methoxyaromadendrin, which is greater in the vegetative stage. The antioxidant capacity of sakuranetin has been previously demonstrated [44]. Indeed, here we observed that sakuranetin possesses the greatest reductive capacity of the analyzed samples. In order to evaluate the antioxidant capacity in a biological system, we used the lipid peroxidation model in brain homogenates. Rat brain homogenates exposed to oxygen spontaneously exhibit lipid peroxidation by a mechanism which is independent of superoxide and free hydroxyl radical production and whose initiation step may involve and iron-mediated cleavage of lipid hydroperoxides to yield peroxide or alkoxy radicals [45,46]. In this system, the extracts obtained from the flowering stage effectively inhibited TBARS generation with estimated values (see Table 1). This result could be explained in term of several mechanisms comprising among others, iron chelation, (at the initiation step) or a synergistic antioxidant activity (at the propagation step). In addition, previous studies demonstrated the metal chelation properties of polyphenols [47,48]. The present results suggest that *Ageratina havanensis* could be represent a source of antioxidants with potential neuroprotective actions. In summary, these results show for first time the antioxidant potential of the extracts obtained from the species *Ageratina havanensis*.

4. Materials and Methods

4.1. General

Analytical-grade *n*-hexane, ethyl acetate (EtOAc), *n*-butanol (*n*-BuOH), ethanol (EtOH) and UPLC/MS-grade methanol (Sigma Aldrich, St. Luis, MO, USA) were used. HPLC-grade water was prepared using a Milli-Q purification system (Millipore, Burlington, MA, USA). The RP18 cartridge was a Phenomenex Strata C18-E. Sakuranetin and 7-methoxyaromadendrin (standards) were previously isolated from the leaves of *Ageratina havanensis* (Kunth) R. M. King & H. Robinson [17]. They were identified and standardized by spectroscopic techniques (^{1}H-NMR, ^{13}C-NMR, 2D NMR, MS). The stability was evaluated by NMR.

4.2. Plant Material and Extraction

Ageratina havanensis (Kunth) R. M. King & H. Robinson (Asteraceae) as authenticated by Prof. Iralys Ventosa, Instituto de Ecología y Sistemática, Havana, Cuba (voucher herbarium specimen number HAC-42498) was collected in Havana (East Havana, Alamar neighbourhood) during 2012 in flowering and vegetative stage. The secondary metabolites were extracted as previously reported [17,18].

4.3. Cytotoxicity and P-glycoprotein Activity Assays

The study was conducted using 4T1 cells (ATCC, Manasssas, VA, USA) cultured in RPMI-1640 medium containing 10% fetal bovine serum, 1% penicillin-streptomycin and glutamine (2 mmol/L) at 37 °C in 5% CO_2 humidified incubator.

Cytotoxicity was measured using the MTT reduction assay [49]. After extracts exposure, cells were washed and a 100 µL/well of MTT reagent (5 mg/mL) was added. After a 4 h incubation period at 37 °C, supernatants were discarded. The dye was extracted with dimethyl sulfoxide and optical density was read at 540 nm. The inhibition of reduction of MTT was expressed as the percentage of viable cells referred to control cells, those incubated in presence of the vehicle only (100% viability value). IC_{50} values were calculated.

P-glycoprotein (P-gp) activity was evaluated by the Rhodamine-123 (Rho-123) accumulation assay [13]. Cells (4×10^4/well) were treated for 24 h with sub-toxic concentrations of the extracts (10–200 µg/mL) or verapamil (20 µM), an inhibitor of P-gp activity (positive control). Cells were washed and incubated with 5 µg/mL Rho-123 for 2 h. Afterwards, the cells were lysed with 0.1% Triton X-100. In cell lysates fluorescence intensity was measured at the 485 nm excitation and 535 nm emission wavelengths. Data were expressed as percentage of fluorescence relative to control cells.

4.4. Antioxidant Capacity Assays

The free radicals scavenging capacity of the extracts was determined [50]. For it, an ethanolic solution of 130 mM 2,2-diphenyl-1-picrylhydrazyl (DPPH•, Sigma Aldrich, St. Luis, MO, USA) was mixed with the extracts (2–1000 µg/mL). Ascorbic acid (Sigma) 50 µg/mL was employed as standard. The reaction mixtures were incubated in the dark at room temperature for 30 min and the absorbance was measured at 515 nm. The inhibition percent of DPPH• radical was calculated by:

$$\text{Inhibition (\%)} = (\text{D.O. control} - \text{D.O. sample})/\text{D.O. control} \times 100 \tag{1}$$

The concentration required to scavenge 50% of DPPH (IC50) was determined.

The reducing capacity of the plant extracts was measured according to the method of Benzie and Strain (1996) [51]. Briefly, acetate buffer (300 mM, pH = 3.6), TPTZ (2, 4, 6-tripyridyl-s-triazine; Sigma) 10 mM in 40 mM HCl and $FeCl_3 \times 6H_2O$ (20 mM) were mixed in the ratio of 10:1:1 to obtain FRAP reagent. The extracts (20 µL) were mixed with 900 µL of FRAP reagent. The mixtures were incubated at room temperature for 4 min and absorbances were measured at 593 nm. Ascorbic acid (100 µM) was used as standard.

To evaluate the inhibition of brain phospholipid peroxidation, rat brains were excised after decapitation, weighed and washed with 0.9% NaCl ice cold solution. Tissue homogenates were prepared in a ratio of 1 g of wet tissue to 9 mL of phosphate buffer (50 mM, pH 7.4), by using a tissue homogenizer (Qiagen). The homogenates were centrifuged at 800× *g* in a Sigma centrifuge at −4 °C during 15 min and the supernatants were kept at −70 °C until analysis. Thiobarbituric reactive substances (TBARS) measurement assay was carried out as previously described [52]. Brain homogenates (25 mL) were incubated with different extracts (5–125 µg/mL). Incubations were stopped by the addition of 350 mL of cold acetic acid 20% pH 3.5. Malondialdehyde (MDA) levels were determined by the addition of 600 mL of TBA 0.5% in acetic acid 20% pH 3.5. The mixtures were incubated at 90 °C for 1 h. Then, 50 mL of sodium dodecyl sulfate (SDS) were added, and samples were centrifuged at 500× *g* during 15 min at room temperature. The absorbance was measured at 532 nm.

All the values are means of three determinations. Trolox-C (0.5–75 µg/mL), was used as standard. The extract concentration which is needed to achieve the 50% of inhibition of lipid peroxidation (IC50) was calculated.

4.5. Statistical Analysis

Values were expressed as mean ± standard error of mean (SEM). Statistical analysis was performed with SPSS 18.0 (SPSS Inc., Chicago, IL, USA). For multiple comparisons, one-way ANOVA was used followed by Dunnett post-hoc test. Values of $p < 0.05$ were considered statistically significant.

4.6. Sample Preparation for UPLC-ESI-MS/MS Analysis

A solution of each extract (MeOH/H_2O 8:2 *v/v*, 1 mg/mL) was submitted to the solid-phase extraction using RP18 cartridge, eluted with MeOH/H_2O 8:2 (*v/v*). After drying, 1 mg was dissolved in 1 mL of MeOH/H_2O 8:2 (*v/v*) solution (solution A) and an aliquot was diluted with MeOH/H_2O 8:2 (*v/v*) to reach a final volume of 1 mL (150 µg/mL), and was filtered through a 0.22 µm nylon filter membrane. The final solution was used for quantification analysis. For PCA, the solution A was diluted with MeOH/H_2O 8:2 (*v/v*) to reach a final concentration of 1 µg/mL. The sample preparations were triplicated.

Standard Solutions Preparation for Quantification Analysis

Sakuranetin and 7-methoxyaromadendrin were dissolved in 1 mL of MeOH/H_2O 8:2 (*v/v*) solution (1 mg/mL) and filtered through a 0.22 µm nylon filter membrane. An aliquot was diluted with MeOH/H_2O 8:2 (*v/v*) up to a volume of 1 mL (100 ppm, solution A). The solution A was diluted to obtain the solutions patterns between 1 and 50 µg/mL (three replicas for each concentration).

4.7. UPLC-ESI-MS Analysis of the Extracts

Analysis was performed on a Waters® Acquity UPLC system coupled with a XevoTqD® mass spectrometer (Waters Corp., Milford, MA, USA). The analytical column used was an ACQUITY™ UPLC X bridge C18 (2.1 × 50 mm, 2.5 µm). Analysis was carried out with water containing 0.1% formic acid (A) and methanol (B) at a flow rate of 400 µL/min during 10 min. A gradient program was used for quantification as follows: 0–8 min, 47% B isocratic; 8–10 min, 47–100% B linear and for PCA: 0–3.2 min, 40% B isocratic; 3.2–4 min, 40–60% B linear; 4–8.2 min, 60% B isocratic; 8.2–10 min, 60–100% B linear. The injection volume was 5 µL in quantification analysis and 10 µL in PCA analysis. Mass spectrometric detection was in negative mode. The MS conditions were as follows: capillary temperature 200 °C; capillary voltage 3.5 kV; Cone voltage 39 kV; desolvation temperature 200 °C; Source gas flow: desolvation 400 L/h. Selected reaction monitoring mode was used for quantification. The monitored transitions included the following: sakuranetin (285 > 165) and 7-methoxyaromadendrin (301 > 165). All data were acquired and processed using the Masslynx™ V4.1 software (Waters Corporation, Milford, MA, USA).

4.7.1. Quantification Method Validation

Linearity, LDQ and LOQ

Calibration curves were generated by using 1/x-weighted least-square linear regression. Concentrations of the flavonoids were calculated by linear interpolation from the calibration curves. LDQ was determined by the following calculation: $(Y_{bl} + 3S_{bl})/b$, while LOQ was calculated multiplying Sbl by 10 [53].

Matrix Effect and Recovery

Matrix effects were determined by comparing the peak area of standards in the extracts (A), after evaluation of a sample target, with that of analyte standard solutions (B). The recoveries of the analytes were determined by comparing the peak area of analytes standard solution (8 ppm) after solid phase extraction (SPE) with that of the analytes' standard solution (8 ppm) before SPE. The ratio (after SPE/before SPE) × 100 was determined.

Precision and Accuracy of the System

Precision and accuracy were assessed on three consecutive days by using mixtures containing low, medium, or high concentrations of the analytes' standard solution. Precision was expressed as the RSD %, and accuracy (% RE) was calculated using the following equation:

$$[(\text{mean measured concentration}-\text{concentration of standard solutions})/ \tag{2}$$
$$(\text{concentration of standard solutions})] \times 100.$$

4.7.2. PCA of Extracts

The software Markerlynx^{XS} (Waters Corporation, Milford, MA, USA) was used to generate a matrix containing the *m/z* ratio of ions detected in each sample and the area under the curve of each peak in the chromatogram. PCA calculation was performed using Past 2.14 software (Waters Corporation). PC to be analyzed were selected according to the significance of the eigenvalues of each component. The loads were considered to evaluate the impact of the original variables on the new components, while percent of variance explained of the new PC selected were used to evaluate similarities and differences between the extracts studied.

5. Conclusions

In this work, a rapid and sensitive method was developed to quantify the major flavonoids present in eleven *Ageratina havanensis* extracts obtained from two phenological states of *Ageratina havanensis*. The phenological state of the plant influences the concentration of sakuranetin, 7-methoxyaromadendrine and glycosides with *m/z* 447 in its extracts; in fact, the content of these compounds is higher in the vegetative state. In addition, the antioxidant potential of *Ageratina havanensis* (Kunth) R. M. King & H. Robinson extracts and its relationship with the concentration of major flavonoids were demonstrated for the first time. The results obtained in this study also highlight that this plant could be a source of new potential inhibitors of drug efflux mediated by P-gp. However, other in vitro and in vivo studies must be conducted to confirm the potential pharmacological or therapeutic relevance of these findings.

Supplementary Materials: The following are available online. Table S1: Equations for calibration curves, limit of detection (LDQ) and limit of quantitation (LOQ) by UPLC/ESI/TQD/MS^n. Table S2: Summary of precision and accuracy results by UPLC/ESI/TQD/MS^n, Table S3: Principal components selected for the PCA, Table S4: Most influential variables in PC. Figure S1: Chromatogram of sakuranetin at 25 µg/mL, Figure S2: Chromatogram of 7-methoxyaromadendrin at 25 µg/mL, Figure S3: MRM chromatogram of 7-methoxyaromadendrin and sakuranetin in the ethyl acetate extract of *Ageratina havanensis* leaves.

Author Contributions: Conceptualization, I.R., W.V., I.S. and L.R.; methodology, T.H.G., I.S. and L.R.; software, L.D.-R.; validation, I.S., C.Q.d.R., I.R. and M.T.P.L.; formal analysis, L.D.-R., Y.Á. and C.C.; investigation, T.H.G., C.Q.d.R., I.H.; resources, I.S. and L.R.; data curation, W.V.; writing—original draft preparation, T.H.G. and C.Q.d.R.; writing—review and editing, G.A. and L.R.; visualization, G.A. and L.R.; supervision, I.S. and L.R.; project administration, I.R., I.S. and L.R.; funding acquisition, I.S., L.D.-R., I.R., and M.T.P.L. All authors have read and agreed to the published version of the manuscript.

Funding: This research was funded by Project CAPES-MES "Sustainable use of Cuban and Brazilian biodiversity: Potentially bioactive: Natural Products from higher plants" (Process No. 122/11) and Visiting Research Program (PVE-Research Project, No. 400768/2014-3), CNPq, Brazil.

Conflicts of Interest: The authors declare no conflict of interest. The funders had no role in the design of the study; in the collection, analyses, or interpretation of data; in the writing of the manuscript, or in the decision to publish the results.

References

1. Procházková, D.; Boušová, I.; Wilhelmová, N. Antioxidant and prooxidant properties of flavonoids. *Fitoterapia* **2011**, *82*, 513–523. [CrossRef] [PubMed]
2. Medini, F.; Fellah, H.; Ksouri, R.; Abdelly, C. Total phenolic, flavonoid and tannin contents and antioxidant and antimicrobial activities of organic extracts of shoots of the plant *Limonium delicatulum*. *J. Taibah Univ. Sci.* **2014**, *8*, 216–224. [CrossRef]
3. Jallali, I.; Megdiche, W.; M'Hamdi, B.; Oueslati, S.; Smaoui, A.; Abdelly, C.; Ksouri, R. Changes in phenolic composition and antioxidant activities of the edible halophyte *Crithmum maritimum* L. with physiological stage and extraction method. *Acta Physiol. Plant.* **2012**, *34*, 1451–1459. [CrossRef]
4. Bansal, T.; Awasthi, A.; Jaggi, M.; Khar, R.K.; Talegaonkar, S. Pre-clinical evidence for altered absorption and biliary excretion of irinotecan (CPT-11) in combination with quercetin: Possible contribution of P-glycoprotein. *Life Sci.* **2008**, *83*, 250–259. [CrossRef]
5. Ozben, T. Mechanisms and strategies to overcome multiple drug resistance in cancer. *FEBS Lett.* **2006**, *22*, 2903–2909. [CrossRef]
6. Borska, S.; Sopel, M.; Chmielewska, M.; Zabel, M.; Dziegiel, P. Quercetin as a potential modulator of P-glycoprotein expression and function in cells of human pancreatic carcinoma line resistant to daunorubicin. *Molecules* **2010**, *15*, 857–870. [CrossRef]
7. Spengler, G.; Ocsovszki, I.; Tönki, Á.S.; Saijo, R.; Watanabe, G.; Kawase, M.; Molnár, J. Fluorinated β-Diketo Phosphorus Ylides Are Novel Inhibitors of the ABCB1 Efflux Pump of Cancer Cells. *Anticancer Res.* **2015**, *35*, 5915–5919.
8. Wang, Z.; Wong, I.L.; Li, F.X.; Yang, C.; Liu, Z.; Jiang, T.; Jiang, T.F.; Chow, L.M.; Wan, S.B. Optimization of permethyl ningalin B analogs as P-glycoprotein inhibitors. *Bioorg. Med. Chem.* **2015**, *23*, 5566–5573. [CrossRef]
9. Wong, I.L.; Wang, B.C.; Yuan, J.; Duan, L.X.; Liu, Z.; Liu, T.; Li, X.M.; Hu, X.; Zhang, X.Y.; Jiang, T.; et al. Potent and Nontoxic Chemosensitizer of P-Glycoprotein-Mediated Multidrug Resistance in Cancer: Synthesis and Evaluation of Methylated Epigallocatechin, Gallocatechin, and Dihydromyricetin Derivatives. *J. Med. Chem.* **2015**, *58*, 4529–4549. [CrossRef]
10. Gottesman, M.M.; Ling, V. The molecular basis of multidrug resistance in cancer: The early years of P-glycoprotein research. *FEBS Lett.* **2006**, *580*, 998–1009. [CrossRef]
11. Bansal, T.; Jaggi, M.; Khar, R.K.; Talegaonkar, S. Emerging Significance of Flavonoids as P Glycoprotein Inhibitors in Cancer Chemotherapy. *J. Pharm. Pharmaceut. Sci.* **2009**, *12*, 46–78. [CrossRef] [PubMed]
12. Brand, W.; Schutte, M.E.; Williamson, G.; van Zanden, J.J. Flavonoid-mediated inhibition of intestinal ABC transporters may affect the oral bioavailability of drugs, food-borne toxic compounds and bioactive ingredients. *Biomed. Pharmacother.* **2006**, *60*, 508–519. [CrossRef] [PubMed]
13. Chieli, E.; Romiti, N.; Rodeiro, I.; Garrido, G. In vitro effects of *Mangifera indica* and polyphenols derived on ABCB1/P-glycoprotein activity. *Food Chem. Toxicol.* **2009**, *47*, 2703–2710. [CrossRef] [PubMed]
14. Chieli, E.; Romiti, N.; Rodeiro, I.; Garrido, G. In vitro modulation of ABCB1/P-glycoprotein expression by polyphenols from *Mangifera indica*. *Chem. Biol. Interact.* **2010**, *186*, 287–294. [CrossRef] [PubMed]
15. Silva, N.; Salgueiro, L.; Fortuna, A.; Cavaleiro, C. P-glycoprotein mediated efflux modulators of plant origin: A Short Review. *Nat. Prod. Commun.* **2016**, *11*, 699–704. [CrossRef] [PubMed]
16. Tolosa, L.; Rodeiro, I.; Donato, M.T.; Herrera, J.A.; Delgado, R.; Castell, J.V.; Gómez-Lechón, M.J. Multiparametric evaluation of the cytoprotective effect of the Mangifera indica L. stem bark extract and mangiferin in Hep-G2 cells. *J. Pharm. Pharmacol.* **2013**, *65*, 1073–1082. [CrossRef]
17. del Barrio, G.; Spengler, I.; García, T.H.; Roque, A.; Álvarez, A.L.; Calderón, J.S.; Parra, F. Antiviral activity of *Ageratina havanensis* and major chemical compounds from the most active fraction. *Braz. J. Pharmacog.* **2011**, *21*, 915–920. [CrossRef]
18. García, T.H.; Quintino da Rocha, C.; Dias, M.J.; Pino, L.L.; del Barrio, G.; Roque, A.; Pérez, C.E.; Campaner dos Santos, L.; Spengler, I.; Vilegas, W. Comparison of the Qualitative Chemical Composition of Extracts from *Ageratina havanensis* Collected in Two Different Phenological Stages by FIA-ESI-IT-MS^n and UPLC/ESI-MS^n: Antiviral Activity. *Nat. Prod. Commun.* **2017**, *12*, 31–34. [CrossRef]

19. Hosu, A.; Cristea, V.M.; Cimpoiu, C. Analysis of total phenolic, flavonoids, anthocyanins and tannins content in Romanian red wines: Prediction of antioxidant activities and classification of wines using artificial neural networks. *Food Chem.* **2014**, *150*, 113–118. [CrossRef]

20. Lee, L.-S.; Choi, E.-J.; Kim, C.-H.; Sung, J.-M.; Kim, Y.-B.; Seo, D.-H.; Choi, H.-W.; Choi, Y.-S.; Kum, J.-S.; Park, J.-D. Contribution of flavonoids to the antioxidant properties of common and tartary buckwheat. *J. Cereal. Sci.* **2016**, *68*, 181–186. [CrossRef]

21. Ben Sghaier, M.; Skandrani, I.; Nasr, N.; Franca, M.G.; Chekir-Ghedira, L.; Ghedira, K. Flavonoids and sesquiterpenes from *Tecurium ramosissimum* promote antiproliferation of human cancer cells and enhance antioxidant activity: A structure-activity relationship study. *Environ. Toxicol. Pharmacol.* **2011**, *32*, 336–348. [CrossRef] [PubMed]

22. Huang, D.; Ou, B.; Prior, R.L. The chemistry behind antioxidant capacity assays. *J. Agric. Food Chem.* **2005**, *53*, 1841–1856. [CrossRef] [PubMed]

23. Ebrahimzadeh, M.A.; Pourmorad, F.; Bekhradnia, A.R. Iron chelating activity screening, phenol and flavonoid content of some medicinal plants from Iran. *Afr. J. Biotechnol.* **2008**, *7*, 3188–3192.

24. Sirivibulkovit, K.; Nouanthavong, S.; Sameenoi, Y. Paper-based DPPH Assay for Antioxidant Activity Analysis. *Anal. Sci.* **2018**, *34*, 795–800. [CrossRef] [PubMed]

25. Dehpour, A.A.; Ebrahimzadeh, M.A.; Fazel, N.S.; Mohammad, N.S. Antioxidant activity of methanol extract of *Ferula assafoetida* and its essential oil composition. *Oils Fats* **2009**, *60*, 405–412.

26. Halliwell, B.; Gutteridge, J. Antioxidant defences: Endogenous and diet derived. *Free Radic. Biol. Med.* **2007**, *4*, 79–186.

27. Badmus, J.A.; Adedosu, T.O.; Fatoki, J.O.; Adegbite, V.A.; Adaramoye, O.A.; Odunola, O.A. Lipid peroxidation inhibition and antiradical activities of some leaf fractions of *Mangifera indica*. *Acta Pol. Pharm.* **2011**, *68*, 23–29.

28. De Santis, C.E.; Bray, F.; Ferlay, J.; Lortet-Tieulent, J.; Anderson, B.O.; Jemal, A. International variation in female breast cancer incidence and mortality rates. *Cancer Epidemiol. Biomark. Prev.* **2015**, *10*, 1495–1506. [CrossRef]

29. Bradley, G.; Ling, V. P-glycoprotein, multidrug resistance and tumor progression. *Cancer Metastasis Rev.* **1994**, *13*, 223–233. [CrossRef]

30. Varma, M.V.; Ashokraj, Y.; Dey, C.S.; Panchagnula, R. P-glycoprotein inhibitors and their screening: A perspective from bioavailability enhancement. *Pharmacol. Res.* **2003**, *48*, 347–359. [CrossRef]

31. Aszalos, A. Role of ATP-binding cassette (ABC) transporters in interactions between natural products and drugs. *Curr. Drug Metab.* **2008**, *9*, 1010–1018. [CrossRef] [PubMed]

32. Chen, X.W.; Sneed, K.B.; Pan, S.Y.; Cao, C.; Kanwar, J.R.; Chew, H.; Zhou, S.F. Herb-drug interactions and mechanistic and clinical considerations. *Curr. Drug Metab.* **2012**, *13*, 640–651. [CrossRef] [PubMed]

33. Banerjee, K.; Basu, S.; Das, S.; Sinha, A.; Biswas, M.K.; Choudhuri, S.K. Induction of intrinsic and extrinsic apoptosis through oxidative stress in drug-resistant cancer by a newly synthesized Schiff base copper chelate. *Free Radic. Res.* **2016**, *50*, 426–446. [CrossRef] [PubMed]

34. Hong, H.; Lu, Y.; Ji, Z.N.; Liu, G.Q. Up-regulation of P-glycoprotein expression by glutathione depletion-induced oxidative stress in rat brain microvessel endothelial cells. *J. Neurochem.* **2006**, *98*, 1465–1473. [CrossRef] [PubMed]

35. Qosa, H.; Lichter, J.; Sarlo, M.; Markandaiah, S.S.; McAvoy, K.; Richard, J.P.; Jablonski, M.R.; Maragakis, N.J.; Pasinelli, P.; Trotti, D. Astrocytes drive up-regulation of the multidrug resistance transporter ABCB1 (P-glycoprotein) in endothelial cells of the blood-brain barrier in mutant superoxide dismutase 1-linked amyotrophic lateral sclerosis. *Glia* **2016**, *64*, 1298–1313. [CrossRef] [PubMed]

36. Stanković, T.; Dankó, B.; Martins, A.; Dragoj, M.; Stojković, S.; Isaković, A.; Wang, H.C.; Wu, Y.C.; Hunyadi, A.; Pešić, M. Lower antioxidative capacity of multidrug-resistant cancer cells confers collateral sensitivity to protoflavone derivatives. *Cancer Chemother. Pharmacol.* **2015**, *76*, 555–565. [CrossRef]

37. Wartenberg, M.; Fischer, K.; Hescheler, J.; Sauer, H. Redox regulation of P-glycoprotein-mediated multidrug resistance in multicellular prostate tumor spheroids. *Int. J. Cancer* **2000**, *85*, 267–274. [CrossRef]

38. Wartenberg, M.; Hoffmann, E.; Schwindt, H.; Grünheck, F.; Petros, J.; Arnold, J.R.; Hescheler, J.; Sauer, H. Reactive oxygen species-linked regulation of the multidrug resistance transporter P-glycoprotein in Nox-1 overexpressing prostate tumor spheroids. *FEBS Lett.* **2005**, *579*, 4541–4549. [CrossRef]

39. Hussain, S.A.; Sulaiman, A.A.; Alhaddad, H.; Alhadidi, Q. Natural polyphenols: Influence on membrane transporters. *J. Intercult. Ethnopharmacol.* **2016**, *5*, 97–104. [CrossRef]

40. Michalak, K.; Wesolowska, O. Polyphenols counteract tumor cell chemoresistance conferred by multidrug resistance proteins. *Anticancer Agents Med. Chem.* **2012**, *12*, 880–990.

41. Reyes-Esparza, J.; Gonzaga, A.I.; González-Maya, L.; Rodríguez-Fragoso, L. (-)-Epigallocatechin-3-gallate modulates the activity and expression of P-glycoprotein in breast cancer cells. *J. Pharmacol. Clin. Toxicol.* **2015**, *3*, 1044–1051.

42. Pandey, K.B.; Rizvi, S.I. Plant polyphenols as dietary antioxidants in human health and disease. *Oxid. Med. Cell Longev.* **2009**, *2*, 270–278. [CrossRef] [PubMed]

43. Scalbert, A.; Johnson, I.T.; Saltmarsh, M. Polyphenols: Antioxidants and beyond. *Am. J. Clin. Nutr.* **2005**, *81*, 215S–217S. [CrossRef] [PubMed]

44. Sakoda, C.P.P.; de Toledo, A.C.; Perini, A.; Pinheiro, N.M.; Hiyane, M.I.; Grecco, S.D.S.; de Fátima Lopes Calvo Tibério, I.; Câmara, N.O.S.; de Arruda Martins, M.; Lago, J.H.G.; et al. Sakuranetin reverses vascular peribronchial and lung parenchyma remodeling in a murine model of chronic allergic pulmonary inflammation. *Acta Histochem.* **2016**, *118*, 615–624. [CrossRef]

45. Arai, H.; Kogure, K.; Sugioka, K.; Nakano, M. Importance of two iron-reducing systems in lipid peroxidation of rat brain: Implications for oxygen toxicity in the central nervous system. *Biochem. Int.* **1987**, *14*, 741–749.

46. Halliwell, B. Reactive oxygen species and the central nervous system. *J. Neurochem.* **1992**, *59*, 1609–1623. [CrossRef]

47. Hider, R.C.; Liu, Z.D.; Khodr, H.H. Metal chelation of polyphenols. *Methods Enzymol.* **2001**, *335*, 190–203.

48. Perron, N.R.; Brumaghim, J.L. A review of the antioxidant mechanisms of polyphenol compounds related to iron binding. *Cell Biochem. Biophys.* **2009**, *53*, 75–100. [CrossRef]

49. Mosmann, T. Rapid colorimetric assay for cellular growth and survival: Application to proliferation and cytotoxicity assays. *J. Immunol. Methods* **1983**, *65*, 55–63. [CrossRef]

50. Tabart, J.; Kevers, C.; Pincemail, J.; Defraigne, J.O.; Dommes, J. Comparative antioxidant capacities of phenolic compounds measured by various tests. *Food Chem.* **2009**, *113*, 1226–1233. [CrossRef]

51. Benzie, I.F.; Strain, J.J. The ferric reducing ability of plasma (FRAP) as a measure of "antioxidant power": The FRAP assay. *Anal. Biochem.* **1996**, *239*, 70–76. [CrossRef] [PubMed]

52. Ohkawa, H.; Ohishi, N.; Yagi, K. Assay for lipid peroxides in animal tissues by thiobarbituric acid reaction. *Anal. Biochem.* **1979**, *95*, 351–358. [CrossRef]

53. Shrivastava, A.; Gupta, V.B. Methods for the determination of limit of detection and limit of quantitation of the analytical methods. *Chron. Young Sci.* **2011**, *2*, 21. [CrossRef]

Sample Availability: Samples of the compounds are not available from the authors.

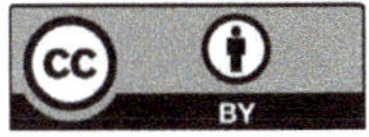

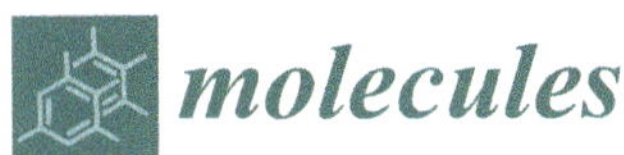 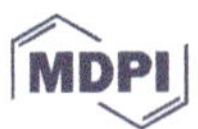

Article

Zingerone [4-(3-Methoxy-4-hydroxyphenyl)-butan-2] Attenuates Lipopolysaccharide-Induced Inflammation and Protects Rats from Sepsis Associated Multi Organ Damage

Adil Farooq Wali [1,*], Muneeb U Rehman [2], Mohammad Raish [3], Mohsin Kazi [3], Padma G. M. Rao [4], Osamah Alnemer [3], Parvaiz Ahmad [5] and Ajaz Ahmad [2,*]

[1] Department of Pharmaceutical Chemistry, RAK College of Pharmaceutical Sciences, RAK Medical and Health Science University, Ras Al Khaimah 11171, UAE

[2] Department of Clinical Pharmacy, College of Pharmacy, King Saud University, Riyadh 11451, Saudi Arabia; mrehman1@ksu.edu.sa

[3] Department of Pharmaceutics, College of Pharmacy, King Saud University, Riyadh 11451, Saudi Arabia; mraish@ksu.edu.sa (M.R.); mkazi@ksu.edu.sa (M.K.); usamah-14@hotmail.co.uk (O.A.)

[4] Department of Clinical Pharmacy and Pharmacology, RAK College of Pharmaceutical Sciences, RAK Medical and Health Science University, Ras Al Khaimah 11172, UAE; padma@rakmhsu.ac.ae

[5] Department of Botany and Microbiology, College of Science, King Saud University, Riyadh 11451, Saudi Arabia; parvaizbot@yahoo.com

* Correspondence: farooq@rakmhsu.ac.ae (A.F.W.); aajaz@ksu.edu.sa (A.A.)

Academic Editors: Raffaele Pezzani and Sara Vitalini
Received: 19 October 2020; Accepted: 1 November 2020; Published: 4 November 2020

Abstract: The present investigation aimed to evaluate the protective effect of Zingerone (ZIN) against lipopolysaccharide-induced oxidative stress, DNA damage, and cytokine storm in rats. For survival study the rats were divided into four groups (n = 10). The control group was treated with normal saline; Group II received an intraperitoneal (i.p) injection (10 mg/kg) of LPS as disease control. Rats in Group III were treated with ZIN 150 mg/kg (p.o) 2 h before LPS challenge and rats in Group IV were given ZIN only. Survival of the rats was monitored up to 96 h post LPS treatment. In another set, the animals were divided into four groups of six rats. Animals in Group I served as normal control and were treated with normal saline. Animals in Group II were treated with lipopolysaccharide (LPS) and served as disease control. Group III animals were treated with ZIN 2 h before LPS challenge. Group IV served as positive control and were treated with ZIN (150 mg/kg orally). The blood samples were collected and used for the analysis of biochemical parameters like alanine transaminase (ALT), alkaline phosphatase (ALP), aspartate transaminase (AST), blood urea nitrogen (BUN), Cr, Urea, lactate dehydrogenase (LDH), albumin, bilirubin (BIL), and total protein. Oxidative stress markers malondialdehyde (MDA), glutathione peroxidase (GSH), myeloperoxidase (MPO), and (DNA damage marker) 8-OHdG levels were measured in different organs. Level of nitric oxide (NO) and inflammatory markers like TNF-α, IL-1ß, IL-1α, IL-2, IL-6, and IL-10 were also quantified in plasma. Procalcitonin (PCT), a sepsis biomarker, was also measured. ZIN treatment had shown significant ($p < 0.5$) restoration of plasma enzymes, antioxidant markers and attenuated plasma proinflammatory cytokines and sepsis biomarker (PCT), thereby preventing the multi-organ and tissue damage in LPS-induced rats also confirmed by histopathological studies of different organs. The protective effect of ZIN may be due to its potent antioxidant potential. Thus ZIN can prevent LPS-induced oxidative stress as well as inflammatory and multi-organ damage in rats when administered to the LPS treated animals.

Keywords: zingerone; lipopolysaccharide; inflammation; anti-oxidant; cytokine storm; procalcitonin; histopathology

---

1. Introduction

Natural compounds have been used as treatments by ancient civilizations in drinks and flavorings. One of the most popular herbs, ginger, is used as a traditional medicine worldwide [1]. Ginger (*Zingiber officinale*) belongs to the family Zingiberaceae. Ginger is a perennial herb used for medicinal and culinary purposes. Ginger is used to treat a variety of ailments around the globe due to its varied phytochemical nature and health benefits [1]. Numerous phytoconstituents are present in ginger which have been divided in to volatile and non-volatile compounds [2]. During drying of ginger, Zingerone is produced directly and by thermal degradation. Zingerone (ZIN) [4-(3-methoxy-4-hydroxyphenyl)-butan-2-one] (Figure 1) is a vanillyl acetone which is a member of phenolic alkanone group [3]. ZIN is present in a significant amount in ginger and it is believed that the pharmacological activities of ginger is due to ZIN. It has a potent antioxidant, anti-inflammatory, anticancer, antidiabetic, antihypertensive, antimicrobial, antithrombotic, anxiolytic, anti-ulcer, and appetite stimulant properties [2].

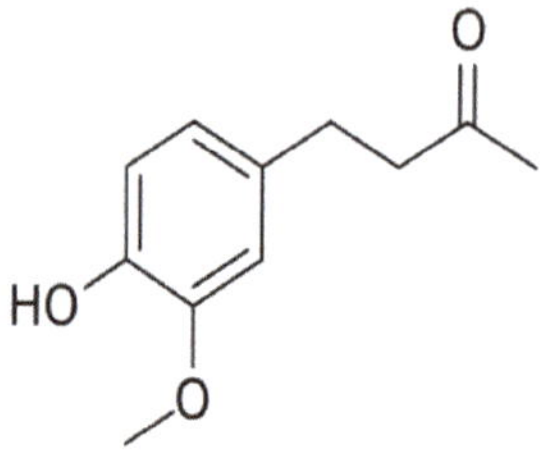

Figure 1. Chemical structure of Zingerone [4-(3-methoxy-4-hydroxyphenyl)-butan-2-one].

Lipopolysaccharide (LPS) is a compound that forms part of Gram-negative bacteria, and is a major pathogenic factor in systemic inflammation or sepsis [4]. Gram-negative bacteria are the only species in existence that contain the endotoxic portion of LPS, and lipid. In septic conditions, LPS can activate the innate immunity as a pathogen-associated molecular pattern (PAMP), which mediates an inflammatory response locally or systemically. Also, LPS can activate non-immune cells and start the inflammatory process which is typically detrimental [5,6]. LPS releases inflammatory cytokines in numerous cell types, causing acute inflammatory response towards pathogens [7]. High doses of LPS triggers the release of pro-inflammatory cytokines which causes a detrimental condition known as oxidative stress [8]. Oxidative stress plays a major role in LPS-induced systemic inflammation and is believed to promote the production of reactive oxygen species (ROS). ROS are believed to be involved in the LPS toxicity mechanism [9,10]. The increased ROS level further encourages inflammatory processes and elevate pro-inflammatory cytokines [11]. The first line of ROS mediated inflammation defense mechanism includes multiple antioxidant enzymes, such as: Myeloperoxidase (MPO) and glutathione peroxidase (GSH). Biological compounds (quercetin, resveratrol, curcumin, thymoquinone, and lycopene) with antioxidant properties can help protect against LPS-induced ROS in the tissues and organs [12]. ZIN is one the natural phytoconstituent considered to be reducing oxidative stress due to its potent antioxidant potential [2,13]. Despite of its antioxidant capacity, ZIN can be used to treat these diseases as an efficient medicine. This characteristic owes its potential to scavenge free oxidative radicals. ZIN can therefore suppress ROS and preserve the antioxidant properties. Thus the aim of the present investigation is to study the protective effect of zingerone against LPS-induced oxidative stress, DNA damage, cytokine storm, and histopathological alterations of different organs in rats.

2. Results

2.1. Effect of ZIN on Survival Rate of Animals

The survival rate of animals was monitored up to 96 h and is illustrated in Figure 2. Zingerone treatment increases the animal survival rate (70%) in lipopolysaccharide (LPS)-challenged animals.

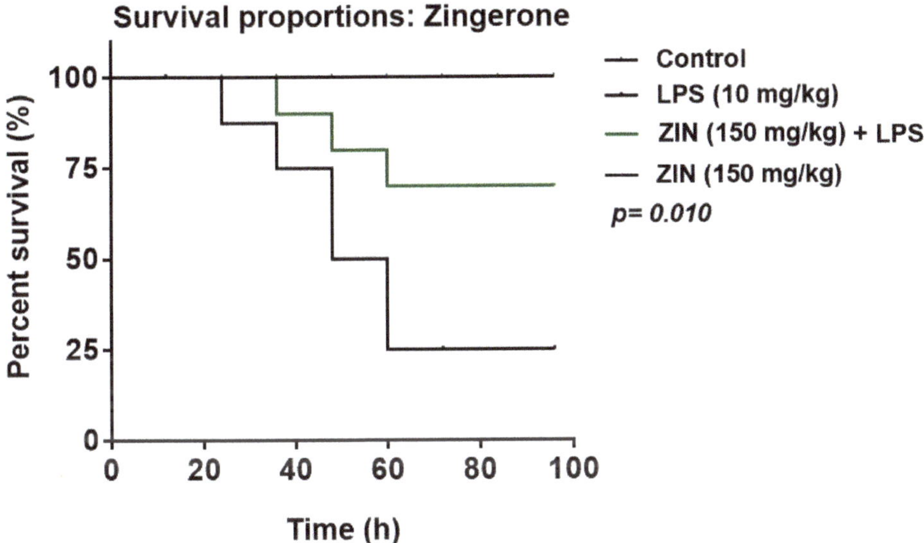

Figure 2. Kaplan–Meier survival plot (n = 10 rats per group). Effect of zingerone (ZIN) 150 mg/kg on survival rate of LPS induce systemic inflammation in rats.

2.2. Effect of ZIN on Biochemical Markers

Zingerone treatment exhibit minor changes in the biochemical parameters in the rats as compared with normal rats (Table 1). Animals in the endotoxemia (LPS) group showed significant abnormalities in different organ function markers as apparent by enhanced biochemical marker levels. The hepatic injury markers ALT (145.02 ± 3.84, U/L), ALP (186.54 ± 8.76, U/L) and AST (206.49 ± 11.45, U/L) levels were significantly higher in LPS group as compared to the control group ALT (27.69 ± 3.20, U/L), ALP (64.24 ± 4.32, U/L), and AST (57.65 ± 3.76, U/L), respectively. ZIN treatment decreases hepatic marker levels significantly from ALT (145.02 ± 3.84 to 74.99 ± 6.69 U/L, $p < 0.05$), ALP (186.54 ± 8.76 to 91.29 ± 5.34 U/L, $p < 0.05$) and AST (206.49 ± 11.45 to 87.35 ± 8.29 U/L, $p < 0.05$). General tissue damage of rats was confirmed from serum LDH levels in LPS group, a significantly increase in LDH levels were observed (972.75 ± 20.74 U/L), and these levels were decreased with ZIN treatment (656.59 ± 7.46 U/L $p < 0.05$). Similarly, a reduction in CK (553.83 ± 19.61 U/L $p < 0.05$), SCr (0.38 ± 0.05 mg/dL $p < 0.05$) and, BUN (67.71 ± 2.27 mg/dL $p < 0.05$) were observed in ZIN treated groups as compared to the animals in LPS group CK (855.47 ± 18.84 U/L), SCr (0.59 ± 0.09 mg/dL), and BUN (153.18 ± 7.34 mg/dL), respectively. Also, albumin levels were also increased with the ZIN treatment (3.18 ± 0.013 g/dL $p < 0.05$) as compared to the animals in the LPS group (2.36 ± 0.12 g/dL).

Table 1. List of plasma biochemical levels of different groups.

S.No.	Parameters	Control	LPS (10 mg/kg)	ZIN (150 mg/kg) + LPS	ZIN Only (150 mg/kg)
1	Creatinine Kinase (U/L)	68.32 ± 3.92	855.47 ± 18.84 *	553.83 ± 19.61 *#	66.67 ± 3.22
2	Serum Creatinine (mg/dL)	0.30 ± 0.03	0.59 ± 0.09 *	0.38 ± 0.05 *#	0.27 ± 0.01
3	BUN (mg/dL)	42.93 ± 1.92	153.18 ± 7.34 *	67.71 ± 2.27 *#	41.05 ± 0.59
4	LDH (U/L)	307.61 ± 12.27	972.75 ± 20.74 *	656.59 ± 7.46 *#	279.28 ± 7.50
5	ALT (U/L)	27.69 ± 3.20	145.02 ± 3.84	74.99 ± 6.69 *#	30.23 ± 1.43
6	ALP (U/L)	64.24 ± 4.32	186.54 ± 8.76 *	91.29 ± 5.34 *#	61.91 ± 2.65
7	AST (U/L)	57.65 ± 3.76	206.49 ± 11.45 *	87.35 ± 8.29 *#	52.24 ± 3.56
8	BIL (µmol/L)	1.69 ± 0.52	8.55 ± 1.07 *	4.56 ± 0.76*#	1.56 ± 0.75
9	GGT (U/L)	1.34 ± 0.24	3.89 ± 0.65 *	2.16 ± 0.66 *#	1.22 ± 0.34
10	Albumin (g/dL)	3.33 ± 0.12	2.36 ± 0.12 *	3.18 ± 0.013 *#	3.37 ± 0.05

Results are represented as mean ± SEM of six rats/group. * $p < 0.05$ vs. control; # $p < 0.05$ vs. LPS group. BUN: Blood urea Nitrogen; LDH: Lactate dehydrogenase; ALT: Alanine transaminase; ALP: Alkaline phosphatase; AST: Aspartate transaminase; BIL: Bilirubin; GGT: Gamma-glutamyl transferase.

2.3. Effect of ZIN on Oxidative Stress and Antioxidant Enzyme Markers

The LPS injection elicited levels of NO (97.08 ± 3.64 µM), which was significantly diminished in ZIN treated animals (57.36 ± 3.50 µM $p < 0.05$). 8-OHdG an indicator of DNA damage, the levels were significantly enhanced in the LPS treated groups (10.02 ± 0.84 ng/mL) and this was decreased with ZIN treatment (5.26 ± 0.40 ng/mL $p < 0.05$), respectively (Figure 3). Oxidative stress markers in different tissues e.g., brain, kidney, lung, and liver were measured in terms of glutathione (GSH), malondialdehyde (MDA), and myeloperoxidase (MPO) levels (Figures 4–6). MPO an enzyme of activated Polymorphonuclear (PMN) were used as an indication of tissue neutrophil accumulation. ZIN treatment in all tissues showed a significant ($p < 0.05$) reduction of these oxidative markers which was increased in LPS treated animals.

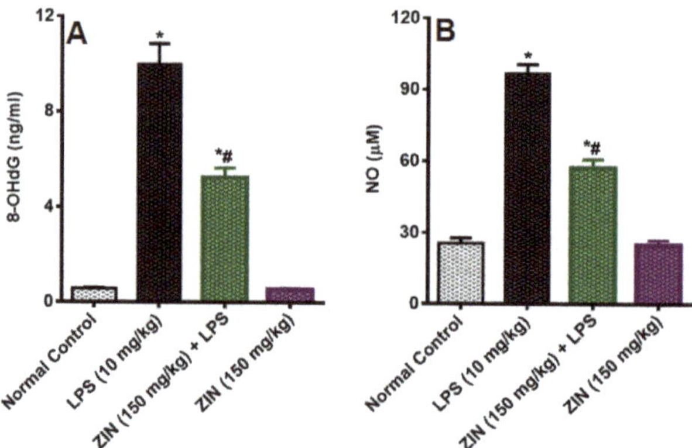

Figure 3. Effect of zingerone (ZIN) on LPS-induced DNA damage and oxidative stress marker. (**A**) 8-OHdG levels (ng/mL), (**B**) Nitric Oxide (NO) levels (µM). Results are represented as mean ± SEM of six rats/group. * $p < 0.05$ vs. control; # $p < 0.05$ vs. LPS group.

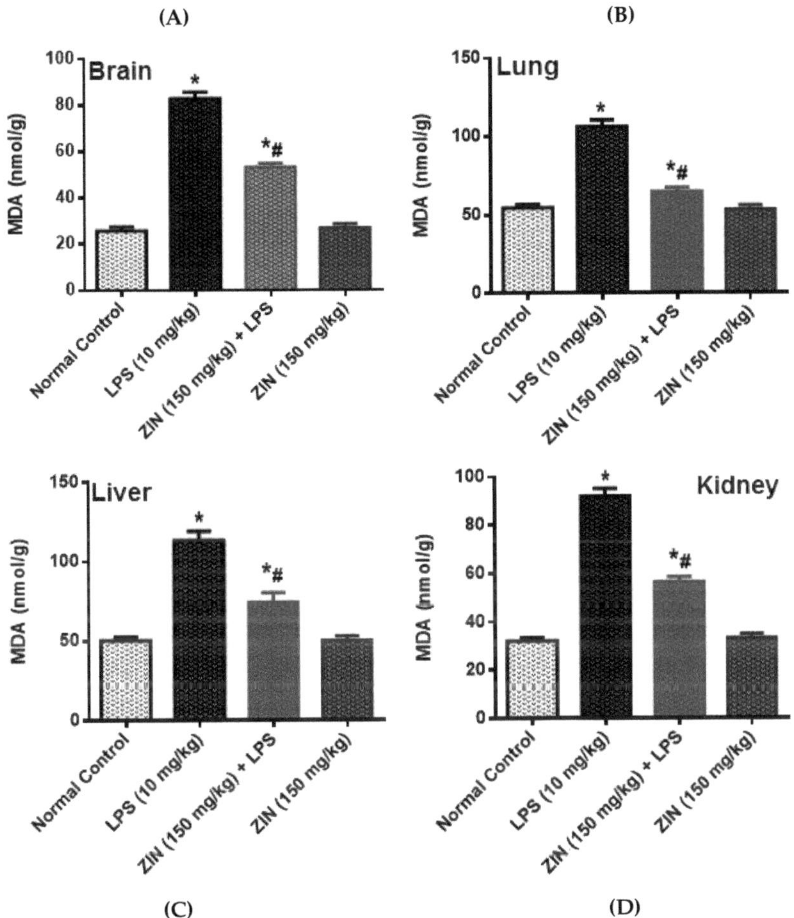

Figure 4. Effect of zingerone (ZIN) on LPS-induced oxidative stress as malondialdehyde (MDA) (nmol/kg). (**A**) Brain, (**B**) lung, (**C**) liver, and (**D**) kidney. Results are represented as mean ± SEM of six rats/group. * $p < 0.05$ vs. control; # $p < 0.05$ vs. LPS group.

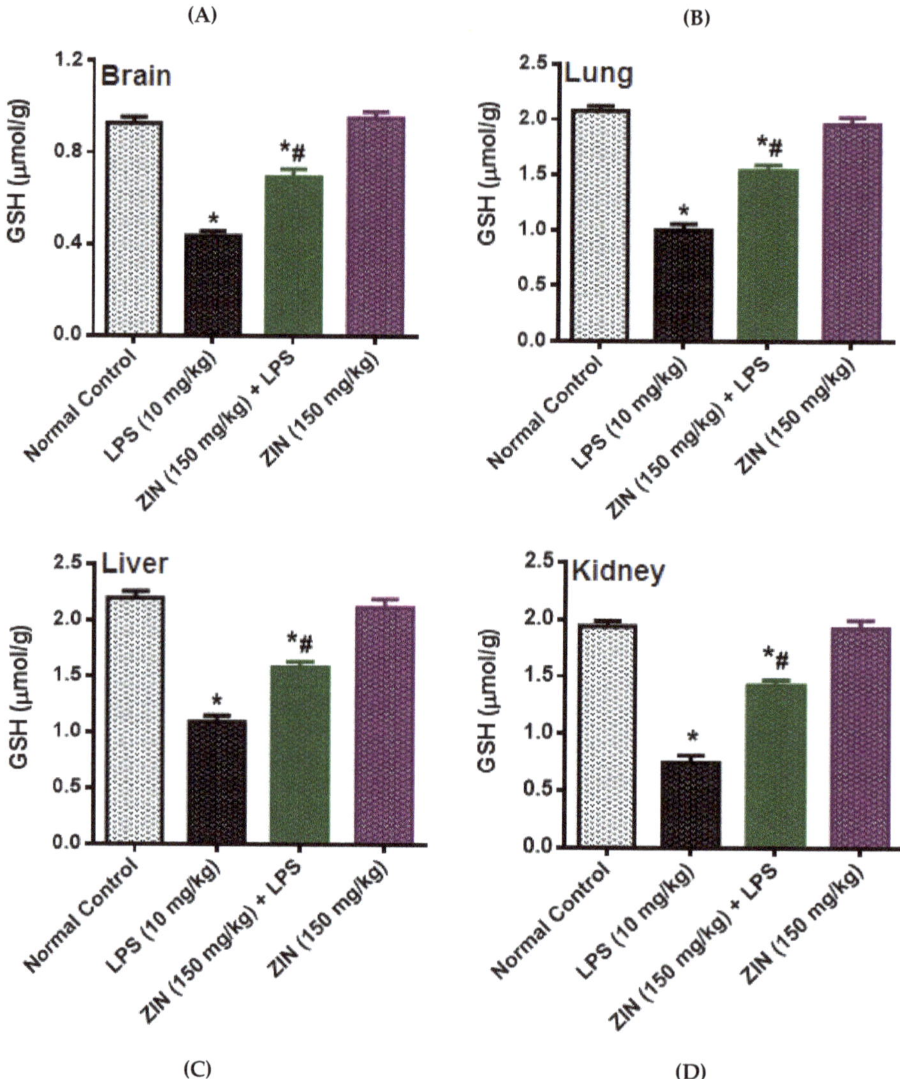

Figure 5. Effect of zingerone (ZIN) on LPS-induced oxidative stress as GSH (μmol/kg). (**A**) Brain, (**B**) Lung, (**C**) Liver and (**D**) Kidney. Results are represented as mean ± SEM of six rats/group. * $p < 0.05$ vs. control; # $p < 0.05$ vs. LPS group.

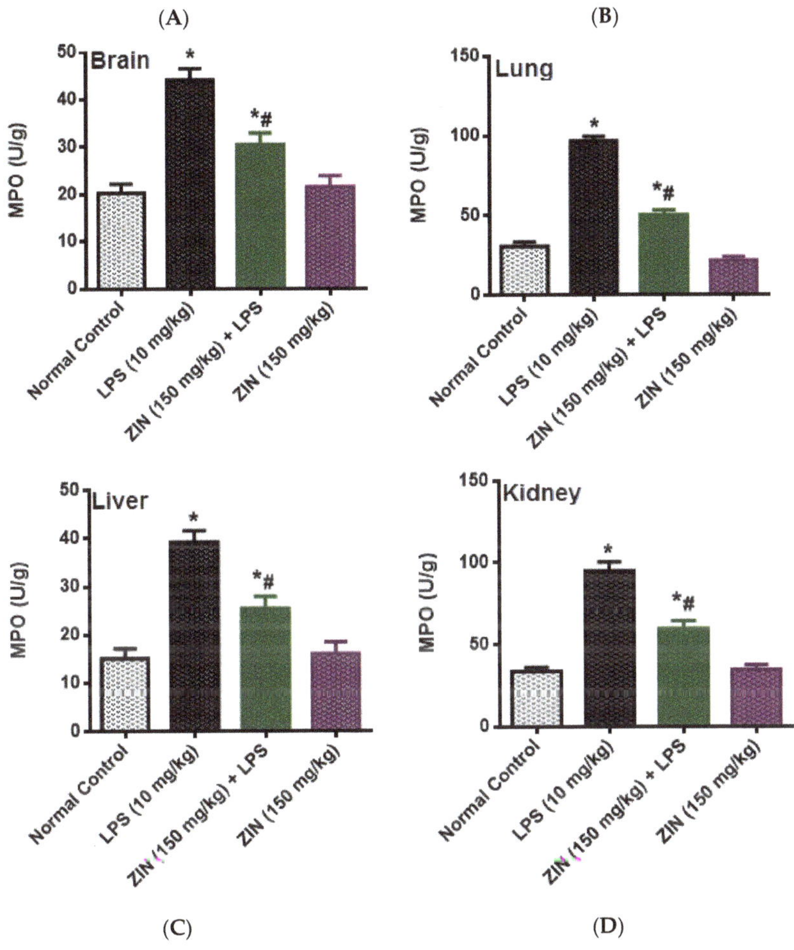

Figure 6. Effect of zingerone (ZIN) on LPS-induced oxidative stress as MPO (U/g). (**A**) Brain, (**B**) lung, (**C**) liver, and (**D**) kidney. Results are represented as mean ± SEM of six rats/group. * $p < 0.05$ vs. control; # $p < 0.05$ vs. LPS group.

2.4. Effect of ZIN on Cytokines and Inflammatory Markers

The inflammatory changes in the LPS-induced animals were determining as their cytokine levels (Figure 7). LPS-induced rats demonstrated a significant increase in the plasma levels of TNF-α (135.56 ± 4.17 pg/mL), IL-1α (509.12 ± 17.79 pg/mL), IL-1ß (1166.01 ± 27.54 pg/mL), IL-2 (20.67 ± 1.70 pg/mL), IL-6 (106.56 ± 3.44 pg/mL) and IL-10 (1037.49 ± 31.65 pg/mL). Zingerone treated animals showed reduced levels of these cytokines as compared to the disease control animals TNF-α (60.16 ± 3.52 pg/mL $p < 0.05$), IL-1α (235.49 ± 10.07 pg/mL $p < 0.05$), IL-1ß (739.78 ± 25.57 pg/mL $p < 0.05$), IL-2 (14.19 ± 1.77 pg/mL $p < 0.05$), IL-6 (61.60 ± 3.21 pg/mL $p < 0.05$) and IL-10 (665.90 ± 14.17 pg/mL $p < 0.05$). PCT levels were determined in the plasma of rats and were significantly increased in the LPS treated animals (2351.65 ± 39.75 pg/mL $p < 0.05$) compared to the normal rats (1053.03 ± 49.49 pg/mL). ZIN treatment significantly diminish the plasma PCT levels (1626.83 ± 86.70 pg/mL $p < 0.05$) Figure 7G.

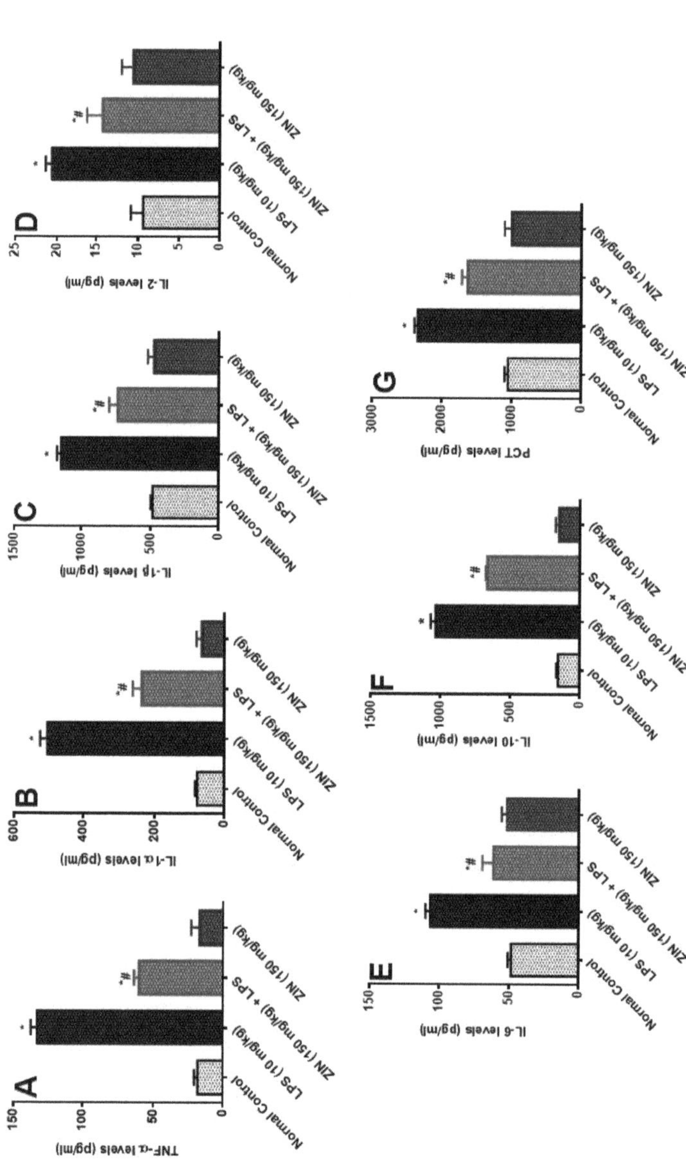

Figure 7. Effect of zingerone (ZIN) on LPS-induced Proinflammatory cytokines and sepsis biomarker PCT (pg/mL). (**A**) TNF-α, (**B**) IL-1α, (**C**) IL-2, (**D**) IL-6, (**E**) IL-8, (**F**) IL-10, and (**G**) procalcitonin (PCT). Results are represented as mean ± SEM of six rats/group. * $p < 0.05$ vs. control; # $p < 0.05$ vs. LPS group.

2.5. Effect of ZIN on Histoarchitecture of Different Organs

As depicted in Figure 8, the tissue sections from normal control group of different organs (brain, lung, liver, and kidney) exhibit normal architecture. Brain, lung, liver, and kidney tissues from LPS group exhibited the pathological alterations comprising widespread inflammation, portal inflammation, and hepatic cell necrosis, infiltration of inflammatory cells, severe hemorrhage, and thickening of alveolar septa, emphysema, and infiltration of leukocytes in walls alveoli and neuronal loss and condensed nucleus. However, treatment with ZIN 150 mg/kg significantly prevented the LPS-induced pathological changes and restored the histological architecture.

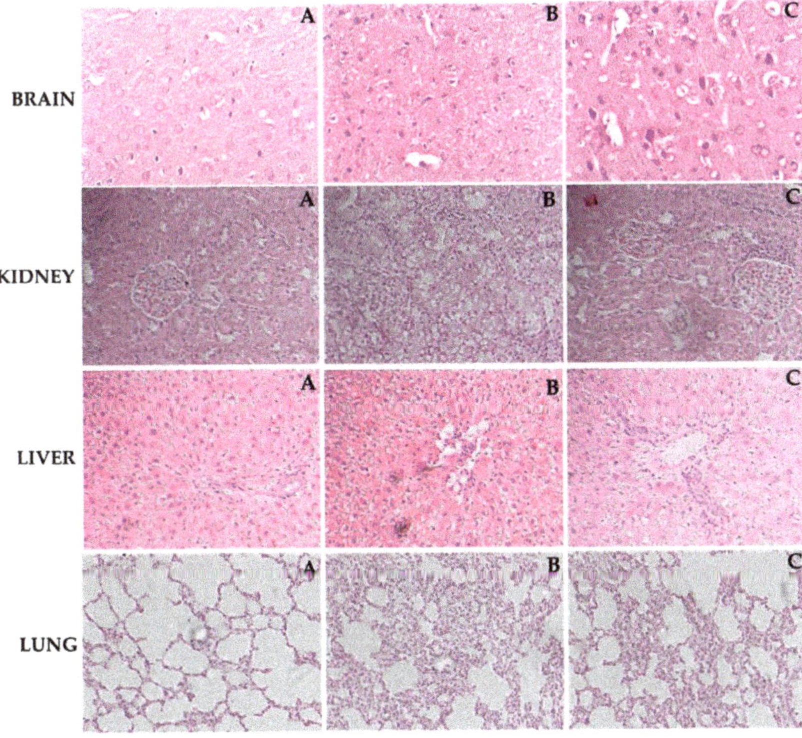

Figure 8. Light histograms of different rat organs (hematoxylin and eosin stains, magnification 40× and scale bar of 100 μm). Effect of ZIN in LPS intoxicated rats. Brain (**A**) normal control group: Showing normal histological structure with intact neurons, (**B**) LPS treated rats: Showing neuronal loss with condensed nuclei, (**C**) Rats treated with (ZIN 150 mg/kg + LPS: Showing decrease in neuronal loss with presence of intact neurons. Kidney (**A**) normal control group: Showing normal histological structure of the glomeruli and tubules at the cortex with absence of histopathological alterations, (**B**) LPS treated rats: Showing marked inflammatory cell aggregation in between the tubules, marked degeneration in the lining epithelium of all the tubules, and blood vessel congestion, (**C**) Rats treated with (ZIN 150 mg/kg + LPS: Showing absence of histopathological alterations. Liver (**A**) Normal control group: Showing normal histological structure of the central vein and intact hepatocytes, (**B**) LPS treated rats: Showing severe loss of hepatic architecture with multiple focal necrosis, ballooning degeneration in the hepatocytes, (**C**) Rats treated with ZIN 150 mg/kg + LPS: Showing absence of histopathological alterations. Lung (**A**) Normal control group showing normal morphology, (**B**) LPS treated rats: Showing moderate to severe hemorrhage, thickening of alveolar septa, emphysema, and infiltration of leukocytes in walls alveoli, (**C**) Rats treated with ZIN 150 mg/kg + LPS: Showing absence of histopathological changes.

3. Discussion

LPS is a significant component of Gram-negative bacteria's outer membrane and can induce inflammatory reactions by penetrating into the bloodstream that can trigger pain and eventually to death [14]. In the current investigation LPS caused impairment of kidney and liver function markers used for the determination of respective organ injuries. This increase in biochemical markers by LPS has been previously reported [15]. LPS has been suggested to generate NO and other ROS which causes peroxidation and cell alterations which further leads to the disruption of cell membrane and subsequent release of cytosolic contents [16]. Moreover, albumin levels were decreased in the in the present investigation which are corroborated with the reports of Amin et al., 2020 [12]. Bilirubin levels in LPS-induced animals were increase 4 fold compared to the normal control animals. ZIN treatment markedly mitigated the alterations induced by LPS by diminishing the levels of CK, Scr, alanine transaminase (ALT), alkaline phosphatase (ALP), aspartate transaminase (AST), blood urea nitrogen (BUN), and bilirubin (BIL) and increasing levels of albumin which is supported by the previous results of Amin et al., 2020 [15].

LPS treatment causes increase in the circulating nitrite levels in LPS intoxicated rats as compare to normal control animals. It is well known that LPS causes' significant increase in the nitrite levels because of over expression of inducible nitric oxide (iNOS) [17]. The endothelial cells are responsible for the increasing circulating levels of NO at the site of infection in response to pathogen [18]. NO is producing a potent oxidant peroxynitrite ($ONOO^-$) by reacting with superoxide anion ($O2^-$) which increases the lipid peroxidation and causes oxidative damages in different tissues [19]. The ZIN treatment was found to have protective effect against LPS-induced inflammation as evident by the significant decrease in circulating NO levels. These results were in agreement with the results of Alkharfy and colleagues in 2015, reported that thymoquinone significantly decrease the plasma levels of nitric oxide and the survival in animal model of sepsis [20]. Oxidative stress is characterized as an imbalance between free radical development and antioxidant defense. Superoxide ($O2^-$), hydroxyl (OH^-) and nitric oxide (NO^-) are among the most common reactive oxygen species. Antioxidants immediately reverse oxidative stress by enzymes, such as GSH, and MPO as well as by plant derived flavonoids [21], GSH (tripeptide thiol), found in cells is the most important anti-oxidant molecule and serves as a protecting agent against pathogen induced ROS and RNS [22] and regulates the cell proliferation, and apoptosis [23]. GSH depletion is an important pathological event in many tissues [24]. MPO is an enzyme located predominantly in the primary neutrophil granules and its key function is to destroy the pathogens, although in some circumstances it yields high amount of oxidants which further leads to tissue damage [25]. ROS destroys the cell membrane, DNA damage to cells, causing oxidation of lipid bilayer releasing MDA as the end product [26,27]. MDA, a lipid peroxidation marker used to evaluate the lipid peroxidation due to oxidative stress [28]. ZIN has an exceptional ability of scavenging reactive oxygen species (ROS), free radicals and other damaging oxidants by inhibiting the enzyme xanthine oxidase [13]. Zingerone has also know to exert beneficial effect and protects DNA damage against stannous chloride induced oxidative damage [13]. Zingerone administration has been shown to suppress the mitochondrial injury and lipid peroxidation and mitigates proapoptotic proteins like BAX, and caspases [29]. These findings suggest that zingerone is a potent antioxidant, which was further supported by the fact that ZIN had shown high antioxidant potential as compared to the ascorbic acid [13]. ZIN has shown antioxidant activity against superoxide and NO generated peroxynitrite causing damage to the cells [30]. The plasma levels of these oxidative markers were markedly increased in LPS-induced rats and were significantly reduced with ZIN treatment, suggesting the anti-oxidant potential of ZIN [2,15]. 8-OHdG is one of the principal forms of free radical-induced DNA damage by oxidation, thus been extensively used as an oxidative stress DNA biomarker [31,32]. The increased levels of 8-OHdG were suggested that DNA oxidation was aggravated by LPS administration. ZIN treatment has been found to prevent the LPS-induced oxidative DNA damages as evident by the decreased levels of 8-OHdG.

Elevated cytokines are recognized as inflammatory biomarkers in endotoxin-related pathogenesis [33,34]. TNF-α, IL-β, IL-α, IL-2, IL-6, and IL-10 are known as the key mediators of inflammation and TNF-α among them is considered to be a principal cytokine regulator [35,36]. Many research studies have identified the function of TNF-α and IL-1 in systemic inflammation, including both animal models of septic shock and in human sepsis trials [37,38]. Once released both TNF-α and IL-1 target on different cells e.g., macrophages, neutrophils and endothelial cells. TNF-α contributed to improved macrophage development which stimulates macrophage activation, differentiation and survival of these cells and thus enhances proinflammatory responses in infection [39]. TNF-α and IL-1 enhance inflammatory cascade by activating macrophages to release certain proinflammatory cytokines such as IL-6 and IL-8, ROS/RNS, and lipid mediators which are essential to sepsis-induced organ failure [40]. Increased IL-2 plasma levels with gram-negative bacteria can serve as a septic shock prognostic catalogue. IL-2 receptors are often released from T and B lymphocytes in biological fluids and tend to contribute to sepsis pathogensis. Inflammatory response of IL-6 is likely to be an effective mediator [41]. Endogenous IL-10 is an important anti-inflammatory cytokine, prevents animals from death in sepsis and has been recognized as a key approach for dealing several inflammatory disorders [42]. IL-10 has been reported to be beneficial in various inflammatory diseases other than sepsis or systemic inflammation such as inflammatory bowel disorder, arthritis, sclerosis [41]. In the present study, ZIN treatment to LPS treated rats showed the marked reduction in plasma cytokine levels significantly as compared to LPS treated rats. It has also been observed that the treatment with ZIN in normal control rats does not alter the physiological state. PCT is deemed one of the best biomarkers for sepsis and endotoxemia [43]. LPS toxicity is followed by its binding to lipopolysaccharide binding protein (LBP), which facilitates binding to the CD14 co-receptor, activating cell responses through TLR4 signaling. Reducing the circulating endotoxin in animals handled with ZIN indicates this flavonoid has the potential to enhance LPS clearance. Endotoxin removal occurs in the liver Kupffer and parenchyma cells where it is catabolized. The involvement of ZIN against LPS-induced inflammation and oxidative damage in governing this protective activity further supports this possibility.

LPS-induced rats exhibiting enhanced levels of biochemical parameters were accompanied by enhanced pathological alterations of brain, lung, liver, and kidney. Staining of the brain cortex in the LPS group showed degenerated neurons with hyperchromatic nuclei and increased vacuoles which were prevented by ZIN treatment. The hepatic tissues from the normal control animals exhibited normal cellular and lobular architecture. Liver tissue from the LPS group exhibited prominent pathological alterations comprising widespread portal inflammation, hepatic cell necrosis, and infiltration of inflammatory cells. However, ZIN significantly ameliorated the LPS-induced pathological alterations as demonstrated by the reduced cell infiltration and restored lobular architecture. Kidney tissues from ZIN-treated rats showed gradual but sustained recovery in cortex and medulla structure. Although the recovery is not full, it is easily noticeable in morphology. The thick descending and ascending parts of Henle loops and collecting coils of small caliber and reduction of interstitial tissue can be seen. The tubules show considerably lower cubic epithelium tubules were gaining normal morphology when treated with ZIN. The histopathological evaluation of lung samples indicated a moderate to severe hemorrhage, thickening of alveolar septa, emphysema, and infiltration of leukocytes in alveoli walls in the LPS group. Treatment with ZIN ameliorated these aberrations in the architecture of lung tissues. The improvement in histology is attributed to antioxidant and anti-inflammatory potential of ZIN as suggested by earlier reports [29,44]. Therefore, this research indicates that ZIN, in addition to its antioxidant and anti-inflammatory effects, may reduce the amount of circulating endotoxin from circulation and thereby alleviate the related multi-organ dysfunction syndrome (MODS) when administered to the animals subjected to LPS-induced sepsis.

4. Materials and Methods

4.1. Chemicals and Reagents

ZIN (99% pure) and LPS were purchased from Sigma-Aldrich. Biochemical estimation kits like ALT, ALP, AST, BUN, Cr, Urea, and CKMB were obtained from Human diagnostics. Oxidative stress markers MDA (K739), GSH (K464), MPO (K747), and (DNA damage marker) 8-OHdG (K4160) were purchased from (BioVision, Inc. Milpitas, CA, USA). Nitric oxide (NO) was obtained from Booster Bio, USA. Tumor necrosis factor-alpha (TNF-α, K1052-100), Interleukin (IL) IL-1β (K4796-100), IL-1α (E4804-100), IL-2 (E4831-100), IL-6 (K4145-100) were procured from (Bio-Vision, Milpitas, CA, USA), IL-10 (MBS355232) and Procalcitonin (PCT, MBS162052), a septic biomarker was purchased from (My BioSource, San Diego, CA, USA). All other chemicals were of analytical grade.

4.2. Animals

Six-week-old male Wistar rats (180–200 g) were obtained from an animal facility. The rats were housed in plastic cages at room temperature (25 °C) and humidity of 10% along with 12:12 light–dark cycle. The rats were given free access to water and food. The study was approved by the ethical committee. The study protocol was approved by the Institutional Review Board (No. RAKMHSU-REC-08-2019-F-P).

4.3. LPS-Induced Endotoxemia and Survival Study

The rats were divided into four groups (n = 10). The control group was treated with normal saline; Group II received an intraperitoneal (i.p) injection (10 mg/kg) of LPS as disease control. Rats in Group III were treated with ZIN 150 mg/kg (p.o) 2 h before LPS challenge. Animals in Group IV were treated with ZIN 150 mg/kg p.o only. Survival of the rats was monitored up to 96 h post LPS treatment.

4.4. Experimental Model

The animals were divided into four groups of six rats in each group. Animals in Group I served as normal control and were treated with normal saline. Animals in Group II served as disease control and IV were treated with LPS (10 mg/kg, i.p). Group III animals were treated with ZIN 150 mg/kg p.o 2 h before LPS challenge. Group IV served as positive control and were treated with ZIN 150 mg/kg p.o.

4.5. Determination of Biochemical, Oxidative Stress and Inflammatory Markers

Animals were euthanized with isoflurane after six hours of LPS challenge and blood samples were collected in sterilized EDTA tubes. Different organs like liver, lung, kidney, and brain tissues were harvested. The plasma samples were stored at −80 °C for biochemical, oxidative, and inflammatory marker analyses. Biochemical parameters like ALT, ALP, AST, BUN, Cr, Urea, LDH, Albumin, bilirubin, total protein, and CKMB were assessed. Oxidative stress markers MDA, GSH, MPO, and (DNA damage marker) 8-OHdGlevels were measure by ELISA technique as per the manufacturer details. Levels of nitric oxide (NO) were measured in plasma by Griess reaction method. The color intensity was recorded at 540 nm using ELISA plate reader. Inflammatory markers like TNF-α, IL-1β, IL-1α, IL-2, IL-6, and IL-10 were quantified using ELISA kits as per their manufacturer protocol. The plasma procalcitonin, a septic biomarker was determined using ELISA kits obtained according to the manufacturer's instructions.

4.6. Histological Evaluation

The tissues of liver, lung, kidney, and brain from each animal were extracted and fixed in 12% formalin for histopathological evaluation. The tissues were gradually dehydrated and embedded in paraffin, cut into 4 μm sections, and were stained with Hematoxylin and Eosin for histological examination [45].

4.7. Statistical Analysis

Animal survival study was checked using Kaplan–Meier analysis plot. The values are represented as mean ± SEM and the analysis of variance was checked with Dennett's post hoc test. The analysis was carried out by using GraphPad Prism. $p < 0.05$ was considered significant.

5. Conclusions

The present investigation reported the effect of ZIN against LPS-induced oxidative stress, DNA damage, and cytokine storm on various organs by evaluating the biochemical, inflammatory, oxidant-antioxidant markers, and histopathological changes. ZIN in regulating its preventive effect against systemic inflammation further encourages the need to improve it as a more successful treatment. Since several of the novel, creative approaches to treating sepsis target particular biomarkers, better strategies to improve the effectiveness of these new treatment methods would benefit. The results have demonstrated that LPS-induced toxicity and ZIN protects and balances the oxidant-antioxidant status and regulate the generation of cytokine storm. Therefore, ZIN can be beneficial in MODS.

Author Contributions: Conceptualization, A.A. and A.F.W.; Data curation, M.U.R. and M.R.; Investigation, A.F.W.; Methodology, A.F.W. and P.G.M.R.; Project administration, A.F.W.; Software, M.U.R., M.R., O.A. and P.A.; Visualization, O.A.; Writing—original draft, M.U.R. and A.A.; Writing—review and editing, A.F.W., M.R., M.K., P.G.M.R., P.A. and A.A. All authors have read and agreed to the published version of the manuscript.

Funding: Deanship of Scientific Research (RG-1438-069), King Saud University.

Acknowledgments: The authors extend their appreciation to the Deanship of Scientific Research at King Saud University for funding this work through Research Group Number (RG-1438-069). The authors also wish to thank RAK Medical and Health Sciences University, Ras Al Khaimah, United Arab Emirates, for their support through RAKMHSU-REC-08-2019-F-P.

Conflicts of Interest: The authors declare no conflict of interest.

Abbreviations

Lipopolysaccharide (LPS); Zingerone (ZIN); Alanine Transaminase (ALT); Alkaline Phosphatase (ALP); Aspartate Transaminase (AST); Gamma-glutamyl transferase (GGT); Blood urea Nitrogen (BUN); Creatinine (Cr); Lactate Dehydrogenase (LDH); Bilirubin (BIL); Malondialdehyde (MDA); Myeloperoxidase (MPO); Glutathione (GSH); Nitric Oxide (NO); Reactive Oxygen Species (ROS); 8-Hydroxy-2′-deoxyguanosine (8-OHdG); Tumor Necrosis Factor (TNF); Interleukins (IL); procalcitonin (PCT).

References

1. El-Seedi, H.R.; Khalifa, S.A.; Yosri, N.; Khatib, A.; Chen, L.; Saeed, A.; Efferth, T.; Verpoorte, R. Plants mentioned in the Islamic Scriptures (Holy Qur'ân and Ahadith): Traditional uses and medicinal importance in contemporary times. *J. Ethnopharmacol.* **2019**, *243*, 112007. [CrossRef]

2. Ahmad, B.; Rehman, M.U.; Amin, I.; Arif, A.; Rasool, S.; Bhat, S.A.; Afzal, I.; Hussain, I.; Bilal, S.; Mir, M.U.R. A Review on Pharmacological Properties of Zingerone (4-(4-Hydroxy-3-methoxyphenyl)-2-butanone). *Sci. World J.* **2015**, *2015*, 816364. [CrossRef] [PubMed]

3. Takizawa, M.; Sato, M.; Kusuoku, H.; Sakasai, M. Lipolysis Stimulator. U.S. Patent US008197859B2, 12 June 2012.

4. Moran, A.P.; Prendergast, M.M.; Appelmelk, B.J. Molecular mimicry of host structures by bacterial lipopolysaccharides and its contribution to disease. *FEMS Immunol. Med. Mic.* **1996**, *16*, 105–115. [CrossRef] [PubMed]

5. Frantz, S.; Kobzik, L.; Kim, Y.-D.; Fukazawa, R.; Medzhitov, R.; Lee, R.T.; Kelly, R.A. Toll4 (TLR4) expression in cardiac myocytes in normal and failing myocardium. *J. Clin. Investig.* **1999**, *104*, 271–280. [CrossRef] [PubMed]

6. Tavener, S.A.; Long, E.M.; Robbins, S.M.; McRae, K.M.; Van Remmen, H.; Kubes, P. Immune Cell Toll-Like Receptor 4 Is Required for Cardiac Myocyte Impairment during Endotoxemia. *Circ. Res.* **2004**, *95*, 700–707. [CrossRef]

7.   Sweet, M.J.; Hume, D.A. Endotoxin signal transduction in macrophages. *J. Leukoc. Biol.* **1996**, *60*, 8–26. [CrossRef]

8.   Di Penta, A.; Moreno, B.; Reix, S.; Fernandez-Diez, B.; Villanueva, M.; Errea, O.; Escala, N.; Vandenbroeck, K.; Comella, J.X.; Villoslada, P. Oxidative Stress and Proinflammatory Cytokines Contribute to Demyelination and Axonal Damage in a Cerebellar Culture Model of Neuroinflammation. *PLoS ONE* **2013**, *8*, e54722. [CrossRef] [PubMed]

9.   Victor, V.M.; Rocha, M.; De La Fuente, M. Immune cells: Free radicals and antioxidants in sepsis. *Int. Immunopharmacol.* **2004**, *4*, 327–347. [CrossRef]

10.   Kallapura, G.; Pumford, N.R.; Hernandez-Velasco, X.; Hargis, B.; Tellez, G. Mechanisms Involved in Lipopolysaccharide Derived ROS and RNS Oxidative Stress and Septic Shock. *J. Microbiol. Res. Rev.* **2014**, *2*, 6–11.

11.   Sena, L.A.; Chandel, N.S. Physiological Roles of Mitochondrial Reactive Oxygen Species. *Mol. Cell* **2012**, *48*, 158–167. [CrossRef] [PubMed]

12.   Forni, C.; Facchiano, F.; Bartoli, M.; Pieretti, S.; Facchiano, A.; D'Arcangelo, D.; Norelli, S.; Valle, G.; Nisini, R.; Beninati, S.; et al. Beneficial Role of Phytochemicals on Oxidative Stress and Age-Related Diseases. *BioMed Res. Int.* **2019**, *2019*, 8748253. [CrossRef]

13.   Rajan, I.; Narayanan, N.; Rabindran, R.; Jayasree, P.R.; Kumar, P.R.M. Zingerone Protects Against Stannous Chloride-Induced and Hydrogen Peroxide-Induced Oxidative DNA Damage in Vitro. *Biol. Trace Element Res.* **2013**, *155*, 455–459. [CrossRef] [PubMed]

14.   Mu, E.; Ding, R.; An, X.; Li, X.; Chen, S.; Ma, X. Heparin attenuates lipopolysaccharide-induced acute lung injury by inhibiting nitric oxide synthase and TGF-β/Smad signaling pathway. *Thromb. Res.* **2012**, *129*, 479–485. [CrossRef]

15.   Amin, I.; Hussain, I.; Rehman, M.U.; Mir, B.A.; Ganaie, S.A.; Ahmad, S.B.; Mir, M.U.R.; Shanaz, S.; Muzamil, S.; Arafah, A.; et al. Zingerone prevents lead-induced toxicity in liver and kidney tissues by regulating the oxidative damage in Wistar rats. *J. Food Biochem.* **2020**, e13241. [CrossRef]

16.   Kaur, G.; Tirkey, N.; Chopra, K. Beneficial effect of hesperidin on lipopolysaccharide-induced hepatotoxicity. *Toxicology* **2006**, *226*, 152–160. [CrossRef]

17.   Kamisaki, Y.; Wada, K.; Ataka, M.; Yamada, Y.; Nakamoto, K.; Ashida, K.; Kishimoto, Y. Lipopolysaccharide-induced increase in plasma nitrotyrosine concentrations in rats. *Biochim. Biophys. Acta (BBA) Mol. Basis Dis.* **1997**, *1362*, 24–28. [CrossRef]

18.   Sethi, S.; Dikshit, M. Modulation of Polymorphonuclear Leukocytes Function by Nitric Oxide. *Thromb. Res.* **2000**, *100*, 223–247. [CrossRef]

19.   Pacher, P.; Beckman, J.S.; Liaudet, L. Nitric Oxide and Peroxynitrite in Health and Disease. *Physiol. Rev.* **2007**, *87*, 315–424. [CrossRef]

20.   Alkharfy, K.M.; Ahmad, A.; Raish, M.; Vanhoutte, P.M. Thymoquinone modulates nitric oxide production and improves organ dysfunction of sepsis. *Life Sci.* **2015**, *143*, 131–138. [CrossRef]

21.   Halliwell, B. Oxidative stress and neurodegeneration: Where are we now? *J. Neurochem.* **2006**, *97*, 1634–1658. [CrossRef]

22.   van Klaveren, R.J.; Demedts, M.; Nemery, B. Cellular glutathione turnover in vitro, with emphasis on type II pneumocytes. *Eur. Respir. J.* **1997**, *10*, 1392–1400. [CrossRef]

23.   Luppi, F.; Aarbiou, J.; Van Wetering, S.; Rahman, I.; I De Boer, W.; Rabe, K.F.; Hiemstra, P. Effects of cigarette smoke condensate on proliferation and wound closure of bronchial epithelial cells in vitro: Role of glutathione. *Respir. Res.* **2005**, *6*, 140. [CrossRef]

24.   Vargas, M.R.; Johnson, D.A.; Johnson, J.A. Decreased glutathione accelerates neurological deficit and mitochondrial pathology in familial ALS-linked hSOD1G93A mice model. *Neurobiol. Dis.* **2011**, *43*, 543–551. [CrossRef] [PubMed]

25.   Ma, Z.; Ji, W.; Fu, Q.; Ma, S.-P. Formononetin Inhibited the Inflammation of LPS-Induced Acute Lung Injury in Mice Associated with Induction of PPAR Gamma Expression. *Inflammation* **2013**, *36*, 1560–1566. [CrossRef]

26.   Mills-Davies, N.; Butler, D.; Norton, E.; Thompson, D.; Sarwar, M.I.; Guo, J.; Gill, R.; Azim, N.; Coker, A.R.; Wood, S.P.; et al. Structural studies of substrate and product complexes of 5-aminolaevulinic acid dehydratase from humans, *Escherichia coli* and the hyperthermophile *Pyrobaculum calidifontis*. *Acta Crystallogr. Sect. D Struct. Biol.* **2017**, *73*, 9–21. [CrossRef]

27. Sarker, S.; Vashistha, D.; Sarker, M.S.; Sarkar, A. DNA damage in marine rock oyster (Saccostrea Cucullata) exposed to environmentally available PAHs and heavy metals along the Arabian Sea coast. *Ecotoxicol. Environ. Saf.* **2018**, *151*, 132–143. [CrossRef]

28. Torun, A.N.; Kulaksizoglu, S.; Kulaksizoglu, M.; Pamuk, B.O.; Isbilen, E.; Tutuncu, N.B. Serum total antioxidant status and lipid peroxidation marker malondialdehyde levels in overt and subclinical hypothyroidism. *Clin. Endocrinol.* **2009**, *70*, 469–474. [CrossRef]

29. Vaibhav, K.; Shrivastava, P.; Tabassum, R.; Khan, A.; Javed, H.; Ahmed, E.; Islam, F.; Safhi, M.M.; Islam, F. Delayed administration of zingerone mitigates the behavioral and histological alteration via repression of oxidative stress and intrinsic programmed cell death in focal transient ischemic rats. *Pharmacol. Biochem. Behav.* **2013**, *113*, 53–62. [CrossRef]

30. Shin, S.-G.; Kim, J.Y.; Chung, H.Y.; Jeong, J.-C. Zingerone as an Antioxidant against Peroxynitrite. *J. Agric. Food Chem.* **2005**, *53*, 7617–7622. [CrossRef]

31. Valavanidis, A.; Vlachogianni, T.; Fiotakis, C. 8-hydroxy-2′ -deoxyguanosine (8-OHdG): A Critical Biomarker of Oxidative Stress and Carcinogenesis. *J. Environ. Sci. Health Part C* **2009**, *27*, 120–139. [CrossRef]

32. Haldar, S.; Dru, C.; Choudhury, D.; Mishra, R.; Fernández, A.; Biondi, S.; Liu, Z.; Shimada, K.; Arditi, M.; Bhowmick, N.A. Inflammation and Pyroptosis Mediate Muscle Expansion in an Interleukin-1β (IL-1β)-dependent Manner. *J. Biol. Chem.* **2015**, *290*, 6574–6583. [CrossRef]

33. Ghezzi, P.; Cerami, A.; Corti, A. Tumor Necrosis Factor as a Pharmacological Target. *Tumor Necrosis Factor* **2004**, *98*, 1–8. [CrossRef]

34. Faix, J.D. Biomarkers of sepsis. *Crit. Rev. Clin. Lab. Sci.* **2013**, *50*, 23–36. [CrossRef]

35. Kany, S.; Vollrath, J.T.; Relja, B. Cytokines in Inflammatory Disease. *Int. J. Mol. Sci.* **2019**, *20*, 6008. [CrossRef]

36. Parameswaran, N.; Patial, S. Tumor Necrosis Factor-α Signaling in Macrophages. *Crit. Rev. Eukaryot. Gene Expr.* **2010**, *20*, 87–103. [CrossRef] [PubMed]

37. Cannon, J.G.; Tompkins, R.G.; Gelfand, J.A.; Michie, H.R.; Stanford, G.G.; Van Der Meer, J.W.M.; Endres, S.; Lonnemann, G.; Corsetti, J.; Chernow, B.; et al. Circulating Interleukin-1 and Tumor Necrosis Factor in Septic Shock and Experimental Endotoxin Fever. *J. Infect. Dis.* **1990**, *161*, 79–84. [CrossRef]

38. Michie, H.R.; Manogue, K.R.; Spriggs, D.R.; Revhaug, A.; O'Dwyer, S.; Dinarello, C.A.; Cerami, A.; Wolff, S.M.; Wilmore, D.W. Detection of Circulating Tumor Necrosis Factor after Endotoxin Administration. *N. Engl. J. Med.* **1988**, *318*, 1481–1486. [CrossRef]

39. Conte, D.; Holcik, M.; Lefebvre, C.A.; Lacasse, E.; Picketts, D.J.; Wright, K.E.; Korneluk, R.G. Inhibitor of Apoptosis Protein cIAP2 Is Essential for Lipopolysaccharide-Induced Macrophage Survival. *Mol. Cell. Biol.* **2006**, *26*, 699–708. [CrossRef] [PubMed]

40. Cohen, J. The immunopathogenesis of sepsis. *Nat. Cell Biol.* **2002**, *420*, 885–891. [CrossRef]

41. Pestka, S.; Krause, C.D.; Sarkar, D.; Walter, M.R.; Shi, Y.; Fisher, P.B. Interleukin-10 and Related Cytokines and Receptors. *Annu. Rev. Immunol.* **2004**, *22*, 929–979. [CrossRef]

42. Zhou, X.; Schmidtke, P.; Zepp, F.; Meyer, C.U. Boosting Interleukin-10 Production: Therapeutic Effects and Mechanisms. *Curr. Drug Targets-Immune Endocr. Metab. Disord.* **2005**, *5*, 465–475. [CrossRef]

43. Vijayan, A.L.; Ravindran, S.; Saikant, R.; Lakshmi, S.; Kartik, R. Procalcitonin: A promising diagnostic marker for sepsis and antibiotic therapy. *J. Intensiv. Care* **2017**, *5*, 51. [CrossRef]

44. Badawy, G.M.; Atallah, M.N.; Sakr, S.A. Effect of gabapentin on fetal rat brain and its amelioration by ginger. *Heliyon* **2019**, *5*, e02387. [CrossRef]

45. Kaid, F.; AlAbsi, A.M.; Al-Afifi, N.; Ali-Saeed, R.; Al-Koshab, M.A.; Ramanathan, A.; Ali, A.M. Histological, Biochemical, and Hematological Effects of Goniothalamin on Selective Internal Organs of Male Sprague-Dawley Rats. *J. Toxicol.* **2019**, *2019*. [CrossRef]

Publisher's Note: MDPI stays neutral with regard to jurisdictional claims in published maps and institutional affiliations.

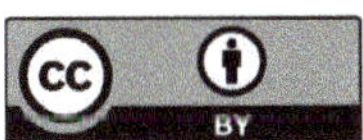

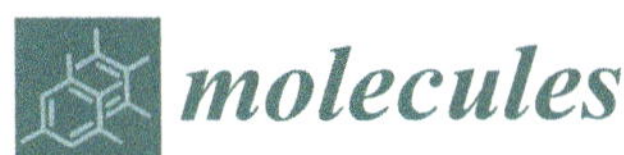 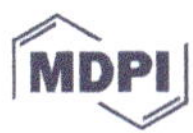

Article

Juglone Suppresses LPS-induced Inflammatory Responses and NLRP3 Activation in Macrophages

Nam-Hun Kim, Hong-Ki Kim, Ji-Hak Lee, Seung-Il Jo, Hye-Min Won, Gyeong-Seok Lee, Hyoun-Su Lee, Kung-Woo Nam, Wan-Jong Kim and Man-Deuk Han *

Department of Life Science and Biotechnology, College of Natural Sciences, Soonchunhyang University, Asan, Chuncheongnam-do 31538, Korea; sem5603@gmail.com (N.-H.K.); pgswkt@naver.com (H.-K.K.); marong932@naver.com (J.-H.L.); 309cho@naver.com (S.-I.J.); whm1223@naver.com (H.-M.W.); ssm4914@sch.ac.kr (G.-S.L.); lhs21c77@hanmail.net (H.-S.L.); kwnam1@sch.ac.kr (K.-W.N.); wjkim56@sch.ac.kr (W.-J.K.)
* Correspondence: mdhan@sch.ac.kr; Tel.: +82-41-530-4702

Academic Editors: Raffaele Pezzani and Sara Vitalini
Received: 19 June 2020; Accepted: 5 July 2020; Published: 7 July 2020

Abstract: The NLRP3 (NACHT, LRR and PYD domains-containing protein 3) inflammasome has been implicated in a variety of diseases, including atherosclerosis, neurodegenerative diseases, and infectious diseases. Thus, inhibitors of NLRP3 inflammasome have emerged as promising approaches to treat inflammation-related diseases. The aim of this study was to explore the effects of juglone (5-hydroxyl-1,4-naphthoquinone) on NLRP3 inflammasome activation. The inhibitory effects of juglone on nitric oxide (NO) production were assessed in lipopolysaccharide (LPS)-stimulated J774.1 cells by Griess assay, while its effects on reactive oxygen species (ROS) and NLRP3 ATPase activity were assessed. The expression levels of NLRP3, caspase-1, and pro-inflammatory cytokines (IL-1β, IL-18) and cytotoxicity of juglone in J774.1 cells were also determined. Juglone was non-toxic in J774.1 cells when used at 10 μM ($p < 0.01$). Juglone treatment inhibited the production of ROS and NO. The levels of NLRP3 and cleaved caspase-1, as well as the secretion of IL-1β and IL-18, were decreased by treatment with juglone in a concentration-dependent manner. Juglone also inhibited the ATPase activities of NLRP3 in LPS/ATP-stimulated J774.1 macrophages. Our results suggested that juglone could inhibit inflammatory cytokine production and NLRP3 inflammasome activation in macrophages, and should be considered as a therapeutic strategy for inflammation-related diseases.

Keywords: juglone; NLRP3 inflammasome; caspase-1; IL-1β; IL-18

---

1. Introduction

Innate immune cells, including macrophages and dendritic cells, play crucial roles in the initiation of inflammatory immune responses upon activation of inflammasome complexes that induce the maturation of inflammatory cytokines [1]. Pattern-recognition receptors (PRRs) recognize pathogen-associated molecular patterns (PAMPs) and damage-associated molecular patterns (DAMPs), initiating signaling cascades that lead to inflammation and release of inflammatory cytokines [2,3]. Toll-like receptors (TLRs) and NOD-like receptors (NLRs) called PRR are membrane-bound and cytoplasmic receptors, respectively, which recognize PAMPs and DAMPs [4]. The immune responses initiated by the interaction between TLRs and PAMPs are mediated through MyD88-dependent and TRIF-dependent pathways [2,3,5]. When TLRs recognize and bind lipopolysaccharides (LPS) or other extracellular PAMPs, the transcription factor nuclear factor (NF)-κB is activated and induces the expression of several pro-inflammatory cytokines, including interleukin (IL)-1β and IL-18 [6]. On the other hand, NLRs, PRRs found in the cytoplasm, are activated by DAMPs, including adenosine triphosphate (ATP), monosodium urate crystals, β-amyloid, and nigericin [7].

P2X7, a membrane-bound PPR that recognizes DAMP, is a membrane-bound receptor that binds extracellular ATP, promoting the release of K^+ [8,9], and subsequently, inducing the formation of inflammasomes after binding of NLRP3 (NACHT, LRR and PYD domains-containing protein 3) to ASC (apoptosis-associated speck-like protein containing a C-terminal caspase recruitment domain) and pro-caspase-1. The formation of NLRP3 inflammasomes activates pro-caspase-1, which induces pyroptosis by cleaving pro-IL-1β and pro-IL-18 into their active forms, which initiate the innate immune response [7]. In addition, intracellular danger signals, such as mitochondrial damage and reactive oxygen species (ROS) production, can promote assembly and activation of NLRP3 inflammasomes [10–12]. Inflammatory factors and cytokines can also prime NLRP3 inflammasomes, and ROS inhibitors have been reported to suppress NLRP3 priming [13]. Therefore, the treatment of macrophages with potent antioxidative agents has emerged as a promising strategy to block NLRP3 inflammasome priming.

Juglone (5-hydroxy-1,4-naphthoquinone) is a natural phenolic compound isolated from the roots, stems, and leaves of walnut trees [14]. Juglone is produced during allelopathy and inhibits the germination or growth of surrounding plants by inhibiting specific enzymes necessary for metabolic function, mitochondrial respiration, and photosynthesis [15]. Recent studies have reported that juglone has a variety of pharmacological effects, including anti-inflammatory, antioxidative, anticancer, and antimicrobial effects, by inhibiting ROS-producing enzymes and preventing oxidative stress [14,16–21]. However, the effect of juglone on NLRP3 inflammasome formation and activation remains elusive. The aim of this study was to investigate the potential of juglone to inhibit the NLRP3 inflammasome-mediated inflammatory effects of LPS and ATP.

2. Results

2.1. Effects of Juglone on Cell Viability

To determine the juglone concentration range that is non-toxic to J774.1 cells, cells were treated with increasing concentrations of juglone (3.1–50 μM), followed by 3-(4,5-dimethylthiazol-2-yl)-2,5-diphenyltetrazolium bromide (MTT) assay. When juglone was used at 10 μM or less, no significant cytotoxic effects were observed ($p > 0.05$; Figure 1). Therefore, juglone was used at 2.5, 5, or 10 μM in subsequent experiments.

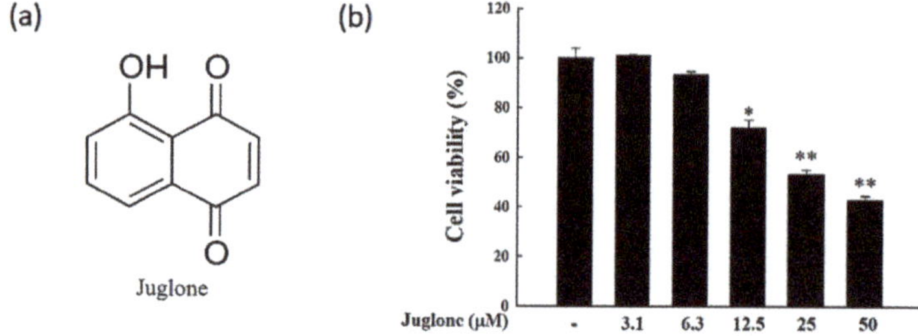

Figure 1. Assessment of the cytotoxic effects of juglone in J774.1 cells using the 3-(4,5-dimethylthiazol-2-yl)-2,5-diphenyltetrazolium bromide (MTT) assay. (**a**) Chemical structure of juglone. (**b**) J774.1 cells were treated with increasing concentrations of juglone (3.1–50 μM) for 24 h, followed by quantification of cell viability using the MTT assay. Data are presented as mean ± standard deviation (SD) of three independent experiments. * $p < 0.05$; ** $p < 0.01$; vs. control.

2.2. Effects of Juglone on Reactive Oxygen Species (ROS) Production

ROS have a strong oxidative capacity and are essential mediators of NLRP3 (NACHT, LRR and PYD domains-containing protein 3) inflammasome activation. To determine the ability of juglone to inhibit lipopolysaccharide (LPS)-induced ROS production in J774.1 cells, we used the cell-permeable

ROS-sensitive dye DCFH-DA, which is non-fluorescent in a reduced state and emits fluorescence upon oxidation by ROS. We found that treatment with LPS enhanced ROS production in J774.1 cells. However, when cells were treated with 10 μM juglone, ROS production was significantly impaired (Figure 2a). The fluorescence intensity in LPS-treated cells was approximately 120%, while the fluorescence intensity in juglone-treated (10 μM) cells after LPS stimulation was only 84.5%. Thus, juglone may exert anti-inflammatory effects by suppressing ROS generation by macrophages during inflammation.

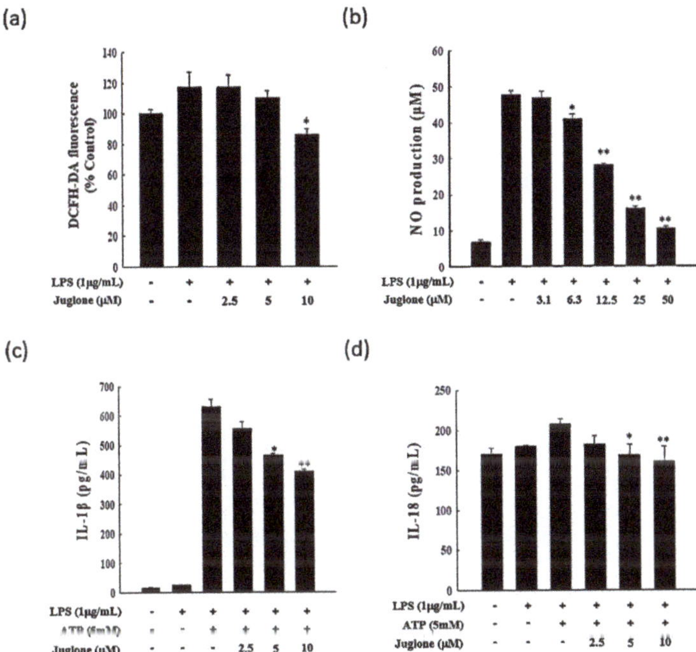

Figure 2. Effects of juglone on the production of inflammatory mediators. (**a**) reactive oxygen species (ROS) production in J774.1 cells treated with lipopolysaccharide (LPS). Cells were treated with different concentrations of juglone (2.5, 5, and 10 μM) for 2 h, followed by treatment with 1 μg/mL LPS for an additional 24 h. (**b**) NO production in J774.1 cells treated with LPS. Cells were treated with increasing concentrations of juglone (3.1–50 μM or 0 μM control) for 2 h, followed by treatment with 1 μg/mL LPS for an additional 24 h. The levels of NO in the cell culture media were measured using Griess reagent. (**c,d**) Effects of juglone on the LPS/ATP-induced secretion of interleukin-1β (IL-1β) and IL-18 in J774.1 cells. J774.1 macrophages were treated with different concentrations of juglone for 2 h, followed by treatment with 1 μg/mL LPS for 6 h and treatment with 5 mM ATP for 1 h. The levels of IL-1β and IL-18 secreted in the culture medium were analyzed by enzyme-linked immunosorbent assay (ELISA). Data are presented as mean ± SD of three independent experiments. * $p < 0.05$; ** $p < 0.01$ vs. LPS or LPS + ATP cells, respectively.

2.3. Effects of Juglone on Nitric Oxide (NO) Production

Inflammatory mediators, such as reactive nitrogen species and ROS, are essential mediators of inflammatory responses, especially in the initial stages of inflammation. Therefore, we assessed the effects of juglone in LPS-induced NO production. We found that even though LPS treatment resulted in a significant increase in NO production in J774.1 cells, juglone treatment suppressed LPS-induced NO production in a dose-dependent manner ($p < 0.05$; Figure 2b).

2.4. Effects of Juglone on the Secretion of the Pro-Inflammatory Cytokines IL-1β and IL-18

Inflammatory cytokines are important mediators of immune responses and orchestrate the initial stages of inflammation. The pro-inflammatory cytokines IL-1β and IL-18 are known to mediate the first steps of an inflammatory immune response [22]. Therefore, targeting these upstream mediators of inflammation has emerged as a promising approach to treat inflammation-related diseases. Thus, we sought to investigate whether juglone could affect the levels of mRNA, protein, or extracellular secretion of IL-18 and IL-1β. We found that treatment with juglone suppressed the induction of IL-18 and IL-1β at the mRNA and protein level in response to LPS and ATP in J774.1 cells (Figure 3 and Figure S1). The secretory inhibition of pro-inflammatory cytokines (IL-1β and IL-18) of juglone on murine macrophage cells was studied and the results are shown Figure 2c,d. Treatment of macrophage cells with juglone caused a concentration-dependent reduction in their IL-1β (5 μM, * $p < 0.05$) and IL-18 (10 μM, ** $p < 0.01$). Juglone-treated cell was reduced 25.9% of IL-1β secretion (5 μM, * $p < 0.05$) and 22.6% of IL-18 secretion (10 μM, ** $p < 0.01$) compared to the LPS plus STP-primed control group. These results suggested that juglone could inhibit the initial steps of the inflammatory immune response by suppressing the expression and secretion of the pro-inflammatory cytokines IL-1β and IL-18 in macrophages.

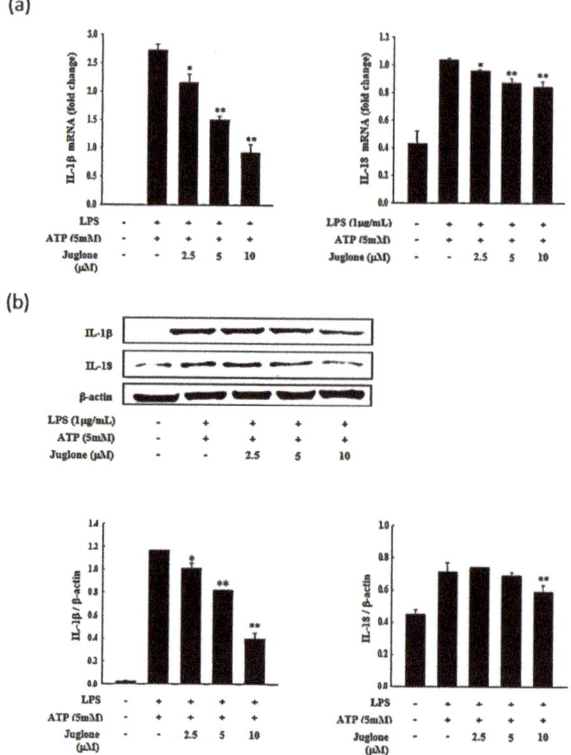

Figure 3. Effects of juglone on IL-1β and IL-18 expression in LPS-treated J774.1 cells. J774.1 macrophages were treated with different concentrations of juglone (2.5, 5, and 10 μM) for 2 h, followed by treatment with 1 μg/mL LPS for 6 h and 5 mM ATP for 1 h. (**a**) The mRNA levels of IL-1β and IL-18 in J774.1 cells were determined with RT-qPCR. Glyceraldehyde 3-phosphate dehydrogenase gene (GAPDH) was used as a reference gene. (**b**) The protein levels of IL-1β and IL-18 in J774.1 cells were assessed by Western blotting and are presented as relative to β-actin intensity. Data are presented as mean ± SD. * $p < 0.05$; ** $p < 0.01$ vs. LPS + ATP treated cells.

2.5. Effects of Juglone on NLRP3 and Caspase-1 Expression

We then assessed the effects of juglone treatment on the mRNA and protein levels of NLRP3 and caspase-1. We found that even though NLRP3 was induced in J774.1 cells following stimulation with LPS and ATP, treatment with juglone suppressed the LPS/ATP-mediated NLRP3 induction at the mRNA level in a dose-dependent manner. The mRNA levels of caspase-1 were not significantly affected by juglone treatment (Figure 4a). Importantly, juglone treatment suppressed the LPS/ATP-mediated NLRP3 ATPase upregulation at the protein level in J774.1 macrophages (Figure 4b and Figure S2). Juglone also reduced the levels of cleaved caspase-1 in a concentration-dependent manner (Figure 4b). These results suggested that juglone could inhibit the interaction of NLRP3 and apoptosis-associated speck-like protein containing a C-terminal caspase recruitment domain (ASC) and subsequent NLRP3 inflammasome formation by downregulating the expression of NLRP3. Moreover, the decreased NLRP3 expression might impair ASC speck formation, leading to reduced cleavage and subsequent activation of the downstream signaling mediator, caspase-1.

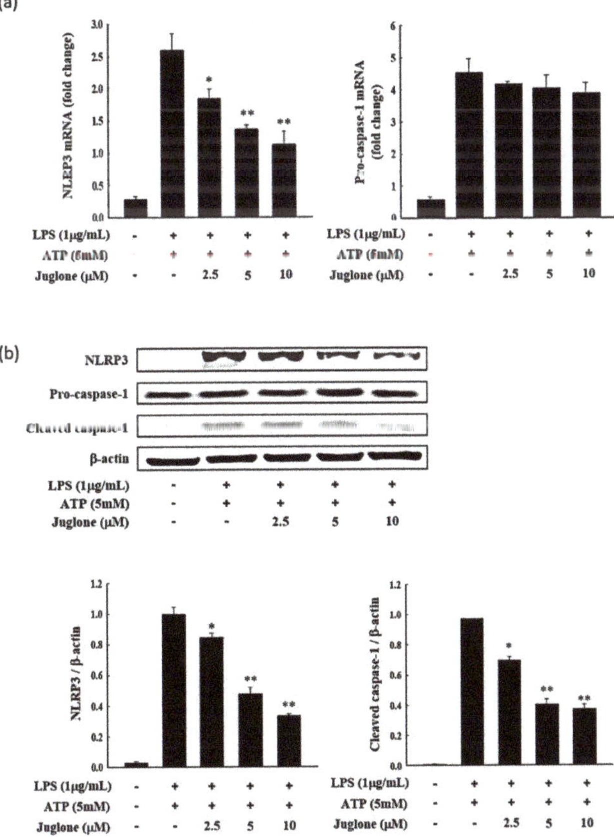

Figure 4. J774.1 cells were treated with various concentrations of juglone for 2 h and then treated with 1 µg/mL LPS for 24 h. (**a**) The mRNA levels of NACHT, LRR and PYD domains-containing protein 3 (NLRP3) and caspase-1 in J774.1 cells were determined by RT-qPCR. GAPDH was used as a reference gene. (**b**) The relative protein levels of NLRP3, procaspase-1, and cleaved caspase-1 were assessed by Western blotting and are presented as relative to β-actin intensity. Data are presented as the mean ± SD. * $p < 0.05$; ** $p < 0.01$ vs. LPS + ATP treated cells.

2.6. Effects of Juglone on the ATPase Activity of NLRP3

The pyrin ATP-binding domain of NLRP3 exhibits ATPase activity, which is essential for NLRP3 inflammasome oligomerization. Therefore, we investigated the effects of juglone treatment on the ATPase activity of NLRP3 in J774.1 cells. Treatment with LPS and ATP in J774.1 macrophages increased the ATPase activity of NLRP3 (Figure 5). However, treatment with 10 μM of juglone significantly reduced the ATPase activity of NLRP3 ($p < 0.05$).

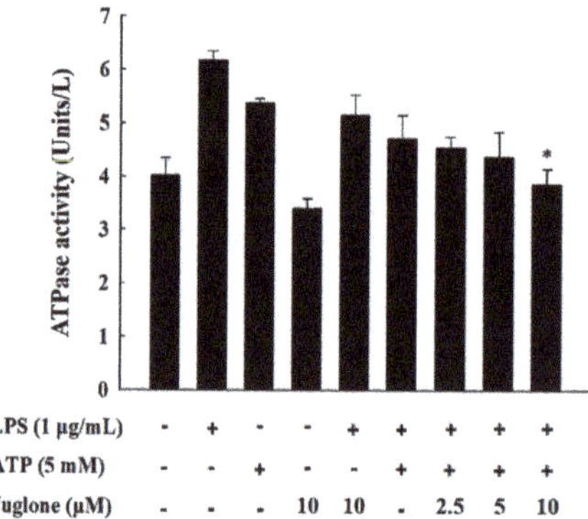

Figure 5. Effects of juglone on the ATPase activity of NLRP3 in LPS/ATP-treated J774.1 cells. J774.1 macrophages were treated with different concentrations of juglone for 2 h, followed by treatment with 1 μg/mL LPS for 6 h and 5 mM ATP for an additional hour. Analysis of the ATPase activity of NLRP3 was performed using a reaction mixture containing 40 mM Tris, 80 mM NaCl, 8 mM MgAc2, 1 mM EDTA, and 4 mM ATP, pH 7.5. Data are presented as mean ± SD of three independent experiments. * $p < 0.05$ vs. LPS/ATP treated cells.

3. Discussion

The NLRP3 (NACHT, LRR and PYD domains-containing protein 3) inflammasome can be activated by a broad range of stimuli that belong either to pathogen-associated molecular patterns (PAMPs) released during viral, bacterial, fungal, or protozoa infection [23] or to danger-associated molecular patterns (DAMPs) of endogenous or exogenous origin, like extracellular ATP and reactive oxygen species (ROS) [24]. The present study demonstrates that juglone inhibits IL-1b and IL-18 secretion in activated macrophages by suppressing various pro-inflammatory signaling molecules and pathways.

Juglone has been reported to have potent antioxidative effects and prevent various oxidative stress-related diseases by inhibiting ROS-producing enzymes [25,26]. Additionally, juglone has been suggested to have anticancer effects, which are least partly mediated by inhibition of NF-κB signaling and NF-κB-mediated expression of inflammatory cytokines [27,28]. However, the effects of juglone NLRP3 inflammasome formation in macrophages are understudied.

IL-1β, IL-18, and NO have been highlighted by numerous studies as essential mediators of inflammation and have been implicated in autoimmune diseases and other inflammatory conditions [29]. LPS, a major component of Gram-negative bacteria, can induce the expression of inflammatory cytokines and NO. Herein, we reported that juglone treatment inhibited the production of NO in LPS-stimulated J774.1 cells in a concentration-dependent manner. ROS are also involved in inflammatory immune responses and have been shown to induce formation and activation of the NLRP3 inflammasome in response to various exogenous stimuli [30]. In addition, excessive intracellular ROS levels can lead to apoptosis or necrosis [31]. To investigate the effects of juglone on ROS production by macrophages, a DCFH-DA assay was performed in J774.1 cells treated with LPS. Our results suggested that LPS stimulation induced ROS production and that juglone could suppress LPS-induced ROS generation in a dose-dependent manner. Therefore, by reducing ROS production in macrophages, juglone could potentially inhibit activation of the NLRP3 inflammasome.

ATP-induced P2X7R activation promotes the rapid production of large amounts of ROS, which, in turn, stimulates activation of the NLRP3 inflammasome [32]. It has been previously reported that inhibition of the ATPase activity of NLRP3 could decrease the self-oligomerization of NLRP3, as well as its interaction with ASC, which is critical for inflammasome activation [31].

In this study, we found that juglone treatment suppresses not only the expression of NLRP3 but also the ATPase activity of NLRP3, and these were followed by the inhibition of active caspase-1 (Figure 6). These results suggest that juglone could potentially impair the formation of NLRP3 inflammasome, and, thus, the inhibition of pro-caspase-1 activation in macrophages. We also found that treatment with juglone could suppress the LPS/ATP-mediated induction of IL-1β and IL-18 in J774.1 cells, both at the mRNA and protein levels. These correspond to the previous research results that juglone inhibits pro-inflammatory cytokines (TNF-α, IL-1 β, and IL-6) and adhesion molecules (VCAM-1 and ICAM-1) expression through the inhibition of IκB-phosphorylation-mediated NF-κB activation [17,33].

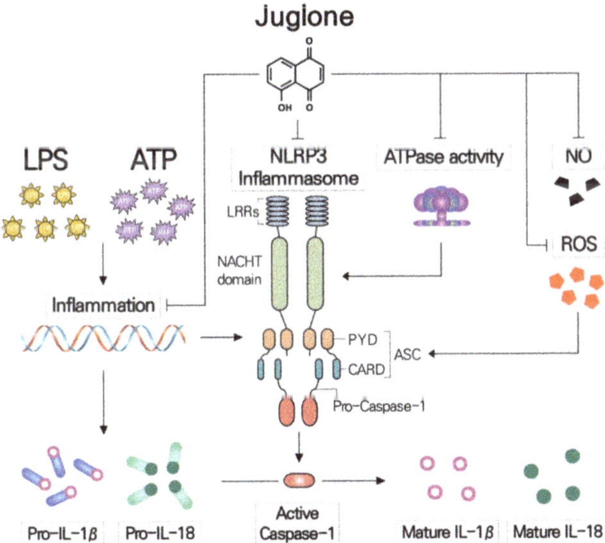

Figure 6. Proposed mechanism underlying the anti-inflammatory effects of juglone in macrophages. Pre-treatment of macrophages with juglone suppressed ATP-induced IL-1β, IL-18 and NLRP3 secretion in LPS-primed J774.1 mouse macrophages. Juglone also caused downregulation of ATPase activity and ROS and NO production. Juglone also reduced the mRNA expression and activation of IL-1β, IL-18, NLRP3 and caspase-1. The results show that juglone inhibits IL-1β and IL-18 secretion and NLRP3 formation in activated macrophages.

Furthermore, our extended study results showed that the secretion levels of IL-1β and IL-18 in macrophages were inhibited by juglone treatment in a dose dependent manner. Of note, pro-IL-1β and pro-IL-18 are cleaved to their active forms by caspase-1 upon activation by NLRP3 inflammasome. The expression of IL-18 showed relatively small change rather than that of IL-1β. It may be due to distinct regulation for Il-1β and IL-18. It is reported that there are distinct licensing requirements for processing of IL-1β and IL-18 activation by NLRP3 inflammasome in mice [34]. Considering that juglone is natural product, it is valuable that juglone shows anti-inflammatory effects in 10 μM of concentration. Because juglone might be categorized as a potential anticancer compound based on the criteria established by the National Cancer Institute [35] that any compound with IC_{50} value of

≤4 µg/mL has the potential to be an anticancer compound. In view of these present findings and the existing reports of its use in traditional folk medicine as an anti-inflammatory agent, juglone deserves further studies to justify its potential as an anti-inflammatory agent, using a spectrum of preclinical models. Hence, our results indicate that juglone treatment could reduce the production of mature inflammatory cytokines IL-1β and IL-18 by suppressing their transcription and translation levels as well as caspase-1-mediated cleavage to their active forms. Therefore, our findings suggest that juglone could be used as a potential therapeutic compound for treating inflammatory diseases in the future.

4. Materials and Methods

4.1. Chemical Compounds

Juglone (5-hydroxy-1,4-naphthoquinone; purity > 97%) was purchased from Merck (Darmstadt, Germany). Adenosine 5′-triphosphate (ATP) and lipopolysaccharide (LPS) were purchased from Sigma-Aldrich, Inc. (St. Louis, MO, USA).

4.2. Cell Cultures

J774.1 cells were purchased from the Korean Collection for Type Cultures and maintained in DMEM (Gibco BRL, Gaithersburg, MD, USA) supplemented with 10% fetal bovine serum (Gibco BRL), 100 µg/mL streptomycin, and 100 U/mL penicillin (Gibco BRL). Cells were incubated at 37 °C in a humidified 5% CO_2 incubator. J774.1 cells were subjected to the following treatments: (i) control; (ii) LPS (Escherichia coli O111:b4) + ATP; (iii) 2.5 µM juglone + LPS + ATP; (iv) 5 µM juglone + LPS + ATP; (v) 10 µM juglone + LPS + ATP. For these treatments, cells were incubated in the presence of juglone for 2 h, followed by treatment with LPS (1 µg/mL) for 6 h and ATP (5 mM) for 1 h. After treatment, cells were harvested for further analyses.

4.3. Cell Viability

The cytotoxic effects of juglone were assessed by 3-(4,5-dimethylthiazol-2-yl)-2,5-diphenyltetrazolium bromide (MTT) assay. Briefly, J774.1 cells were seeded in 24-well plates (2×10^5 cells/well) in 500 µL of cell culture medium and incubated in a 37 °C and 5% CO_2 incubator for 12 h to allow for cell adhesion. After incubation, cells were treated with increasing concentrations of juglone (3.1–50 µM) for 24 h. Subsequently, the cell culture medium was replaced with phenol red-free medium, and 50 µL of 5 mg/mL MTT solution was added to each well. Cells were incubated with MTT for an additional 4 h in a 37 °C and 5% CO_2 incubator. The supernatant was removed, and 200 µL dimethyl sulfoxide (DMSO) was added to each well to dissolve the MTT crystals. Optical absorbance was measured at 450 nm using a microplate reader (Marshall Scientific, Hants, UK). Cell viability was calculated, according to the following Formula (1):

$$\text{Cell viability (\%)} = (\text{Abs 450 nm of untreated cells} - \text{Abs 450 nm of treated cells/Abs 450 nm of untreated cells}) \times 100 \tag{1}$$

4.4. Measurement of Nitric Oxide (NO)

To evaluate the anti-inflammatory effects of juglone in macrophages, NO production was measured in J774.1 cells. The amount of NO produced in response to LPS stimulation was measured using the Griess test, which determines the amount of nitrite (NO_2^-) generated. J774.1 cells were seeded in 24-well plates (2×10^5 cells/well) and incubated at 37 °C for 12 h to allow for cell adhesion. After incubation, the cell culture medium was replaced with phenol red-free medium. Cells were treated with different concentrations of juglone for 2 h, followed by stimulation with LPS (1 µg/mL) for 24 h at 37 °C and 5% CO_2. After incubation, 200 µL of the cell culture solution and 50 µL of Griess reagent [1% (*w/v*) sulfanilamide and 0.1% N-1-naphthylethylene diamine in 2.5% (*v/v*) phosphoric acid] were mixed in a 96-well plate. After a 10 min incubation at room temperature, the absorbance was measured at 540 nm. The standard calibration curve was obtained by measuring the optical absorbance of serial dilutions of sodium nitrate ($NaNO_2$). The amount of NO produced was determined using the standard calibration curve.

4.5. Measurement of the Antioxidative Capacity of Juglone

The antioxidative capacity of juglone was measured using the hydrophilic peroxyl radical scavenging capacity (PSC) assay [36]. To measure ROS in J774.1 cells, 2,7-Dichlorodihydrofluorescein diacetate (DCFH-DA, Sigma, St. Louis, MO, USA) was used. The cells were seeded into 24-well plates (2×10^5 cells/well) and incubated for 12 h. Cells were treated with 2.5, 5, and 10 µM juglone. After 2 h of incubation, cells were exposed to 1 µg/mL LPS for 24 h in a 37 °C and 5% CO_2 incubator. After incubation, the cells were washed twice with cold phosphate-buffered saline (PBS) and incubated with 10 µM of DCFH-DA for 30 min at 37 °C. The fluorescence intensity was measured on a fluorescence microplate reader (Marshall Scientific) using an excitation wavelength of 485 nm and an emission wavelength of 535 nm.

4.6. Measurement of Cytokine Release

The amounts of IL-1β and IL-18 produced by J774.1 cells were measured using enzyme-linked immunosorbent assay (ELISA). Briefly, cells were seeded into a 24-well plate (1×10^6 cells/well) and incubated for 12 h in a 37 °C and 5% CO_2 incubator. Subsequently, cells were treated with 2.5, 5, and 10 µM of juglone for 2 h, followed by LPS treatment (1 µg/mL) for 6 h and ATP treatment (5 mM) for 1 h. The production of pro-inflammatory cytokines was assessed using commercial ELISA kits (mouse IL-1β: R&D Systems, Minneapolis, MN, USA; mouse IL-18: Cloud-Clone Co., Katy, TX, USA) according to the manufacturer's instructions. The absorbance was measured at 540 nm. All experiments were performed in triplicate.

4.7. RNA Isolation and cDNA Synthesis

Total cellular RNA from J774.1 cells was isolated using the RNeasy Midi Kit (Qiagen GmbH, Hilden, Germany) according to the manufacturer's instructions. Samples were treated with RNase-free DNase I (Takara, Dalian, China) at 37 °C for 30 min to avoid any DNA contamination. The quality and quantity of the RNA samples were measured using a bioanalyzer (Agilent 2100; Agilent Technologies, Santa Clara, CA, USA). RNAs with RNA integrity values ≥ 8.0 were used. Complementary DNA was synthesized from 1 µg total RNA using the iScript cDNA synthesis kit (Bio-Rad Laboratories, Hercules, CA, USA). cDNA synthesis was performed at 46 °C for 20 min, followed by enzyme inactivation at 95 °C for 1 min.

4.8. Real-Time Reverse Transcriptase Quantitative Polymerase Chain Reaction (RT-qPCR)

Total RNA was extracted using TRIzol reagent (Life Technologies, Carlsbad, CA, USA) according to the manufacturer's instructions. RT-qPCR was performed on a CFX96 Real-time PCR (Bio-Rad Laboratories Inc., Hercules, CA, USA). RT-qPCR reactions were prepared using 1 µL cDNA, 10 µL SYBR Green master mix (Bio-Rad Laboratories, Inc.), and 2 µL of primer mix in a total volume of 20 µL. Thermocycling conditions were as follows: 3 min at 95 °C, 35 cycles of denaturation (15 s at 95 °C), and combined annealing/extension (30 s at 60 °C). GAPDH was used as a housekeeping gene. Primer sequences and their respective PCR fragment lengths were as follows: NLRP3 (NACHT, LRR and PYD domains-containing protein 3), forward 5′-GTGGAGATCCT AGGTTTCTCTG-3′ and reverse 5′-CAGGATCTCATTCTCTTGGATC-3′; Caspase-1, forward 5′-GAGCTGATGTT GACCTCAGAG-3′ and reverse 5′-CTGTCAGAAGTCTTGTGCTCTG-3′; IL-1β, forward 5′-GTGGAGATCCTAGGTTTCTCTG-3′ and reverse 5′-CAGGATCTCATTCTCTTGGATC-3′; IL-18, forward 5′-AGGACACTTTCTTGCTTGCC-3′, and reverse 5′-CACAAACCCTCCCCACCTAA-3′, GAPDH forward 5′-GTGGGGCGCCCCAGGCACCA-3′ and reverse 5′-CTCCTTAATGTCA CGCACGATTTC-3′. After amplification, a melting curve (0.01 °C/s) was used to confirm product purity. Relative mRNA content was normalized to GAPDH content.

4.9. Western Blot Analysis

Cells were seeded into 6-well plates (2×10^6 cells/well) and incubated in a 37 °C and 5% CO_2 incubator for 12 h. Cells were then treated with different concentrations of juglone for 2 h, followed by treatment with LPS (1 µg/mL) for 6 h and ATP (5 mM) for 1 h. Cells were then washed with cold PBS and lysed with RIPA buffer (Thermo Scientific, Waltham, MA, USA). Protein concentration was quantified using a BCA protein assay kit (Sigma). Proteins (40 µg) were separated by SDS-PAGE (10% and 15% gels) and transferred onto polyvinylidene difluoride membranes using a Mini Tran-Blot Electrophoretic Transfer Cell (Bio-Rad Laboratories). Membranes were blocked with 5% skimmed milk at room temperature for 2 h, and washed three times with 1× TBST buffer (20 mM Tris-HCl, 150 mM NaCl, and 5% Tween 20, pH 7.6). Membranes were incubated with the primary antibodies (1:1000 dilution) at 4 °C for at least 10 h. After three washes with 1 × TBST buffer, membranes were incubated with mouse or rabbit IgG-horseradish peroxidase conjugated secondary antibodies at room temperature for 2 h. Westsave ECL detection reagent and a chemiluminescent Western blot imaging instrument (Labgear Australia, Milton, Australia) were used to visualize the signal intensities. NLRP3 (NACHT, LRR and PYD domains-containing protein 3; #13158), and caspase-1 antibody (#24232) were purchased from Cell Signaling (Danvers, MA, USA). IL-1β (sc-7884) and β-Actin (sc-130656) antibody were bought from Santa Cruz Biotechnology (Dallas, TX, USA). IL-18 antibody (A16737) was purchased from ABclonal (Woburn, MA, USA). Mouse anti-rabbit secondary antibody (sc 2357)/or anti-mouse IgG HRP secondary antibody (sc516102) were bought from bought from Santa Cruz Biotechnology (Dallas, TX, USA). All antibodies were used at a dilution of 1:1000.

4.10. ATPase Activity Measurement

J774.1 cells were seeded into 6-well plates (2×10^6 cells/well) and incubated at 37 °C for 12 h. Cells were then treated with juglone for 2 h, followed by treatment with LPS (1 µg/mL) for 6 h and ATP (5 mM) for 1 h. After washing twice with 0.9% NaCl, lysis buffer (40 mM Tris, 80 mM NaCl, 8 mM MgAc2, and 1 mM EDTA, pH 7.5) was used to lyse the cells. Cells were centrifuged at 15,000 rpm for 15 min at 4 °C. After pushing the cell lysate through a 25-gauge needle, the aqueous layer was collected and analyzed using the ATPase activity assay kit (Sigma), according to the manufacturer's instructions.

4.11. Statistical Analysis

All the data were analyzed using SPSS Statistics 25 software (International Business Machines, Armonk, NY, USA). Data are expressed as mean ± standard deviation. Statistical significance was determined using one-way ANOVA, and $P < 0.05$ was considered statistically significant; * $p < 0.05$ and ** $p < 0.01$

5. Conclusions

Increased ROS, NO, and NLRP3 ATPase activity by LPS and/or ATP treatment causes activation of the NLRP3 inflammasome in macrophages. Juglone treatment reduced the production of ROS and NO, and inhibited the ATPase activity of NLRP3 in J774.1 macrophages. Moreover, juglone treatment suppressed NLRP3 expression and inhibited NLRP3 inflammasome activation, thereby inhibiting the cleavage of caspase-1. Secretion of the pro-inflammatory cytokines IL-1β and IL-18 was also decreased by juglone in a concentration-dependent manner. Thus, juglone should be considered as a therapeutic strategy for inflammation-related diseases.

Supplementary Materials: The following are available online. Figure S1: Original images for Western blots of IL-1β, IL-18 and β-actin., Figure S2: Original images for Western blots of NLRP3, pro-caspase and cleaved caspase-1.

Author Contributions: Conceptualization, N.-H.K. and M.-D.H.; methodology, H.-K.K. and S.-I.J.; formal analysis, H.-K.K., J.-H.L., S.-I.J and H.-M.W.; investigation, N.-H.K.; resources, N.-H.K.; data curation, G.-S.L., H.-S.L., K.-W.N. and W.-J.K.; writing—original draft preparation, N.-H.K. and M.-D.H.; writing—review and editing, G.-S.L., H.-S.L., K.-W.N. and W.-J.K.; visualization, N.-H.K.; supervision, K.-W.N. and M.-D.H.; project administration, M.-D.H.; funding acquisition, M.-D.H. All authors have read and agreed to the published version of the manuscript.

Funding: This research received no external funding.

Acknowledgments: This study was supported by the Soonchunhyang University Research Fund.

Conflicts of Interest: The authors declare no conflict of interest.

References

1. Takeuchi, O.; Akira, S. Pattern Recognition Receptors and Inflammation. *Cell* **2010**, *140*, 805–820. [CrossRef] [PubMed]
2. Kumar, H.; Kawai, T.; Akira, S. Pathogen Recognition by the Innate Immune System. *Int. Rev. Immunol.* **2011**, *30*, 16–34. [CrossRef] [PubMed]
3. Takeda, K.; Kaisho, T.; Akira, S. Toll-Likereceptors. *Annu. Rev. Immunol.* **2003**, *21*, 335–376. [CrossRef] [PubMed]
4. Schroder, K.; Tschopp, J. The Inflammasomes. *Cell* **2010**, *140*, 821–832. [CrossRef] [PubMed]
5. Ozinsky, A.; Underhill, D.M.; Fontenot, J.D.; Hajjar, A.M.; Smith, K.D.; Wilson, C.B.; Schroeder, L.; Aderem, A. The repertoire for pattern recognition of pathogens by the innate immune system is defined by cooperation between Toll-like receptors. *Proc. Natl. Acad. Sci. USA* **2000**, *97*, 13766–13771. [CrossRef] [PubMed]
6. Sahoo, M.; Ceballos-Olvera, I.; Del Barrio, L.; Re, F. Role of the Inflammasome, IL-1β, and IL-18 in Bacterial Infections. *Sci. World J.* **2011**, *11*, 2037–2050. [CrossRef] [PubMed]
7. Martinon, F.; Mayor, A.; Tschopp, J. The Inflammasomes: Guardians of the Body. *Annu. Rev. Immunol.* **2009**, *27*, 229–265. [CrossRef]
8. Perregaux, D.; Gabel, C.A. Interleukin-1 beta maturation and release in response to ATP and nigericin. Evidence that potassium depletion mediated by these agents is a necessary and common feature of their activity. *J. Boil. Chem.* **1994**, *269*, 15195–15203.
9. Walev, I.; Klein, J.; Husmann, M.; Valeva, A.; Strauch, S.; Wirtz, H.; Weichel, O.; Bhakdi, S. Potassium Regulates IL-1β Processing Via Calcium-Independent Phospholipase A2. *J. Immunol.* **2000**, *164*, 5120–5124. [CrossRef]
10. Zhou, R.; Yazdi, A.S.; Menu, P.; Tschopp, J. A role for mitochondria in NLRP3 inflammasome activation. *Nature* **2010**, *469*, 221–225. [CrossRef]
11. Sorbara, M.T.; Girardin, S.E. Mitochondrial ROS fuel the inflammasome. *Cell Res.* **2011**, *21*, 558–560. [CrossRef] [PubMed]
12. Heid, M.E.; Keyel, P.A.; Kamga, C.; Shiva, S.; Watkins, S.C.; Salter, R.D. Mitochondrial reactive oxygen species induces NLRP3-dependent lysosomal damage and inflammasome activation. *J. Immunol.* **2013**, *191*, 5230–5238. [CrossRef]
13. Bauernfeind, F.; Bartok, E.; Rieger, A.; Franchi, L.; Núñez, G.; Hornung, V. Cutting edge: Reactive oxygen species inhibitors block priming, but not activation, of the NLRP3 inflammasome. *J. Immunol.* **2011**, *187*, 613–617. [CrossRef] [PubMed]
14. Aithal, B.K.; Kumar, M.S.; Rao, B.N.; Udupa, N.; Rao, B.S. Juglone, a naphthoquinone from walnut, exerts cytotoxic and genotoxic effects against cultured melanoma tumor cells. *Cell Boil. Int.* **2009**, *33*, 1039–1049. [CrossRef]
15. Soderquist, C.J. Juglone and allelopathy. *J. Chem. Educ.* **1973**, *50*, 782. [CrossRef]
16. Seetha, A.; Devaraj, H.; Sudhandiran, G. Indomethacin and juglone inhibit inflammatory molecules to induce apoptosis and colon cnacer cells. *J. Biochem. Mol. Toxicol.* **2020**, *34*, e22433. [CrossRef]
17. Peng, X.; Nie, Y.; Wu, J.; Huang, Q.; Cheng, Y. Juglone prevents metabolic endotoxemia-induced hepatitis and neuroinflammation via suppressing TLR4/NF-κB signaling pathway in high-fat diet rats. *Biochem. Biophys. Res. Commun.* **2015**, *462*, 245–250. [CrossRef] [PubMed]
18. Reese, S.; Vidyasagar, A.; Jacobson, L.; Acun, Z.; Esnault, S.; Hullett, D.; Malter, J.S.; Djamali, A. The Pin 1 inhibitor juglone attenuates kidney fibrogenesis via Pin 1-independent mechanisms in the unilateral ureteral occlusion model. *Fibrogenesis Tissue Repair* **2010**, *3*, 1. [CrossRef]

19. Zhang, X.-B.; Zou, C.-L.; Duan, Y.-X.; Wu, F.; Li, G. Activity guided isolation and modification of juglone from *Juglans regia* as potent cytotoxic agent against lung cancer cell lines. *BMC Complement. Altern. Med.* **2015**, *15*, 396. [CrossRef]

20. Tan, D.T.C.; Osman, H.; Mohamad, S.; Kamaruddin, A.H. Synthesis and antibacterial activity of juglone derivatives. *J. Chem. Chem. Eng.* **2012**, *6*, 84–89.

21. Zakavi, F.; Hagh, L.G.; Daraeighadikolaei, A.; Sheikh, A.F.; Daraeighadikolaei, A.; Shooshtari, Z.L. Antibacterial effect of *Juglans regia* bark against oral pathologic bacteria. *Int. J. Dent.* **2013**, *2013*, 1–5. [CrossRef]

22. Kandasamy, M.; Mak, K.-K.; Devadoss, T.; Thanikachalam, P.V.; Sakirolla, R.; Choudhury, H.; Pichika, M.R. Construction of a novel quinoxaline as a new class of Nrf2 activator. *BMC Chem.* **2019**, *13*, 117. [CrossRef] [PubMed]

23. Mariathasan, S.; Weiss, D.S.; Newton, K.; McBride, J.; O'Rourke, K.; Roose-Girma, M.; Lee, W.P.; Weinrauch, Y.; Monack, D.M.; Dixit, V.M. Cryopyrin activates the inflammasome in response to toxins and ATP. *Nature* **2006**, *440*, 228–232. [CrossRef] [PubMed]

24. Benko, S.; Philpott, D.J.; Girardin, S.E. The microbial and danger signals that activate Nod-like receptors. *Cytokine* **2008**, *43*, 368–373. [CrossRef]

25. Galas, M.; Dourlen, P.; Bégard, S.; Ando, K.; Blum, D.; Hamdane, M.; Buée, L. The Peptidylprolylcis/ trans-Isomerase Pin1 Modulates Stress-induced Dephosphorylation of Tau in Neurons. *J. Boil. Chem.* **2006**, *281*, 19296–19304. [CrossRef] [PubMed]

26. Zhou, D.-J.; Mu, D.; Jiang, M.-D.; Zheng, S.-M.; Zhang, Y.; He, S.; Weng, M.; Zeng, W.-Z. Hepatoprotective effect of juglone on dimethylnitrosamine-induced liver fibrosis and its effect on hepatic antioxidant defence and the expression levels of α-SMA and collagen III. *Mol. Med. Rep.* **2015**, *12*, 4095–4102. [CrossRef]

27. Sugie, S.; Okamoto, K.; Rahman, K.; Tanaka, T.; Kawai, K.; Yamahara, J.; Mori, H. Inhibitory effects of plumbagin and juglone on azoxymethane-induced intestinal carcinogenesis in rats. *Cancer Lett.* **1998**, *127*, 177–183. [CrossRef]

28. Dinarello, C.A. Interleukin 1 and interleukin 18 as mediators of inflammation and the aging process. *Am. J. Clin. Nutr.* **2006**, *83*, 447S–455S. [CrossRef]

29. Martinon, F. Signaling by ROS drives inflammasome activation. *Eur. J. Immunol.* **2010**, *40*, 616–619. [CrossRef]

30. Valencia, A.; Morán, J. Reactive oxygen species induce different cell death mechanisms in cultured neurons. *Free Radic. Boil. Med.* **2004**, *36*, 1112–1125. [CrossRef] [PubMed]

31. Sharif, H.; Wang, L.; Wang, W.L.; Magupalli, V.G.; Andreeva, L.; Qiao, Q.; Hauenstein, A.V.; Wu, Z.; Núñez, G.; Mao, Y.; et al. Structural mechanism for NEK7-licensed activation of NLRP3 inflammasome. *Nature* **2019**, *570*, 338–343. [CrossRef] [PubMed]

32. Cruz, C.M.; Rinna, A.; Forman, H.J.; Ventura, A.L.M.; Persechini, P.; Ojcius, D.M. ATP activates a reactive oxygen species-dependent oxidative stress response and secretion of proinflammatory cytokines in macrophages. *J. Boil. Chem.* **2006**, *282*, 2871–2879. [CrossRef] [PubMed]

33. Costantino, S.; Paneni, F.; Lüscher, T.F.; Cosentino, F. Pin1 inhibitor Juglone prevents diabetic vascular dysfunction. *Int. J. Cardiol.* **2016**, *203*, 702–707. [CrossRef] [PubMed]

34. Schmidt, R.L.; Lenz, L.L. Distinct Licensing of IL-18 and IL-1β Secretion in Response to NLRP3 Inflammasome Activation. *PLoS ONE* **2012**, *7*, e45186. [CrossRef]

35. Pisha, E.; Chai, H.; Lee, I.-S.; Chagwedera, T.E.; Farnsworth, N.R.; Cordell, G.A.; Beecher, C.W.W.; Fong, H.H.; Kinghorn, A.D.; Brown, D.M.; et al. Discovery of betulinic acid as a selective inhibitor of human melanoma that functions by induction of apoptosis. *Nat. Med.* **1995**, *1*, 1046–1051. [CrossRef]

36. Adom, K.K.; Liu, R.H. Rapid Peroxyl Radical Scavenging Capacity (PSC) Assay for Assessing both Hydrophilic and Lipophilic Antioxidants. *J. Agric. Food Chem.* **2005**, *53*, 6572–6580. [CrossRef] [PubMed]

Sample Availability: Sample compound (juglone) is available from the authors or Merck (Darmstadt, Germany).

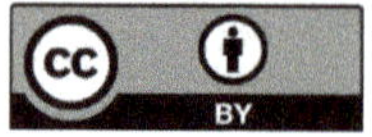

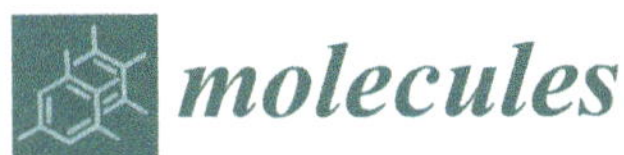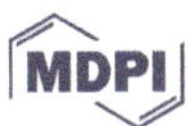

Article

Nootkatone Inhibits Acute and Chronic Inflammatory Responses in Mice

Lindaiane Bezerra Rodrigues Dantas [1], Ana Letícia Moreira Silva [1], Cícero Pedro da Silva Júnior [2], Isabel Sousa Alcântara [2], Maria Rayane Correia de Oliveira [2], Anita Oliveira Brito Pereira Bezerra Martins [2], Jaime Ribeiro-Filho [3], Henrique Douglas Melo Coutinho [4], Fabíolla Rocha Santos Passos [5], Lucindo José Quintans-Junior [5], Irwin Rose Alencar de Menezes [2], Raffaele Pezzani [6,7] and Sara Vitalini [8,*]

[1] Departamento de Saúde, Centro Universitário Dr. Leão Sampaio-UNILEÃO, Av. Leão Sampaio, 400-Lagoa Seca, Juazeiro do Norte 63040-000, Ceará, Brazil; lindaianebrd@gmail.com (L.B.R.D.); leticia-drt@hotmail.com (A.L.M.S.)

[2] Laboratory of Pharmacology and Molecular Chemistry, Department of Biological Chemistry, Regional University of Cariri, Rua Coronel Antônio Luis 1161, Pimenta, Crato 63105-000, Ceará, Brazil; juninhocatolico@hotmail.com (C.P.d.S.J.); isabel-alcantara-@hotmail.com (I.S.A.); rayaneoliveirabio@gmail.com (M.R.C.d.O.); anitaoliveira24@yahoo.com.br (A.O.B.P.B.M.); irwin.alencar@urca.br (I.R.A.d.M.)

[3] Gonçalo Moniz Institute, Oswaldo Cruz Foundation, Salvador 45500-000, Bahia, Brazil; jaimeribeirofilho@gmail.com

[4] Microbiology and Biology Molecular Laboratory, Department of Chemical Biology, Regional University of Cariri, Crato 63105-000, Ceara, Brazil; hdmcoutinho@gmail.com

[5] Graduate Program in Health Sciences, Federal University of Sergipe, Aracaju, Sergipe 49100-000, Brazil; fabiollarsp@hotmail.com (F.R.S.P.); lucindojr@gmail.com (L.J.Q.-J.)

[6] O.U. Endocrinology, Department of Medicine (DIMED), University of Padova, via Ospedale 105, 35128 Padova, Italy; raffaele.pezzani@gmail.com

[7] AIROB, Associazione Italiana per la Ricerca Oncologica di Base, 35128 Padova, Italy

[8] Department of Agricultural and Environmental Sciences, Milan State University, via G. Celoria 2, 20133 Milan, Italy

* Correspondence: sara.vitalini@unimi.it; Tel.: +39-02-50316766

Academic Editor: Massimo Bertinaria

Received: 8 April 2020; Accepted: 5 May 2020; Published: 7 May 2020

Abstract: Nootkatone (NTK) is a sesquiterpenoid found in essential oils of many species of *Citrus* (Rutaceae). Considering previous reports demonstrating that NTK inhibited inflammatory signaling pathways, this study aimed to investigate the effects of this compound in mice models of acute and chronic inflammation. Murine models of paw edema induced by carrageenan, dextran, histamine, and arachidonic acid, as well as carrageenan-induced peritonitis and pleurisy, were used to evaluate the effects of NTK on acute inflammation. A murine model of granuloma induced by cotton pellets was used to access the impact of NTK treatment on chronic inflammation. In the acute inflammation models, NTK demonstrated antiedematogenic effects and inhibited leukocyte recruitment, which was associated with decreased vascular permeability, inhibition of myeloperoxidase (MPO), interleukin (IL)1-β, and tumor necrosis factor (TNF)-α production. In silico analysis suggest that NTZ anti-inflammatory effects may also occur due to inhibition of cyclooxygenase (COX)-2 activity and antagonism of the histamine receptor type 1 (H_1). These mechanisms might have contributed to the reduction of granuloma weight and protein concentration in the homogenates, observed in the chronic inflammation model. In conclusion, NTK exerted anti-inflammatory effects that are associated with inhibition of IL1-β and TNF-α production, possibly due to inhibition of COX-2 activity and antagonism of the H1 receptor. However, further studies are required to characterize the effects of this compound on chronic inflammation.

Keywords: nootkatone; anti-inflammatory; acute inflammation; granuloma

---

1. Introduction

Inflammation is the body's response against tissue damage triggered by a variety of endogenous and exogenous stimuli. Its purpose is to remove the harmful agent and restore tissue integrity. The inflammatory reaction involves a series of tissue changes, such as vasodilation with increased blood flow, increased vascular permeability with plasma exudation and protein extravasation, and recruitment of leukocytes in response to cytokines and chemokines. In this context, neutrophils and macrophages, which play critical roles in the early phase of inflammation, also contribute to the development of many chronic inflammatory diseases [1,2].

Inflammatory mediators include a great diversity of lipids (e.g., eicosanoids), proteins (e.g., cytokines, chemokines, and adhesion molecules) and other chemically related substances that orchestrate various cellular and tissue changes through binding to receptors on leukocytes, endothelial cells, and many other cell types [3]. Some of these mediators are preformed and stored in cytoplasmic granules of mast cells, basophils, and platelets while others circulate as inactive precursors in the plasma. However, most of them are produced directly in response to inflammatory stimuli that may cause severe tissue damage related to the activation of autolytic pathways [4,5]. Persistence of the stimulus, as well as continuous production of inflammatory mediators, cause significant tissue damage, which is associated with morphological and functional changes observed in the pathogenesis of several chronic diseases [6].

Cytokines are notable chemical mediators associated with the development of uncountable inflammatory events. These molecules are produced from gene transcription in immune and non-immune cells, exerting crucial roles in the host defense against pathogens; however, especially in response to severe tissue damage, intense production of cytokines can be potentially harmful [7].

In this context, the tumor necrosis factor (TNF)-α and interleukin (IL) and IL-1 have remarkable local and systemic effects. These cytokines are capable of activating leukocytes and other cell types, stimulating the production of chemical mediators that amplify the inflammatory response [7,8].

Anti-inflammatory compounds, either synthetic or naturally occurring, are substances capable of inhibiting inflammatory events by interfering with signaling cascades associated with the production or action of inflammatory mediators. In most cases, their mechanism of action involves inhibition of enzymes (such as cyclooxygenase (Cox) -2 and 5- lipoxygenase (LO)), receptors or gene transcription. Corticosteroids and Non-Steroidal Anti-inflammatory Drugs (NSAIDs) are the main drug classes used to treat inflammatory symptoms. Nevertheless, they cause severe side effects, indicating the importance of developing novel, safe, and effective anti-inflammatory drugs [6,9].

(+)–Nootkatone (NTK) is a ketone terpenoid belonging to the largest subclass of sesquiterpenes (Figure 1) [10]. This naturally occurring organic compound is found as a component of aromatic species such as Alaskan cedar (*Cupressus nootkatensis* D.Don) and Java (*Cyperus rotundus* L.), as well as in essential oils of *Citrus* (Rutaceae), *Alpinia* (Zingiberaceae), *Chrysopogon* (Poaceae) and many other genera [11]. Due to its pleasant fragrance, this compound, as well as its biogenetic precursor valencene, have been industrially used in the chemical, food, and cosmetic sectors [11,12]. Nevertheless, studies have demonstrated that other components of citrus fruits, such as flavonoids, mainly due to their antioxidant and anti-inflammatory activities, contribute to the relevance of *Citrus* species as sources of natural products with both industrial and medicinal use. Additionally, as flavonoids are abundant in fruit juices, the consumption of these products represents an easy way to take advantage of the therapeutic properties of these compounds [12].

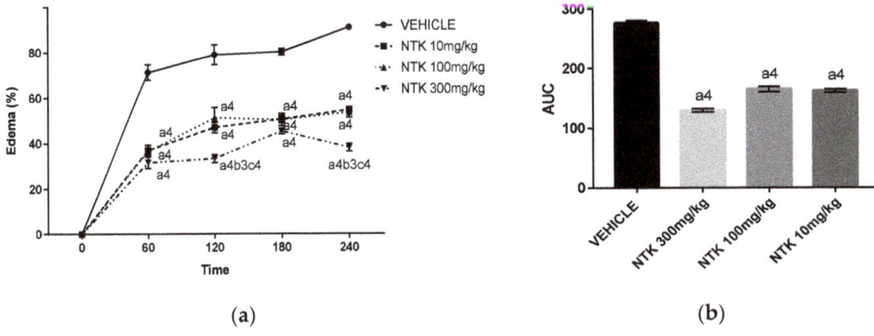

Figure 1. (+)-Nootkatone (NTK) [8].

Previous studies demonstrated that plant extracts containing NTK presented anti-inflammatory effects. Tsoyi and collaborators demonstrated that NTK and valencene inhibited nitric oxide (NO) production by inhibiting NO synthase [13]. It was also found that the compound inhibited platelet activation [14] and lipid peroxidation, in addition to inhibiting systemic oxidative stress, as well as preventing DNA damage by activating nuclear factor erythroid-derived 2-like 2 and heme oxygenase 1 [15].

Considering the pharmacological properties of NTK, this study aimed to investigate its effects in mice models of acute and chronic inflammation.

2. Results

2.1. NTK Inhibits Paw Edema Induced by Different Inflammatory Agents

Because edema is one of the first inflammatory cardinal signs in acute responses, we investigated the effects of NTK on paw edema induced by different triggering agents. Initially, we analyzed the effect of a single oral pre-treatment with varying doses of NTK (10, 100, and 300 mg/kg) at different time points after challenge with carrageenan (Figure 2a) or dextran (Figure 2c). These treatments caused significant inhibition of the edema caused by both agents at all evaluated time-points. In addition, as demonstrated by the analysis of the area under the curve (AUC) (Figure 2b,d), no significant difference among the doses was observed. Therefore, the lower dose (10 mg/kg) was used throughout the experiments.

(a)   (b)

Figure 2. *Cont.*

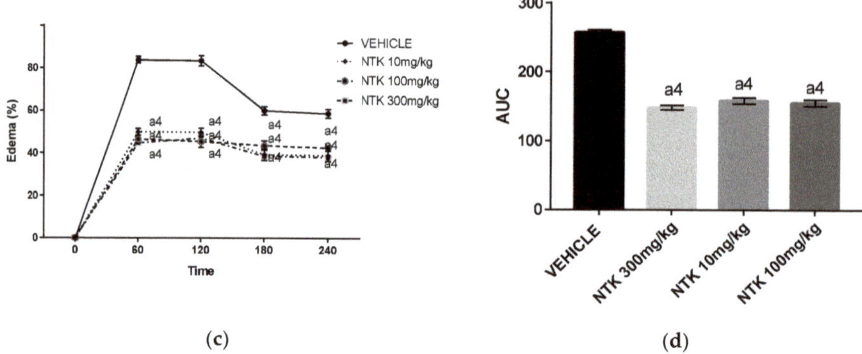

(c)

(d)

Figure 2. Time-point analysis of treatment with different NTK doses on paw edema formation induced by carrageenan (**a**) or dextran (**c**). These data are also represented as area under the curve (AUC) ((**b,d**), respectively). a4 = $p < 0.0001$ vs. saline; b3 = $p < 0.001$ vs. NTK 100 mg/kg group; c4 = $p < 0.0001$ vs. NTK 10 mg/kg group. Statistical significance was determined with two-way ANOVA (**a,c**) and post hoc Tukey test.

Histamine and arachidonic acid (AA)-derived lipid mediators are crucially involved in edema formation during inflammatory conditions [16]. Therefore, we investigated the participation of these mediators on NKT-mediated edema inhibition. As shown in Figure 2a, a single oral pre-treatment with NTK (10 mg/kg) inhibited paw edema formation at 30 and 60 min after challenge in comparison with vehicle pre-treatment. Promethazine (PTZ) (6 mg/kg), a histamine receptor antagonist, caused similar inhibition of the edema, suggesting that NTK-mediated antiedematogenic effects may involve, at least partially, inhibition of histamine vascular actions. Accordingly, the most significant antiedematogenic effect of NTK was observed in AA-stimulated mice (Figure 3b). Moreover, indomethacin (IND), an NSAID used as a positive control, caused comparable inhibition at all evaluated time-points, suggesting that the antiedematogenic effects of NTK might involve arachidonic acid metabolism inhibition.

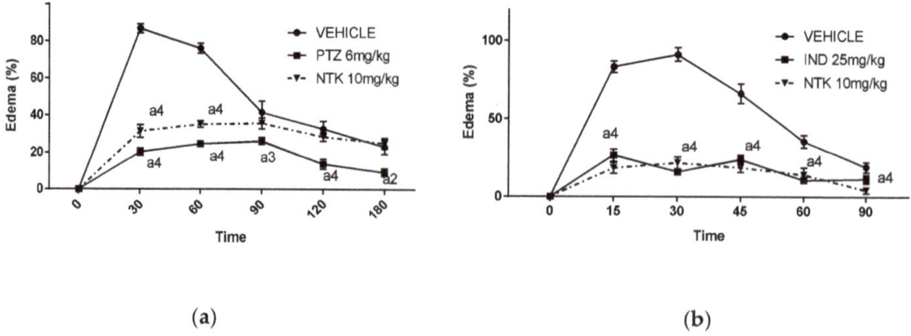

(a)

(b)

Figure 3. Potential mechanisms associated with NTK-mediated paw edema inhibition. The antiedematogenic effect is expressed as a percentage of edema induced by histamine (**a**) or arachidonic acid (**b**). a4 = $p < 0.0001$ vs. saline; a3 = $p < 0.001$ vs. saline and a2 = $p < 0.01$ vs. saline. Statistical significance was determined with two-way ANOVA and post hoc Tukey test.

2.2. The Effects of NTK on Carrageenan-Induced Peritonitis

The intraperitoneal administration of carrageenan (1%) induced an intense influx of leukocytes associated with elevated myeloperoxidase (MPO) and albumin levels into the peritoneal cavity of mice

4 h after challenge (Figure 4a–c), indicating the development a peritoneal inflammation associated with leukocyte migration and activation, and increased vascular permeability. The animals treated with NTK (10 mg/kg) or indomethacin (25 mg/kg) presented a significant reduction in all these inflammatory parameters, demonstrating that the treatments exerted anti-inflammatory effects in mice.

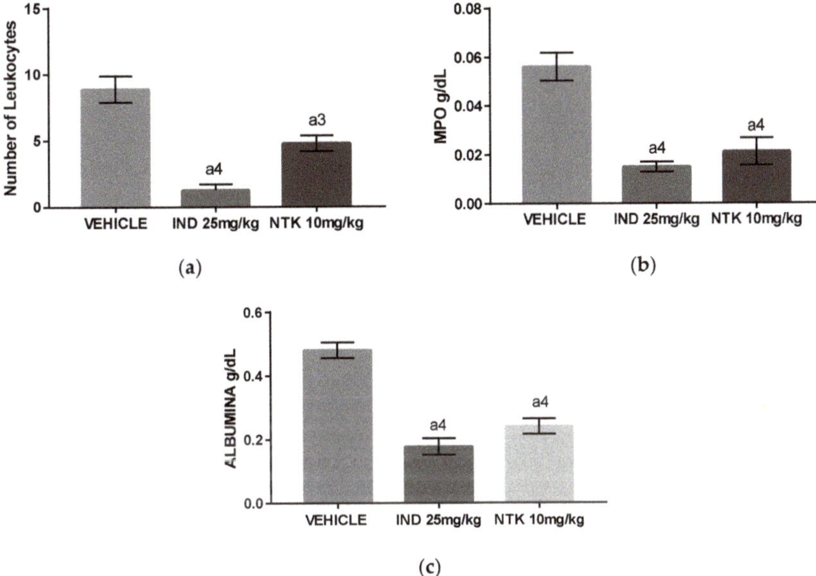

Figure 4. The effects of NTK on carrageenan-induced peritonitis. (**a**) The number of total leukocytes; (**b**) concentrations of myeloperoxidase (MPO), and (**c**) concentrations of albumin in the peritoneal fluid of mice. a4 = $p < 0.0001$ vs. saline and a3 = $p < 0.001$ vs. saline. Statistical significance was determined with one-way ANOVA and post hoc Tukey test.

2.3. NTK Inhibits Leukocyte Recruitment and Cytokine Production on Carrageenan-Induced Pleurisy

Interleukin (IL)-1β and Tumor Necrosis Factor (TNF)-α have critical roles in the development of acute inflammation [17]. The group of mice challenged with carrageenan and pre-treated with NTK (10 mg/kg) presented a significantly reduced number of total leukocytes associated with lower concentrations of IL1-β and TNF-α in the pleural lavages in comparison with untreated animals (Figure 5a–c), indicating that inhibition of cytokine production is potentially related with NTK anti-inflammatory mechanisms.

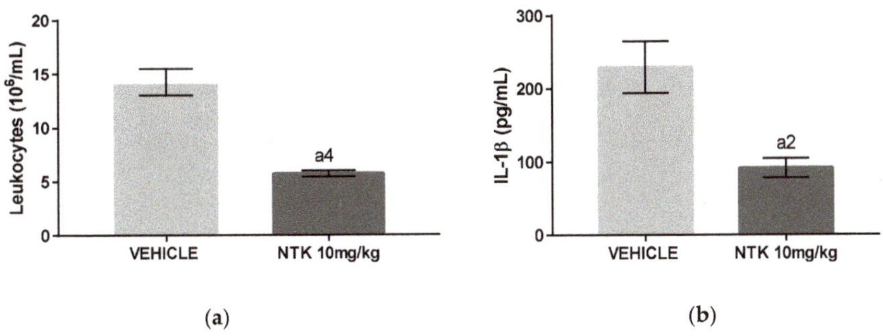

Figure 5. *Cont.*

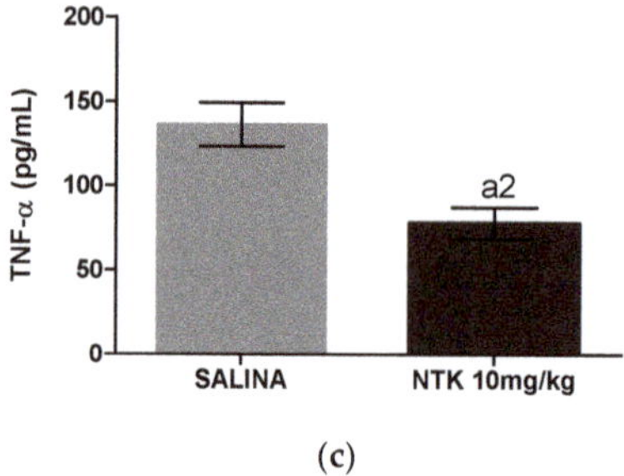

(c)

Figure 5. The effects of NTK on carrageenan-induced pleurisy. (**a**) The number of total leukocytes; (**b**) concentrations of Interleukin (IL)-1β, and (**c**) concentrations of Tumor Necrosis Factor (TNF)-α in the pleural lavages of mice. a4 = $p < 0.0001$ vs. saline and a2 = $p < 0.01$ vs. saline. Statistical significance was determined with one-way ANOVA and post hoc Tukey test.

2.4. Investigation of NTK-Mediated COX-2 and H_1 Inhibition in Silico

In the present study, the docking procedure was validated by removing and repositioning each ligand into the binding site. The root-mean-square deviation (RMSD) resulting from the X-ray crystallography structures found conformations of 0.87Å and 0.32Å (for COX-2 and histamine, respectively), demonstrating convergence in the calculated complex formation and attesting the performance of the docking protocol. The results of docking analysis determine how closely the lowest energy pose (binding conformation) from the COX-2 enzyme and the H_1 receptor.

The docked ligands showed score energies of −8.6 kcal/mol to diclofenac and −8.0 kcal/mol for nootkatone in the COX-2 binding site. Considering the H_1 receptor, the score energies were −11.5 kcal/mol for doxepin and −8.1 kcal/mol for nootkatone. Of note, these data were useful to analyze the hydrophobic and polar interactions in the binding site of the complexes. The best conformation of nootkatone into COX-2 enzyme and H_1 receptor binding sites indicate a favorable interaction with both proteins (Figure 6a,b), as well as their respective control ligands diclofenac and doxepin, suggesting a link between COX-2 and H_1 inhibition and the NTK-mediated anti-inflammatory effects (Figure 7a–d).

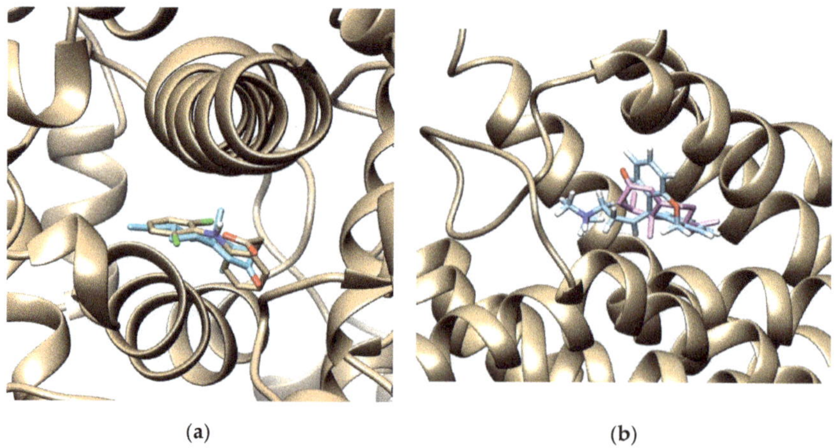

(**a**)   (**b**)

Figure 6. The binding poses of best stability between NTK and diclofenac into the cyclooxygenase (COX)-2 enzyme binding site (**a**) and between NTK and doxepin into the binding site of the H_1 receptor (**b**).

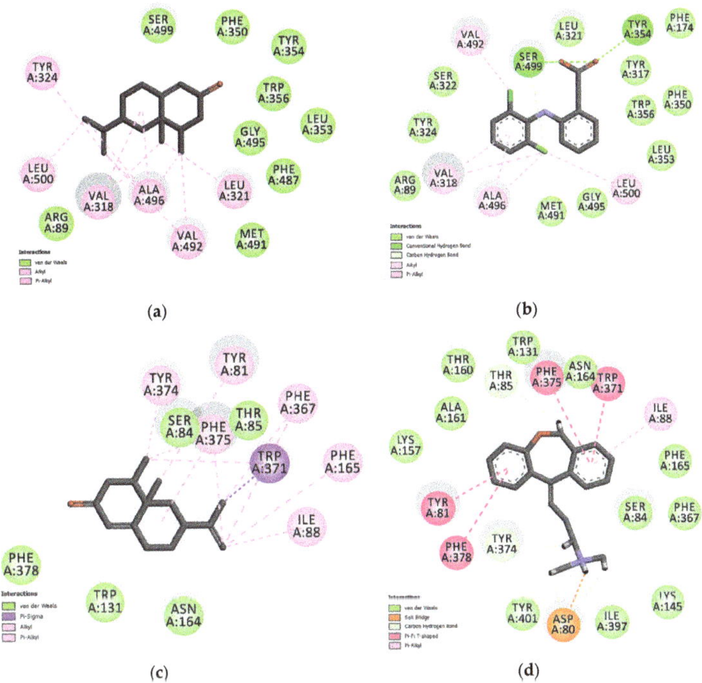

Figure 7. Maps of amino acid residues within the binding pocket of COX-2 (**a**,**b**) and the H1 receptor (**c**,**d**). The interactions of NKT (**a**,**c**), Diclofenac (**b**), and Doxepin (**d**) with these amino acids is illustrated.

2.5. The Effects of NTK on Cotton Pellet-Induced Granuloma

The cotton pellet-induced granuloma model was used to evaluate the effects of NTK on chronic inflammation. Administration of NTK (10 mg/kg) to mice decreased both granuloma weight (Figure 8a) and concentration of proteins in the homogenates (Figure 8b) in comparison with untreated mice, indicating that the treatment inhibited, at least partially, the inflammatory response in this model.

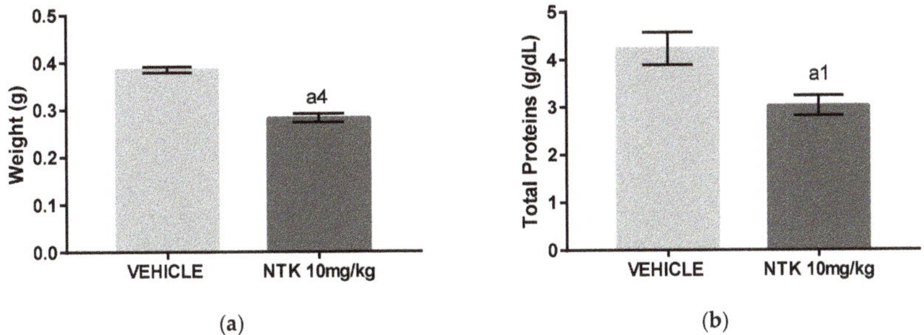

Figure 8. The effects of NTK treatment on cotton pellet-induced granuloma in mice. (**a**) Final weight of the granuloma. (**b**) Protein concentration in the homogenates. a4 = $p < 0.0001$ vs. saline and a1 = $p < 0.05$ vs. saline. Statistical significance was determined with T test.

3. Discussion

The present study demonstrated the anti-inflammatory effects of NTK, an aromatic sesquiterpenoid widely found in the plant kingdom. A screening evaluating the effect of different doses of this compound on paw edema induced by carrageenan or dextran, demonstrated significant antiedematogenic effects at 10, 100, or 300 mg/kg in mice. Therefore, we chose the lower dose for the following analysis. Carrageenan and dextran are phlogistic agents that act by triggering an inflammatory reaction characterized by the release of chemical mediators, such as prostaglandins (e.g., PGE_2) and vasoactive amines (e.g., histamine), which increase the vascular permeability and cause the biochemical, cellular, and vascular changes observed in acute inflammation [18].

Considering the involvement of vasoactive amines and lipid mediators on edema induction, we investigated the effects of NTK pre-treatment on edema triggered by histamine and AA challenge. It was shown that the compound partially inhibited paw edema formation triggered by histamine administration and promethazine, a histamine receptor antagonist, caused comparable inhibition, suggesting that NTK-mediated antiedematogenic effects may involve, at least partially, inhibition of histamine vascular actions. NTK Pre-treatment significantly inhibited edema formation in AA-stimulated mice. Accordingly, indomethacin, an NSAID used as the positive control, caused comparable inhibition at all evaluated time-points, suggesting that the effects of NTK in acute inflammation might involve arachidonic acid metabolism inhibition, possibly through interference with the enzymatic activity of cyclooxygenase (COX), lipoxygenase (LO), or phospholipase A_2 (PLA_2), or even by antagonizing the effects of bioactive eicosanoids on tissue receptors. Nevertheless, the similarity in magnitude between the effect of NTK and indomethacin, suggests a common action on the COX pathway [19,20]. Our findings are corroborated by previous research demonstrating that NTK concentration-dependently inhibited platelet activation induced by AA in vitro. Since prostaglandins significantly mediate AA-induced platelet activation, we hypothesized that NTK could be acting through inhibition of COX activation in platelets [14].

To investigate the involvement of COX-2 and H_1 receptor inhibition on NTZ-mediated anti-inflammatory effects, we performed in silico analysis by molecular docking. The COX-2 binding site shows two important regions of interaction with inhibitors: the hydrophobic pocket formed by Tyr324, Trp356, Phe487, Phe350, Ala496, Tyr317, and Leu321, and the hydrogen bond pocket formed by Ser-499 and Tyr-354. The Alkyl and Alkyl-pi stacking interactions work as "anchors", favoring the van der Waals interactions and contributing to the formation of a stable bond in the COX-2/NTK complex. Our results demonstrated a complementarity between the ligands and the active site of COX-2. The relative contribution of van der Waals interactions has demonstrated to be relevant for both NTK and diclofenac. In addition, 15 similar interaction points with hydrophobic and hydrophilic cavities were found between NTK and diclofenac. However, the control drug had relatively better docking energy, in part, generated by hydrogen bonds. Previous studies with other terpenes derivatives have demonstrated that these compounds interacted similarly, although no involvement of hydrogen bonds was shown [21,22]. In the H_1 receptor binding site, NTK showed potential Van der Waals interactions with Ser84, Thr 85, Phe 378, Trp 131, Asn 164 (Figure 7). However, other interactions such as alkyl, π-sigma, and π-alkyl, contribute to the stabilization of the interaction, as well as to the formation of the lipophilic pocket in the binding site. According to Keserű, G. M. et al. (2004), taking part in the lipophilic pocket formation is crucial for the antagonist activity in the binding cavity. The interactive map shows nine similar stabilization points between the NTK/H_1 and the doxepin/H_1 complex at the binding site. Therefore, NTK shows favorable docking with the COX-2 enzyme and the H_1 receptor. These amino acid similarities support the hypothesis that NTK occupies the active site in both targets, corroborating our experimental data using in vivo models.

Carrageenan-induced pleurisy and peritonitis are well-established models used for evaluation of the systemic anti-inflammatory properties of natural and synthetic drugs. A single oral pre-treatment with NTK (10 mg/kg) caused significant inhibition of leukocyte recruitment associated with decreased concentrations of albumin, MPO, IL1-β, and TNF-α, demonstrating that the compound inhibited hallmark parameters of acute systemic inflammation. The decreased albumin levels found in NTK-treated animals indicates an inhibitory action by this compound on carrageenan-mediated increased vascular permeability. Accordingly, the lower concentrations of IL-1β and TNF-α found in the NTK group justify, at least partially, the inhibitory effects of this compound on all acute inflammation parameters demonstrated by this study, since these cytokines were shown to exert multiple inflammatory actions, leading to increased vascular permeability and leukocyte recruitment and activation [22]. In this context, in addition to presenting a reduced number of leukocytes in both pleural and peritoneal lavages, the NTK-treated mice showed significantly reduced MPO levels, indicating inhibition of leukocyte activity.

In order to evaluate the effects of NTK against a chronic stimulus, we used the cotton pellet-induced granuloma model in mice. NTK treatment for 10 consecutive days showed positive effects, reducing both granuloma weight and total proteins in the homogenates. These findings suggest a possible inhibitory action of the treatment on macrophage migration and activation as well as of the proliferative response, corroborating the effects of NTK on cytokine production and leukocyte activity. Importantly, because NTK was found to reduce several inflammatory parameters induced by different noxious stimuli in different mice models of acute systemic inflammation, we suggest that this sesquiterpene may be used for further research aimed at the development of new anti-inflammatory drugs.

The results obtained in the present research are corroborated by the findings of previous studies. Choi et al. [20] demonstrated in vitro that NTK suppressed the expression of chemokines such as thymus and activation-regulated chemokine (TARC/CCL17) and macrophage-derived chemokine (MDC/CCL22) in HaCaT cells, by inhibiting the mitogen-activated protein kinases (MAP kinases) PKC and p38. Since these kinases participate in signaling pathways involved in the activation of the transcriptional nuclear factor-kappaB (NF-κB) transcriptional factor, these findings suggest that NKT could modulate the inflammatory response at multiple levels, since NF-κB stimulates the transcription of numerous genes from cytokines, chemokines and adhesion molecules, supporting the findings of the present study. According to Qi and collaborators [23], the NKT treatment reduced the levels of TNF-α, IL-1β, and IL-6 in models of cognitive impairment and dementia in rats, corroborating the data from our pleurisy model. Moreover, NKT significantly reduced the activities of inflammatory enzymes such as superoxide dismutase (SOD), glutathione S-transferase (GST), cyclooxygenase-2 (COX-2), and inducible nitric oxide synthase (iNOS) and levels of glutathione (GSH), in addition to decreasing the total antioxidant capacity (T-AOC), as well as concentrations of malondialdehyde (MDA) and nitric oxide (NO) through inhibition of the Toll-like receptor 4/NF-κB/domains-containing-protein-3-inflammasome (TLR4/NF-κB/NLRP3) pathway [23]. NTK (90 mg Kg) was also shown to reduce the anti-inflammatory effects of cigarette vapor [24], as well as inhibit lung inflammation parameters via NF-κB inhibition [19]. Nevertheless, the mechanisms underlying the effects of NTK as an anti-inflammatory compound remain to be fully characterized. Therefore, we will carry out in vitro studies to analyze the impact of NTK on COX-1 and COX-2 expression and activity, which will be correlated with the levels of PGE$_2$ in the supernatants of macrophage cultures. Additionally, we will use mast cell cultures will to analyze the effects of NTK on histamine release in vitro, which will be correlated with the activity of this compound in combination with agonists and antagonists of the H$_1$ receptor in vivo.

Finally, Kurdi and colleagues demonstrated that NTK (10 mg/kg) treatment exerted hepatoprotective and antifibrotic effects by suppressing the carbon tetrachloride (CCL4)-induced lesion, which is characterized by expression of pro-inflammatory cytokines, such as TNF-α, monocyte chemotactic protein (MCP)-1 and IL-1β in liver tissues. In the same study, histopathological findings revealed that NTK reduced fibrosis, steatosis, hepatocyte necrosis and leukocyte infiltration [25], providing evidence that NTK could be useful in the management of chronic inflammation, as indicated by our findings in the cotton pellet-induced granuloma. However, further research is required to characterize better the anti-inflammatory effects of NTK, as well as its mechanism of action on chronic inflammation. To this end, we will carry out experiments to characterize the cell populations, as well as the expression of chronic inflammation markers in the granuloma model.

In conclusion, NTK presented anti-inflammatory effects in mice models of acute and chronic inflammation. In acute inflammation, the antiedematogenic effects, as well as leukocyte recruitment inhibition, may be associated with decreased vascular permeability and inhibition of MPO, IL1-β, and TNF-α production, possibly due to inhibition COX-2 activity and antagonism of the H1 receptor. These mechanisms might have contributed to the anti-inflammatory effects displayed by NTK on the granuloma model. However, further studies are required to characterize the effects of this compound on chronic inflammation.

4. Materials and Methods

4.1. Drugs and Reagents

Compound NTK, all inflammatory agents (carrageenan, dextran, histamine, and arachidonic acid), ELISA kits from eBioscience and compound o-dianisidine (used for myeloperoxidase assay) were purchased from Sigma-Aldrich (New York, NY, USA); the kits for albumin and total proteins quantification were supplied by Labtest (Lagoa Santa, Brazil), ketamine was purchased by the VETNIL (São Paulo, Brazil), and xylazine was purchased by CEVA (São Paulo, Brazil).

4.2. Animals

Swiss mice (Mus musculus) of both sexes, weighing 20–30 g, were randomly assigned into groups and maintained in polypropylene cages at 22 ± 3 °C, under a 12 h light/dark cycle and with free access to water and food (Labina, Purina®, Euskirchen, Germany). The research was carried out in accordance with the guidelines animal testing (Guide for the care and use of laboratory animals, from NIH—National Institute of Health—USA, 1996; Federal Law No. 11,794/2008 and National Experiment Control Council—CONCEA). The protocols used in this study were approved by the local institutional review board for animal experimentation (CEUA, Regional University of Cariri, protocol number 100/2019.2).

4.3. Evaluation of the Anti-Inflammatory Activity

The effects of NTK on acute inflammation were evaluated using the following mice models: carrageenan-induced peritonitis, carrageenan-induced pleurisy, and paw edema induced by either carrageenan, dextran, histamine, or arachidonic acid (AA). In all these protocols, the mice received a single oral treatment one hour before the challenge. Each challenge was performed through a single administration of an inflammatory agent (carrageenan, histamine, dextran, or AA) to the mice, triggering an acute inflammatory response, which was monitored immediately after the challenge at specific time-points, according to standard protocols. The paw edema models were used to evaluate the local inflammatory response, while pleurisy and peritonitis were used to analyze systemic inflammatory parameters. In the chronic inflammation protocol, the animals were treated daily for ten consecutive days, after surgically receiving a persistent stimulus (cotton pellets). This protocol induces the formation of granuloma, which is considered as a parameter of chronic inflammation.

4.3.1. Evaluation of the Antiedematogenic Activity

The animals ($n = 6$ per group) were randomly assigned into groups and orally treated with NTK (10, 100, or 300 mg/kg), vehicle (0.9% saline, negative control) or control drugs (promethazine, 10 mg/kg or indomethacin, 25 mg/kg) 1 h before challenge with 20 µL of carrageenan, dextran, histamine, or AA at 1% (w/v). Each inflammatory agent used in the challenge was administered in the hind right paw and an equal volume of saline was administered in the hind left paw. The volume of both paws was measured at different time-points according to the type of challenge, using a plethysmometer and the results were expressed as a percentage of edema, considering the difference between the hind and left paw of the untreated group as 100% [19,21,22].

4.3.2. Carrageenan-Induced Peritonitis

The mice ($n = 6$) were orally pre-treated with the vehicle, NTK (10 mg/kg), or indomethacin (25 mg/kg) 1 h before receiving an intraperitoneal injection of 1 mL of 1% carrageenan (challenge).

Four hours after challenge, these animals were euthanized by CO_2 inhalation, the peritoneal cavity was washed with 3 mL of heparinized PBS (10 IU/mL), and the peritoneal lavage was collected for leukocyte counting and quantification of MPO and total proteins [26]. Total leukocyte counts were performed using the SDH-20 model automatic counter and the differential counts were performed by optical microscopy, on slides stained using the panoptic method.

4.3.3. Carrageenan-Induced Pleurisy

The mice (n = 6) were orally pre-treated with the vehicle, NTK (10 mg/kg), or indomethacin (25 mg/kg) 1 h before receiving an intrathoracic injection of 1% carrageenan (challenge). Four hours later, the animals were anesthetized with ketamine (8 mg/kg) and xylazine (8 mg/kg) and euthanized by cervical dislocation. The pleural cavity was washed with 1 mL of saline containing 0.9% Ethylenediaminetetraacetic acid (EDTA, Sigma, New York, NY, USA). The pleural lavages were centrifuged (5000 rpm, 5 min, at room temperature), and supernatants were stored (at −80 °C) for further analysis. The precipitate was added with 1 mL of PBS, and leukocytes were counted under light microscopy after diluting the pleural lavage samples in Turk fluid (2% acetic acid) [27].

4.3.4. Quantification of MPO and Total Proteins

Samples of the peritoneal lavage were centrifuged at 6000 RPM for 2 min. Albumin quantification in the supernatants was performed using a Labtest kit (Lagoa Santa, Brazil) and used as a parameter of protein extravasation due to increased vascular permeability. In this method, the absorbance of bromocresol green, which specifically binds albumin, is proportional to the concentration of the protein in the sample. The readings were performed using a spectrophotometer with absorbance adjusted between 600 and 640 nm. Leukocyte activity was determined by quantifying the MPO enzyme. To this end, a tube was added with 40 µL of the supernatant of the pleural lavage and 1960 µL of the o-dianisidine and H_2O_2 reagent in PBS (pH = 6.0). The readings were performed using a spectrophotometer at 450 nm.

4.3.5. Cytokine Quantification

The concentrations of TNF-α and IL-1β were determined using enzyme-linked immunosorbent assay (ELISA) kits (Invitrogen®, California, CA, USA) according to the manufacturer's instructions. Briefly, supernatants of pleural lavages were diluted 1:1 (*w/w*) in the diluent solution provided by the ELISA kit, and the readings were performed at 450 nm using a microplate reader (ASYS®, New York, NY, USA). The concentrations were obtained by interpolation from a standard curve and data were expressed as pg/mL.

4.3.6. Cotton Pellet-Induced Granuloma

Mice (n = 6) previously anesthetized with ketamine (80 mg/kg) and xylazine (20 mg/kg) had four cotton pellets (0.01 g each) implanted through a small dorsal incision. Twenty-four hours later, the animals were treated orally with vehicle or NTK (10 mg/kg) for ten consecutive days. On day 11, the animals were euthanized, and the pellets, as well as the surrounding tissue, were removed, dried at 37 °C for 24 h, and weighed. The results were expressed as the difference between the final weight and the initial weight [28].

For total protein quantification, the pellets were placed in test tubes and homogenized with 1 mL of 0.9% saline. The concentration of total proteins was determined using a specific kit (Labtest, Lagoa Santa, Brazil) that is based on the reaction with copper ions in an alkaline medium, creating a violet color complex whose absorbance is proportional to the concentration of proteins in the sample. The readings were performed at 550 nm using a spectrophotometer.

4.4. In Silico Analysis of COX-2 Inhibition

Docking simulations were carried out for ligand-bound protein complexes, obtained from the Protein Data Bank (PDB, ID. 1PXX and 3RZE). The complexed structures were adjusted using a protein preparation tool provided by the Chimera package, the 3D structures of ligands were obtained using the corina® 3D structure generator and minimization of energy was achieved using the UCSF Chimera structure build module. The binding region was defined by a 10 Å × 10 Å × 10 Å box set at the centroid of the co-crystallized ligand in the crystal complex to explore a large region of the enzyme structure. The docking analysis was carried out using the UCSF Chimera and AutoDock Vina software based on the Iterated local search global optimizer. Proteins and ligands were maintained flexible during the docking process. The selection of flexible residues from proteins was based on the active site at 4.0 Å from the co-crystallized ligands. The most favorable binding free energy was represented by clustering the positional RMSD results with not more than 1.0 Å. The final docked complexes were analyzed using Discovery Studio 3.1 visualizer [29].

4.5. Statistical Analyses

Data were analyzed by one-way ANOVA or two-way ANOVA and Tukey post hoc test or T test using GraphPad Prism software version 7.00 (GraphPad, San Diego, CA, USA, 2016). Values are expressed as means ± SEM. Statistical significance was considered when $p < 0.05$.

Author Contributions: Conceptualization, H.D.M.C., I.R.A.d.M., R.P., and S.V.; methodology, L.B.R.D., A.L.M.S., I.S.A., A.O.B.P.B.M., and F.R.S.P.; validation, C.P.d.S.J.; formal analysis, M.R.C.d.O.; resources, L.J.Q.-J.; writing—original draft preparation, J.R.-F., writing—review and editing, J.R.F. and L.B.R.D. supervision, H.D.M.C., I.R.A.d.M., R.P., and S.V. All authors have read and agreed to the published version of the manuscript.

Funding: This work was supported by Coordenação de Aperfeiçoamento de Pessoal de Nível Superior-Brasil (CAPES), Fundação Cearense de Apoio ao Desenvolvimento Científico e Tecnológico (FUNCAP) and Conselho Nacional de Desenvolvimento Científico e Tecnológico (CNPq)–finance code 304291/2017-0 and Financiadora de Estudos e Projetos-Brasil (FINEP).

Acknowledgments: The authors would like to thank the support and resources provided by the Leão Sampaio University Center (Juazeiro do Norte, Brazil).

Conflicts of Interest: The authors declare no conflict of interest.

References

1. Buckley, C.D.; Gilroy, D.W.; Serhan, C.N. Proresolving lipid mediators and mechanisms in the resolution of acute inflammation. *Immunity* **2014**, *40*, 315–327. [CrossRef] [PubMed]
2. Prame Kumar, K.; Nicholls, A.J.; Wong, C.H.Y. Partners in crime: Neutrophils and monocytes/macrophages in inflammation and disease. *Cell Tissue Res.* **2018**, *371*, 551–565. [CrossRef] [PubMed]
3. Hannoodee, S.; Nasuruddin, D.N. *Acute Inflammatory Response*; StatPearls Publishing LLC.: Treasure Island, FL, USA, 2020.
4. Rahmati, M.; Mobasheri, A.; Mozafari, M. Inflammatory mediators in osteoarthritis: A critical review of the state-of-the-art, current prospects, and future challenges. *Bone* **2016**, *85*, 81–90. [CrossRef] [PubMed]
5. Rai, R.C. Host inflammatory responses to intracellular invaders: Review study. *Life Sci.* **2020**, *240*, 117084. [CrossRef]
6. Nathan, C.; Ding, A. Nonresolving Inflammation. *Cell* **2010**, *140*, 871–882. [CrossRef]
7. John, O.; Massimo, G.; Richard, M.S. Cytokines and Cytokine Receptors. In *Clinical Immunology; Principles and Practice*, 5th ed.; Elsevier: San Diego, CA, USA, 2019.
8. Peter, J.D.; Seamus, J.M.; Dennis, R.B. *Roitt's Essential Immunology*; John Wiley & Sons: West Sussex, UK, 2017.
9. Robb, C.T.; Regan, K.H.; Dorward, D.A.; Rossi, A.G. Key mechanisms governing resolution of lung inflammation. *Semin. Immunopathol.* **2016**, *38*, 425–448. [CrossRef]
10. Leonhardt, R.-H.; Berger, R.G. Nootkatone. In *Biotechnology of Isoprenoids*; Springer: Berlin, Germany, 2015; pp. 391–404.
11. Rana, V.S.; Blazquez, M.A. Compositions of the Volatile Oils of *Citrus macroptera* and *C. maxima. Nat. Prod. Commun.* **2012**, *7*, 1271–1372. [CrossRef]

12. Harapu, C.D.; Miron, A.; Cuciureanu, M.; Cuciureanu, R. Flavonoids-bioactive compounds in fruits juice. *Rev. Med. Chir. Soc. Med. Nat. Iasi* **2010**, *114*, 1209–1214.

13. Tsoyi, K.; Jang, H.J.; Lee, Y.S.; Kim, Y.M.; Kim, H.J.; Seo, H.G.; Lee, J.H.; Kwak, J.H.; Lee, D.-U.; Chang, K.C. (+)-Nootkatone and (+)-valencene from rhizomes of *Cyperus rotundus* increase survival rates in septic mice due to heme oxygenase-1 induction. *J. Ethnopharmacol.* **2011**, *137*, 1311–1317. [CrossRef]

14. Seo, E.J.; Lee, D.-U.; Kwak, J.H.; Lee, S.-M.; Kim, Y.S.; Jung, Y.-S. Antiplatelet effects of *Cyperus rotundus* and its component (+)-nootkatone. *J. Ethnopharmacol.* **2011**, *135*, 48–54. [CrossRef]

15. Nemmar, A.; Al-Salam, S.; Beegam, S.; Yuvaraju, P.; Ali, B.H. Thrombosis and systemic and cardiac oxidative stress and DNA damage induced by pulmonary exposure to diesel exhaust particles and the effect of nootkatone thereon. *Am. J. Physiol. Circ. Physiol.* **2018**, *314*, H917–H927. [CrossRef] [PubMed]

16. Serhan, C.N. Resolution phase of inflammation: Novel endogenous anti-inflammatory and proresolving lipid mediators and pathways. *Annu. Rev. Immunol.* **2007**, *25*, 101–137. [CrossRef] [PubMed]

17. Cook, A.D.; Christensen, A.D.; Tewari, D.; McMahon, S.B.; Hamilton, J.A. Immune cytokines and their receptors in inflammatory pain. *Trends Immunol.* **2018**, *39*, 240–255. [CrossRef]

18. Eze, F.I.; Uzor, P.F.; Ikechukwu, P.; Obi, B.C.; Osadebe, P.O. In vitro and in vivo models for anti-inflammation: An evaluative review. *INNOSC Theranostics Pharmacol. Sci.* **2019**, *2*, 3–15. [CrossRef]

19. Nemmar, A.; Al-Salam, S.; Beegam, S.; Yuvaraju, P.; Hamadi, N.; Ali, B.; Nemmar, A.; Al-Salam, S.; Beegam, S.; Yuvaraju, P.; et al. In vivo protective effects of nootkatone against particles-induced lung injury caused by diesel exhaust is mediated via the NF-κB pathway. *Nutrients* **2018**, *10*, 263. [CrossRef] [PubMed]

20. Choi, H.-J.; Lee, J.-H.; Jung, Y.-S.; Choi, H.-J.; Lee, J.-H.; Jung, Y.-S. (+)-Nootkatone inhibits tumor necrosis factor α/interferon γ-induced production of chemokines in HaCaT cells. *Biochem. Biophys. Res. Commun.* **2014**, *447*, 278–284. [CrossRef]

21. Singh, S.; Pandey, V.P.; Naaz, H.; Singh, P.; Dwivedi, U.N. Structural modeling and simulation studies of human cyclooxygenase (COX) isozymes with selected terpenes: Implications in drug designing and development. *Comput. Biol. Med.* **2013**, *43*, 744–750. [CrossRef]

22. de Santana Souza, M.T.; Almeida, J.R.G.D.S.; de Souza Araujo, A.A.; Duarte, M.C.; Gelain, D.P.; Moreira, J.C.F.; dos Santos, M.R.V.; Quintans-Júnior, L.J. Structure-activity relationship of terpenes with anti-inflammatory profile: A systematic review. *Basic Clin. Pharmacol. Toxicol.* **2014**, *115*, 244–256. [CrossRef]

23. Qi, Y.; Cheng, X.; Jing, H.; Yan, T.; Xiao, F.; Wu, B.; Bi, K.; Jia, Y. Combination of schisandrin and nootkatone exerts neuroprotective effect in Alzheimer's disease mice model. *Metab. Brain Dis.* **2019**, *34*, 1689–1703. [CrossRef]

24. Ali, B.H.; Al-Salam, S.; Adham, S.A.; Al Balushi, K.; Al Za'abi, M.; Beegam, S.; Yuvaraju, P.; Manoj, P.; Nemmar, A. Testicular toxicity of water pipe smoke exposure in mice and the effect of treatment with nootkatone thereon. *Oxid. Med. Cell. Longev.* **2019**, *2019*, 1–10. [CrossRef]

25. Kurdi, A.; Hassan, K.; Venkataraman, B.; Rajesh, M. Nootkatone confers hepatoprotective and anti-fibrotic actions in a murine model of liver fibrosis by suppressing oxidative stress, inflammation, and apoptosis. *J. Biochem. Mol. Toxicol.* **2018**, *32*, e22017. [CrossRef] [PubMed]

26. Lapa, A. *Métodos de Avaliação da Atividade Farmacológica de Plantas Medicinais*; Sociedade Brasileira de Plantas Medicinais: Botucatu, Brazil, 2003.

27. Fereidoni, M.; Ahmadiani, A.; Semnanian, S.; Javan, M. An accurate and simple method for measurement of paw edema. *J. Pharm. Toxicol. Methods* **2000**, *43*, 11–14. [CrossRef]

28. Lalitha, K.G.; Sethuraman, M.G. Anti-inflammatory activity of roots of *Ecbolium viride* (Forsk) Merrill. *J. Ethnopharmacol.* **2010**, *128*, 248–250. [CrossRef] [PubMed]

29. BS Biovia. BIOVIA Discovery. Available online: https://www.3dsbiovia.com/products/collaborative-science/biovia-discovery-studio/ (accessed on 3 April 2020).

Sample Availability: Samples of the compounds are not available from the authors.

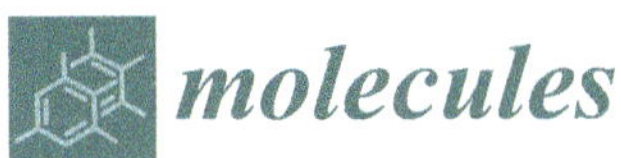 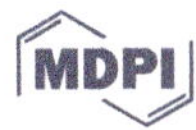

Article

A Lanosteryl Triterpene (RA-3) Exhibits Antihyperuricemic and Nephroprotective Effects in Rats

Nomadlozi Blessings Hlophe [1], Andrew Rowland Opoku [1], Foluso Oluwagbemiga Osunsanmi [2], Trayana Georgieva Djarova-Daniels [1], Oladipupo Adejumobi Lawal [3] and Rebamang Anthony Mosa [4,*]

[1]   Department of Biochemistry and Microbiology, University of Zululand, KwaDlangezwa 3886, South Africa; nomadlozih4@gmail.com (N.B.H.); opokuA@unizulu.ac.za (A.R.O.); trayana.djarova@gmail.com (T.G.D.-D.)

[2]   Department of Agriculture, University of Zululand, KwaDlangezwa 3886, South Africa; alafin21@yahoo.com

[3]   Products Research Unit, Department of Chemistry, Lagos State University, 102101 Lagos, Nigeria; jumobi.lawal@lasu.edu.ng

[4]   Department of Biochemistry, Genetics and Microbiology, Division of Biochemistry, University of Pretoria, Hatfield 0028, South Africa

*   Correspondence: rebamang.mosa@up.ac.za; Tel.: +27-21-420-2906

Received: 19 June 2020; Accepted: 24 July 2020; Published: 2 September 2020

Abstract: Considering the global health threat posed by kidney disease burden, a search for new nephroprotective drugs from our local flora could prove a powerful strategy to respond to this health threat. In this study we investigated the antihyperuricemic and nephroprotective potential of RA-3, a plant-derived lanosteryl triterpene. The antihyperuricemic and nephroprotective effect of RA-3 was investigated using the adenine and gentamicin induced hyperuricemic and nephrotoxicity rat model. Following the induction of hyperuricemia and nephrotoxicity, the experimental model rats (Sprague Dawley) were orally administered with RA-3 at 50 and 100 mg/kg body weight, respectively, daily for 14 days. Treatment of the experimental rats with RA-3, especially at 100 mg/kg, effectively lowered the serum renal dysfunction (blood urea nitrogen and creatinine) and hyperuricemic (uric acid and xanthine oxidase) biomarkers. These were accompanied by increased antioxidant status with decrease in malondialdehyde content. A much improved histomorphological structure of the kidney tissues was also observed in the triterpene treated groups when compared to the model control group. It is evident that RA-3 possesses the antihyperuricemic and nephroprotective properties, which could be vital for prevention and amelioration of kidney disease.

Keywords: RA-3; nephrotoxicity; triterpene; antioxidant; hyperuricemia

---

1. Introduction

The recent massive hike of kidney disease on the global rankings of disease burden signals public health crisis [1]. Kidney disease (nephropathy) is a product of multiple factors that inflict damage to nephron, renal parenchyma, and subsequent renal failure, if diagnosis and treatment are delayed [2]. Amongst various risk factors such as diabetes, hypertension, hyperuricemia, and infections, drug-induced nephrotoxicity is considered one of the significant contributors to both acute and chronic kidney disease [3]. This is attributable to increased exposure of the general population to a large number of prescribed and over-the-counter drugs as well as a variety of other ingested foodstuff and environmental intoxicants [4]. Hyperuricemia, a condition characterized by abnormally elevated uric acid levels in the blood, is considered an independent risk factor of kidney disease [5,6]. The underlying kidney damaging effects of uric acid are associated with tubular toxicity, vasoconstriction, oxidative stress, and inflammation [6,7].

Though nephropathy is harmful, with early diagnosis it is treatable to prevent end-stage renal failure. Depending on the underlying cause and stage of the injury, there are various drugs currently in clinical use against hyperuricemia and nephropathy. These drugs include captopril, allopurinol, and some diuretics (loop and thiazide). Despite efficacy of these drugs, they are also associated with some adverse reactions such as hypersensitivity syndrome, acute interstitial nephritis, and electrolyte imbalances [8,9]. The discovery of new nephroprotective drugs with improved safety profile and tolerance are encouraged. Since tissue damages are commonly prone to oxidative stress and excessive inflammatory response [10], new therapeutic drugs with strong antioxidant and anti-inflammatory activities would be preferred.

There is substantial evidence on potential role of various medicinal plants, as crude extracts or pure isolated compounds [2,11–13], in protecting the kidney from various insults thus, maintaining its integrity and functions. Even though methyl-3β-hydroxylanosta-9,24-dien-21-oate (RA-3), a lanosteryl triterpene from *Protorhus longifolia* (Bernh) Engl., has displayed significant various bioactivities such as antihyperlipidemic [14], antihyperglycemic [15], and cardioprotective [16] effects, its nephroprotective potential has not been reported. However, the triterpenes from this plant have previously exhibited lack of cytotoxic effects on human embryonic kidney cell lines [17]. To continue exploring potential significant bioactivities of this plant-derived bioactive compound, the current study investigated its antihyperuricemic and nephroprotective potential in adenine-gentamicin induced hyperuricemic and nephrotoxicity rat model. Adenine and gentamicin induced kidney damage is characterized by increased renal tubular cell death and increased blood urea nitrogen (BUN), creatinine (Cr), and uric acid (UA). All these parameters are commonly observed in human clinical subjects of nephropathy.

2. Results

2.1. Confirmation of the Isolated Lanosteryl Triterepene (RA-3)

RA-3 was routinely isolated and purified from the chloroform extract of *P. longifolia* stem bark using chromatographic techniques. The physical (white crystals, >95% pure, melting point 204–205 °C) and spectral data (IR (KBr) v_{max} = 3469, 1683 cm^{-1}, molecular formula $C_{31}H_{50}O_3$) of this compound were in agreement with previous reports from our laboratory [14,18]. The expected chemical structure of the compound was confirmed as methyl-3β-hydroxylanosta-9,24-dien-21-oate (Figure 1).

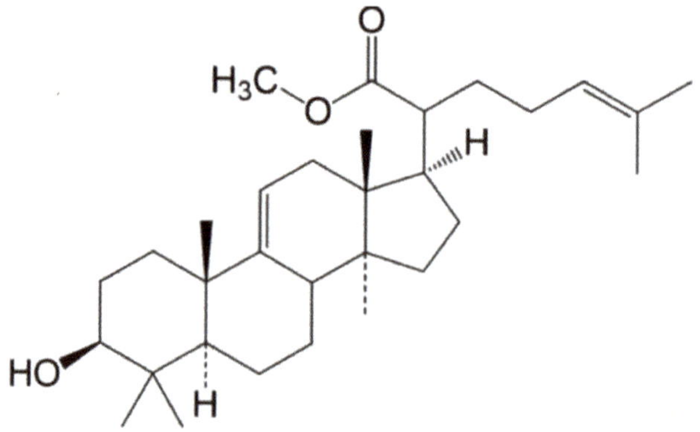

Figure 1. Methyl-3β-hydroxylanosta-9,24-dien-21-oate (RA-3), a lanosteryl triterpene from *P. longifolia*.

2.2. Body Weight Changes

Body weights of the rats were monitored for the duration of the study. A normal increase in body was observed in the normal. However, the model group showed a slow increase in body when compared to the normal rats. A slight difference in body weight increase was also observed in the RA-3 and allopurinol treated rats (Table 1).

Table 1. Body weight changes of the rats after 28 days of the experiment.

Group	Initial Body Weight (g)	Final Body Weight (g)	Body Weight Changes (g)
Normal	192.3 ± 9.33	215.0 ± 4.71	22.7 *
Model control	165.8 ± 14.06	176.9 ± 10.32	11.1
Allopurinol (10 mg/kg)	155.2 ± 21.68	173.1 ± 7.77	17.9 *
RA-3 (50 mg/kg)	179.1 ± 6.20	193.7 ± 15.49	14.6
RA-3 (100 mg/kg)	159.6 ± 10.18	176.8 ± 20.17	17.2

Data were expressed as mean ± SD ($n = 5$). * $p < 0.05$ vs. model control group.

2.3. Changes on Serum Levels of Some Renal Dysfunction Biomarkers

Changes in serum levels of some common renal dysfunction biomarkers were analyzed following treatment of the ailing rats with RA-3. Elevated levels of serum creatinine (Cr, 4.8 ± 1.78 mg/dL), angiotensin converting enzyme (ACE, 138.0 ± 39.61 U/L), and blood urea nitrogen (BUN, 22.5 ± 1.11 mg/dL), were observed in the model control group (MC). However, treatment of the rats with RA-3, especially at 100 mg/kg, effectively lowered these renal dysfunction biomarkers (Cr, 0.92 ± 0.23 mg/dL; ACE 75.5 ± 10.9 U/L; BUN 5.75 ± 0.29 mg/dL) near to the values of the normal control group (Figure 2). The results (Cr and BUN) obtained from RA-3 (100 mg/kg) treated groups were also comparable to the group treated with allopurinol.

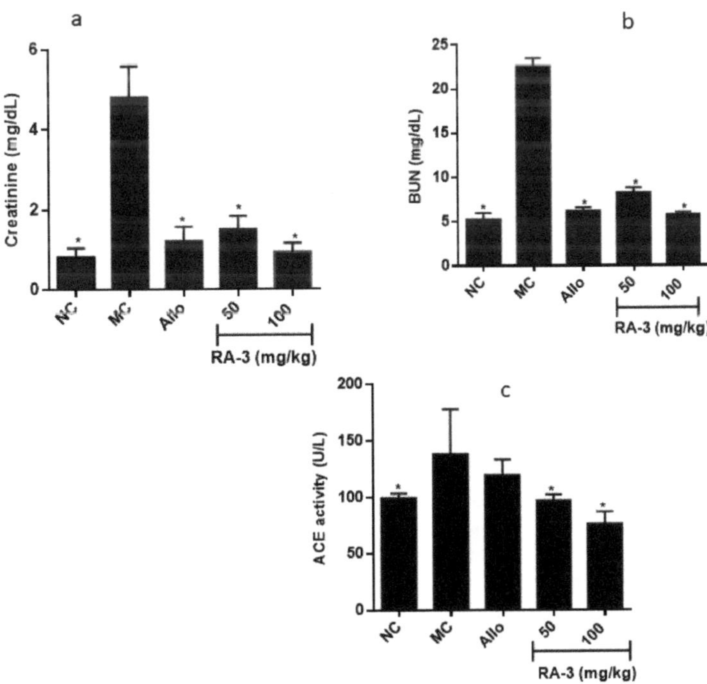

Figure 2. Effect of RA-3 on serum levels of creatinine (**a**), blood urea nitrogen (BUN) (**b**), and angiotensin converting enzyme (ACE) (**c**). Data were expressed as mean ± SD ($n = 5$), * $p < 0.05$ vs. MC group. NC—normal control, MC—model control, Allo—allopurinol.

2.4. Serum Levels of Xanthine Oxidase, Uric Acid and Interleukin-6

While higher serum levels of UA (0.61 ± 0.10 mg/dL), xanthine oxidase (XO, 1.48 ± 0.22 mU/mL), and interleukin-6 (IL-6, 0.71 ± 0.28 pg/mL) were observed in the model control group when compared to the normal control, RA-3, in a concentration dependent manner, significantly decreased the serum levels of UA (0.34 ± 0.08; 0.16 ± 0.02 mg/dL, $p < 0.01$) and XO (0.62 ± 0.12; 0.44 ± 0.08 mU/mL, $p < 0.05$). Though the difference was not significant, a relatively lower serum levels of IL-6 were also observed in the RA-3 treated groups when compared to the model control. Similar results were observed in the allopurinol (a known XO inhibitor and hypouricemic drug) treated group (Figure 3) in which a significant decrease in the serum levels of AU and XO were observed.

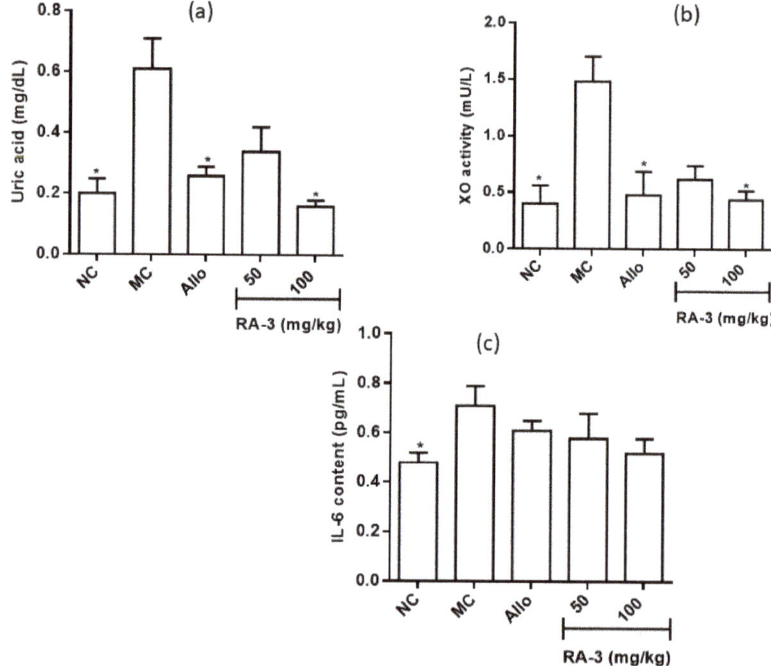

Figure 3. Effect of RA-3 on the serum levels of uric acid (**a**), xanthine oxidase (XO) (**b**) and interleukin-6 (IL-6) (**c**). Data were expressed as mean ± SD ($n = 5$), * $p < 0.05$ vs. MC group. NC—normal control, MC—model control, Allo—allopurinol.

2.5. Serum Biomarkers of Oxidative Stress

Decreased serum levels of superoxide dismutase (SOD) activity, reduced glutathione (GSH) content and thus total antioxidant status along with increased malondialdehyde (MDA) content were observed in the untreated group (model control) when compared to the normal, RA-3, and allopurinol treated groups (Table 2), an indication of oxidative stress. Nevertheless, treatment of the animals with RA-3 at both concentrations (50 and 100 mg/kg) improved the levels of the antioxidants while decreasing the MDA content.

Table 2. Effect of RA-3 on the serum levels of oxidative stress markers in the rats.

Group	GSH (nmol/mL)	SOD (Units/mL)	Total Antioxidant Status (mM)	MDA (nmol/µL)
Normal	0.91 ± 0.31 *	71 ± 0.14 *	1.94 ± 0.17 *	0.17 ± 0.06 *
Model control	0.22 ± 0.06	14.3 ± 0.06	0.34 ± 0.02	1.04 ± 0.03
Allopurinol (10 mg/kg)	1.20 ± 0.68 *	21.0 ± 0.03	1.00 ± 0.55	0.20 ± 0. 44 *
RA-3 (50 mg/kg)	0.74 ± 0.22	24. 7± 0.15 *	1.40 ± 0.40 *	0.16 ± 0.04 *
RA-3 (100 mg/kg)	0.80 ± 0.18 *	55.0 ± 0.17 *	1.87 ± 0.20 *	0.14 ± 0.02 *

Data were expressed as mean ± SD ($n = 5$). * $p < 0.05$ vs. model control group.

2.6. Histological Analysis of the Kidney Tissues

The results of histological analysis are presented in Figure 4. The sections of kidneys from the normal group showed a normal architecture with intact glomerulus and renal tubules. A marked damage to the kidney indicated by robust display of glomerular congestion, dilated renal tubules and epithelial degeneration was observed on the kidney sections from the model control group. However, kidney sections from the rats treated with RA-3, especially at 100 mg/kg showed a much improved histomorphological structure of the kidney (Figure 4v), characterized by minimal renal tubular dilation and necrosis, indicative of recovery.

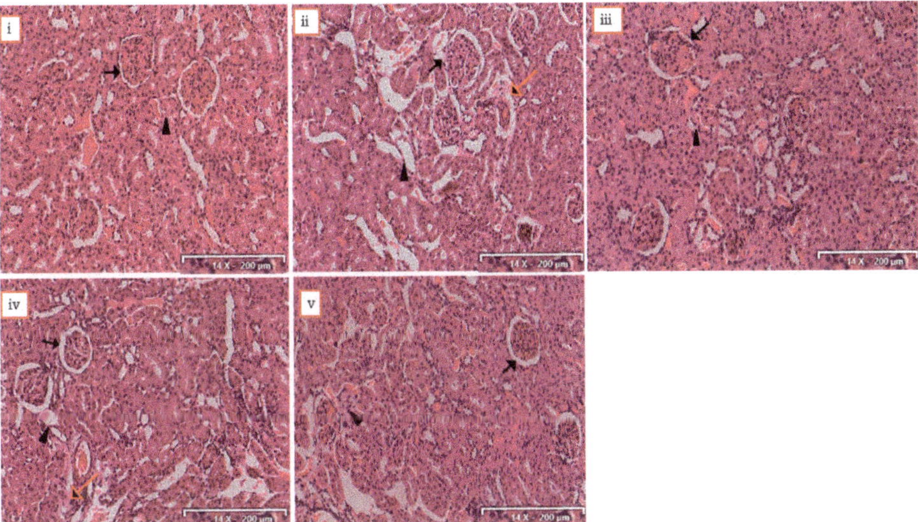

Figure 4. Photomicrographs of the kidney sections of the rats. (**i**) Section of kidney from normal group, showing normal kidney architecture with intact glomerulus (black arrow) and renal tubules (black triangle); (**ii**) section from model control group, showing glomerular congestion, dilated renal tubules, and epithelial degeneration (red arrow), (**iii**) section from group treated with allopurinol, showing minimal improved renal architecture; (**iv**) section from group treated with RA-3 (50 mg/kg), showing regeneration of epithelium, (**v**) section from group treated with RA-3 (100 mg/kg), showing improved renal architecture characterized by epithelial regeneration and reduced glomerular congestion. The indicator size for each image is 14X-200 μm (H&E).

3. Discussion

Considering the global health threat posed by kidney disease burden, a search for new nephroprotective drugs from our local flora could prove a powerful strategy to respond to this health threat. Potential of plant-derived triterpenes as new nephroprotective agents has been demonstrated using various animal models [13,19].

This study investigated the antihyperuricemic and nephroprotective potential of RA-3, a lanosteryl triterpene from *P. longifolia*. The increased serum levels of these biomarkers along with a robust display of glomerular congestion and epithelial degeneration in the kidney samples from the MC group confirmed the induction of hyperuricemia and nephrotoxicity in the rats. It was interesting to observe the significant decrease in serum levels of these biomarkers (UA, BUN, Cr) with improved histomorphology of the kidney tissues from the rats treated with RA-3 at both concentrations. The results served as an indication of the hypouricemic and nephroprotective potential of the triterpene. Substantial experimental evidence has also demonstrated the significant nephroprotective properties of some other plant-derived triterpenes [13,19,20].

While renal toxicity of gentamicin is strongly linked to oxidative stress [3], adenine's toxicity is associated with renal tubular obstruction and hyperuricemic effect [21]. Hyperuricemia is considered an independent risk factor of kidney disease [5]. Blood UA levels are physiologically regulated by XO activity, an enzyme that catalyzes the formation of UA from xanthine. The XO catalyzed reaction also generates reactive oxygen species (ROS) which can trigger inflammatory reactions and consequent tissue damage [22]. The reduced serum levels of UA along with decreased XO activity in the triterpene treated groups supported the antihyperuricemic effect of RA-3. These observations were also similar to those of the group treated with allopurinol, a standard hyporuricemic drug. Experimental evidence has shown that antihyperuricemic compounds do possess nephroprotective effect [19,23].

Hyperuricemia is known to cause, among others, vascular smooth muscle cell proliferation, endothelial dysfunction, and increased IL-6 synthesis, all of which may contribute to the progression of chronic kidney disease [9]. Though there was no significant difference between the model control and the treated nephrotoxic groups, the relatively lower serum levels of IL-6 in the RA-3 and allopurinol treated groups were observed. This could further be correlated with the suppressed XO activity in these groups. Since XO activity is known to trigger inflammatory reactions and consequent tissue damage [22], the observed results further indicated the tissue protective potential of the triterpene.

It has further been demonstrated that even mild elevations in serum UA can cause hypertension and renal microvascular disease without causing urate crystal deposition in kidneys [24]. The hypertensive effect of elevated serum UA has been associated with activation of the renin-angiotensin system (RAS) [7]. The vasoconstrictive effect of RAS is mediated by ACE, an enzyme that catalyzes conversion of angiotensin I to a bioactive angiotensin II. The observed lower ACE activity in the lanosteryl triterpene treated groups further suggests the potential role of RA-3 in management of hypertension, another important risk factor of nephropathy [25]. The role of ACE inhibitors in prevention of renal function deterioration is well-established [26,27]. The hypouricemic effect exhibited by RA-3 may also be vital in the prevention of other ailments known to be associated with hyperuricemia [28–30].

Furthermore, despite the ROS-mediated renal toxicity of gentamicin and adenine, the improved serum total antioxidant status, GSH and SOD along with reduced MDA content in the rats treated with RA-3 indicated its tissue protective potential against oxidative damage. It is interesting to note from these results that the ability of RA-3 to enhance endogenous antioxidant defense while inhibiting lipid peroxidation has previously been demonstrated in streptozotocin (STZ)-induced diabetes and isoproterenol (ISO)-induced myocardial injury in rat models [15,16]. It is also worth noting that similar to gentamicin induced renal tubular toxicity, the necrotic toxicity of STZ and ISO are also associated with oxidative stress [31,32]. Since inflammation and oxidative tissue damage are common culprits in various pathophysiologies including nephropathy, nephroprotective drugs with both anti-inflammatory and antioxidant properties are highly desired. The nephroprotective potential of most medicinal plant extracts and their derived compounds has been associated with their antioxidant and anti-inflammatory activities [11,33].

4. Materials and Methods

4.1. Reagents

Glutathione assay kit (catalog number: CS0260), xanthine oxidase assay kit (catalog number: MAK078), superoxide dismutase assay kit (catalog number: 19160), antioxidant assay status kit (catalog number: CS0790), malondialdehyde assay kit (catalog number: MAK085), rat interleukin-6 assay kit (catalog number: RAB0333). All the commercial assay kits used were purchased from Sigma Aldrich (St. Louis, MO, USA)

4.2. Plant Extraction and Isolation of the Lanosteryl Triterpene (RA-3)

Plant extract was prepared from stem bark of *P. longifolia* collected from KwaHlabisa, KwaZulu-Natal, South Africa. The plant material (voucher specimen number RA01UZ) was identified and confirmed by Dr. NR Ntuli from Botany Department, University of Zululand. The targeted compound (RA-3) was routinely isolated and purified from the chloroform extract using the method well established in our laboratory [18]. The lanosteryl triterpene was isolated over silica gel chromatography and the pure compound was recrystallized in 100% ethyl acetate. Melting point and spectroscopic data analysis were used, in comparison with literature data [14,18], to confirm chemical structure of the isolated pure (>95%) lanosteryl triterpene.

4.3. Animals

The University of Zululand Research Ethics Committee (UZREC) granted ethical clearance (UZREC 171110-030 PGM 2016/321) for use of laboratory animals (Sprague Dawley rats). Sprague Dawley rats ($n = 30$) were collected from the animal unit of the Department of Biochemistry, University of Zululand. The animals were housed in standard cages (maximum of four rats per cage) and maintained at room temperature (23–25 °C; relative humidity ~50%) with a 12:12-h light/dark cycle as per stipulated national guidelines for the care and use of animals. All the rats were in good state of health and were allowed to acclimatize to the experimental set-up for a week before the experiment was conducted. Unless stated otherwise, all the animals had free access to drinking water and normal rat feed throughout the experimental period.

4.4. Preparation of RA-3 Solution

Fresh working solutions of RA-3 (50 and 100 mg/kg body weight) were prepared in 2% Tween 20. These concentrations were based on our previous studies on the compound [14–16].

4.5. Investigation of the Antihyperuricemic and Nephroprotective Potential of RA-3

The adenine and gentamicin induced hyperuricemia and nephrotoxicity rat model, slightly modified from that described by Meng et al. [34] was used to evaluate the antihyperuricemic and nephroprotective effect of the triterpene (RA-3). Sprague Dawley rats of either sex (150–200 g) were randomly divided into two major groups; normal and model groups. The rats in the model group were orally administered with adenine (150 mg/kg body weight) and intraperitoneally injected with gentamicin (40 mg/kg body weight) daily for fourteen days to induce hyperuricemia and nephrotoxicity.

Following induction of nephrotoxicity, the animals in the model group were randomly divided into four groups (II-V) of at least five rats per group ($n = 5$). The normal control (I) and model control (II) groups received drinking water and 2% Tween 20 (vehicle, p.o), respectively, throughout the experimental period. While the positive control group (III) received allopurinol (10 mg/kg, body weight, p.o), the experimental groups IV and V were orally administered with RA-3 at 50 and 100 mg/kg, respectively. The respective drugs were administered daily for a further fourteen days period. All drug administrations were performed between 8:00 and 9:00 AM and the animals were treated in the same order throughout the experimental period. At the end of the experimental period, the rats were fasted for eight hours and euthanized under anesthesia (Pentobarbital at 30 mg/kg body weight, ip). A complete loss of sensation was confirmed by pedal withdrawal reflex before any procedure could be conducted on the rats. The rats were quickly dissected, blood and kidney samples were immediately collected. The collected tissues samples were used for estimation of some biochemical parameters and histopathological indications, respectively.

4.5.1. Biochemical Analysis

The collected blood samples were separately allowed to clot and centrifuged at 1200 rpm for 10 min. Serum was collected and used for estimation of some selected biochemical parameters. The serum levels of total antioxidant status, GSH, SOD, XO, and MDA were estimated using commercial activity assay kits (Sigma Aldrich, St. Louis, MO, USA). The total antioxidant status assay kit non-specifically measures the total concentration of the antioxidant molecules (small molecules and proteins) in a biological sample (serum, cell and tissue lysate etc.). The serum IL-6 content was measured with ELISA kit (Sigma Aldrich, St. Louis, MO, USA). Standard laboratory procedures (Global Clinical & Viral Laboratory, Kwazulu Natal, South Africa) were followed to estimate the serum levels of Cr, UA, ACE, and BUN.

4.5.2. Histological Analysis of Kidney Tissues

Kidney tissues, preserved in 10% neutral buffered formalin, were embedded in paraffin and sectioned according to standard procedures. The sectioned tissues were subjected to Hematoxylin and Eosin staining for routine histopathological examination (Department of Physiology Department, University of KwaZulu-Natal, Kwazulu Natal, South Africa).

4.6. Data Analysis

Data were expressed as mean ± standard deviation (SD) of the mean. The results were analyzed by Kruskal-Wallis test followed by Dunn's post hoc multiple comparison test using GraphPad Prism software (version 6). The statistical differences were considered significant at $p < 0.05$.

5. Conclusions

The results of the current study have indicated and confirmed the antihyperuricemic and nephroprotective potential of RA-3. The ACE inhibitory effect and hypouricemic potential displayed by the triterpene are not only crucial in renal protection, but in other related complications such as cardiovascular disease, hypertension and gout arthritis as well. Investigation of the molecular basis of its nephroprotective potential will provide an insight into the triterpene's therapeutic mechanism.

Author Contributions: Investigation, analysis, and writing—original draft preparation, N.B.H.; spectral analysis and confirmation of structure, O.A.L.; data analysis and manuscript editing, F.O.O., T.G.D.-D.; conceptualization, methodology, supervision, and manuscript editing, A.R.O., R.A.M. All authors have read and agreed to the published version of the manuscript.

Funding: This research received no external funding. The work was supported by the University of Zululand Research and Innovation Department (S956/16). The APC was funded by the University of Zululand.

Acknowledgments: The authors are grateful to N.R. Ntuli for confirmation of the plant material, Z. Yuroukova (Ex Officio, St Ekaterina Hospital, Department of Pathology, Medical University, Sofia, Bulgaria) for her expertise in histological analysis of the photomicrographs of the kidney sections, and the South African National Research Foundation (SA-NRF) for the scholarship awarded to N.B.H.

Conflicts of Interest: The authors declare no conflict of interest.

References

1. Wang, H.; Naghavi, M.; Allen, C.; Barber, R.M.; Bhutta, Z.A.; Carter, A.; Casey, D.C.; Charlson, F.J.; Chen, A.Z.; Coates, M.M.; et al. Global, regional, and national life expectancy, all-cause mortality, and cause-specific mortality for 249 causes of death, 1980–2015: A systematic analysis for the Global Burden of Disease Study 2015. *Lancet* **2016**, *388*, 1459–1544. [CrossRef]

2. Gong, Q.; He, L.L.; Wang, M.L.; Ouyang, H.; Gao, H.W.; Feng, Y.L.; Yang, S.L.; Du, L.J.; Li, J.; Luo, Y.Y. Anemoside B4 protects rat kidney from adenine-induced injury by attenuating inflammation and fibrosis and enhancing podocin and nephrin expression. *Evid. Based Complement. Alternat. Med.* **2019**. [CrossRef] [PubMed]

3. Siddama, A.; Suneel, I.M. Drug induced kidney disease. *Open Acc. J. Toxicol.* **2017**. [CrossRef]

4. Dhodi, D.K.; Bhagat, S.B.; Pathak, D.; Patel, S.B. Drug-induced nephrotoxicity. *Int. J. Basic. Clin. Pharmacol.* **2014**, *3*, 591–597. [CrossRef]

5. Franklin, B.S.; Mangan, M.S.; Latz, E. Crystal formation in inflammation. *Annu. Rev. Immunol.* **2016**, *34*, 173–202. [CrossRef] [PubMed]

6. Xu, X.; Hu, J.; Song, N.; Chen, R.; Zhang, T.; Ding, X. Hyperuricemia increases the risk of acute kidney injury: A systematic review and meta-analysis. *BMC Nephrol.* **2017**, *18*, 27. [CrossRef]

7. Hahn, K.; Kanbay, M.; Lanaspa, M.A.; Johnson, R.J.; Ejazd, A.A. Serum uric acid and acute kidney injury: A mini review. *J. Adv. Res.* **2017**, *8*, 529–536. [CrossRef]

8. Shah, P.B.; Soundararajan, P.; Sathiyasekaran, B.W.C.; Sanjeev, C.; Hegde, S.C. Diuretics for people with chronic kidney disease. *Cochrane Database Syst. Rev.* **2014**, *2014*. [CrossRef]

9. Kim, S.; Kim, H.J.; Ahn, H.S.; Oh, S.W.; Han, K.H.; Um, T.H.; Cho, C.R.; Han, S.Y. Renoprotective effects of febuxostat compared with allopurinol in patients with hyperuricemia. A systematic review and meta analysis. *Kidney Res. Clin. Pract.* **2017**, *36*, 274–281. [CrossRef]

10. Tucker, P.S.; Scanlan, A.T.; Dalbo, V.J. Chronic kidney disease influences multiple systems: Describing the relationship between oxidative stress, inflammation, kidney damage, and concomitant disease. *Oxid. Med. Cell Longev.* **2015**, *2015*, 806358. [CrossRef]

11. Torres-González, L.; Cienfuegos-Pecina, E.; Perales-Quintana, M.M.; Alarcon-Galvan, G.; Muñoz-Espinosa, L.E.; Pérez-Rodríguez, E.; Cordero-Pérez, P. Nephroprotective effect of *Sonchus oleraceus* extract against kidney injury induced by ischemia-reperfusion in Wistar Rats. *Oxid. Med. Cell Longev.* **2018**, *2018*, 9572803. [CrossRef] [PubMed]

12. Chinnappan, S.M.; George, A.; Thaggikuppe, P.; Choudhary, Y.K.; Choudhai, V.K.; Ramani, Y.; Dewangan, R. Nephroprotective effect of herbal extract *Eurycoma longifolia* on paracetamol-induced nephrotoxicity in rats. *Evid. Based Complement Alternat. Med.* **2019**, *2019*, 4916519. [CrossRef]

13. Lee, S.; Jung, K.; Lee, D.; Lee, S.R.; Lee, K.R.; Kang, K.S.; Kim, K.H. Protective effect and mechanism of action of lupane triterpenes from *Cornus walteri* in cisplatin-induced nephrotoxicity. *Bioorg. Med. Chem. Lett.* **2015**, *25*, 5613–5618. [CrossRef] [PubMed]

14. Machaba, K.E.; Cobongela, S.Z.Z.; Mosa, R.A.; Lawal, O.A.; Djarova, T.G.; Opoku, A.R. In vivo anti-hyperlipidemic activity of the triterpene from the stem bark of *Protorhus longifolia* (Benrh) Engl. *Lipids Health Dis.* **2014**. [CrossRef] [PubMed]

15. Mabhida, S.E.; Mosa, R.A.; Penduka, D.; Osunsanmi, F.O.; Dludla, P.V.; Djarova, T.G.; Opoku, A.R. A lanosteryl triterpene from *Protorhus longifolia* improves glucose tolerance and pancreatic beta cell ultrastructure in type 2 diabetic rats. *Molecules* **2017**, 1252. [CrossRef]

16. Mosa, R.A.; Hlophe, N.B.; Ngema, N.T.; Dambudzo, P.; Lawal, O.A.; Opoku, A.R. Cardioprotective potential of a lanosteryl triterpene from *Protorhus longifolia*. *Pharm. Biol.* **2016**, *54*, 3244–3248. [CrossRef] [PubMed]

17. Mosa, R.A.; Oyedeji, O.A.; Shode, F.O.; Singh, M.; Opoku, A.R. Triterpenes from the stem bark of *Protorhus longifolia* exhibit anti-platelet aggregation activity. *Afri. J. Pharm. Pharmacol.* **2011**, *5*, 2698–2714.

18. Mosa, R.A.; Naidoo, J.J.; Nkomo, F.S.; Mazibuko, S.E.; Muller, C.J.; Opoku, A.R. In vitro antihyperlipidemic potential of triterpenes from stem bark of *Protorhus longifolia*. *Planta Med.* **2014**, *80*, 1685–1691. [CrossRef]

19. Prakash, B.; Surendran, A.; Chandraprabha, V.R.; Pettamanna, A.; Nair, H.N.R. Betulinic acid, natural pentacyclic triterpenoid prevents arsenic-induced nephrotoxicity in male Wistar rats. *Comp. Clin. Path.* **2018**, *27*, 37–44. [CrossRef]

20. Pai, P.G.; Nawarathna, S.C.; Kulkarni, A.; Habeeba, U.; Reddy, S.C.; Teerthanath, S.; Shenoy, J.P. Nephroprotective effect of ursolic acid in a murine model of gentamicin-induced renal damage. *Int. Sch. Res. Not.* **2012**, *2012*, 410902. [CrossRef]

21. Nomura, J.; Busso, N.; Ives, A.; Tsujimoto, S.; Tamura, M.; So, A.; Yamanaka, Y. Febuxostat, an inhibitor of xanthine oxidase, suppresses lipopolysaccharide-induced MCP-1 production via MAPK phosphatase-1-mediated inactivation of JNK. *PLoS ONE* **2013**, *8*, e75527. [CrossRef] [PubMed]

22. Xu, W.H.; Wang, H.; Sun, Y.; Xue, Z.; Liang, M.; Su, W. Antihyperuricemic and nephroprotective effects of extracts from *Orthosiphon stamineus* in hyperuricemic mice. *J. Pharm. Pharmacol.* **2020**, *72*, 551–560. [CrossRef]

23. Isaka, Y.; Takabatake, Y.; Takahashi, A.; Saitoh, T.; Yoshimo, T. Hyperuricemia-induced inflammasome and kidney diseases. *Nephrol. Dial. Transpl.* **2016**, *31*, 890–896. [CrossRef]

24. Kang, D.H.; Nakagawa, T.; Feng, L.; Watanabe, S.; Han, L.; Mazzali, M.; Truong, L.; Harris, R.; Johnson, R.J. A role for uric acid in the progression of renal disease. *J. Am. Soc. Nephrol.* **2002**, *13*, 2888–2897. [CrossRef]

25. Nwankwo, E.A.; Wudiri, W.W.; Akinsola, A. Risk factors for the development of chronic kidney disease among Nigerians with essential hypertension. *J. Med. Sci.* **2007**, *7*, 579–584.

26. Orth, S.; Nowicki, M.; Wiecek, A.; Ritz, E. Nephroprotective effect of ACE inhibitors. *Drugs* **1993**, *46*, 189–196. [CrossRef] [PubMed]

27. Hsu, F.Y.; Lin, F.J.; Ou, H.T.; Huang, S.H.; Wang, C.C. Renoprotective effect of angiotensin-converting enzyme inhibitors and angiotensin II receptor blockers in diabetic patients with proteinuria. *Kidney Blood Press. Res.* **2017**, *42*, 358–368. [CrossRef] [PubMed]

28. Kivity, S.; Kopel, E.; Maor, E. Association of serum uric acid and cardiovascular disease in healthy adults. *Am. J. Cardiol.* **2013**, *111*, 1146–1151. [CrossRef] [PubMed]

29. Giordano, C.; Karasik, O.; King-Morris, K.; Asmar, A. Uric acid as a marker of kidney disease: Review of the current literature. *Dis. Markers* **2015**, *2015*, 382918. [CrossRef]

30. Nile, S.H.; Ko, E.Y.; Kim, D.H.; Keum, Y.S. Screening of ferulic acid related compounds as inhibitors of xanthine oxidase and cyclooxygenase-2 with anti-inflammatory activity. *Rev. Bras. Farmacogn.* **2016**, *26*, 50–55. [CrossRef]

31. Al Nahdi, A.M.T.; John, A.; Haider Raza, H. Elucidation of molecular mechanisms of streptozotocin-induced oxidative stress, apoptosis, and mitochondrial dysfunction in Rin-5F pancreatic β-cells. *Oxid. Med. Cell Longev.* **2017**, *2017*, 7054272. [CrossRef] [PubMed]

32. Kumar, H.S.; Anandan, R.; Devaki, T.; Kumar, M.S. Cardioprotective effects of *Picrorrhiza kurroa* against isoproterenol-induced myocardial stress in rats. *Fitoterapia* **2001**, *72*, 402–405. [CrossRef]

33. Ojha, S.; Venkataraman, B.; Kurdi, A.; Mahgoub, E.; Sadek, B.; Mohanraj Rajesh, M. Plant-derived agents for counteracting cisplatin-induced nephrotoxicity. *Oxid. Med. Cell Longev.* **2016**, *2016*, 4320374. [CrossRef] [PubMed]

34. Meng, Z.; Yan, Y.; Tang, Z.; Guo, C.; Li, N.; Huang, W.; Ding, G.; Wang, Z.; Xiao, W.; Yang, Z. Anti-hyperuricemic and nephroprotective effects of Rhein in hyperuricemic mice. *Planta Med.* **2015**, *81*, 279–285. [CrossRef] [PubMed]

Sample Availability: Sample of the compound is available from the authors.

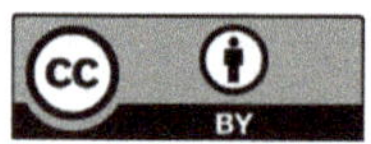

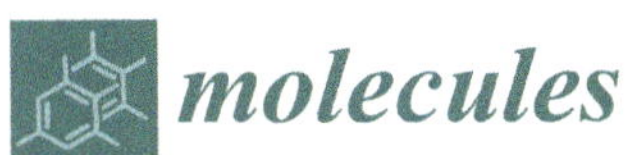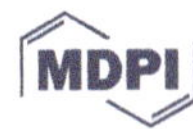

Article

New Sustainable Process for Hesperidin Isolation and Anti-Ageing Effects of Hesperidin Nanocrystals

Danijela Stanisic [1], Leticia H. B. Liu [1], Roney V. dos Santos [1], Amanda F. Costa [1], Nelson Durán [2,3] and Ljubica Tasic [1,*]

1. Biological Chemistry Laboratory, Organic Chemistry Department, Institute of Chemistry, University of Campinas (UNICAMP), Campinas 13083-970, SP, Brazil; dacici.stanisic@gmail.com (D.S.); leticia.bacellar@gmail.com (L.H.B.L.); torroney@gmail.com (R.V.d.S.); amanda.fc92@gmail.com (A.F.C.)
2. Laboratory of Urogenital Carcinogenesis and Immunotherapy, Department of Structural and Functional Biology, University of Campinas, Campinas 13083-862, SP, Brazil; nelsonduran1942@gmail.com
3. Nanomedicine Research Unit (Nanomed), Federal University of ABC (UFABC), Santo André 09210-580, SP, Brazil
* Correspondence: ljubica@unicamp.br; Tel.: +55-19-3521-1106

Academic Editor: Federica Pellati
Received: 31 August 2020; Accepted: 28 September 2020; Published: 3 October 2020

Abstract: Hesperidin, a secondary orange (*Citrus sinensis*) metabolite, was extracted from orange bagasse. No organic solvents or additional energy consumption were used in the clean and sustainable process. Hesperidin purity was approximately 98% and had a yield of 1%. Hesperidin is a known supplement due to antioxidant, chelating, and anti-ageing properties. Herein, hesperidin application to eliminate dark eye circles, which are sensitive and thin skin regions, was studied. In addition, the proposed method for its aqueous extraction was especially important for human consumption. Further, the most effective methods for hesperidin nanonization were explored, after which the nanoemulsions were incorporated into a cream formulation that was formulated for a tropical climate. Silky cream formulations (oil in water) were tested in vitro on artificial 3D skin from cultured cells extracted from skin residues after plastic surgery. The proposed in vitro assay avoided tests of the different formulations in human volunteers and animals. It was shown that one of the nanonized hesperidin formulations was the most skin-friendly and might be used in cosmetics.

Keywords: hesperidin; new-clean process extraction; nanocrystals; antioxidant; anti-ageing

---

1. Introduction

Hesperidin (HSD) is a secondary plant metabolite and one of the principal bioflavonoids of citrus fruits. This flavanone and its aglycone form, hesperetin (HST), are present in relatively high quantities (1–2%), especially in sweet immature oranges (*Citrus sinensis*) [1,2]. HSD is known for valuable bioactivity and can act as an antioxidant [3–10], anti-inflammatory [3,9,10], hypolipidemic [8], vasoprotective [3,4,8,11], and anticancerogenic [3,9] agent. The great majority of flavanones are glycosylated mainly with rutinose and neohesperidose [1,12]. HSD (Figure 1) is proposed, after different in vitro studies, as a plant defense molecule and a potent antioxidant [7,13]. It is water soluble just at high pH, dimethyl sulfoxide, and pyridine, giving yellow and clear solutions. HSD is partially soluble in methanol and glacial acetic acid, and almost insoluble in acetone, chloroform, and benzene [12,14].

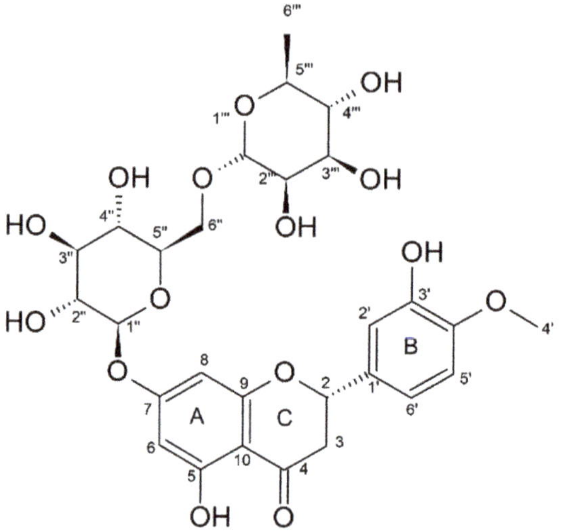

Figure 1. Chemical structure of hesperidin (2*S*)-5-hydroxy-2-(3-hydroxy-4-methoxyphenyl)-7-[(2*S*,3*R*, 4*S*,5*S*,6*R*)-3,4,5-trihydroxy-6-[[(2*R*,3*R*,4*R*,5*R*,6*S*)-3,4,5-trihydroxy-6-methyloxan-2-yl]oxymethyl]oxan-2-yl]oxy-2,3-dihydrochromen-4-one). HSD carbon atoms are numbered, and A–C rings are shown.

1.1. Antioxidant Activity of Hesperidin

Bioflavonoids have been known for a long time because of their noticeable antioxidant potential that mitigates the harmful impact of free radical and reactive oxygen species. Hydroxyl, alkoxyl, peroxyl, and peroxyl nitrite radicals induce ageing, tissue damage, and contribute to many disease developments like cancer, hypertension, atherosclerosis, amyloidosis, and senile dementia. Nevertheless, the cited free radicals are produced in everyday life and neutralized as well by enzymes [1]; with ageing and increased radical production, their nocive effects are enlarged and become far more potent. The radical scavenging property inherent to natural bioflavonoids is related to their structure and in HSD, hydroxyl groups at positions 3′- and 5- demonstrate mild antioxidant activities [15,16]. Hesperetin (HST) has an additional hydroxyl group (7-), thus showing a stronger antioxidant activity compared to HSD. Disaccharide in the HSD structure affects its capacity for electronic delocalization and decreases its antioxidant activity [6]. For example, HSD nano-loaded lipid carrier showed antioxidant effects in concentrations of 45 µM in 2,2-diphenyl-1-picrylhydrazyl (DPPH) assay, and without any toxic effects on several cell lines [17].

1.2. Hesperidin and Hesperetin Use in Cosmetics as Anti-Ageing Active Components

Hesperidin and hesperetin are the foci of intensive research for topical application. For example, sulfonated, acetylated, or phosphorylated HSD derivatives are potent inhibitors of hyaluronidase. Moreover, HSD can also act on superoxide in electron transfer as well as proton transfer in vivo. HSD might act as a topical UV-protective agent, by protecting phosphatidylcholine liposomes from UV irradiation-induced peroxidation. The neohesperidin, for example, demonstrates the capacity to extend yeast's chronical lifespan, individually or in synergism with the HST, for 10 different aging factors, such as scavenging ROS effects, regulation of stress-related enzymes, and maintaining pH cellular value, favorable for life extension of yeast cells [18]. Hesperidin was also proved as a potent anti-photoageing factor, through regulation of metalloproteinases MMP-9 via mitogen activation protein kinase (MAPK) signaling pathways. In the same study, Lee and colleagues [19] approved the positive effect of the hesperidin on wrinkle depth on a mouse dorsal skin model, and reduction in UVB-induced hydration changes and trans-epidermal water loss [20]. Different studies demonstrate accelerated cutaneous diabetic or venous wounds healing and ameliorate skin epidermal barrier function already after 7 days of HSD application [20]. On the other side, HST was found to penetrate through the *stratum corneum* [5] and assays conducted in vitro showed that the presence of lecithin and d-limonene in formulations may aid towards faster hesperetin penetration into the skin [21]. Additionally, in vitro studies of the *stratum corneum* have demonstrated that flavonoids show differences in penetration capacities, which depend in a large part on the ingredients/vehicles present in the formulation. Therefore, the penetration rate of flavonoids, such as catechin, rutin, quercetin, and others, is influenced by moisturizing ingredients (glycerol, glycols, polyglycols, ethoxylated methyl glucoside, and urea) and by the type of cosmetic formulation (hydrogel, emulsion, microemulsion, and micellar system) [6]. For example, the water in oil microemulsion formulations significantly enhances quercetin skin penetration up to 12 h after application [22–24]. HSD-loaded nanostructured lipid vehicles show burst release in the beginning and further sustained bioflavonoid release from the lipid nanocarrier [17]. Despite their interesting and beneficial skin effects, bioflavonoids are very demanding for making effective formulations. In addition, their insolubility in water complicates their use in cosmetic products and influences greatly on their extraction from fruits and plants that is usually performed by the use of organic solvents.

Many different protocols are described and used for the extraction of hesperidin from various starting materials, including maceration [12,25–27], Soxhlet extraction [26,28], assisted extraction with ultrasound [25], high hydrostatic pressure and microwave assisted extraction [29,30], enzymatic process [14], and supercritical fluids extraction [31]. All the aforementioned extraction methods require the use of organic solvents, energy, and/or high-pressure, which makes those processes unfavorable for an ecologically clean way of treating orange peel. Herein, a new and green method, without using organic solvents and with low energy consumption, was implemented for the extraction of hesperidin from fresh orange bagasse. Hesperidin extracted in this manner is safe to use and biocompatible for topical application.

2. Results

2.1. Yield of Hesperidin Extracted from Humid Orange Peel—Green Method

The obtained hesperidin was pale yellow amorphous powder (Supplementary Information Figure S1). The yield of HSD extracted in this manner was ~1.2% calculated per dry orange peel bagasse. The same method was repeated varying calcium(II) chloride solution concentrations—5% and 10%—but HSD yields were significantly lower when compared to one obtained with 7.5% calcium(II) chloride solution. In addition, the color of the solution with 7.5% calcium(II) chloride was much darker than obtained with the other two solutions (Figure S1, Supplementary Information). In the case of 5%, there are not enough calcium(II) ions to react the pectin and disrupt interaction of HSD with the macromolecule, and in the case of 10% of the solution, calcium(II) interactions with HSD are due to their ability to chelate metal ions.

2.2. Spectral Data and Characterization of Obtained HSD

The chemical structure and purity of the obtained HSD were analyzed applying High-field Nuclear Magnetic Resonance (NMR) (Supplementary Information Figures S2 and S3), Fourier Transform-Infrared (FT-IR) spectroscopy and Ultra High-Performance Liquid Chromatography (UPLC, Supplementary Information Figure S3) techniques. All HSD NMR peak assignments of proton and carbon signals were in accordance with the literature [32]. From the ^{1}H NMR spectrum of the obtained HSD, typical flavanone structure signals could be assigned at δ 12.02 (1H, s, 5-OH) and δ 9.09 (1H), which originate from two hydroxyl groups attached to an aromatic ring, further δ 5.51 (1H, dd, J = 12.1, 3.3 Hz, H-2), from protons of the 1,3,4-trisubstitued ring at δ 6.91 (3H, m), protons of rhamnose and glucose at δ 4.98 (1H, d, J = 7.3 Hz) and 4.53 (H, m), one methoxy group peak at δ 3.80 (3H, s), and one methyl group peak at δ 1.09 (4H, d, J = 6.2 Hz). The acquired Heteronuclear Single Quantum Coherence (HSQC) spectra (Figure S2) and Heteronuclear Multiple Bond Coherence (HMBC) spectra (Figure S3) of the extracted HSD were used to confirm its structure. HSD was monitored by UV maximum at 284 nm, caused by the conjugation of the keto group and the other oxygen atoms with the aromatic ring systems. HSD purity was determined utilizing Ultra High-Performance Liquid chromatography (UHPLC) with the reverse stationary phase (C18, length 10 cm, 5 µm). HSD analytical standard (Sigma-Aldrich, 97% of purity) was used for calibration curve construction from the injection of aliquots of 1, 2, 4, 6, 8, and 10 µL of standard HSD solution in methanol (concentration 100 ppm). Calibration curves and the analysis of the sample from the extraction were performed in triplicate. A solution of 100 ppm of HSD in methanol (HPLC grade of purity) was analyzed in UHPLC as to obtain the area of the peak and to determine the relative concentration of HSD, comparing to the Sigma-Aldrich standard of HSD with grade purity > 97%. The peak with the retention time of 6.877 min was assigned to HSD (Figure S3) as the same procedure was done with the standard for HSD (>97%, Sigma-Aldrich). The determined purity was 97.2%, m/m, when compared to the Sigma-Aldrich analytical standard (> 97%). Therefore, the applied extraction process was adequate and a high HSD yield was achieved, while purity of the extracted HSD was high. It was observed that low impurities coming from naringin were present (Supplementary Information Figures S2–S4).

2.3. Chelation Properties of Hesperidin

Hesperidin and copper(II) acetate were dissolved in methanol and mixed to obtain hesperidin-copper complex. Likewise, with other compounds with a similar structure, HSD possesses chelation potential when it is mixed with metal(II) ions [33]. Figure 2 presents the FT-IR spectra of hesperidin, copper(II) acetate, and hesperidin–copper complex.

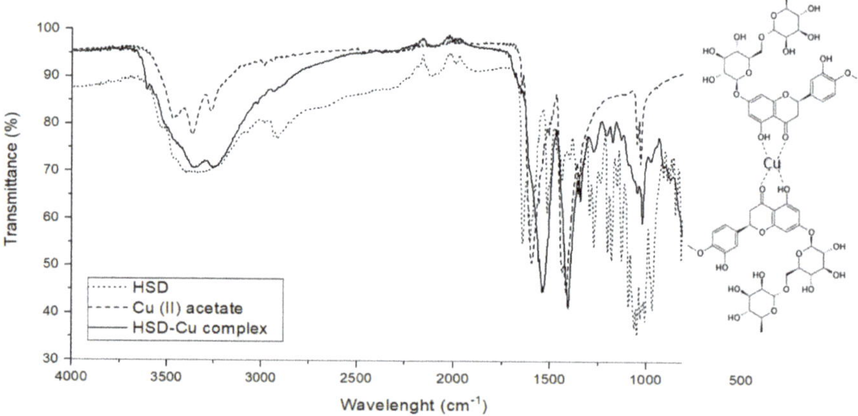

Figure 2. Fourier transform infrared (FT-IR) spectra of hesperidin (HSD, dotted line), copper(II) acetate (Cu(II), dashed line), and HSD–Cu(II) complex (full line) on a Cary 630 FT-IR spectrometer equipped with a monolithic design diamond Attenuated Total Reflectance (ATR) accessory (Agilent Technologies Inc.). Hesperidin is a chelating agent of metal multivalent ions (Me^{2+}). The creation of the complex involves -OH groups in ortho- positions that coordinate with divalent cations [1].

The FT-IR spectra of HSD, copper(II) acetate, and the HSD–Cu(II) complex showed HSD band shift upon complexation with a metal ion [33]. For example, the vibration stretching for -C=O in HSD at 1644 cm^{-1} was shifted to 1515 cm^{-1} in the HSD–Cu(II) complex, due to the coordination with the metal ion. The absorption bands in HSD for C-O at 1297, 1275, 1242, 1206, 1184, 1154, 1132, 1095, 1054, 1037, and 1009 cm^{-1} were suppressed, probably because of the Cu(II) bonding with -OH groups. Therefore, there is a strong indication that hesperidin formed a complex with Cu(II) ions.

2.4. HSD Interacts with Collagenase

Collagenase enzymes are a group of metalloproteinases responsible for the degradation of collagen and may cause an ageing effect in skin when present in higher levels in extracellular matrix. Figure 3 presents suppression of fluorescence quenching—observed for collagenase (*Clostridium histolyticum*, Sigma-Aldrich) by the addition of hesperidin in different concentrations (DMSO solution). Hesperidin, as other flavonoids, can reduce the intensity of tryptophan or other fluorophores of enzyme fluorescence emissions. Hesperidin chelates zinc(II) ion, which is in the catalytic site of the enzyme, and changes the conformation of the protein. There are already various studies in which it has been proven that flavonoids have an inhibitory effect on metalloproteinase (collagenase, elastases, and hyaluronidases) by chelating their metal ions. Additionally, the temperature of the experiment was varied as to evaluate and calculate the thermodynamic values of enthalpy (ΔH) and entropy (ΔS) of collagenase–hesperidin interaction.

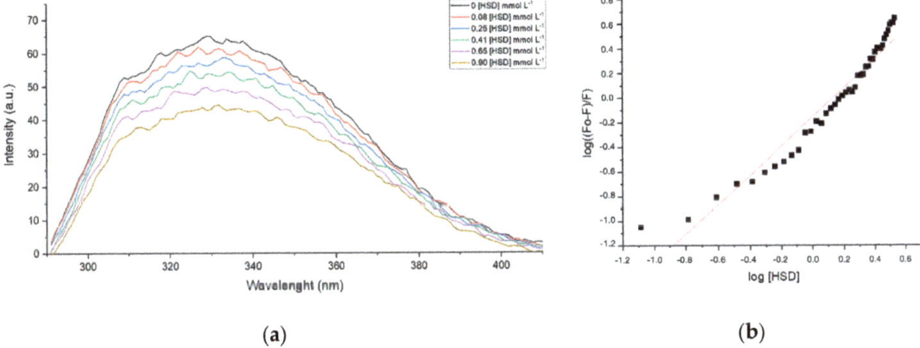

Figure 3. Illustration of fluorescence spectroscopy data: (**a**) Collagenase (*Clostridium hystolicum*) at 37 °C upon addition of HSD (in DMSO) at concentrations from 0.08 to 0.90 mmol L^{-1}. (**b**) Diagram of $\log((F_0-F)/F)$ in function of $\log[\text{HSD}]$.

The mechanism of fluorescence suppression can be explained through collision quenching between the excited enzyme and suppressor (Q), defined by bimolecular quenching constant Kq according to Stern–Volmer [34]. The reduction in the intensity of the fluorescence emission (F) in relation to the intensity observed in the absence of suppressor (F_0) is given by Equation (1):

$$(F_0/F) = 1 + K_q\tau_0[Q] = 1 + K_S[Q] \tag{1}$$

[Q] is a concentration of HSD, τ_0 is 10^{-8} s, and Kq is the association constant, 0.29×10^{-3} mol^{-1} L, 0.32×10^{-3} mol^{-1} L, or 0.15×10^{-3} mol^{-1} L obtained for collagenase–HSD at 25 °C, 30 °C, and 37 °C, respectively. The active site number was estimated at n = 1.2 (1.26, 1.24, and 1.19 for collagenase–HSD interaction at 25 °C, 30 °C, and 37 °C, respectively). It was possible to calculate Gibbs free energy, entropy, and enthalpy, ref [35] for collagenase–HSD at 25 °C, 30 °C, and 37 °C, as shown in Table 1.

Table 1. Thermodynamic parameters of collagenase–HSD interaction.

	Temperature °C	ΔG (kJ mol^{-1})	ΔH (kJ mol^{-1})	ΔS (J mol^{-1} K^{-1})
Collagenase–Hesperidin	25	20.0	−14.5	−19.0
	30	22.2		
	37	22.6		

According to the data (Table 1) and as well to Ross and Subramanian [35], the interaction between collagenase and HSD is a partial immobilization. This interaction occurs when protein and ligand are leaving the state from which the two are separated and when they are hydrophobically associated. Further, this type of association contributes to the decrease in the ΔS and ΔG values.

2.5. Characterization of HSD Nanocrystals

The obtained HSD was pre-milled and further nanonized on a homogenizer or ultrasound of high potency. The effectiveness of pre-milling was clearly revealed by the reduction in particle size distribution observed after applying different analytical methodologies for HSD nanonization. The average size, zeta potential, and polydispersity index of the HSD nanoparticles are shown in Table 2.

Table 2. Mean size, zeta potential, and polydispersity (PdI) of nanoparticles from different formulations prepared with various techniques, measured by a Malvern Zetasizer and a NanoSight LM20 microscope.

Formulation	Dynamic Light Scattering (DLS)			Nanoparticle Tracking Analysis (NTA)		
	Mean Size [nm]	Zeta Potential [mV]	PdI	Mean [nm]	Standard Deviation [nm]	Conc. of Particles [E8/mL]
I	148.0	−36.2	0.181	109.0	39.0	2.03
II	1126	−29.6	0.579	157.0	59.0	0.14
III	265.7	−4.81	0.332	226.0	55.0	0.63
IV	259.7	−32.7	0.370	73.0	15.0	0.27
V	335.6	−30.1	0.375	63.0	18.0	0.43
VI	367.2	−33.6	0.332	111.0	47.0	5.65
VII	287.7	−19.0	0.433	76.0	15.0	2.34
VIII	485.4	−51.6	0.506	33.0	4.00	2.48

The results were obtained after 6 months of preparation of the emulsions. The sizes of the HSD nanoparticles, after passing through the homogenizer and ultrasound, reduced from 600 to 150–350 nm, depending on the type, concentration of the polymer, and technique used for preparation. Zeta potentials were very variable, and it was not possible to obtain the desired stability for all nanoemulsions (for example, III, Table 2) with the best zeta potential being around −30 ± 6 mV. Part of the particles had sizes up to 400 nm as measured using the Dynamic Light Scattering (DLS) and will not affect their permeation via *stratum corneum*.

Scanning and transmission electron micrographs obtained for the formulations I, II, and IV–VIII are presented in Figure 4 and show particles whose sizes are in accordance with the sizes measured by (DLS) and NanoTracking Analysis (NTA) techniques. Nanoparticles of formulation I were around 200 nm in size, as shown in Table 2 and Figure 4. The formulation II contained bigger particles, around 1 μm, probably because of sodium-carboxyl methyl cellulose as surfactant (image not shown). Formulation IV (Figure 4) had particles with sizes of 250 nm (DLS and NTA), probably due to the aggregation of poloxamer around the hesperidin particles, whereas NTA experiments showed the presence of smaller particles of 50–100 nm.

Formulations V and VI were prepared utilizing the technique NANOEDGE[like], where hesperidin was dissolved in small amounts of propylene glycol and glycerol, respectively. SEM experiments were not adequate to characterize the VI formulation and it was necessary to apply atomic force microscopy (AFM) to perform such characterization. The particles were in the size range of 50–200 nm, and in the image of formulation VI, nanofibers of nanocellulose could be seen. Formulations V and VI showed above average stability for 6 months without any precipitation of the nanoparticles. Their stability was achieved mostly because of the significant amount of nanocellulose used for their production, while good dispersibility of hesperidin was achieved because of propylene glycol and glycerol used in their formulation. As the formulations were prepared in aqueous solutions, there was no observed HSD binding with CNF, which was also especially important from the point of view of skin permeation. The stability of the prepared nanoemulsions (I–VIII) was very good (up to 6 months), which despite showing a small percentage of agglomerates, returned to the initial state by a process involving the use of an ultrasound bath (5 min).

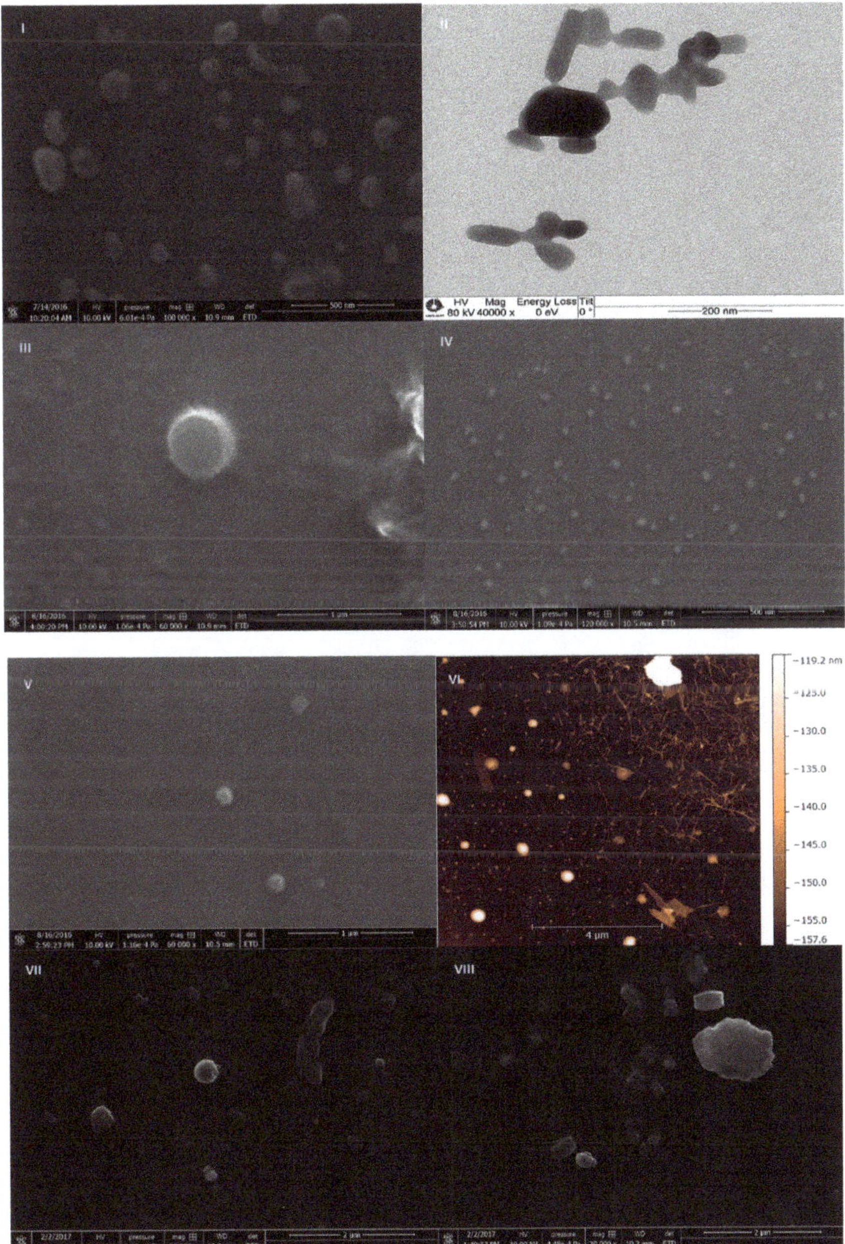

Figure 4. Scanning electron micrographs (**left**; scale bar = 500 nm) of formulation **I** and transmission electron micrographs (**right**; scale bar = 200 nm) of formulation **I**. Scanning electron micrographs of formulation **III** (**left**; scale bar = 1 μm) and formulation **IV** (**right**; scale bar = 500 nm), respectively. Scanning electron micrographs of formulation **V** (**left**; scale bar = 1 μm) and atomic force micrographs of formulation **VI** (**right**; scale bar = 4 μm). Scanning electron micrographs of formulations **VII** and **VIII** (**left**; scale bar = 2 μm).

2.6. Stability of HSD Cream Formulations

The stability tests for HSD incorporated in silky cream formulations, kept in plastic boxes made of polypropylene at 4 °C and at room temperature, were carried out 72 h, 30 days, and 12 months after manufacture. Organoleptic tests included appearance, color, brightness, consistency, and homogeneity of the creams, evaluated by visual observation. Applied and sensory characteristics of samples, such as spreadability, absorption, stickiness, and fat film on the skin were assessed after applying the cream on the skin. Shortly after preparation, creams were homogenous, bright, and easily spreadable on the skin. During the following 12 months, their consistency did not change, and the cream formulations maintained odor and color as well. Measurement of the pH value was carried out potentiometrically, by direct immersion of the glass electrode into the tested samples of creams at room temperature. Values of the pH were in the range from 5 to 6, as is recommended by pharmacopoeia.

2.7. Evaluation of Toxicity of HSD Nanoemulsions and Cream

Full thickness skin (FTS) models for the toxicity (corrosion) test of hesperidin cream formulations were synthesized in the Laboratory of Biology of the Skin, Faculty of Pharmaceutical Sciences, University of Sao Paulo. As the experiment is quite complicated and expensive, just some of the HSD cream formulations were tested.

Figure 5 presents photomicrographs of histological analysis—eosin stain (samples in paraffin) of the FTS skin model after the cream application assay (24 h). This model was synthesized from the fibroblast and keratinocytes isolated from normal human skin cells-donated foreskin samples. The model was composed from two main skin layers-epidermis and dermis-and used for the evaluation of the toxicity of cosmetic and other preparations. Epidermis was composed from five layers: stratum corneum, stratum lucidum, stratum granulosum, stratum spinosum, and stratum basale. The last one was formed from the undifferentiated cells, with a full metabolic activity, which was lost in later proliferation of the cells and formation of the corneocytes. It is important to mention that macrophage and Langerhans cells were not present, which are the first defensive line of the skin [36].

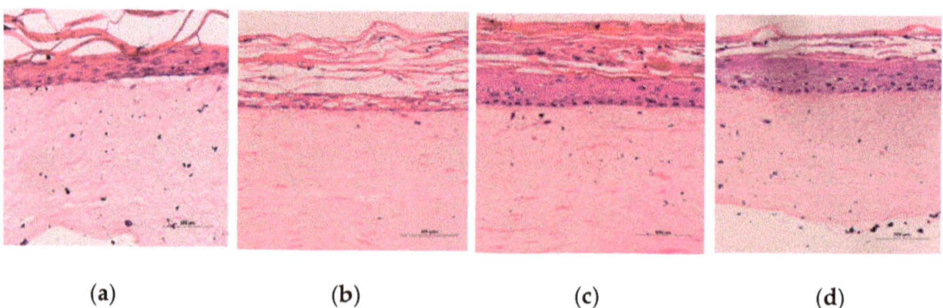

(a)   (b)   (c)   (d)

Figure 5. Photomicrographs of Histological Analysis—Eosin stain (sample in paraffin) of the full thickness skin (FTS) equivalent skin model after the cream application assay (**a**) negative control: sodium chloride 0.9%; (**b**) positive control: HSD-DMSO, (**c**) A1 cream, and (**d**) A2 cream. The skin models were generated using primary human keratinocytes and fibroblasts—the FTS model; (Scale bar = 500 μm).

In the negative control sample (Figure 5a) photomicrograph, epidermis and dermis layers were preserved and there was no presence of vacuolization in the stratum basale. After application of the A1 cream (without HSD-nanoemulsion), the basal layer was preserved, with remaining proliferation despite some vacuoles' presence (Figure 5b). The stratum corneum of this sample was preserved and thicker, and the cream demonstrated good moisturizing effects. HSD in 10% DMSO showed corrosive and cytotoxic effects on the FTS skin model, and led to complete degradation of the basal layer (Figure 5b). Further, the formulation with even a small percentage of DMSO was avoided. Application of nanoemulsion VI showed an irregular basal layer and elevated stratum corneum; therefore, a slight corrosive effect for this formulation was observed (Figure 5d). Nanoemulsion VII demonstrated less cytotoxic effects, inclusively in the basal membrane, compared to the A2 cream. The corrosion test with the A2 and A3 creams (data not shown) showed moderate hydration effects on the FTS skin model, probably due to the hygroscopic effect of some of their ingredients. As this skin model is a living organ, some of the ingredients of the nanoemulsion or the surfactant alone could have led to lower vitality of the cells and prevented their further proliferation. The A2 cream contained only a Pluronic-F127 as a hygroscopic compound, and therefore, the viability of the cells was much higher than in the case of the A3 cream. Nanoemulsions VI and VII demonstrated corrosive effects on the skin model (data not shown) due to the dilution of the buffer solution as well as the inadequate environment for the development and proliferation of cells. It is important to mention that the generated FTS skin model does not contain macrophages or Langerhans cells, which are the first defense of the skin tissue's immunity, which makes it much more sensitive than normal skin tissue.

3. Discussion

A new, water-based, eco-friendly extraction was performed to yield hesperidin (HSD, 1.2%) with approximate purity of 98%. This new method explored the use of calcium(II) and changes in the pH as to isolate HSD from orange peel. The use of calcium(II) enabled the complexation of pectin within the bagasse and release of HSD, which dissolved at high pH values. NaOH solution at pH ~11.5 deprotonated phenol HSD groups and promoted its better solubility. The next step counted on HSD protonation (HCl), which caused HSD precipitation on pH ~4.2. Pale yellow powder was obtained and characterized using different spectroscopic techniques. HSD is usually extracted with organic solvents [30,32] or by supercritical fluid extraction [31]. The organic solvent extraction for hesperidin extraction was performed by Cypriano and colleagues [37] in a 1.2% yield, following Ikan's method [12]. The method suggested in this work is energy- and organic solvents-free, and calcium(II) and pH-triggered. The use of calcium(II) facilitated complexation of pectin polysaccharide and at the same time, liberation of hesperidin from orange bagasse. The suggested process is longer but facilitates the extraction of hesperidin with greater purity compared to the Sigma-Aldrich analytical standard.

Observing the structure of HSD (Figure 1), it is evident that its B-ring is electron richer than the A-ring due to the contribution of the ortho methoxy group. The first site of oxidation in HSD is the 3'-phenoxyl group in a one-electron reduction [8,38]. The pKa of HSD -OH groups is 8.9 and 11.2, respectively. However, the pKa of the hydroxyl radical in the 3' position drops to a value around 4–5. Due to this, HSD acts as antioxidant in the pH range of 7 to 10. Therefore, the mechanism of HSD oxidation involves the transfer of one electron and one proton. The reduction potential of the phenolate radical is strongly affected by substituents in the B-ring [8]. HSD has an electron-donating group (methoxy) attached to the B-ring, which elevates its reduction potential (E = 0.72 V) when compared to other flavonoids with catechol groups in the B-ring (E value from 0.5 to 0.7 V). Nevertheless, its reduction potential is still smaller than those from alkyl peroxyl radicals (E = 1.05 V) and superoxide radicals (E = 0.94 V), which confirms that HSD can scavenge and inactivate these harmful radical species in the organism [8,39–51]. HSD high chemical reactivity can prevent injuries caused by free radicals through direct interaction with radical oxygen species (ROS), or indirectly by inducing antioxidant enzymes activation, chelating of metal ions, reduction in α-tocopherol radicals, inhibition of oxidases, reduction in NO oxidative [4,38] stress, and increases in antioxidant effects of low molecular antioxidants [9,39].

Many other polyphenols, such as phenolic acid, flavonoids, coumarins, stilbenes, and lignans, are the most important polyphenols used in traditional and modern cosmetic and dermatologic products [3,52,53]. The antioxidant, anti-ageing, anti-inflammatory, antimicrobial, and anticancer properties of flavonoids are frequently deployed in skincare products. Their antiradical functions, as well as the ability to inhibit some enzymes, are some of the most important effects. Flavonoids have an influence on skin microcirculation and can be used as ingredients in creams for vascular, oily, and/or atypical skin [3]. Dermal bioavailability and antioxidant activity [54,55] of glycosides is beneath when compared to their aglycon forms, due to their low permeability [3]. One of the interesting physical-chemical properties of bioflavonoids is their ability to absorb ultraviolet radiation due to the presence of the conjugated double bonds in their structure. They may absorb UV radiations in the range of 550–300 and 285–240 nm, resulting from phenolic electron-donating substituents, as well as inter- and intramolecular hydrogen bonds and steric effects. The polyphenol concentrations used in cosmetics cannot replace conventional UV filters. Moreover, they can act as co-adjuvants in erythema and skin burns reduction caused by exposures to UVB radiation and IR rays of sunlight [3]. The anti-ageing properties of flavonoids are associated with their effect on the modulation of matrix metalloproteinases activities, which are dependent on the Zn^{2+} ion and involved in connective tissue remodeling. Equally, by sequestering metal ions or the effects on the expression of endogenous protein tissue inhibitors of metalloproteinase (TIMPs) [9], flavonoids can act protectively. Flavonoids' skin whitening activity relates to their modulation of tyrosinase activity, through their chelating of calcium(II), in the formation of L-dopaquinone, which is a part of the melanogenesis process [56]. This ability is common to quercetin, cyanidin, and kaempferol, while their glycoside forms have not shown this capability [3]. Hyaluronic acid, which is an integral part of the dermis and blood vessel wall, is degraded by the activity of the enzyme hyaluronidase, which can be inhibited by the protective roles of flavonoids [3]. Additionally, phenolic compounds may have antimicrobial properties and assist in the preservation of cosmetic products against secondary infections [3].

Low drug permeability through human epidermis can be ameliorated using penetration enhancers (compounds such as surfactants, terpenes, lipophilic solvent, and fatty acids), which modify the permeability of the skin barrier reversibly. Rutin, catechin, epicatechin, and quercetin have a limited penetration. Quercetin shows poor permeability even in the presence of the enhancers, due to its absolute insolubility in water [35]. Several authors suggested that the permeability of this compound can be increased by uploading flavonoids in liposomes or other kinds of carrier systems. It can also be affected by the presence of promoters of permeability, such as glycerin and propylene glycol [3]. In the skin, HSD may significantly stimulate epidermal hyperplasia and improve epidermal permeability through epidermal proliferation, osteoblasts differentiation, and lipid secretion. Different skin layers and skin proteins can respond differently to HSD treatment. Involucrin, present in the stratum spinosum, does not respond to HSD treatment. Filaggrin and loricrin (located in the stratum granulosum and stratum spinosum) expressions are increased. These beneficial effects that improve epidermal permeability and regulate filaggrin can be useful in the treatment of certain skin disorders, such as cutaneous inflammation and atopic dermatitis [52]. In vitro, HSD can inhibit the tyrosinase in melanocytes and reduce the process of melanogenesis, or influence melanocytes proliferation. Therefore, the possibility of affecting tyrosinase activity, and the practical application thereof in the field of anti-ageing preparations designed to prevent lentigo senilis and lentigo solaris makes HSD remarkably interesting for skin whitening [3]. Daily topical applications of HSD microemulsion have shown a significant skin whitening effect, reduction in trans-epidermal water loss, and inhibition of irritation effect after exposure to UV rays after four weeks. In their study, Kim et al. [56] showed that HSD had a depigmentation effect by blocking the melanophilin, a tripartite protein complex which is a response for transport of the melanosome into the melanocytes. This was proven by melanosome aggregation tests in cells. HSD did not inhibit melanin production in melanoma cells, but reduced skin pigmentation in the reconstruction of human epidermal skin [56]. HSD may also affect polyoxygenase, cyclooxygenase, hyaluronidase, collagenase, elastase, and tyrosinase; thus, it can contribute to the reduction in modifications in the skin's connective tissue remodeling [3]. Hyaluronidase plays a significant role in regulating the permeability of capillary walls and supporting tissues by causing the breakdown of hyaluronic acid and increasing the permeability of the tissue [5]. The HSD's ability to chelate multivalent metals such as iron(III), iron(II), copper(II), zinc(II), and manganese(II) is as relevant to the inhibition of enzymes, which contain metal ions in their reaction center or require metal cations cofactors, as to the inhibition of inflammatory processes and function of vascular vessels [3,15,57,58]. Chelation properties of HSD are particularly important for skin bleaching activities, as well as HSD interaction with the tyrosinase during catalytic production of melanin. Tyrosinase has copper(II) in the active site, which is responsible for tyrosinase oxidation activities [9].

4. Materials and Methods

4.1. Materials

Oranges (*Citrus sinensis*) and orange peel bagasse were purchased from a local supermarket in Campinas (Sao Paulo, Brazil). Hesperidin standard was bought from Sigma-Aldrich (St. Louis, MA, USA) at analytical grade (>97%). Calcium(II) chloride, copper(II) acetate, sodium hydroxide, and hydrochloric acid were from Labsynth (Diadema, Sao Paulo, Brazil) at practical grade. Deuterated solvent (DMSO-d_6) was purchased from Sigma-Aldrich (St. Louis, MA, USA). Methanol and phosphoric acid for the UHPLC assays were analytical grade (Avantor "Performance Materials", Mexico®, Ecatepec de Morelos, Mexico). ABIL® Care 85 (Bis-PEG/PPg-16/16 PEG/PPG16/16 Dimethicone; Caprylic/Capric Triglyceride) were sampled from the EVONIK® group (Essen, Germany). Muru muru (*Astrocaryum murumuru* Seed Butter), Cupuaçu butter (*Theobroma grandiflorum* Seed Butter), and Andiroba oil (*Carapa Guianensis* Seed Oil) were sampled from Amazon oil industry; Glyceryl monostearate, Mineral oil, Carbopol ULTREZ 10, Triethanolamine, and Vit E-acetate (α-Tocopheryl acetate) were bought from Fagron® (Rotterdam, The Netherlands).

4.2. Extraction of HSD from Humid Orange Bagasse

The fresh chopped orange peel (*Citrus sinensis*, 100 g) was milled in a blender and immersed in 300 mL of aqueous CaCl$_2$ solution (7.5%). The mixture was left to stand for 24 h, then, a NaOH 1 mol L^{-1} solution was added dropwise until a pH of 11.50 was reached. It was set to stand for 24 h, the pH was measured, and it dropped to 9.66 overnight. Then, the suspension was filtered, and the pellet was much harder when compared with the starting material, probably because of the interactions between calcium(II) ions and pectin. Concentrated HCl was then added to the solution, and pH was lowered to 4.35. The solution was left to stand at 4 °C for 2 days. After 24 h, crystals were formed at the bottom of the glass. However, for the best yields, two days of precipitation is recommended. After 48 h, HSD was filtered onto a MILIPORE® (Burlington, MA, USA) apparatus, using a 0.45 μm pore filter, and dried for 2 h in drying oven (60 °C).

4.3. Nuclear Magnetic Resonance—NMR

Nuclear Magnetic Resonance spectra were acquired on a Bruker *AVANCE III* 600 MHz spectrometer (Bruker Biospin, Karlsruhe, Germany) equipped with a 5 mm Triple Resonance Broadband Inverse (TBI) probe at 25 °C. ^{1}H NMR (1D, 600.173 MHz) spectra were acquired using a f1 pre-saturation sequence with 32 transient scanning, 64 k data points, and 13 kHz bandwidth. ^{13}C NMR spectra were obtained using the 1D sequence with power decoupling. Isolated HSD was dissolved in DMSO-d_6 (20 mg mL^{-1}). Two-dimensional spectra (Heteronuclear Single Quantum Coherence—HSQC) were acquired using the 600.17 MHz frequency domain spectrometer F2 and 150.91 MHz in the F1 domain with a free induction decay size (FID) of 4096 (F2) and 256 (F1) data points and 16 "ghost" scans were used. HSQC (*hsqcedetgpsp.*) spectra were recorded with an acquisition time of 2.129 × 10^{-1} s (F2) and 4.437 × 10^{-3} s (F1) pulse sequence. The Heteronuclear Multiple Bond Correlations (HMBC) were acquired using the 600.17 MHz frequency domain spectrometer F2 and 150.91 MHz in the F1 domain with a free induction decay size (FID) of 2048 (F2) and 256 (F1) data points and 16 "ghost" scans were used. HMBC spectra were acquired with an acquisition time of 2.130 × 10^{-1} s (F2) and 4.437 × 10^{-3} s (F1), using the *hmbcgplpndgf.* pulse sequence. The spectra were processed in MestreNova software, using LB = 1.00 for F2 and LB = 0.30 for F1.

4.4. Fourier Transform Infrared Spectroscopy—FT-IR

The Fourier transform infrared spectrum (FT-IR) of HSD was obtained on a Cary 630 FT-IR spectrometer equipped with a monolithic diamond attenuated total reflection (ATR) accessory (Agilent Technologies Inc., Santa Clara, CA, USA). The spectra were recorded accumulating 128 scans at a resolution of 4 cm^{-1} in the range from 4000 to 400 cm^{-1}.

4.5. UHPLC—Purity of Extracted Hesperidin

The HSD purity was determined utilizing Ultra-High-Performance Liquid (UHPLC—Waters, Milford, MA, USA) with the reverse stationary phase (Zorbax Eclipse C18, length 10 cm, 5 μm, Agilent Technologies Inc., Santa Clara, CA, USA). The mobile phase was prepared with methanol and water (60:40 v/v) with the addition of phosphoric acid (0.1%). A hesperidin analytical standard (Sigma-Aldrich, >97% of purity, St. Louis, MO, USA) was used for calibration curve construction from the injection of aliquots of 1, 2, 4, 6, 8, and 10 μL of standard solution, HSD in methanol (100 ppm). Calibration curves and the analysis of the sample from the extraction were performed in triplicate. The following method was adapted from Weon et al. (2012) [59].

4.6. Chelation Properties of Hesperidin

Chelation properties of HSD were tested through the interaction of HSD with copper(II), following the procedure in Selvaraj et al. [58]. For the experiment, HSD (1 mmol L^{-1}) was dissolved in 50 mL of methanol, mixed with 0.199 g of copper(II) acetate in 25 mL of double distilled water and stirred for 6 h at room temperature. The pale green insoluble precipitate was obtained and filtered and washed with water and methanol to remove the excess of HSD and copper(II) acetate. The product was then air-dried. The greenish precipitate obtained was vacuum dried and characterized.

4.7. Fluorescence Suppression—Quenching

The measurements were performed on a Varian spectrofluorometer (Cary Eclipse model, Agilent Technologies Inc., Santa Clara, CA, USA) by applying a wavelength of 278 nm for excitation of the collagenase, excitation and emission slits were 5 nm wide, and acquisition of emission spectra occurred in the range of 300–450 nm, with the sample compartment with a thermostat at 25, 30, and 37 °C. A 10×10 mm optical path quartz (Hellma, Mülheim, Germany) cuvette was used. To obtain spectra, 2 mL of collagenase (Sigma-Aldrich) in concentration 0.065 mg mL^{-1} (water solution) were titrated with hesperidin solution in DMSO (0.10 mg mL^{-1} concentration). Additions of aliquots of HSD were as follow: 0.5 μL up to 4 μL, 1.0 μL up to 50 μL, and 5 μL up to a volume of 110 μL, reaching the final concentrations of 5.68 mg mL^{-1} of HSD in solution.

4.8. Preparation of Hesperidin Nanocrystals

HSD was utilized to formulate nanoemulsions. Polymers utilized in preparations were poloxamer (Pluronic F127, Sigma Aldrich, St. Louis, MO, USA) and nanocellulose, which served as stabilizers and showed different capacities regarding the preservation of hesperidin nanostructure. These were dissolved in water and mixed with an Ultra Turrax mixer for 15 min at a speed of 14,000 rpm min^{-1}. Pre-milling with the mixer avoided blocking the homogenizing gap of the homogenizer present in the prepared formulation. Hereupon, the formulations I, II, and VII were processed through the homogenizer (Gea Niro Soavi, Model NS 1001L—Panda 2k, Dusseldorf, Germany) at high pressure (600 bar) for 5 cycles. During the homogenization process, a pressure decrease was observed, especially after the third cycle. The process utilized for HSD nanonization for formulations III, IV, V, and VI was based on the technology NANOEDGE™, where HSD was solubilized in a minimum quantity of solvent (or homogenous mixture of complex composition). The resulting solution was added to a mixture of purified water and stabilizers and it underwent a homogenization process with high-potency ultrasound (Ultronique, Model: DESRUPTOR; Freq. US: 20 kHz; Potency US: 750 W, Indaiatuba SP,

Brazil), 70% potency for 30 min. Formulations V and VI were prepared through a NANOEDGE-like technique, where initially HSD was dissolved in the mixture of essential oil (orange peels) and glycerol and added into the solution of purified water and nanocellulose; afterwards, it was sonicated. Formulations prepared using two nano-techniques and their ingredients were as follows:

I—H69, combination of pre-milling with an Ultra Turrax and high-pressure homogenization, ingredients used: hesperidin and water;

II—H69, combination of pre-milling in an Ultra Turrax and high-pressure homogenization, ingredients used: hesperidin, DMSO, glycerol, sodium-carboxyl methyl cellulose, and water;

III—NANOEDGE-like, combination of microprecipitation and ultrasound, used ingredients: hesperidin, DMSO, glycerol, poloxamer (Pluronic F127), and water;

IV—NANOEDGE-like, combination of microprecipitation and ultrasound, used ingredients: hesperidin, DMSO, orange oil, poloxamer (Pluronic F127), and water;

V—NANOEDGE-like, combination of microprecipitation and ultrasound, used ingredients: hesperidin, propylene glycol, nanocellulose, and water;

VI—NANOEDGE-like, combination of microprecipitation and ultrasound, used ingredients: hesperidin, glycerol, nanocellulose, and water;

VII—H69, combination of pre-milling in an Ultra Turrax and high-pressure homogenization: hesperidin, glycerol, orange oil, poloxamer (Pluronic F127), and water;

VIII—Milling in an Ultra Turrax, ingredients used: hesperidin, glycerol, orange oil, poloxamer (Pluronic F127), and water.

4.9. Formulation of the Silky Cream

Oil-in-water silky cream formulations were prepared following the protocols of the EVONIK® group (Essen, Germany), for use of the surfactant ABIL® Care 85 (Bis-PEG/PPg-16/16 PEG/PPG16/16 Dimethicone; Caprylic/Capric Triglyceride) and presented in Table 3. Muru muru (*Astrocaryum murumuru* Seed Butter), Cupuaçu butter (*Theobroma grandiflorum* Seed Butter), and Andiroba oil (*Carapa Guianensis* Seed Oil) were sampled from Amazon oil industry; Glyceryl monostearate, Mineral oil, Carbopol ULTREZ 10, Triethanolamine, and Vit E-acetate (α-Tocopheryl acetate) were from Fagron®. Emulsifier ABIL® Care 85 that gives a velvety-silky skin feel was sampled from EVONIK® and was used in exceptionally low usage concentration. Ethylhexylglycerin and Phenoxyethanol (Fagron®) were used for formulation preserving in exceptionally low concentration, instead of the commercial paraben's components.

Table 3. Silky velvet cream formulations prepared for application of hesperidin nanoemulsions.

Phase	Name	A1 (%, g g^{-1})	A2 (%, g g^{-1})	A3 (%, g g^{-1})
A	Bis-PEG/PPG-16/16 PEG/PPG-16/16 Dimethicone; Caprylic/Capric Triglyceride	1.0	1.0	1.0
	Muru muru butter	1.0	1.0	1.0
	Cupuaçu butter	1.0	1.0	1.0
	Andiroba oil	3.0	3.0	3.0
	GMS	2.0	2.0	2.0
	Cetostearyl alcohol	3.0	3.0	3.0
	Mineral oil	5.0	5.0	5.0
B	Carbopol ULTREZ 10	0.2	0.2	0.2
	Aqua (Purified Water)	79.8	-	-
	Nanoemulsion	-	79.8	79.8
C	Triethanolamine	5 *gtts	5 *ggts	5 *ggts
B	Vit E-acetate	0.5	0.5	0.5
E	Ethylhexylglicerin, Phenoxyethanol	0.5	0.5	0.5

*gtts is drops.

Ingredients of the phases A and B were measured, transferred into two beakers, and heated to 50 °C. When the oil phase was homogenized and all the ingredients were molten, phase A was added into phase B. The mixture was stirred and homogenized until it cooled down to a temperature of 25 °C. Ingredients of the phases C and E were added at room temperature, along with stirring. A whitish cream, oil-in-water, silky, with soft consistency, and easy to apply with no greasy film leftovers after applying was obtained. Nanoemulsion VI was used for the preparation in the A2 cream and Nanoemulsion VII was used for preparation in the A3 cream formulation.

4.10. Skin Model USP-FTS Skin Corrosion Test of Cream Formulations

Full thickness skin models (FTS) for the toxicity test of hesperidin cream formulations were prepared in the Laboratory of Biology of the Skin, coordinated by Prof. Silvya Stuchi Maria-Engler, Faculty of Pharmaceutical Sciences, University of Sao Paulo. Fibroblast and keratinocytes were isolated from the normal human skin cells, from donated foreskin samples obtained from the University of Sao Paulo Hospital (Sao Paulo, Brazil). Performed assays were under the approval of the local Ethics Committee (HU CEP Case No. 943/09 and CEP FCF/USP 534). Isolated cells were seeded on top of the collagen I matrix model in a 6-well plate containing enough specific medium mixture for the FTS model as to maintain the skin at the air–liquid interface, as it is described by Catarino et al. [32]. For the corrosion tests, the following system was used: 100 µg mL^{-1} of hesperidin in 10% DMSO, cream without the hesperidin nanoemulsion (A1), two formulations of hesperidin nanoemulsions (Nanoemulsion VI and Nanoemulsion VII), and the last two in the cream formulations as A2 and A3 creams. As a negative control, 0.9% sodium-chloride solution was used. The 100 µg mL^{-1} of hesperidin in 10% DMSO were tested by adding 5 mL in the well plate, and the 0.5 mL of cream formulations were applied over epidermis. Samples were left over night for incubation (37 °C, 5% CO_2). All tests were performed in duplicate. After 24 h, skins were washed with 0.9% of sodium-chloride solution and preserved in paraffin for further microscopic tests.

4.11. Diffraction Light Scattering and Zeta Potential

Mean size, polydispersity, and zeta potential of nanoparticles from each formulation were determined using diffraction light scattering technique (Nano ZS Zetasizer—Malvern, PANalytical Almelo, The Netherlands). Known also as Photon Correlation Spectroscopy—PCS, this is the technique that was used to measure the hydrodynamic diameter of particles in a range from microns up to 1 nm.

4.12. Nanoparticle Tracking Analysis—NTA Analysis

Analysis (NTA) was performed with a NanoSight LM20 microscope (NanoSight, Amesbury, UK), equipped with a 640 nm laser sample camera and a fluoroelastometer. Samples were diluted and injected with sterile syringes 57 (BD Discardit II, Jersey, USA) until the liquid reached the tip of the mouthpiece. All measurements were performed at room temperature, with live monitoring of thermal stresses. The software used to capture and analyze the data was NTA 2.0 Build 127. The samples were captured with 60 s time using the parameters predetermined by the manual.

4.13. Electronic Microscopy—Transmission, Scanning, and Atomic Force

Utilizing the microscope SEM JEOL JSM-6360 LV (JEOL, Akishima, Tokyo, Japan) and an atomic force microscope (Shimadzu, SPM 9500J3), the size of the nanoparticles in the nanoemulsions was verified. The sonicated hesperidin nanoemulsion was dropped onto a sample holder, dried at room temperature, and coated with gold or platinum using a MED 020 Sputter (BalTech, Balzers, Liechtenstein). The images were obtained using an acceleration voltage of 10 kV and a secondary electron detector.

5. Conclusions

Hesperidin (HSD) was obtained from citrus peels through a pH-triggered precipitation method conducted just in water. The extracted hesperidin purity and yield were excellent when compared to standard methods of its extraction and a commercially available compound. HSD showed chelating activity toward bivalent ions and interacted with collagenase. HSD was used for the formulation of a promising anti-ageing face cream. Upon nanonizing, HSD nanoparticles (150 to 400 nm) were employed into up to 12 months stable nanoemulsions, whose applicability was tested in vitro on artificial skin. No nocive effects were observed, and the best face cream formulation (cream A2) showed good results in reducing the black circles in the under eye region. Moreover, daily topical applications of hesperidin nanoemulsion have shown a significant skin whitening effect, reduction in trans-epidermal water loss, and inhibition of an irritation effect after exposure to UV rays. This way, a clean cream active ingredient is proposed, and a promising cosmeceutical was formulated starting from agro-industrial waste.

Supplementary Materials: The following are available online, Figure S1. Steps of hesperidin water extraction: (a) squeezing orange peel, alkaline medium solution; (b) acidic solution and first precipitate of hesperidin; (c) precipitated hesperidin after 7 days at 4 °C; (d) filtration of precipitated hesperidin; (e) dried yellow powder of hesperidin. Figure S2. HSQC contour plot of hesperidin (20 mg mL^{-1}) in DMSO-d$_6$ (2.50 ppm; 39.50 ppm) as a solvent, on Bruker *AVANCE* III 600 MHz equipment at 25 °C. Figure S3. HMBC contour plot of hesperidin (20 mg mL^{-1}) in DMSO-d$_6$ (2.50 ppm; 39.50 ppm) as a solvent, on Bruker *AVANCE* III 600 MHz equipment at 25 °C. Figure S4. Chromatogram obtained from injection of the extracted hesperidin sample by separation through ultra-high-performance liquid chromatography (UHPLC) with reverse phase C18; the peak with the retention time at 6.877 min corresponds to hesperidin. Figure S5. Fluorescence suppression - quenching effect of hesperidin solution in DMSO (concentration from 0.00 to 5.09 mmol L^{-1}) on collagenase (*Clostridium histolyticum*, Sigma-Aldrich) at 37 °C. Figure S6. Fluorescence suppression—quenching effect of hesperidin solution in DMSO (concentration from 0.00 to 5.22 mmol L^{-1}) on collagenase (Clostridium histolyticum, Sigma-Aldrich) at 30 °C.

Author Contributions: Conceptualization, D.S. and L.T.; methodology, D.S., R.V.d.S., A.F.C., L.H.B.L.; formal analysis, D.S., R.V.d.S., A.F.C. and L.H.B.L.; investigation, D.S.; resources, L.T.; data curation, D.S., N.D. and L.T.; writing—original draft preparation, D.S.; writing—review and editing, D.S., N.D. and L.T.; supervision, L.T. All authors have read and agreed to the published version of the manuscript.

Funding: This research received funding from CAPES (code 01), CNPq (Grant number: 140837/2015-3), FUNCAMP-CITROSUCO (Grant Number 5417).

Acknowledgments: Authors acknowledge the Laboratory of Biology of the Skin, coordinated by Silvya Stuchi Maria-Engler, Faculty of Pharmaceutical Sciences, University of Sao Paulo for the artificial skin tests performed.

Conflicts of Interest: The authors declare no conflict of interest.

References

1.   Tasic, L.; Mandic, B.; Barros, C.H.N.; Cypriano, D.Z.; Stanisic, D.; Schultz, L.G.; da Silva, L.L.; Mariño, M.A.M.; Queiroz, V.L. *Citrus Fruits: Productions, Consumption and Health Benefits*; Simons, D., Ed.; Nova Science Publishers: New York, NY, USA, 2016; Chapter 2; pp. 27–70.

2.   Stanisic, D.; Costa, A.F.; Cruz, G.; Durán, N.; Tasic, L. *Studies in Natural Products Chemistry*; Rahman, A.-U., Ed.; Elsevier Science: Amsterdam, The Netherlands, 2018; Chapter 6; Volume 58, pp. 161–210.

3.   Ratz-Lyko, A.; Arct, J.; Majewski, S.; Pytkowska, K. Influence of polyphenols on the physiological processes in the skin. *Phytother. Res.* **2015**, *29*, 509–517. [CrossRef] [PubMed]

4.   Chanet, A.; Milenkovic, D.; Manach, C.; Mazur, A.; Morand, C. Citrus Flavanones: What Is Their Role in Cardiovascular Protection? *J. Agric. Food Chem.* **2012**, *60*, 8809–8822. [CrossRef] [PubMed]

5.   Garg, A.; Garg, S.; Zaneveld, L.J.D.; Singla, A.K. Chemistry and pharmacology of the citrus bioflavonoid Hsd. *Phytother. Res.* **2001**, *15*, 655–669. [CrossRef] [PubMed]

6.   Heim, K.E.; Tagliaferro, A.R.; Bobilya, D.J. Flavonoid antioxidants: Chemistry, metabolism and structure-activity relationships. *J. Nutr. Biochem.* **2002**, *13*, 572–584. [CrossRef]

7.   Parhiz, H.; Ali, R.; Soltani, F.; Rezaee, R.; Iranshahi, M. Antioxidant and anti-inflammatory properties of the citrus flavonoid's hesperidin and hesperetin: An updated review of their molecular mechanisms and experimental models. *Phytother. Res.* **2015**, *29*, 323–331. [CrossRef] [PubMed]

8. Jovanovic, S.V.; Steenken, S.; Tosic, M.; Marjanovic, B.; Simic, M.G. Flavonoids as antioxidants. *J. Am. Chem. Soc.* **1994**, *116*, 4846–4851. [CrossRef]

9. Roohbakhsh, A.; Parhiz, H.; Soltani, F.; Rezaee, R.; Iranshahi, M. Molecular mechanisms behind the biological effects of hesperidin and hesperetin for prevention of cancer and cardiovascular diseases. *Life Sci.* **2014**, *124*, 67–74. [CrossRef]

10. Chen, M.; Gu, H.; Ye, Y.; Lin, B.; Sun, L.; Deng, W.; Zhang, J.; Liu, J. Protective effects of hesperidin against oxidative stress of tert-butyl hydroperoxide in human hepatocytes. *Food Chem. Toxicol.* **2010**, *48*, 2980–2987. [CrossRef]

11. Calderone, V.; Chericoni, S.; Martinelli, C.; Testai, L.; Nardi, A.; Morelli, I.; Breschi, C.M.; Martinotti, E. Vasorelaxing effects of flavonoids: Investigation on the possible involvement of potassium channels. *Naunyn-Schmiedebergs Arch. Pharmacol.* **2004**, *370*, 290–298.

12. Ikan, R. *Natural Products: A Laboratory Guide*, 2nd ed.; Academic Press: San Diego, CA, USA, 1991.

13. Raw, L.; Sastry, P.G. Glycosides of citrus fruits. I. Oranges. *Indian J. Appl. Chem.* **1962**, *25*, 86–95.

14. Yu, L.; Huang, H.; Yu, L.L.; Wang, T.T.Y. Utility of hesperidinase for food function research: Enzymatic digestion of botanical extracts alters cellular antioxidant capacities and anti-inflammatory properties. *J. Agric. Food Chem.* **2014**, *62*, 8640–8647. [CrossRef]

15. Dragicevic, N.; Maibach, H.I. *Percutaneous Penetration Enhancers—Chemical Methods in Penetration Enhancement Drug—Manipulation Strategies and Vehicle Effects*; Springer: Berlin/Heidelberg, Germany, 2015.

16. Duran, N.; Duran, M.; Tasic, L.; Marcato, P.D. Nanocrystal technology in Pharmaceuticals. *Quim. Nova* **2010**, *33*, 151–158.

17. Duran, N.; Costa, A.F.; Stanisic, D.; Bernardes, J.S.; Tasic, L. Nanotoxicity and Dermal Application of Nanostructured Lipid Carrier Loaded with Hesperidin from Orange Residue. *J. Phys. Conf. Ser.* **2019**, *1323*, 012021. [CrossRef]

18. Guo, C.; Zhang, H.; Guan, X.; Zhou, Z. The Anti-Aging Potential of Neohesperidin and Its Synergistic Effects with Other Citrus Flavonoids in Extending Chronological Lifespan of *Saccharomyces Cerevisiae* BY4742. *Molecules* **2019**, *24*, 4093. [CrossRef]

19. Lee, H.J.; Im, A.-R.; Kim, S.-M.; Kang, H.-S.; Lee, J.D.; Chae, S. The flavonoid hesperidin exerts anti-photoaging effect by downregulating matrix metalloproteinase (MMP)-9 expression via mitogen activated protein kinase (MAPK)-dependent signaling pathways. *BMC Complem. Altern. Med.* **2018**, *18*, 1–20. [CrossRef]

20. Man, M.-Q.; Yang, B.; Elias, P.M. Benefits of Hesperidin for Cutaneous Functions. *Evid.-Based Complementary Altern. Med.* **2019**, *2019*, 2676307. [CrossRef]

21. Saija, A.; Tomaino, A.; Trombetta, D.; Giacchi, M.; Pasquale, A.; de Bonina, F. Influence of different penetration enhancers on in vitro skin permeation and in vivo photoprotective effect of flavonoids. *Int. J. Pharm.* **1998**, *175*, 85–94. [CrossRef]

22. Vicentini, F.; Simi, T.; Del Ciampo, J.; Wolga, N.; Pitol, D.; Iyomasa, M.; Bentley, V.; Fonseca, M. Quercetin in w/o microemulsion: In vitro and in vivo skin penetration and efficacy against UVB-induced skin damages evaluated in vivo. *Eur. J. Pharm. Biopharm.* **2008**, *69*, 948–957. [CrossRef]

23. Barel, A.O.; Paye, M.; Maibach, H.I. *Handbook of Cosmetic Science and Cosmetology*, 3rd ed.; Taylor and Francis Group: Boca Raton, FL, USA, 2009.

24. Barel, A.O.; Paye, M.; Maibach, H.I. *Handbook of Cosmetic Science and Cosmetology*, 4th ed.; Taylor and Francis Group: Boca Raton, FL, USA, 2014.

25. Sharma, P.; Pandey, P.; Gupta, R.; Roshan, S.; Garg, A.; Shulka, A.; Pasi, A. Isolation and characterization of hesperidin from orange peel. *Indo Am. J. Pharm. Res.* **2013**, 2231–6876.

26. Hendrickstone, R.; Kesterstone, J.W. Purification of crude hesperidin. *Annu. Meet. Fla. State Hort. Soc.* **1995**, *3*, 121–124.

27. Londoño-Londoño, J.; de Lima, V.R.; Lara, O.; Gil, L.; Crecsynski Pasa, T.B.; Arango, G.J.; Pineda, J.R. Clean recovery of antioxidant flavonoids from citrus peel: Optimizing an aqueous ultrasound-assisted extraction method. *Food Chem.* **2010**, *119*, 81–87. [CrossRef]

28. Manach, C.; Morand, C.; Gil-Isquierdo, A.; Bouteloup-Demange, C.; Rémésy, C. Bioavailability in humans of the flavones hesperitin and narirutin after the ingestion of two doses of orange juice. *Eur. J. Clin. Nutr.* **2003**, *57*, 235–242. [CrossRef]

29. Lahmer, N.; Belboukhari, N.; Cheriti, A.; Sekkoum, K. Hesperidin and hesperitin preparation and purification from *Citrus sinensis* peels. *Der Pharma Chem.* **2015**, *7*, 1–4.

30. Rezzadori, K.; Benedetti, S.; Amante, E.R. Proposals for the residues recovery: Orange waste as raw material for new products. *Food Bioprod. Process.* **2012**, *90*, 606–614. [CrossRef]

31. Cheigh, C.; Chung, E.-Y.; Chung, M.-S. Enhanced extraction of flavanones hesperidin and narirutin from Citrus unshiu peel using subcritical water. *J. Food Eng.* **2012**, *110*, 472–477. [CrossRef]

32. Berger, S.; Sicker, D. *Classics in Spectroscopy. Isolation and Structure Elucidation of Natural Products*; Wiley-VCH Verlag GmbH & Co. KGaA: Weinheim, Germany, 2009.

33. Morel, L.; Lescoat, G.; Cogrel, P.; Sergent, O.; Pasdeloup, N.; Brisot, P.; Cillard, P.; Cillard, J. Anti-oxidant and iron-chelating activities of the flavonoids catechins, quercetin and diosmetin on iron-loaded rat hepatocyte cultures. *Biochem. Pharmacol.* **1993**, *45*, 13–19. [CrossRef]

34. Moreira, M.B.; Franciscato, D.S.; Toledo, K.C.; de Souza, J.R.B.; Nakatani, H.S.; de Souza, V.R. Investigation of the fluorescence quenching of bovine and human serum albumin by ruthenium complex. *Quim. Nova* **2015**, *38*, 227–232.

35. Ross, P.D.; Subramanian, S. Thermodynamics of protein association reactions: Forces contributing to stability. *Biochemistry* **1981**, *20*, 3096–3102. [CrossRef]

36. Catarino, C.M.; Pedrosa, T.d.N.; Pennacchi, P.C.; de Assis, S.R.; Gimenes, F.; Consolaro, M.E.L.; Barros, S.B.d.M.; Maria-Engler, S.S. Skin corrosion test: A comparison between reconstructed human epidermis and full thickness skin models. *J. Drug Deliv. Sci. Technol.* **2018**, *31*, 72–82. [CrossRef]

37. Cypriano, D.; da Silva, L.L.; Tasic, L. High value-added products from the orange juice industry waste. *Waste Manag.* **2018**, *79*, 71–78. [CrossRef]

38. Saija, A.; Scalese, M.; Lanza, M.; Marzullo, D.; Bonina, F.; Castelli, F. Flavonoids as antioxidant agents: Importance of their interaction with biomembranes. *Free Radic. Biol. Med.* **1995**, *19*, 481–486. [CrossRef]

39. Chen, M.C.; Ye, Y.Y.; Ji, G.; Liu, J.W. Hesperidin upregulates heme oxygenase-1 to attenuate hydrogen peroxide-induced cell damage in hepatic L02 cells. *J. Agric. Food Chem.* **2010**, *58*, 3330–3335. [CrossRef] [PubMed]

40. Elavarasan, J.; Velusamy, P.; Ganesan, T.; Ramakrishnan, S.K.; Rajasekaran, D.; Periandavan, K. Hesperidin-mediated expression of Nrf2 and upregulation of antioxidant status in senescent rat heart. *J. Pharm. Pharmacol.* **2012**, *64*, 1472–1482. [CrossRef]

41. Martinez, M.C.; Fernandez, S.P.; Loscalzo, L.M.; Wasowski, C.; Paladini, A.C.; Marder, M.; Medina, J.H.; Viola, H. Hesperidin, a flavonoid glycoside with sedative effect, decreases brain pERK1/2 levels in mice. *Pharmacol. Biochem. Behav.* **2009**, *92*, 291–296. [CrossRef]

42. Wilmsen, P.K.; Spada, D.S.; Salvador, M. Antioxidant activity of the flavonoid hesperidin in chemical and biological systems. *J. Agric. Food Chem.* **2005**, *53*, 4757–4761. [CrossRef] [PubMed]

43. Fraga, C.G. *Plant Phenolics and Human Health, Biochemistry, Nutrition, and Pharmacology*; Wiley and Sons, Inc.: New York, NY, USA, 2010.

44. Guardia, T.; Rotelli, A.E.; Juarez, A.O.; Pelzer, L.E. Anti-inflammatory properties of plant flavonoids. Effects of rutin, quercetin and hesperidin on adjuvant arthritis in rat. *Il Farmaco* **2001**, *56*, 683–687. [CrossRef]

45. Rotelli, A.E.; Juarez, A.O.; Guardia, T.; La Rocha, N.E.; Pelzer, L.E. Comparative study of flavonoids in experimental models of inflammation. *Pharmacol. Res.* **2003**, *48*, 601–606. [CrossRef]

46. Pan, P.H.; Lai, C.S.; Ho, C.T. Anti-inflammatory activity of natural dietary flavonoids. *Food Funct.* **2010**, *1*, 15–31. [CrossRef]

47. Tanaka, T.; Makita, H.; Ohnishi, K.; Mori, H.; Satoh, K.; Hara, A.; Sumida, T.; Fukutani, K.; Tanaka, K.T.; Ogawa, H. Chemoprevention of 4-nitroquinoline1-oxide induced oral carcinogenesis in rats by flavonoids diosmine and hesperidin, each alone and in combination. *Cancer Res.* **1997**, *57*, 246–252.

48. Tanaka, T.; Makita, H.; Kawabata, K.; Mori, H.; Kakumoto, M.; Satoh, K.; Hara, A.; Sumida, T.; Tanaka, T.; Ogawa, H. Chemoprevention of azoxymethane-induced rat colon carcinogenesis by the naturally occurring flavonoids, diosmine and hesperidin. *Carcinogenesis* **1997**, *18*, 957–965. [CrossRef]

49. Jain, M.; Parmar, H.S. Evaluation of antioxidative and anti-inflammatory potential of hesperidin and naringin on the rat air pouch model of inflammation. *Inflamm. Res.* **2011**, *60*, 483–491. [CrossRef] [PubMed]

50. So, F.V.; Guthrie, N.; Chambers, A.F.; Carroll, K.K. Inhibition of proliferation of estrogen receptor-positive MCF-7 human breast cancer cells by flavonoids in the presence and absence of excess estrogen. *Cancer Lett.* **1997**, *112*, 127–133. [CrossRef]

51. Lentini, A.; Forni, C.; Provenzano, B.; Beninati, S. Enhancement of transglutaminase activity and polyamine depletion in B16-F10 melanoma cells by flavonoids naringenin and hesperetin correlate to reduction of the in vivo metastatic potential. *Amino Acids* **2007**, *32*, 95–100. [CrossRef]

52. Hou, M.; Man, M.; Man, W.; Zhu, W.; Hupe, M.; Park, K.; Crumine, D.; Elias, P.M.; Man, M. Topical hesperidin improves permeability barrier function and epidermal differentiation in normal murine skin. *Exp. Dermatol.* **2012**, *21*, 337–340. [CrossRef]

53. Yi-Hung, T.; Ko-Feng, L.; Yaw-Bin, H.; Chi-Te, H.; Pao-Chu, W. In vitro permeation and in vivo whitening effect of topical hesperetin microemulsion delivery system. *Int. J. Pharm.* **2010**, *388*, 257–262.

54. Brglez, M.E.; Knez, H.M.; Škerget, M.; Knez, Ž.; Bren, U. Polyphenols: Extraction methods, antioxidative action, bioavailability and anticarcinogenic effects. *Molecules* **2016**, *21*, 901. [CrossRef]

55. Hrnčič, M.K.; Španinger, E.; Košir, I.J.; Knez, Ž.; Bren, U. Hop compounds: Extraction techniques, chemical analyses, antioxidative, antimicrobial, and anticarcinogenic Effects. *Nutrients* **2019**, *11*, 257. [CrossRef]

56. Kim, B.; Lee, J.; Lee, H.; Nam, K.; Park, J.; Lee, S.; Kim, J.; Lee, J.; Hwang, J. Hesperidin suppresses melanosome transport by blocking the interaction of Rab27A-Melanophilin. *Biomol. Ther.* **2013**, *21*, 343–348. [CrossRef]

57. An, B.; Kwak, J.; Park, J.; Lee, J.; Park, T.; Son, J.; Jo, C.; Byun, M. Inhibition of enzyme activities and the antiwrinkle effect of polyphenol isolated from the persimmon leaf (*Diospyros kaki folium*) on human skin. *Dermatol. Surg.* **2005**, *31*, 848–854. [CrossRef]

58. Selvajar, S.; Krishnaswamy, S.; Devashya, V.; Sethuraman, S.; Krishnan, U.M. Investigations on the membrane interactions of naringin and its complexes with copper and iron: Implications for their cytotoxicity. *RSC Adv.* **2014**, *4*, 46407–46417. [CrossRef]

59. Weon, J.B.; Ma, J.Y.; Yang, H.J.; Ma, C.J. Simultaneous determination of ferulic acid, hesperidin, 6-gingerol and glycyrrhizin in insampaedok-san by HPLC coupled with diode array detection. *J. Anal. Chem.* **2012**, *67*, 955–959. [CrossRef]

Sample Availability: Samples of the compounds hesperidin, nano sized HSD, facial creams A1 and A2, formulations I-VIII, and hesperidin complex with Cu(II) are available from the authors.

MDPI

St. Alban-Anlage 66

4052 Basel

Switzerland

Tel. +41 61 683 77 34

Fax +41 61 302 89 18

www.mdpi.com

Molecules Editorial Office

E-mail: molecules@mdpi.com

www.mdpi.com/journal/molecules